Nancy Caroline's
Emergency
Care in the Streets

Student Workbook

AAOS

AMERICAN ACADEMY OF ORTHOPAEDIC SURGEONS

Bob Elling, MPA, EMT-P

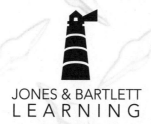

JONES & BARTLETT
LEARNING

World Headquarters
Jones & Bartlett Learning
5 Wall Street
Burlington, MA 01803
978-443-5000
info@jblearning.com
www.jblearning.com

Jones & Bartlett Learning books and products are available through most bookstores and online booksellers. To contact Jones & Bartlett Learning directly, call 800-832-0034, fax 978-443-8000, or visit our website, www.jblearning.com.

Substantial discounts on bulk quantities of Jones & Bartlett Learning publications are available to corporations, professional associations, and other qualified organizations. For details and specific discount information, contact the special sales department at Jones & Bartlett Learning via the above contact information or send an email to specialsales@jblearning.com.

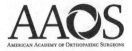

Production Credits
Chief Executive Officer: Ty Field
President: James Homer
SVP, Editor-in-Chief: Michael Johnson
SVP, Chief Marketing Officer: Alison M. Pendergast
Executive Publisher: Kimberly Brophy
Executive Acquisitions Editor—EMS: Christine Emerton
Associate Managing Editor: Amanda Brandt
Production Manager: Jenny L. Corriveau
Associate Production Editor: Nora Menzi

Vice President of Sales, Public Safety Group: Matthew Maniscalco
Director of Sales, Public Safety Group: Patricia Einstein
Director of Marketing: Alisha Weisman
VP, Manufacturing and Inventory Control: Therese Connell
Composition: Cenveo Publisher Services
Cover Design: Kristin E. Parker
Cover Image: © Glen E. Ellman
Rights & Photo Research Associate: Lian Bruno
Printing and Binding: Edwards Brothers Malloy
Cover Printing: Edwards Brothers Malloy

6048

Printed in the United States of America
18 17 16   10 9 8 7 6 5

Contents

EMS Systems

Matching

Match each of the definitions in the left column to the appropriate term in the right column.

_____ **1.** Outlined measure that may be difficult to obtain in a research project.

_____ **2.** A research format that uses a hypothesis to prove one finding from another.

_____ **3.** A computer-generated list of subjects or groups for research.

_____ **4.** A type of study in which the subjects are advised of all aspects of the study.

_____ **5.** A process in which a person, an institution, or a program is evaluated and recognized as meeting certain predetermined standards to provide safe and ethical care.

_____ **6.** The process of granting licensure or certification to a provider from another state or agency.

_____ **7.** Time parameters set during a research project.

_____ **8.** The process used by the medical magazines, journals, and other publications to ensure quality and validity of an article before publishing it; it involves sending the article to subject matter experts for review of the content and research methods.

_____ **9.** The use of practices that have been proven to be effective in improving patient outcomes.

_____ **10.** Medical direction given in real time to an EMS service or provider.

A. Systematic sampling

B. Reciprocity

C. Parameter

D. Inferential

E. Evidence-based practice

F. Unblinded study

G. Certification

H. Peer review

I. Alternative time sampling

J. Online medical control

Multiple Choice

Read each item carefully, and then select the best response.

1. In what year did the National Academy of Science and the National Research Council release the white paper entitled "Accidental Death and Disability: The Neglected Disease of Modern Society"?
   A. 1965
   B. 1967
   C. 1968
   D. 1969

2. Which of the following was NOT an EMS system element during the 1980s and 1990s?
   A. Resource management
   B. Public information and education
   C. Decrease in number of providers
   D. Medical direction

3. What does EMD stand for?
   A. Emergency medical defibrillator
   B. Emergency medical doctor
   C. Emergency management director
   D. Emergency medical dispatcher

4. Which of the following may involve telemetry transmission during patient care?
   A. Off-line medical control
   B. Online medical control
   C. Protocols
   D. Standing orders

5. What type of research is considered a basic observation only, may involve interviews with subjects, and specifies that no alterations occur?
   A. Experimental
   B. Descriptive
   C. Cross-sectional
   D. Qualitative

6. Attributes of professionalism include all of the following, EXCEPT:
   A. communication.
   B. patient advocacy.
   C. empathy.
   D. reciprocity.

7. Which of the following is considered a high-risk activity from a continuous quality improvement point of view?
   A. Taking vital signs
   B. Intravenous therapy
   C. Handing patients off
   D. Basic airway management

8. Who is considered the father of paramedicine?
   A. Dr. David Boyd
   B. Dr. Eugene Nagel
   C. Dr. Jean Larrey
   D. Dr. Peter Safar

9. Who is usually the first EMS professional the public deals with?
   A. EMT
   B. Law enforcement officer
   C. EMD
   D. Paramedic

10. In 2009, which level of EMS was changed to Advanced EMT in the National EMS Education Standards?
    A. EMR
    B. EMT-Basic
    C. EMT-Intermediate
    D. Paramedic

Fill-in-the-Blank

Read each item carefully, and then complete the statement by filling in the missing word(s).

1. In the late 1950s and early 1960s, the _____ _____ _____ _____ were staffed by specially trained physicians.

2. The _____ receives and enters all information on the call, interprets the information received, and relays it to the appropriate resources.

3. When a state grants certification (or licensure) to a provider from another state, it is known as _____.

4. The paramedic who can demonstrate to the patient, the patient's family members, and other health care providers the ability to identify and understand their feelings is showing _____.

5. During scene management, ensuring your own safety and the safety of your crew is your _____ _____.

6. The tool often used to continually evaluate your care is called _____ _____ _____.

7. _____ research is based on a clearly defined problem or question and gathers information as events occur in real time.

Ambulance Calls

The following case scenarios provide an opportunity to explore the concerns associated with patient management and paramedic care. Read each scenario, and then answer each question.

1. You are exiting a theater after watching a movie, when suddenly the woman in front of you falls down on the carpeted floor, landing on her knees and hands. She apparently has tripped in the dark on the steps. As you help her up, you find that she is not responding to you as she should. She says she feels very faint, so you lower her back to the ground. She then loses consciousness, and you lower her all the way to a supine position and make sure her airway is open and she is breathing. You ask your spouse to call 9-1-1 on her cell phone and to find management to bring up the theater lights and get the nearest AED. Your patient is a 60-year-old woman who wakes up and says she is all right and doesn't want anyone making a fuss over her. She just wants to go home.

   a. What information should you give your spouse to tell the dispatcher (EMD)?

   _____

   _____

   _____

   b. What are some reasons this patient should go to the hospital to get checked out?

   _____

   _____

   _____

2. Wow, what an evening at the theater! After your patient has left in an ambulance, you head out the door to go home. Just as you are getting into your vehicle, you hear a woman scream. It seems she has been hit by a small pickup truck that was backing up to get a good parking spot. You run over to find a 40-year-old woman who is conscious and alert. She is sprawled out on the ground. She is screaming about her left leg, which is where the bumper of the pickup impacted her leg. She was knocked to the pavement. The driver of the pickup stopped when he heard the impact and then pulled forward, which caused no more injury to the woman. She has an obvious deformity midthigh on the left leg. An EMT comes running to help because several people have already called 9-1-1. Because you are first on scene and the more highly trained responder, you take charge of this patient.

   a. What is the first thing you should do on this scene?

   _____

   _____

   _____

   b. What steps should you take in treating this patient before the ambulance arrives?

   _____

   _____

   _____

True/False

If you believe the statement to be more true than false, write the letter "T" in the space provided. If you believe the statement to be more false than true, write the letter "F."

   _____ 1. The first documented ambulance service was started in 1869 in New York City out of Bellevue Hospital.

   _____ 2. "The White Paper" provided authority and financial support for the development of basic and advanced life support services.

   _____ 3. An emergency medical dispatcher (EMD) can give simple medical instructions to the caller.

   _____ 4. The primary and backbone level in the EMS system is the EMR.

_____ **5.** In EMS, paramedics constitute the greatest number of trained and certified individuals in the field.

_____ **6.** The first priority of the scene is assessment of the patient.

_____ **7.** Peer review is used as a means of continuous quality improvement.

_____ **8.** Retrospective research uses available data from medical records or PCRs.

_____ **9.** Only the emergency vehicle operator is responsible for restocking the unit after a call.

_____ **10.** Injury prevention in the home is an attribute the paramedic should be comfortable discussing with patients and bystanders.

Short Answer

Complete this section with short written answers using the space provided.

1. Pretend you are a fly on the wall during this scene: A team of paramedics arrives on scene for a routine geriatric call. The woman has fallen and has a broken hip. Her daughter has found her and called 9-1-1. List below the professional attributes the paramedics should demonstrate on this and every call.

a. _____

b. _____

c. _____

d. _____

e. _____

f. _____

g. _____

h. _____

i. _____

j. _____

2. Paramedics follow an important sequence of procedures for every emergency call. List the eight procedures below.

a. _____

b. _____

c. _____

d. _____

e. _____

f. _____

g. _____

h. _____

3. No paramedic service in the United States can perform advanced life support procedures without medical direction. What is medical direction, and why is it necessary?

_____

_____

_____

4. Medical control consists of several different parts. Give an example of each of the following:

a. Online medical control: _____

b. Protocols: _____

c. Standing orders: _____

Workforce Safety and Wellness

Matching

Part I

Stress is a major part of a paramedic's job. Indicate which of the following two types of stress you are more likely to experience in the following scenarios.

A. Eustress   **B.** Distress

_____ **1.** You are running a 10-kilometer road race with your best friend. You have been training to beat her, and she is about 15 steps in front of you.

_____ **2.** You respond to a rollover collision and find out that the unrestrained driver of the vehicle is your 17-year-old son.

_____ **3.** You are assigned to work with Billy Bob for the next month. Billy Bob is not your favorite person and is always criticizing every move you make.

_____ **4.** You are taking your National Registry Paramedic exam next week, and you are studying in hopes of passing the test with an excellent grade the first time you take it.

_____ **5.** You find out the ambulance service that you work for is merging with a larger service. There is talk that your job will be eliminated.

_____ **6.** You are climbing Pikes Peak and you are about to make the summit (your lifelong dream), but you don't feel that you have enough energy left to climb the last 500 feet.

_____ **7.** Your spouse has left a letter explaining to you that he/she is divorcing you and that he/she has already cleaned out the bank accounts.

Part II

Match each psychological defense mechanism with the situation in which it is most likely to be used.

A. Projection   **B.** Denial   **C.** Regression

_____ **1.** Your patient is ignoring the symptoms he has been having over the past few days.

_____ **2.** Your school-aged patient is upset by her injuries and seems to be acting like a toddler.

_____ **3.** Your patient seems to be blaming his symptoms on the bad behaviors of everyone in his family.

Part III

Match each of the definitions in the left column to the appropriate term in the right column.

_____ **1.** A fear reaction in which a person's judgment seems to disappear entirely; it is particularly dangerous because it may precipitate mass panic among others.

A. Defense mechanism

_____ **2.** Pathogenic microorganisms that are present in human blood and can cause disease in humans include, but are not limited to, hepatitis B virus and human immunodeficiency virus.

B. Transmission

_____ **3.** Any disease that can be spread from person to person or from animal to person.

C. Denial

_____ **4.** An event that overwhelms the ability to cope with the experience, either at the scene or later.

D. Blind panic

_____ **5.** Psychological ways to relieve stress; they are usually automatic or subconscious (eg, denial, regression, projection, and displacement).

E. Standard precautions

_____ **6.** An early response to a serious medical emergency in which the severity of the emergency is diminished.

F. Bloodborne pathogens

_____ **7.** Exposure to, or transmission of, a communicable disease from one person to another by physical contact.

G. Direct contact

_____ **8.** A disease that is caused by infection or one that is capable of being transmitted with or without direct contact.

H. Communicable disease

_____ **9.** Protective measures that have traditionally been developed by the CDC for use in dealing with objects, blood, body fluids, or other potential exposure risks of communicable disease.

I. Infectious disease

_____ **10.** The way in which an infectious agent is spread—contact, airborne, by vehicles (eg, food or needles), or by vectors.

J. Critical incident

Multiple Choice

Read each item carefully, and then select the best response.

1. You respond to a 10-year-old boy who has been hit by a car. He is alert, but with a deformity to his lower left leg. The boy "baby talks" as he is answering your questions. This is a form of:
   A. denial.
   B. projection.
   C. regression.
   D. displacement.

2. You respond to a multiple-casualty incident (MCI) involving a collision of a charter bus of senior citizens and a car with four teenagers. At the scene, you find one teen with no obvious injuries. You have to tell him numerous times to sit on the side of the road and stay away from the moving traffic. His judgment seems impaired and he may be suffering from:
   A. conversion hysteria.
   B. projection.
   C. depression.
   D. blind panic.

3. Which of the following would NOT be a symptom of impending paramedic burnout?
   A. Increased interest in hobbies
   B. Chronic fatigue and irritability
   C. Cynical, negative attitude
   D. Decreasing ability to concentrate

4. As a result of the careless nature of your partner, you have been stuck by a needle that was used to start an IV on your patient. Which of the following should be done immediately?
   A. Get a medical evaluation from the ED physician.
   B. Document the negligence of your partner.
   C. Wash the area of the exposure with soap and water.
   D. Get a booster shot for all of your immunizations.

5. According to the CDC, when should a HEPA respirator be worn by the paramedic?
   A. Between patient contacts
   B. When working with a patient who has tuberculosis
   C. When touching mucous membranes
   D. When dealing with blood or body fluids

6. You are on your first "code." As you arrive on scene, you feel stressed. Which of the following management techniques would NOT help you during this call?
   A. Reframing
   B. Controlled breathing
   C. Progressive relaxation
   D. Regression

7. You are on the scene of a major car crash. Your patient is an elderly gentleman who has now accepted the fact that he is really hurt and could be in the hospital for a long time. Which of the following reactions might the patient experience?
   A. Depression
   B. Fear
   C. Anger
   D. All of the above

8. At a vehicle crash, you believe that you have everyone accounted for and taken care of. Suddenly you hear a baby crying and realize there is a child that you have not found yet. Your heart begins to race; this is an example of a/an:
   A. acute stress.
   B. alert response.
   C. defense mechanism.
   D. fight-or-flight response.

9. After being told she might be suffering from a heart attack, an elderly woman hits the paramedic in anger and tells the paramedic he doesn't know what he is talking about. Which defense mechanism relates to this statement?
   A. Displacement
   B. Projection
   C. Alarm reaction
   D. Denial

10. A paramedic who has been on duty for 6 months (without a personal day) begins to show signs of physical and emotional breakdown. He is cynical and doesn't seem to be able to sleep. These are signs of:
    A. eustress.
    B. burnout.
    C. anxiety.
    D. alert response.

Fill-in-the-Blank

Read each item carefully, and then complete the statement by filling in the missing word(s).

1. The following paragraphs describe behaviors of different individuals under stress. For each description, fill in the defense mechanism that the individual is apparently using.
   a. Your partner has been irritable and ill-tempered ever since he arrived at work today. You are doing your best to keep a low profile and not annoy him further, but nonetheless he snaps at you, "You sure are in a lousy mood today." Your partner is showing the mechanism of defense known as _____.
   b. You are called by a very distraught woman to treat her husband, who has been having chest pain. When you reach the patient's house, he says, "I can't understand why my wife called for an ambulance; I'm just having a little indigestion, that's all." His face is gray, and he is sweating profusely. He is using the psychological defense mechanism known as _____.
   c. An 18-year-old woman is extricated from a wrecked automobile in which her boyfriend remains trapped. She says she has lost all sensation in her hands and feet. She does not appear terribly upset about that fact, and you cannot find any signs of injury on her body. She is using the psychological defense mechanism known as _____ _____.
   d. At the scene of a car crash, you are trying to extricate an entrapped front-seat passenger who is seriously injured. The driver, who has not suffered any apparent injury, is giving you a hard time. "Be careful, will you! Don't drop her! Watch what you're doing, you damn idiot!" He is very aggressive toward you, but you realize that his behavior is simply a/an _____ of the anger he feels toward himself for having caused the injury to his passenger.

2. Being a paramedic is a stressful job. For some, the stresses are too much and burnout can occur. The time to start thinking about burnout—and about how to prevent it—is now, during your training. Now is the time to develop strategies that will keep burnout from happening to you. List some of the steps you plan to take to keep from burning out as a paramedic.
   a. _____
   b. _____
   c. _____

d. _____

e. _____

f. _____

g. _____

h. _____

Identify

In the following case study, list the six pertinent negatives with regard to the well-being of your partner, Tommy Jones. Also, identify two stress reactions of the patient.

It is midnight, and Tommy Jones is still awake, watching a horror movie on TV and drinking his last soda out of the six pack that he bought today. You are both on a 24-hour shift today, and he has just been lying around the TV room when he is not on a call. He skipped his workout today so he could watch his favorite soap opera. He is bummed out that he is out of cigarettes and is searching the kitchen for yet another bag of popcorn when the tones go off, indicating another call.

As you head from the bunk room to the ambulance, Tommy is yelling that it is all your fault there is another call. "If you wouldn't have gone to bed, we wouldn't have had another call tonight," he grumbles.

You arrive at the scene to find an elderly woman who has fallen and possibly broken her hip. As you begin your treatment phase, the patient begins to blame you for all of her problems. As you load her into the ambulance, the patient reaches out and pinches your arm as hard as she can.

After you deliver your patient to the hospital, Tommy stops to grab another pack of smokes and a bean burrito. As you pull into the bay, Tommy tells you to restock because he wants to watch the end of the movie. As he heads into the TV room, he tells you his stomach is killing him and he might be your next patient.

1. Pertinent Negatives

   a. _____

   b. _____

   c. _____

   d. _____

   e. _____

   f. _____

2. Stress Reactions

   a. _____

   b. _____

Ambulance Calls

The following case scenarios provide an opportunity to explore the concerns associated with patient management and paramedic care. Read each scenario, and then answer each question.

1. Your unit responds to a call for a 3-month-old boy who is not breathing. When you enter the house, you find a mother holding the boy, who is not breathing and is very pale. You and your partner John begin working the code. You start the steps of CPR, with compressions, while gathering as much information as possible about what has happened. As you arrive at the hospital with the infant, you know in your heart that the child is dead. The code team works further on the child, and finally the doctor calls for the time of death. John storms out of the room and out to the ambulance to begin cleanup. John begins to yell about the fact the child died, and how if he hadn't missed the first IV on the child, he might still be alive. You finish your paperwork and then head back to the station. At the station, John refuses to talk about the call and says he wants to be alone. He ends up sitting at the table just staring off into space for the rest of the afternoon. At the next shift, John is very negative and flies off the

handle at everyone that day. After the shift is over, John heads for the local bar instead of going home to his wife and his 2-month-old son. Two weeks later, John is put on mandatory leave for his mental well-being.

a. Explain how this one incident could have triggered John's decline.

_____

_____

_____

b. What are some steps that EVERY PARAMEDIC can take to reduce stress on the job?

_____

_____

_____

2. A call comes in for a motor vehicle crash involving a pickup truck and a semitruck. It was a head-on collision with both vehicles going 60 mph. Your patient is a 56-year-old man. He was not wearing his seat belt when the crash occurred. He has multiple breaks of both arms and legs. He has a large cut on his forehead that is bleeding profusely. You begin a rapid trauma assessment on him after doing a rapid extrication to a long backboard. In the back of the ambulance, you begin treatment by applying oxygen and starting two large-bore IVs en route to the hospital. The patient is alert and is able to respond to you correctly. His blood pressure is 78/40 mm Hg, and respirations are 32 breaths/min and shallow. Skin is cool and clammy, and you have no pulses in the wrists or the feet. The cardiac monitor is showing sinus tachycardia with multifocal PVCs that are becoming very frequent. You don't hear good lung sounds and you prepare for needle decompression of the right chest. You know that this patient is approaching death and will more than likely turn into a trauma code.

a. Your patient looks up at you and asks, "Am I going to die?" How do you respond to him?

_____

_____

_____

b. What are the five stages that you might witness in this patient, and how will the patient act during these stages?

  1. _____

  2. _____

  3. _____

  4. _____

  5. _____

True/False

If you believe the statement to be more true than false, write the letter "T" in the space provided. If you believe the statement to be more false than true, write the letter "F."

_____ **1.** The USDA 2010 Dietary Guidelines contain five different food groups.

_____ **2.** You should avoid caffeine and keep a regular sleep schedule.

_____ **3.** When lifting, you should use your back, so you don't injure your knees.

_____ **4.** Eustress is a negative type of stress.

_____ **5.** Initial management of stress is to control your breathing.

_____ **6.** Anger is a defense mechanism.

_____ **7.** Blind panic is when a patient will convert anxiety to a bodily dysfunction, such as a paralyzed extremity.

_____ **8.** Burnout is a consequence of chronic, unrelieved stress.

_____ **9.** The stages of death and dying are denial, anger, bargaining, depression, and anxiety.

_____ **10.** Gloves are the absolute essential of every EMS call.

_____ **11.** Gloves are the only PPE needed when suctioning a patient.

_____ **12.** A mask worn by you can protect the patient from your germs.

_____ **13.** Your maximum heart rate during exercise should be 320 minus your age.

_____ **14.** The redirecting of one's emotions from the original source to the paramedic is known as displacement.

Short Answer

Complete this section with short written answers using the space provided.

1. When faced with a perceived threat, the body reacts with a fight-or-flight response. From your own experience, list four signs or symptoms of the fight-or-flight response.

a. _____

b. _____

c. _____

d. _____

2. At times, you are the person who will be dealing with a grieving family. List the six guidelines for helping the family begin the process of coping with their loss.

a. _____

b. _____

c. _____

d. _____

e. _____

f. _____

3. The American Psychiatric Association has identified five categories of reactions to multiple-casualty incidents (MCIs) by the public. They are:

a. _____

b. _____

c. _____

d. _____

e. _____

Problem Solving

Calculate the maximum heart rate and target heart rate for a person with a resting heart rate of 76 beats/min and an age of 46 years.

a. Resting heart rate _____

b. 220 – _____ (age in years) = _____ (Maximum heart rate)

c. _____ (Maximum heart rate) – _____ (Resting heart rate) = _____ × 0.7 = _____ (round up)

d. _____ (Total) + _____ (Resting heart rate) = _____ (Target heart rate)

Public Health

Matching

Match the following prevention methods with the correct situation.

    A. Education
    B. Enforcement
    C. Engineering/environment
    D. Economic incentives

_____ **1.** The road has had new guardrails installed in the area because a lot of crashes have occurred there.

_____ **2.** The EMS agency is holding a free "Learn CPR Week" for residents of the town.

_____ **3.** A vehicle insurance company offers a discount rate to 16-year-olds for taking driver's education.

_____ **4.** The police are stopping students on the way to school and handing out coupons for a free iTunes music download to the students who are wearing their seat belts.

_____ **5.** The car dealership is offering a free child car seat check this weekend.

_____ **6.** My son was stopped in a work zone for speeding and given a ticket that cost him $250.

_____ **7.** The new car seats available have a five-point harness system instead of a bar that holds the child in the seat.

_____ **8.** The ambulance crew will do an inspection of any elderly person's home to determine any potential risk areas. This service is provided free of charge.

_____ **9.** Because of the law, all poisons must be listed on the front of every container that contains products that can cause poisoning.

_____ **10.** We receive a discount on our home insurance because we have a smoke alarm and CO monitor on every floor of the house.

Multiple Choice

Read each item carefully, and then select the best response.

    1. Fred is on the roof trying to reposition the "dish" during the big game. He falls off and hurts his back. This is considered a/an _____ injury.
        A. intentional
        B. unintentional
        C. secondary
        D. environmental

    2. Which of the following is NOT an intentional injury?
        A. Rape
        B. Motor vehicle crash
        C. Suicide
        D. Elder abuse

    3. When choosing objectives as you build an implementation plan, the *S* in SMART stands for:
        A. signs.
        B. swelling.
        C. simple.
        D. success.

4. Which of the following patients could benefit from a "teachable moment"?
   A. An 18-year-old not wearing his seat belt who received cuts and bruises as a result of a motor vehicle crash
   B. A 3-year-old drowning patient
   C. An elderly person suffering from dementia
   D. A 45-year-old woman with a dog bite

5. Which of the following is NOT a primary injury prevention measure?
   A. Wearing your seat belt
   B. Using safe lifting techniques
   C. Smoking a pack a day
   D. Wearing gloves at the scene of a crash

6. When developing a prevention program, what is the second step out of the five steps discussed in the text?
   A. Plan and test interventions.
   B. Conduct a community assessment.
   C. Set goals and objectives.
   D. Define the injury problem.

7. According to the Centers for Disease Control and Prevention (CDC), home injuries to children are most frequently caused by:
   A. abuse.
   B. small toys.
   C. filled bathtubs.
   D. cribs.

8. What is the primary focus for an EMS provider when dealing with prevention?
   A. Primary injury prevention
   B. Secondary injury prevention
   C. Illness prevention
   D. Intervention research

9. Which of the following is NOT a reason EMS should be involved in the prevention field?
   A. EMS providers reflect the composition of the community.
   B. EMS providers are high-profile role models.
   C. EMS personnel are contacted by auto makers for safety recommendations.
   D. EMS providers are welcomed by school systems.

10. What is the leading killer among ages 1 year to 44 years?
    A. Heart disease and congenital defects of the heart
    B. Diabetes
    C. Influenza and pneumonia
    D. Unintentional injuries

Fill-in-the-Blank

Read each item carefully, and then complete the statement by filling in the missing word(s).

1. A/an _____ is a specific prevention measure that increases positive safety and health outcomes.

2. Abuse, suicide, and rape are defined as a/an _____ injury.

3. The four Es of prevention are _____, _____, _____/_____, and _____ _____.

4. The toy manufacturer no longer sews buttons on the teddy bears for eyes; instead it paints on the eyes with non-toxic paint. An automatic protection for our children such as this is known as _____ _____.

5. There are five categories of behaviors that lead to an increased risk for poor health in adolescents. They are _____ use, alcohol and other drug use, sexual behavior leading to _____ _____ _____ and _____ _____, unhealthy dietary behavior leading to obesity, and _____ _____ leading to obesity.

6. When developing a prevention program, the type of objective that declares that all mobile homes will be provided with a smoke alarm and CO monitor is known as a/an _____ _____.

7. Specific, nonjudgmental advice given on a scene to a patient who is receptive to the message is called a/an _____ _____.

Identify

In the following case study, list the pertinent negatives that can lead to injury.

Mrs. M is so tired. She is 6 months pregnant with Katie's new brother. She works a night shift and takes care of curious 3-year-old Katie during the day. Their day starts with a bath for Katie. Mrs. M takes her out, dries her off, and gets her dressed but forgets to pull the plug in the tub because the phone is ringing. Katie runs off to get some breakfast in the kitchen where she finds a pot of hot water for oatmeal boiling on the stove. Meanwhile, Mrs. M is still on the phone with her overbearing mother. Because Katie can't find anything to eat, she decides to go outside and play on the trampoline. Mr. M didn't get the safety net up last night when he put it together. Mrs. M finally gets off the phone with her mother and has a hard time finding Katie. Later on in the day, Mrs. M sneaks a nap while Katie is playing on the floor. Katie decides she wants to play sewing like her mommy and finds the knitting needles and scissors in mommy's bag beside the chair. Luckily, Katie decides to play barbershop instead of doctor on her mommy. When Mrs. M wakes up, she is horrified to find lots of her own hair on the chair. Mrs. M. decides it would be better to take Katie to day care in the mornings while she catches up on her sleep!

1. Pertinent Negatives
   a. _____
   b. _____
   c. _____
   d. _____

Ambulance Calls

The following case scenarios provide an opportunity to explore the concerns associated with patient management and paramedic care. Read each scenario, and then answer each question.

1. Missy and Jake are on duty when the tones go off for a man down. As they respond to the call, they radio dispatch for more information. Dispatch tells them that this is a lifeline call, and they are unable to get any response when they call the residence. Not knowing what they will encounter, Missy and Jake radio for law enforcement backup. When they arrive at the residence and first knock on the door, they can hear shouts for help from inside the house. A police officer shows up to help, and they determine that all doors and windows are locked and there is no way into the house. The officer determines the basement window is the best one to break. Because Missy is the smallest person there, she is chosen to crawl through the basement window. She enters the house and finds an elderly man on the bathroom floor. After checking on the patient, she goes to unlock the front door. Missy and Jake determine that the man fell trying to get from the toilet back to his wheelchair. He has no injuries and doesn't want to go to the hospital. He just needs a hand getting up. After calling a neighbor to come stay with the gentleman until his caregiver gets home, they load up and head back.

   a. Why is it a good idea that Missy and Jake call for an officer before they get to the scene?

   _____

   _____

   b. What equipment should Missy have taken with her when she entered the home through the basement window?

   _____

   _____

   c. During this call, Missy and Jake can apply the teachable moment. What are some things they can teach their patient?

   _____

   _____

2. Courtney and Larry have been called by the local elementary school to do a program for the third and fourth grades. They decide to educate the children on how and why to call 9-1-1. They arrive with a video of a dispatcher taking a "call" from a child. They show all the steps of how and when to call, what the dispatcher will say, and how the ambulance will respond to them. The video shows a child calling 9-1-1 after she finds her grandpa "asleep" on

the floor and is unable to wake him up. Three days later during their shift, Courtney and Larry get a call for a woman who won't wake up. The dispatcher has the woman's 8-year-old son on the phone. When they arrive, they find a woman who won't wake up on the couch and a very upset little boy. With a few good questions, they determine the mom is a diabetic. After getting a low reading on the glucometer, they start an IV and give her D_{50}. The woman wakes up, and after eating a peanut butter and jelly sandwich, her glucose level stabilizes. They stay a little longer to make sure everything is going well and wait for her neighbor to arrive. After receiving medical control approval, they allow her to sign off and not be transported. During this time, they find out the boy, Ryan, was at their demonstration a few days ago.

a. When Larry and Courtney created an implementation plan for their program, they developed their objective with the SMART plan. What does the SMART plan stand for?

S _____

M _____

A _____

R _____

T _____

b. How did their program help Ryan decide to get help for his mother?

_____

_____

True/False

If you believe the statement to be more true than false, write the letter "T" in the space provided. If you believe the statement to be more false than true, write the letter "F."

_____ **1.** Tertiary prevention is defined as reducing the effects of an injury that has already happened.

_____ **2.** Unintentional injuries are the leading cause of death for people between 1 and 44 years of age.

_____ **3.** The three factors used in making a public health model are the host, the event, and the postevent.

_____ **4.** The collection, analysis, and interpretation of injury data are called injury surveillance.

_____ **5.** A risk factor for an intentional injury would be not wearing your seat belt.

_____ **6.** In creating an implementation plan, you need a realistic timeline to complete your project.

_____ **7.** Two of the five steps in developing a prevention plan include conducting a community assessment and setting goals and objectives.

_____ **8.** When using SMART to meet your objectives, the *R* stands for risk.

_____ **9.** Funding for a prevention program can include donations from local media, grants, and sponsorships from different organizations.

_____ **10.** Every EMS call includes a teachable moment.

Short Answer

Complete this section with short written answers using the space provided.

1. What is the difference between primary injury prevention and secondary injury prevention? Give an example of each.

Primary injury prevention: _____

Secondary injury prevention: _____

2. Give three examples of why EMS providers should be active in the prevention field.

a. _____

b. _____

c. _____

3. List the four Es of prevention and explain each one.

a. _____

b. _____

c. _____

d. _____

4. A public health model will help to identify a problem and how to approach the problem. Use this approach to list the three key factors involved in the problem of children and swimming pool drowning deaths.

a. _____

b. _____

c. _____

5. Discuss three of the six risk factors connected with intentional violence.

a. _____

b. _____

c. _____

Fill-in-the-Table

Fill in the missing parts of the table.

Top 10 Causes of Death in 2007
1. _____
2. _____
3. _____
4. Chronic, lower respiratory disease
5. _____
6. _____
7. Diabetes
8. Influenza and pneumonia
9. _____
10. _____

4 Medical, Legal, and Ethical Issues

Matching

Match the following sentences with the correct situation. For questions 1 to 6, indicate whether:

    A. You may treat the patient without obtaining the patient's expressed consent.

    B. You may NOT treat the patient without obtaining the patient's expressed consent.

_____ **1.** A 9-year-old child is struck by a car. He is bleeding profusely. His parents cannot be located.

_____ **2.** A 42-year-old man is injured in a motor vehicle crash in which his car was demolished. He has bruises on his forehead. He seems confused. He says, "I'm all right. Let me alone. Just call me a taxi."

_____ **3.** A 58-year-old man has chest pain. His wife phoned for an ambulance. The man says, "It's nothing, just indigestion." He refuses to be examined or treated.

_____ **4.** A 30-year-old woman is pulled from the beach surf in cardiac arrest.

_____ **5.** A 25-year-old man is injured in a barroom altercation. He is bleeding profusely from his nose and mouth. He smells strongly of alcohol. He is very belligerent and shouts at you, "Leave me alone, you creeps. If you come any closer, I'll knock your teeth in."

_____ **6.** An 80-year-old woman has fainted at home. Her son found her on the floor and called for an ambulance. She is conscious when you arrive. She says to you, "You are all very sweet, but one can't live forever, you know, and I don't fancy hospitals."

For questions 7 to 10, match the following words to the correct situation.

    A. Slander

    B. Defamation

    C. Battery

    D. Assault

_____ **7.** The reporting paramedic wrote in his report that Mr. Paul was obviously drunk. The paramedic made that statement because he has a long-running feud with Mr. Paul and thought this was a great way to pay him back.

_____ **8.** Mrs. O'Malley told the EMT not to touch her. She did not want any help. The EMT went ahead and tried to grab Mrs. O'Malley and put her on the cot.

_____ **9.** Mitch is taking a patient into the hospital. The patient asks about the doctor on staff. Mitch tells the patient, "Sorry, buddy, but I wouldn't want that witch doctor treating me. Good luck, partner."

_____ **10.** Ryan is in the back of the ambulance with his patient Jake, who is 16 years old and has just rolled his car. Jake is really wound up and wants out of the ambulance. Ryan tells Jake that if he doesn't calm down, he is going to strap him down and give him a shot.

Match each of the following items to the appropriate situation.

    E = Ethical   M = Moral   UE = Unethical practice

_____ **11.** The patient's religion determines that no matter how sick the person is, the person will not seek medical attention.

_____ **12.** Our physician feels that Mother is terminal, but he wants to try at least one more medication to see if it can help her.

_____ **13.** My patient has overdosed on crack cocaine, so he is not worth working on.

_____ **14.** Even though my patient, who was drinking and driving, has just killed a family of four in a car crash, I will do my best to provide medical attention to him.

_____ **15.** A 42-year-old woman has tried to commit suicide by overdosing; if she wants to die, let's give her that wish by working this as a "slow code."

_____ **16.** The patient does not want any pain medication because he feels that those medications are considered "drugs."

_____ **17.** This patient obviously doesn't have the money for this ED visit; let's wait until all of the other patients have been taken care of before we work on this welfare case.

_____ **18.** Mark intentionally left out the fact that he gave five times the normal epinephrine dose on the PCR.

_____ **19.** After helping give birth to a premature stillborn child, the paramedic blessed the infant because the mother requested the child be blessed.

_____ **20.** The paramedic gave the apparently "drunk" 18-year-old patient Lasix on the long transport to the hospital. He wanted to teach the patient a lesson. He thought that if the patient wet himself, it would be funny.

Multiple Choice

Read each item carefully, and then select the best response.

1. You have responded to a fender bender, where your patient is conscious and alert. The patient is able to answer all questions correctly and declines treatment. Your overzealous partner starts to put a C-collar on the patient. What could he be charged with?
   A. Assault
   B. Battery
   C. False imprisonment
   D. Libel

2. You are on a volunteer squad in a small town. At the grocery store, your neighbor starts asking you what happened the night before. You proceed to tell her that the local dentist was hitting his wife and you had to take her up to the hospital for a broken jaw. Along the way, you let slide a few of your own opinions about the dentist. Soon the story is all over town. The dentist is pretty upset and contacts a lawyer to initiate a lawsuit against you. What will you be charged with?
   A. Defamation
   B. Libel
   C. Slander
   D. Assault

3. What does HIPAA guarantee the patient?
   A. The hospital cannot transfer a mother in labor.
   B. The paramedic can treat the patient without consent if the paramedic feels the patient has a life-threatening problem.
   C. The paramedic meets minimum qualifications.
   D. The patient's medical information will remain confidential at all times.

4. Which of the following is NOT needed to prove negligence of the paramedic?
   A. The paramedic treated an unconscious patient.
   B. The paramedic had a legal duty to act.
   C. The paramedic breached his or her duty.
   D. The patient was harmed by the paramedic.

5. You arrive at the ED with a patient with chest pain as your pager goes off for the next call of the night. In your hurry to get out of the hospital, you hand off your patient to the ward clerk, knowing that an RN will be coming soon to take over. You are guilty of:
   A. proximate cause.
   B. ordinary negligence.
   C. gross negligence.
   D. abandonment.

6. You are called to the local elementary school for a child who has fallen from the top of the slide. The child is not making any sense and is vomiting. The school is unable to reach her parents. Under what type of consent can you treat and transport this child?
   A. Informed
   B. Implied

C. Expressed

D. Involuntary

7. You respond to a man down. You find a homeless person in an alley. Which of the following findings would allow you to take the man to the hospital under implied consent?

   A. He has not eaten for at least 6 hours.

   B. He is not clean.

   C. His oxygen level is 82%.

   D. His blood glucose level is normal.

8. After transferring care of the homeless man in the preceding question to the nurse, which of the following does NOT belong in your PCR?

   A. The patient was unkempt and stunk badly.

   B. The patient had an oxygen level of 92%.

   C. The patient has not had anything to eat.

   D. The patient's blood glucose was 100 mg/dL.

9. Which of the following patients must be reported?

   A. A 16-year-old girl who refuses to eat

   B. A new mother who is feeling very depressed

   C. A 10-year-old boy who was bitten by a dog

   D. A 25-year-old man who was binge drinking

10. How are most civil cases resolved?

    A. A settlement process

    B. A trial by a judge

    C. A trial by jury

    D. None of the above

11. What is the paramedic's best protection in court?

    A. A voice recording of every call

    B. A complete and accurate patient care report (PCR)

    C. Rewriting the PCR at a later date or time

    D. Video cameras in the back of the units

12. In which of the following situations would you work "the code"?

    A. A woman who was found in rigor mortis in her bathroom

    B. A patient who was decapitated in a car wreck

    C. A 6-year-old child who was under the ice for 20 minutes

    D. A 56-year-old man who has had a tractor crush his chest area and has been trapped for 40 minutes

13. What is the person (or procedure) called when one adult has the legal authority to make the health care decisions for another?

    A. Power of attorney

    B. Parents

    C. Surrogate decision maker

    D. None of the above

14. Which of the following is NOT an advance directive?

    A. The doctor's recommendations

    B. DNR order

    C. A living will

    D. A health care power of attorney

15. In the NAEMT *Code of Ethics for Emergency Medical Technicians*, which of the following is NOT a fundamental responsibility?

    A. Alleviating suffering

    B. Promoting health

    C. Conserving life

    D. Providing moral support

Fill-in-the-Blank

Read each item carefully, and then complete the statement by filling in the missing word(s).

1. Failure to obtain consent before providing medical treatment might give rise to charges of technical assault and battery. What are the requirements for obtaining consent to treat the following?
   a. From a conscious, mentally competent adult, consent must be _____.
   b. To treat a child, consent must be obtained from the _____ _____ or _____ _____.

2. The patient is claiming that he was harmed by the paramedic's actions. In a lawsuit, the patient will be the _____, and the paramedic will be the _____.

3. The paramedic is permitted by the medical director to carry out certain treatments. This is known as the paramedic's _____ _____ _____.

4. A document that expresses the patient's wants, needs, and desires in relation to the patient's future medical care is known as a/an _____ _____.

5. A minor who has been _____ is a minor under legal age, but because of marriage, pregnancy, or active military service is treated as an adult.

6. When determining whether your patient is mentally competent, you will ask a series of questions to make sure the patient is orientated to _____, _____, and _____.

Identify

In the following case study, list the chief complaint, vital signs, and pertinent negatives.

You are called to respond to the local bar and grill for a man not feeling well. When you arrive, you are confronted by a 34-year-old man who is acting very strange. He is yelling that he doesn't need anyone's help and just to leave him alone. All he wants is a sandwich and a beer. The patient refuses any type of help and correctly answers all of your questions. Once again, he says he wants to be left alone. Without consent and with a cranky patient, you don't feel you can treat this patient. As you are ready to leave, the man falls off the bar stool unconscious. You begin treatment by opening his airway and checking for breathing. He is breathing 20 breaths/min with an oxygen saturation level of 97%. The patient moans but makes no other noises. Your partner notices a medical ID bracelet stating the man is a diabetic. You take a blood glucose reading and find it to be 42 mg/dL. Your partner applies oxygen by a nonrebreathing mask and starts an IV on the patient. Vital signs on this patient are as follows: blood pressure is 132/70 mm Hg, pulse is 96 beats/min, lung sounds are clear bilaterally, skin is cool, and pupils are a bit sluggish. You give 25 g of D_{50} by IV. Your patient begins to wake up very quickly and asks what is going on. He tells you he had taken his sugar reading earlier and realized he needed to eat so he stopped for food. He now is competent and does not want to be transported to the ED. After making sure his vital signs are in normal ranges and his blood glucose level has come up to a reading of 118 mg/dL, you discontinue the IV. Your partner writes up a report, and once again you check all of the patient's vital signs and find them normal. The patient again refuses transport after you have determined that he is competent. You have the patient sign off, and you return to your squad to prepare for the next call.

1. Chief complaint: _____

   _____

   _____

2. Vital signs: _____

   _____

   _____

3. Pertinent negatives: _____

   _____

   _____

Ambulance Calls

The following case scenarios provide an opportunity to explore the concerns associated with patient management and paramedic care. Read each scenario, and then answer each question.

1. Described below are six emergency calls. Circle the letter beside those calls in which it is permissible for a paramedic to give treatment without obtaining expressed consent from the patient. In those cases in which you may *not* treat the patient without expressed consent, describe what action you would take.

   a. A 12-year-old boy has fallen at school and sprained his ankle. The school authorities have so far been unable to reach the boy's parents.

   _____

   _____

   b. A middle-aged woman is found in cardiac arrest.

   _____

   _____

   c. A young man called for an ambulance after his 19-year-old girlfriend swallowed a large number of sleeping pills. She is awake and refuses treatment. She says, "Go away and let me die."

   _____

   _____

   d. A 20-year-old man has taken PCP (a psychedelic drug that often induces violent behavior) and has tried to gouge out his eyes. He is bleeding profusely from the face and screaming, "Don't come near me."

   _____

   _____

   e. A 14-year-old boy was knocked from his bicycle and run over by a truck. He is unconscious and bleeding. Both legs appear fractured. Bystanders do not know the boy or his parents.

   _____

   _____

   f. A 43-year-old man has crushing chest pain. His wife called for the ambulance. The man says he doesn't need an ambulance; he just has indigestion. His face is gray, and he is sweating profusely.

   _____

   _____

2. You are called to the scene of a crash in which a pedestrian has been struck by a car. The driver of the car says the pedestrian staggered out into the street in front of him. The pedestrian is now sitting on the curb. He has an obvious bruise on his head. He is unkempt and smells strongly of alcohol. He tells you that he doesn't want to go to the hospital. You suspect that the patient might not be competent to make that decision. List three things you can check to assess his mental competence.

   a. _____

   b. _____

   c. _____

True/False

If you believe the statement to be more true than false, write the letter "T" in the space provided. If you believe the statement to be more false than true, write the letter "F."

_____ 1. You can be sued for slander when you write a false statement in your report.

_____ 2. The discovery period during a lawsuit can take anywhere from a few months to more than 2 years.

_____ 3. You should contact medical control in the case of a physician's orders on a scene if the orders do not fit the emergency situation.

_____ 4. HIPAA protects the patient's right to confidentiality.

_____ 5. Good Samaritan laws are designed to protect all paramedics from lawsuits.

_____ 6. To prove negligence on the part of the paramedic, the plaintiff must prove legal duty, breach of duty, failure to act, and harm.

_____ 7. A DNR order is not considered an advance directive.

_____ 8. You must gain informed consent from every competent adult before beginning treatment.

_____ 9. You must have parental consent even for an emancipated minor.

_____ 10. The paramedic's best defense in a lawsuit is his or her written report on the patient.

_____ 11. Ethics is a code of conduct that is defined by society and religion along with a person's conscience.

_____ 12. The *Code of Ethics for Emergency Medical Technicians* states that EMTs should adhere to standards of personal ethics that reflect credit upon the profession.

_____ 13. You should always place the welfare of your patient ahead of any personal considerations, except for your own safety.

_____ 14. Patient autonomy is the power of attorney making medical decisions for the patient.

_____ 15. A DNR order can be printed on a medical ID bracelet.

_____ 16. Advance directives are usually made once the patient can no longer make the decisions for his or her own health care.

_____ 17. A person who makes health care decisions for another or carries the power of attorney is called a surrogate decision maker.

_____ 18. Your general focus during resuscitation should be to provide at least an hour of your best efforts.

_____ 19. If you witness misconduct by another EMS provider, you should report that person immediately to the chain of command.

_____ 20. You should always work on a SIDS baby, even if the baby is in rigor mortis.

Short Answer

Complete this section with short written answers using the space provided.

1. Every state in the United States defines certain cases as "coroner's cases"—that is, cases of death that you are obliged to report to law enforcement authorities. Although regulations vary somewhat from state to state, there are certain categories of cases that are nearly universally regarded as coroner's cases. List three such categories.

   a. _____

   b. _____

   c. _____

2. Good Samaritan legislation was written to stop any lawsuits being brought against people who tried to assist at an emergency scene. Explain why the Good Samaritan laws would not be a good defense for a paramedic who has a lawsuit brought against him or her.

   _____

   _____

   _____

3. If legal action is taken against a paramedic, the charge most likely to be brought is that of professional negligence, or "malpractice." To prove that the paramedic was negligent, the plaintiff must demonstrate four things. List the four elements required to prove negligence.

   a. _____

   b. _____

   c. _____

   d. _____

4. List at least four types of cases that paramedics or other health care professionals in your state are required to report to the appropriate authorities.

   a. _____

   b. _____

   c. _____

   d. _____

5. (a) What is MOLST, and (b) is it used in your state?

   a. _____

   b. _____

6. Ethics refers to the rules of right and wrong that we live by. Medical ethics are rules of right and wrong that guide behavior of health care professionals. State in one or two sentences what you regard as the guiding principle of your work as a paramedic.

   _____

   _____

   _____

7. How would you handle a senior paramedic who continually makes racist remarks about your patients?

   _____

   _____

   _____

8. Explain the things you would look for in a DNR order when you arrive on scene to find the patient in cardiac arrest.

   _____

   _____

   _____

EMS Communications

Matching

Part I

Indicate whether each of the following questions from a patient interview is:

   O = an open-ended question

   C = a closed-ended question

_____ **1.** What happened today?

_____ **2.** Do you remember the collision?

_____ **3.** What is a normal blood pressure for you?

_____ **4.** Are you pregnant?

_____ **5.** Have you been sick in the last few weeks?

_____ **6.** Do you have asthma?

_____ **7.** What medications do you take?

_____ **8.** What does the pain feel like to you?

_____ **9.** Do you wear contact lenses?

_____ **10.** How much do you weigh?

Part II

For each of the following statements, indicate whether the statement is most applicable to VHF radio, UHF radio, or cellular telephone.

_____ **1.** Best means for calling the base from skyscraper row downtown

_____ **2.** Best means for calling the base from a rural, wooded area

_____ **3.** Best means for sending a 12-lead ECG to medical command

_____ **4.** Best means for calling a patient's family doctor

_____ **5.** FCC-preferred for routine voice communications

_____ **6.** FCC-approved for one-lead ECG transmission

_____ **7.** Can be monitored by someone with a scanner

Part III

The following statements come from a patient's case history. Arrange them in the correct order for transmission by radio to medical command.

   1.

   A. Pulse is 50 beats/min and regular, respirations are 36 breaths/min and deep, and blood pressure is 180/126 mm Hg.

   B. The patient has a history of high blood pressure.

   C. The deep tendon reflexes are hyperactive.

   D. Her daughter says the patient complained of a severe headache before she collapsed.

   E. The patient was still conscious when we arrived, but she rapidly lost consciousness.

   F. The patient is a 60-year-old woman who collapsed in the bathroom while sitting on the toilet.

   G. We are administering supplemental oxygen at 4 L/min by nasal cannula.

   H. The patient's medications include nitroglycerin and Aldomet (methyldopa).

I. Her left pupil is larger than the right and does not react to light.
J. She was apparently well until this morning.
K. Her neck is somewhat stiff.
L. She was hospitalized 6 years ago for an AMI.

(1)_____   (5)_____   (9)_____

(2)_____   (6)_____   (10)_____

(3)_____   (7)_____   (11)_____

(4)_____   (8)_____   (12)_____

Multiple Choice

Read each item carefully, and then select the best response.

1. Which of the following best describes the use of slang terms?
   A. Helpful when communicating with the hospital because of patient confidentiality
   B. Breaks up the stress of the job by interjecting "dark humor"
   C. Unprofessional and disrespectful
   D. Helpful when communicating with other paramedics

2. EMS systems require a large number of personnel to work and communicate together. All of the following are part of this communication, EXCEPT:
   A. emergency medical dispatcher (EMD).
   B. a citizen notifier.
   C. computer-aided dispatch (CAD).
   D. online medical control with base station physician.

3. Federal oversight of emergency medical communication is accomplished by:
   A. civil defense.
   B. the Department of Homeland Security.
   C. the Federal Emergency Management Agency (FEMA).
   D. the Federal Communications Commission (FCC).

4. The transmission of ECGs to hospital base stations is an important component in the evolution of modern-day paramedicine. All of the following can cause a distortion of the signals, EXCEPT:
   A. loose ECG electrodes.
   B. 60-cycle interference.
   C. ventricular fibrillation.
   D. weak batteries and geographic factors.

5. What is the mode of two-way radio transmission that allows users to talk and listen simultaneously by using two separate radio frequencies at once?
   A. Multiplex
   B. Stereoflex
   C. Duplex
   D. Simplex

6. Which of the following is a way to communicate with your patient?
   A. Verbal communication
   B. Body language
   C. Listening to the patient
   D. All of the above

7. What is the best way to develop rapport with your patient?
   A. Have genuine concern for your patient.
   B. Always call the patient by a pet name.
   C. Hug your patient.
   D. Always use medical terminology.

8. Which of the following would suggest a mental impairment when first addressing your patient?
   A. The patient responds with a coherent speech pattern.
   B. The patient does not turn and look at you when you speak.
   C. The patient waits a second before answering your question.
   D. The patient has a meaningful response to your greeting.

9. When dealing with a fearful patient, which of the following will NOT be useful?
   A. Showing concern for the patient
   B. Standing with your arms crossed
   C. Acting like a professional
   D. Telling the patient about his ECG rhythm

10. Which of the following strategies will help you get a useful response from your patient?
   A. Asking questions with specific medical terms
   B. Talking constantly with your patient
   C. Being quiet and letting the patient talk
   D. Speaking calmly and clearly.

11. If you don't understand what the patient is trying to say to you, you should:
   A. just nod and say, "I understand."
   B. let the patient continue until you do catch something you understand.
   C. ask the patient to explain in more detail.
   D. ask the patient a closed-ended question.

12. What is the best way to convey honesty to your patient?
   A. Using frequent and direct eye contact
   B. Patting the patient on the arm
   C. Kneeling on the floor in front of the patient
   D. Always having a smile on your face

13. When assessing a patient's memory, which of the following is NOT a useful tool?
   A. Asking the patient's name
   B. Asking the patient what he or she had for breakfast the day before
   C. Asking the patient where he is
   D. Asking the patient what happened to her

14. Which of the following cultures considers direct eye contact rude?
   A. Islamic
   B. French
   C. Brazilian
   D. Asian

15. When treating a patient from another culture, what is a good rule of thumb?
   A. Always use hand gestures.
   B. Never use hand gestures.
   C. Always use medical terms.
   D. Use pet names for the patient because it makes the patient feel you like him or her.

Fill-in-the-Blank

You have just been appointed Communications Director for your regional EMS system, and you have been asked to draw up plans for an EMS communications system. To do so, you have to figure out who needs to communicate with whom in such a system and what is the best technical means (pager, radio, landline, or cellular phone) to achieve each link in the communications chain. Complete the following statements.

   1. _____ needs to be able to talk with _____. The best technical means of establishing that link is _____.

   2. _____ needs to be able to talk with _____. The best technical means of establishing that link is _____.

3. _____ needs to be able to talk with _____. The best technical means of establishing that link is _____.

4. _____ needs to be able to talk with _____. The best technical means of establishing that link is _____.

5. _____ needs to be able to talk with _____. The best technical means of establishing that link is _____.

6. _____ needs to be able to talk with _____. The best technical means of establishing that link is _____.

7. The act of transmitting information to another person is called _____.

8. When dealing with a crisis, your challenge is to remain _____.

9. Voice _____ is just as important as the words that you say.

10. A/an _____ _____ _____ is a question that does not have a yes or no answer.

11. When using touch to assure your patient, you should touch a _____ part of the patient's body.

12. If your patient is hostile and you are unable to diffuse the patient's anger, you may need to call the _____.

13. When treating a child, _____ are useful tools for bridging the emotional gap with the child.

14. The best offense when dealing with a cross-culture patient is _____.

Identify

After reading the following case history, provide the indicated assessment information.

The patient is a 49-year-old man who called for an ambulance because of chest pain. The pain was "squeezing" in character, radiated to the left shoulder and jaw, and had been present for 2 hours. The pain was accompanied by increasing difficulty in breathing, relieved somewhat by sitting upright. The patient denied nausea, vomiting, sweating, or palpitations. He is known to be a cardiac patient and takes nitroglycerin at home; he took two nitroglycerin today, without relief. He denies any history of hypertension or diabetes. He has been treated for peptic ulcer in the past.

On physical examination, the patient was sitting bolt upright; he appeared alert and apprehensive and was in moderate respiratory distress, breathing shallowly at 30 breaths/min. Pulse was 130 beats/min, weak and regular, and blood pressure was 200/90 mm Hg. His neck veins were distended to the angle of the jaw at 45°. Wet crackles were heard at both lung bases, and auscultation of the heart revealed a gallop rhythm. The abdomen was not distended. There was 1+ presacral and ankle edema.

The patient was given supplemental oxygen by nonrebreathing mask at 12 L/min, a 12-lead ECG, and IV of normal saline, and transported to Mount Fiore Hospital in a semi-Fowler's position. His vital signs remained stable throughout transport.

1. Chief complaint:

   _____

   _____

2. History of the present illness:

   _____

   _____

3. Other medical history:

   _____

   _____

4. General appearance:

   _____

   _____

5. Vital signs:

_____

_____

6. Head-to-toe exam:

_____

_____

7. Treatment given:

_____

_____

8. Pertinent negatives:

_____

_____

Ambulance Calls

Part I

The following case scenarios provide an opportunity to explore the concerns associated with patient management and paramedic care. Read each scenario, and then answer each question.

1. Following is a transcript of a transmission between a paramedic unit in the field and a local hospital. The transmission does *not* follow the guidelines for good radio communications. Read through the transmission, and then list all the errors in it that you can find.

Ambulance: Medic 12 to County Hospital.

Hospital: Who's calling County Hospital?

Ambulance: This is Medic 12.

Hospital: Go ahead, Medic 12.

Ambulance: Be advised that we are en route to your location with Maggie Jones, a lady well endowed with adipose tissue who's complaining of SOB.

Hospital: Could you please 10-9 that chief complaint?

Ambulance: What's the matter, are you deaf or something? S. O. B. S as in silly, O as in old, B as in bag. Stand by for the ECG. [Pause.]

Ambulance: Medic 12 to County Hospital. Did you get the strip?

Hospital: Yes.

Ambulance: Say again.

Hospital: Yes, we received the strip. The doctor wants to know how old the patient is.

Ambulance: She's 58.

Hospital: And does she have any medical history?

Ambulance: Yeah, she's a cardiac patient and takes digitalis, atenolol, potassium chloride, chlorothiazide, and a whole bunch of other stuff here.

Hospital: Did you get any vitals?

Ambulance: That's affirmative. The blood pressure is 180/120 mm Hg, the pulse is 44 beats/min, and the respirations are, let's see, here it is, the respirations are 30 breaths/min.

Hospital: Doctor's orders are to give 1 mg of atropine IV.

Ambulance: That's a 10–4. Will do.

Hospital: What's your ETA?
Ambulance: About 10 minutes.
Hospital: We'll see you then.
Ambulance: Roger. Pop a few doughnuts into the microwave for us, will you?

What's wrong with this transmission?

a. _____

b. _____

c. _____

d. _____

e. _____

f. _____

g. _____

h. _____

2. You are covering for the dispatcher during his lunch break. ("Don't worry about a thing," you tell him as he heads out the door. "This job's a piece of cake.") The dispatcher has no sooner departed than the telephone rings. You answer on the first ring, and a caller blurts out, "There's been a terrible crash. Oh my God, it's terrible, it's terrible," and he starts sobbing. List the questions you will ask this caller, and indicate at what point you will dispatch an ambulance.

_____

_____

_____

Part II

The following case scenarios provide an opportunity to explore the concerns associated with patient management and paramedic care. Read each scenario, and then answer each question.

1. You are called to the scene of a bad motor vehicle crash in which a semitrailer plowed head-on into a passenger car. The driver of the car is pinned inside his vehicle, very seriously injured. You manage to gain access to the patient and start tending to him while you await help in what will be a lengthy extrication procedure. The patient is still conscious, and he asks you, "Am I going to die?" There is, in fact, a high probability that he will die. Describe how you would reply to this patient's question.

_____

_____

_____

2. You are called to a suburban neighborhood where a 22-year-old female diabetic patient is having some problems with her glucose levels. Your assessment determines that you need to start an IV and give the patient D_{50}. How would you explain to your patient what you are about to do?

_____

_____

_____

3. You are dispatched to a call for chest pain. The scene is a large farm in the rural Midwest. Upon your arrival, a man in a pickup truck meets you at the front gate. He waves for you to follow him. He leads you to a large area on the farm where many camper-trailers are parked. As you get out of your ambulance, the driver of the truck approaches you. He introduces himself as the owner of the farm and tells you that the grandmother of his harvest foreman is experiencing chest pain. He also explains that the foreman and his family are migrant farm workers who speak mostly Spanish.

As you enter a camper, a worried Hispanic gentleman meets you, and the farmer introduces you as "el paramedico." The man extends his hand to you to shake it and says, "Gracias, gracias, señor," and gestures for you follow him. You are led to a cramped bedroom, where an elderly Hispanic woman is lying on a bed, propped up with several blankets. There are several Catholic icons on the wall, as well as a statue of the Virgin Mary at the bedside. The woman has a string of beads in her hand. You notice several small candles burning on a dresser next to the bed. The man gestures toward her and says, "Mi abuela." The woman presents with pale complexion, diaphoresis, obvious dyspnea, and has a facial grimace that you associate with severe pain. You have an EMT partner and an EMT student intern riding with you, so you direct your partner to start setting up the ECG monitor and the student to take vital signs. The excited student says, "Yo," and starts to work. Knowing the patient needs oxygen, you bend over and blow out the candles, not wanting the hazard of open flame around the oxygen. This action really seems to upset the woman, who lets out a little cry. You don't speak any Spanish, so you kneel beside the bed and very slowly ask, "What . . . is . . . your . . . name?" The woman looks in confusion to her grandson, who says "nombre." The woman tells you, very proudly, "Mi nombre es Señora Talia Elizabet Cordoba de Castille." You feel around your uniform for your pen to write it down and realize you left it in the ambulance. You find the red pen you have been using to correct the students' reports and begin to write down her name. The woman lets out a hysterical shriek and tries to back away from you on the bed. There is suddenly much excited confusion in the room, and the grandson is trying desperately to calm his grandmother. The woman is very agitated, and the ECG monitor shows you a sinus tachycardia with several PVCs. You tell the EMT student to run and get the cot. He responds with another "yo" and makes the "rock on" sign with his left hand. The woman's eyes get wide and she shrieks again, only this time she faints. The grandson cries out, "Abuela!" and then tearfully asks you to perform last rites. You inform the grandson that his grandmother is not dead but needs to be transported immediately. You really don't like the way this call is progressing and just want to get back in the ambulance.

In the preceding scenario, you not only have a language barrier, but a religious one as well. Hispanic families are very close-knit, and older Hispanics are generally very religious, especially those who have come from the "old country." The majority practice Roman Catholicism and may also be very superstitious. Old World beliefs in the forces of good and evil may be very prevalent, and traditional religious practices may also be interspersed with additional spiritual beliefs. Some of these may include Candomble, which is a mixture of Roman Catholicism and African Voodoo, practiced predominately in the Pan-Caribbean regions and South America; Santeria, which is popular in Cuba, the Caribbean, and South America; espiritismo, which is practiced predominately in Puerto Rico and Central America; and curanderismo, which is found in Mexico and the American Southwest, and still exists in "Old Spain."

In some of these traditions, the color yellow is associated with death, the color red with witchcraft, and white with resisting evil spells. Thus, writing a person's name in red ink may be perceived as an attempt to "cast a spell" and gain power over the individual.

Hispanics generally use two surnames. The first surname listed is from the father, and the second surname listed is from the mother. When speaking to someone, use his or her father's surname. A married woman may attach her husband's surname to the end of hers with a "de." A widow may indicate her widowed status by including "vda" (widow of) in her name as well. Hispanics are very proud of their family names, and a good name is often more important than wealth or status. They also expect to be treated with dignity and respect (familiar theme, no?) and will reciprocate the same. It is very important in the paramedic–patient relationship to treat the Hispanic patient with polite formality and address him or her by title (Mr., Mrs., Señor, Señora). Once rapport is established, the paramedic can gain valuable inroads in the trust factor by politely asking about family members or loved ones. Hispanics, especially older Hispanics, base clinical trust on *individual* perception, not an institutional one.

a. What should you have asked the farmer before you entered the residence?

_____

_____

_____

b. Upon seeing all the religious symbols in the room, what should you have done before blowing out the candles?

_____

_____

_____

c. Why did the student intern upset the woman?

_____

_____

_____

d. Why is a translator so important at this scene?

_____

_____

_____

True/False

If you believe the statement to be more true than false, write the letter "T" in the space provided. If you believe the statement to be more false than true, write the letter "F."

_____ **1.** EMS may use VHF, UHF, and "trunking systems."

_____ **2.** Paramedics skilled in dysrhythmia recognition don't rely heavily on ECG telemetry.

_____ **3.** An EMS base station consisting of a transmitter, receiver, and antenna is usually mounted in the front console of an ambulance for emergency communications.

_____ **4.** To have clarity of transmission there must be a sender, a clear message, a receiver, and a feedback loop.

_____ **5.** Most EMS agencies use radio codes to comply with HIPAA requirements on transmitting patient information over the radio.

_____ **6.** Sometimes it might be more practical to step out of the patient exam room or to speak in a softer tone to provide the history and transfer information to the receiving medical practitioner.

_____ **7.** An EMD is nothing more than a "call taker" that relays the initial dispatch information.

_____ **8.** The description of "feeling what the patient is feeling" is used to describe empathy.

_____ **9.** Saying to the patient, "Please feel welcome to tell me about that" is referred to as facilitation.

_____ **10.** People in a crisis couldn't care less about your nonverbal communications.

_____ **11.** It is okay to use pet names with your patients.

_____ **12.** One of the most important treatments you can provide is reassurance.

_____ **13.** When caring for patients with alcoholism or behavioral problems, you will need to use patience and persistence.

_____ **14.** A paramedic who frowns or smirks during a patient interview is demonstrating empathy.

_____ **15.** You show respect to other cultures when you make an effort to learn their language.

Short Answer

Complete this section with short written answers using the space provided.

1. You are planning a radio system for your ambulance service, which consists of six vehicles serving an area of 150 square miles. List the components you will need, and state the function of each component.

Component	Function

2. To the paramedic knee-deep in mud trying to extricate the patient involved in a motor vehicle crash, the dispatcher's job looks pretty easy. In fact, the job is not easy at all. List four tasks the dispatcher has to perform to ensure that the EMS system operates as it should.

a. _____

b. _____

c. _____

d. _____

3. According to the dictionary, communication is a process by which information is exchanged. In EMS, information must go back and forth in several different channels. Suppose you had to design the communications network for *your* EMS system. Who needs to be connected to whom? Draw a diagram to show those connections or describe who should be in contact with one another.

4. Create a sample radio report for the following patient scenario. Be sure to include all findings, care provided, and status of improvement of the patient.

You are en route to the hospital with a conscious, alert 58-year-old man who appears to be having an acute MI. The ETA is about 20 minutes. With the patient's consent you have mutually decided that the most appropriate facility to treat him has a 24-hour interventional cardiac catheter lab.

The patient's chief complaint is substernal chest pressure that was radiating down his left arm. It began after he started shoveling snow. He describes the pain initially to be 10 on a 10-point scale, with 10 being the worst pain he ever felt. He also states feeling nauseated and appears to be anxious and sweaty.

His previous medical history includes hypertension and hypercholesterolemia. The patient states that he believes that his father had a heart attack when he was in his 40s. The patient is allergic to Novocain (procaine; causes nausea). He takes 81 mg of aspirin daily PO. He also takes atorvastatin (Lipitor). The patient ate lunch 3 hours ago and was directed to self-administer 162 mg of aspirin by the EMD.

The patient's exam includes bilateral crackles in the bases, pulse of 110 beats/min, and a blood pressure of 146/82 mm Hg. His SaO_2 is 96% on high-flow supplemental oxygen via nonrebreathing mask. The 12-lead ECG indicates a sinus tachycardia and elevations in V3 and V4.

The patient has been treated with morphine, oxygen, nitroglycerin, and the self-administered aspirin.

_____

_____

_____

_____

_____

_____

_____

_____

_____

_____

_____

_____

_____

_____

_____

_____

_____

_____

_____

_____

_____

_____

Fill-in-the-Table

Fill in the table with the International Phonetic Alphabet.

A		J		S	
B		K		T	
C		L		U	
D		M		V	
E		N		W	
F		O		X	
G		P		Y	
H		Q		Z	
I		R			

Documentation

Matching

Part I

It does little good to take a careful history and conduct a thorough physical examination if you cannot communicate your findings to others. To do so, you need to know how to organize those findings in such a way that other medical professionals will be able to read your patient care report (PCR) and get a good understanding of your assessment findings and management of the patient.

Label each of the following statements to indicate which part of the PCR pertains to each item:

_____ 1. There was no pedal edema (edema of the ankles).

_____ 2. The patient is allergic to penicillin.

_____ 3. The pain came on while he was watching television.

_____ 4. The blood pressure was 190/110 mm Hg.

_____ 5. He was administered supplemental oxygen by nonrebreathing mask at 12 L/min.

_____ 6. The patient is a 51-year-old man with chest pain.

_____ 7. The chest was clear.

_____ 8. His skin was pale, cold, and sweaty (diaphoretic).

_____ 9. The patient was transported in a semi-Fowler's position.

_____ 10. Nothing seemed to make the pain better or worse.

_____ 11. The pulse was 52 beats/min and full, with an occasional premature beat.

_____ 12. The neck veins were not distended.

_____ 13. There was no cyanosis of the lips.

_____ 14. The patient takes Maalox (alumina/magnesia) and cimetidine (Tagamet) regularly.

_____ 15. He also felt nauseated.

_____ 16. His abdomen was soft and nontender.

_____ 17. His respirations were 20 breaths/min and unlabored.

_____ 18. He was sitting in a chair and appeared to be frightened.

_____ 19. He is under the care of Dr. Tums for an ulcer.

_____ 20. He was alert and oriented to person, place, and day.

_____ 21. He denies any shortness of breath.

_____ 22. An IV was started with normal saline to a KVO rate.

_____ 23. The pain radiates down his left arm.

_____ 24. The blood pressure came down to 170/90 mm Hg during transport.

_____ 25. He describes the pain as squeezing.

_____ 26. Lung sounds were clear.

A. The chief complaint

B. Part of the history of the present illness

C. Part of the patient's other medical history

D. Part of the description of the patient's general appearance

E. Part of the vital signs

F. Part of the head-to-toe physical examination

G. Part of the treatment

H. Part of the patient's condition during transport

27. Now, rearrange the preceding 26 statements into the order in which they should be presented.

(1)_____	(10)_____	(19)_____
(2)_____	(11)_____	(20)_____
(3)_____	(12)_____	(21)_____
(4)_____	(13)_____	(22)_____
(5)_____	(14)_____	(23)_____
(6)_____	(15)_____	(24)_____
(7)_____	(16)_____	(25)_____
(8)_____	(17)_____	(26)_____
(9)_____	(18)_____	

Part II

Now try the same exercise with a patient who has been injured. Keeping in mind what you will need to document on your PCR, label each of the following statements to indicate which part of the PCR pertains to each item.

_____ **1.** The right leg was severely angulated at the mid-femur.

_____ **2.** The pulse was 92 beats/min, somewhat weak, and regular.

_____ **3.** Bystanders say that the car that hit him was traveling very fast.

_____ **4.** He has a medical identification bracelet that says he is a diabetic.

_____ **5.** There is a bruise on the left forehead.

_____ **6.** His skin is pale, cool, and moist.

_____ **7.** He was secured to a long backboard.

_____ **8.** The patient is a middle-aged man who was struck by a car while crossing the street.

_____ **9.** Respirations were 30 breaths/min, deep, and noisy; blood pressure was 160/100 mm Hg.

_____ **10.** The patient was unconscious and did not withdraw from painful stimuli.

_____ **11.** An oropharyngeal airway was inserted, and supplementary oxygen was given by nonrebreathing mask at 12 L/min.

_____ **12.** He apparently staggered into the street without looking, as if he were drunk.

_____ **13.** The chest wall was stable, and breath sounds were equal bilaterally.

_____ **14.** We put the right leg in a traction splint.

_____ **15.** The pupils were equal, midposition, and reactive to light.

_____ **16.** There was no change in his condition during transport.

_____ **17.** There was no blood or fluid draining from his nose or ears.

_____ **18.** His abdomen was soft.

_____ **19.** The dorsalis pedis pulses were equal.

20. Now, arrange the preceding 19 statements in the correct order for presentation.

A. The chief complaint

B. Part of the history of the present illness

C. Part of the patient's other medical history

D. Part of the description of the patient's general appearance

E. Part of the vital signs

F. Part of the head-to-toe physical examination

G. Part of the treatment

H. Part of the patient's condition during transport

(1)_____	(8)_____	(14)_____
(2)_____	(9)_____	(15)_____
(3)_____	(10)_____	(16)_____
(4)_____	(11)_____	(17)_____
(5)_____	(12)_____	(18)_____
(6)_____	(13)_____	(19)_____
(7)_____		

Part III

Sometimes you will be given information, or obtain it in a sequence that needs to be rearranged into the standardized flow of information in which all health care professionals process a case. The following statements come from a patient's case history. Arrange them in the correct order for documentation on the PCR.

1.

  A. Pulse is 50 beats/min and regular, respirations are 36 breaths/min and deep, and blood pressure is 180/126 mm Hg.

  B. The patient has a history of hypertension.

  C. The deep tendon reflexes are hyperactive.

  D. Her daughter says the patient complained of a severe headache before she collapsed.

  E. The patient was still conscious when we arrived, but she rapidly lost consciousness.

  F. The patient is a 60-year-old woman who collapsed in the bathroom while sitting on the toilet.

  G. We are administering supplemental oxygen at 12 L/min by nonrebreathing mask.

  H. The patient's medications include nitroglycerin and Aldomet (methyldopa).

  I. Her left pupil is larger than the right and does not react to light.

  J. She was apparently well until this morning.

  K. Her neck is somewhat stiff.

  L. She was hospitalized 6 years ago for an AMI.

(1)_____   (5)_____   (9)_____

(2)_____   (6)_____   (10)_____

(3)_____   (7)_____   (11)_____

(4)_____   (8)_____   (12)_____

Multiple Choice

Read each item carefully, and then select the best response.

1. Which of the following would NOT be an example of a significant finding that indicates medical necessity for ambulance transport?
   A. Patient is transported in an emergency fashion (Code 3).
   B. Patient needs to be restrained.
   C. Patient has no other means of transport for his doctor's appointment.
   D. Patient has uncontrollable hemorrhage.

2. Patient data include basic patient information collected on a PCR, documenting information like the chief complaint and:
   A. call location.
   B. assessment findings.
   C. arrival time at the hospital.
   D. disposition hospital.

3. A thorough patient refusal should involve documentation on the PCR of each of the following, EXCEPT:
   A. your opinion the patient is a system abuser.
   B. willingness of EMS to return.
   C. evidence the patient is able to make rational, informed decisions.
   D. discussion with medical control according to protocols.

4. The paramedic may be required to provide supplemental reports, aside from the PCR, in the case of:
   A. a patient injured in a car crash.
   B. a cardiac arrest patient.
   C. a child who was abused.
   D. a burn patient.

5. Each of the following is a method used to organize the narrative section of the PCR, EXCEPT:
   A. body systems/parts approach.
   B. AVPU.
   C. CHARTE method.
   D. SOAP method.

6. Proper documentation is an essential job function of a paramedic. Today, in the majority of the jurisdictions in the United States, this formal written report is referred to as a:
   A. trip sheet.
   B. patient care report.
   C. call sheet.
   D. All of the above.

7. PCRs may be used as all of the following, EXCEPT:
   A. a patient description for the media.
   B. legal documents.
   C. quality assurance reviews.
   D. billing documents.

8. Different EMS systems might use a variety of report-writing formats. Which of the following is an example of a report-writing format?
   A. HEARSAY
   B. TALK
   C. SOAP
   D. SAMPLE

9. Patients may have the ability and right to refuse medical care. Which of the following patients would be appropriate for refusing?
   A. A 10-year-old boy injured in a skateboard crash
   B. A 28-year-old woman who fell off a bar stool and struck her head
   C. An 18-year-old woman who is conscious and alert
   D. An elderly man who called for assistance and was found shivering in an unheated house

10. When a paramedic discovers that he or she has made a documentation error on a PCR, it is okay for the paramedic to do which of the following actions?
    A. Erase or "white out" the mistake
    B. Destroy the original report and rewrite the report without the error
    C. Draw a single line through the error, initial it, and insert the corrected information next to it
    D. Have the paramedic's partner write an addendum

Fill-in-the-Blank

Part I

Paramedics use abbreviations frequently when completing the PCR. For each of the following, list the abbreviation or the phrase the abbreviation stands for.

1. Abd = _____
2. ADL = _____
3. AICD = _____
4. BM = _____
5. BS = _____
6. as soon as possible = _____
7. central venous pressure = _____
8. deep venous thrombosis = _____
9. chronic obstructive pulmonary disease = _____
10. history of present illness = _____

Part II

Paramedics use terminology with common prefixes and suffixes frequently when completing the PCR. For each of the following prefixes and suffixes, write the meaning or list the abbreviation or the phrase the abbreviation stands for.

1. cyst(o)- = _____
2. dermat(o)- = _____
3. ortho- = _____
4. brady- = _____

5. hydr(o)- = _____

6. cephal(o)- = _____

7. cerebr(o)- = _____

8. rhin(o)- = _____

9. tri- = _____

10. supra- = _____

11. -lysis = _____

12. -scope = _____

13. -uria = _____

14. -megaly = _____

15. -otomy = _____

Identify

After reading the following case history, provide the indicated information for a PCR.

The patient is a 55-year-old woman who called for an ambulance because of chest pain. The pain was described as a pressure in the center of the chest with numbness of the left arm, and had been present for 30 minutes. The pain was accompanied by difficulty in breathing with no relief. The patient denied vomiting, but has some nausea and has been sweating profusely. She is known to have angina and takes nitroglycerin at home; she took one nitroglycerin today, without relief. She denies any history of hypertension or diabetes. She has been treated for asthma in the past.

On physical examination, the patient was sitting bolt upright; she appeared alert and apprehensive and was in moderate respiratory distress, breathing shallowly at 32 breaths/min. Pulse was 136 beats/min, weak and regular, and blood pressure was 180/82 mm Hg. Her neck veins were distended to the angle of the jaw at 45°. Rales were heard at both lung bases, and auscultation of the heart revealed a gallop rhythm. The abdomen was not distended. There was no pedal edema.

The patient was given supplemental oxygen by nonrebreathing mask at 12 L/min, a 12-lead ECG was acquired and transmitted because there was evidence of a STEMI. She was transported to St. Joseph's Hospital cath lab in a semi-Fowler's position. An IV of normal saline at KVO was started, and she was given morphine, ASA, and nitroglycerin. Her vital signs remained stable throughout transport.

1. Chief complaint:

_____

_____

2. History of the present illness:

_____

_____

3. Other medical history:

_____

_____

4. General appearance:

_____

_____

5. Vital signs:

_____

_____

6. Head-to-toe exam:

_____

_____

7. Treatment given:

_____

_____

8. Pertinent negatives:

_____

_____

True/False

If you believe the statement to be more true than false, write the letter "T" in the space provided. If you believe the statement to be more false than true, write the letter "F."

_____ **1.** Times used to document actions on a PCR generally use Greenwich Mean Time (GMT).

_____ **2.** To document time accurately, paramedics should "synchronize" their watches with the Public Safety Access Point (PSAP).

_____ **3.** Accurate documentation depends on all information being provided, including times, narrative, and check boxes.

_____ **4.** The abbreviation PRN means as is needed.

_____ **5.** The abbreviation for right bundle branch block is RBB.

_____ **6.** When completing a PCR, if you gave magnesium sulfate, abbreviate it to $MgSO_4$.

_____ **7.** The abbreviation "qid" should not be used because it is confusing.

_____ **8.** It is best to write out "greater than" instead of using the symbol > on your PCR.

_____ **9.** Your PCR may be used in legal proceedings against you or someone else and is the only record of the care you provided and why.

_____ **10.** Falsifying information on the PCR may result in suspension and/or revocation of your certification/license.

Short Answer

Complete this section with short written answers using the space provided.

1. An ambulance run report, or trip sheet, must also contain other information besides that contained in a traditional medical history. List at least one other item of information that needs to be recorded on a trip sheet, and explain why that information is important.

a. Information that should be recorded:

_____

_____

_____

b. Why that information is important:

_____

_____

_____

2. Give two reasons why you should make certain that your trip sheet (PCR) is as accurate and complete as possible.

   a.

   _____

   _____

   _____

   b.

   _____

   _____

   _____

3. Give specifics to document for each topic listed below:

   a. Number of patients:

   _____

   _____

   _____

   b. Standard precautions:

   _____

   _____

   _____

   c. MOI/NOI:

   _____

   _____

   _____

   d. Oxygen:

   _____

   _____

   _____

Complete the Patient Care Report (PCR)

This feature will be found in a number of the chapters of this workbook. Read the incident scenario and then complete the following PCR.

You and your partner are posted at the corner of Second Avenue and 14th Street completing the paperwork for a recent diabetic call when the dispatcher calls your unit. "Medic 185" the dispatcher says immediately.

"Medcom 185," you respond.

"Medic 185, Charlie response to 3-5-5 East 16th Street for a male with severe bleeding. Show your time of dispatch at sixteen-fifty-three."

You copy the assignment and slowly roll out into traffic after activating the lights and siren, proceeding to the address about six blocks away.

Five minutes later, you pull up outside a well-kept apartment house with a parking spot right in front of the building and are met by a woman frantically waving her arms.

"Please hurry!" She shouts as you open your door. "My husband was working with an electric saw in the basement and has a real deep cut on his leg. He's bleeding real bad!"

You and your partner grab your bags and walk down a flight of stairs into the basement area where there is a wood shop. The man, whom you estimate to be about 170 pounds, is sitting on a pile of wood, pale and shaking, holding an old bloody t-shirt against his lower left leg; a huge circle of blood is soaking into the wood pile under him.

"Sir, we're from the city ambulance service and we're here to help you," you say, kneeling next to the man. "Can you tell me what happened?"

As the 42-year-old man describes how the saw glanced off of a knot in the shelving he was cutting, sending it deep into the flesh of his leg, you remove the t-shirt from the wound—observing a jagged laceration approximately 9 cm long—and replace it with a wide trauma dressing. Your partner then places a nonrebreathing mask on the patient with the supplemental oxygen set to 15 LPM and begins assessing vitals.

At 1704 hours, your partner reports the patient's vitals as: systolic BP 136; diastolic BP 86; pulse of 128, strong and regular; respirations of 16 with good tidal volume; pale, cool and diaphoretic skin; and a pulse oximetry of 97%.

About 5 minutes after obtaining vitals, you have stopped the bleeding using a pressure bandage and are loading the patient into the ambulance, keeping him covered with a blanket and in the Trendelenburg position.

His wife tells you that he is allergic to amoxicillin and that he has been taking a cholesterol medication called Crestor ever since he suffered a transient ischemic attack in the spring of last year. You thank her for the information and climb into the patient compartment while your partner jumps into the driver's seat. Within a minute you are en route to the Beth Israel emergency department and taking the patient's vitals again.

This time they are: systolic BP 122; diastolic BP 76; pulse of 136, weak and regular; respirations of 20 and shallow but with adequate tidal volume; still pale, cool, and diaphoretic skin; and a pulse oximetry of 94%.

At 1715 you arrive at the ambulance bay of the Beth Israel Medical Center, quickly move the patient inside and transfer his care to the emergency department staff. After giving a full report to the receiving nurse and properly cleaning and preparing the ambulance, you and your partner go back available at 1735.

EMS Patient Care Report (PCR)

Date:	Incident No.:	Nature of Call:		Location:	
Dispatched:	En Route:	At Scene:	Transport:	At Hospital:	In Service:

Patient Information

Age:	Allergies:
Sex:	Medications:
Weight (in kg [lb]):	Past Medical History:
	Chief Complaint:

Vital Signs

Time:	BP:	Pulse:	Respirations:	SpO$_2$:
Time:	BP:	Pulse:	Respirations:	SpO$_2$:
Time:	BP:	Pulse:	Respirations:	SpO$_2$:

EMS Treatment
(circle all that apply)

Oxygen @ _____ L/min via (circle one): NC NRM Bag-Mask Device	Assisted Ventilation	Airway Adjunct	CPR
Defibrillation	Bleeding Control	Bandaging	Splinting	Other

Narrative

CHAPTER 7

Anatomy and Physiology

Matching

Part I

Match the terms as they relate to specific areas of the body.

___J___ 1. Pertaining to the armpit

___E___ 2. Pertaining to the lungs

___B___ 3. Pertaining to the chest

___A___ 4. Pertaining to the inferior posterior region of the head

___G___ 5. Pertaining to the navel

___F___ 6. Pertaining to the bones surrounding the eye

___C___ 7. Pertaining to the thigh

___H___ 8. Pertaining to the breast

___D___ 9. Pertaining to the buttocks

___E___ 10. Pertaining to the skin

A. Occipital

B. Pectoral

C. Femoral

D. Gluteal

E. Cutaneous

F. Orbital

G. Umbilical

H. Mammary

I. Pulmonary

J. Axillary

Part II

Now match the following types of epithelial tissue with their function and/or location in the human body.

___H___ 1. Simple squamous

___D___ 2. Simple cuboidal

___I___ 3. Simple columnar

___G___ 4. Pseudostratified columnar

___B___ 5. Stratified squamous

___C___ 6. Stratified cuboidal

___E___ 7. Stratified columnar

___A___ 8. Transitional

___F___ 9. Glandular

A. Distensibility, protection of the inner urinary bladder lining

B. Protection of the outer layer of the skin

C. Protection of gland ducts, pancreas, and salivary glands

D. Absorption and secretion in the kidney tubule linings

E. Protection and secretion in part of male urethra and parts of pharynx

F. Secretion in the endocrine, salivary, and sweat glands

G. Movement of mucus, protection and secretion in respiratory passage linings

H. Diffusion, filtration, osmosis, covering of surfaces in air sacs of lungs and blood vessels

I. Absorption, protection, and secretion in the intestine, stomach, and uterus lining

Multiple Choice

Read each item carefully, and then select the best response.

1. All of the cells in the body, with the exception of the _____, have between a hundred and a few thousand organelles called _____, which are the powerhouses of the cell.
   A. white blood cells; lysosomes
   B. red blood cells; golgi apparatus
   C. white blood cells; endoplasmic reticulum
   D. red blood cells; mitochondria

2. The movement of a solvent from an area of low solute concentration to one of high concentration through a selective permeable membrane is called:
   A. facilitated diffusion.
   B. osmosis.
   C. active transport.
   D. differentiation.

3. There are 230 joints in the human body. The joints that are the most complex, which allow free movement and are surrounded by an outer layer of ligaments forming a capsule, are called the:
   A. fibrous joints.
   B. cartilaginous joints.
   C. synovial joints.
   D. immovable joints.

4. The kidneys are found in which body cavity?
   A. Thoracic
   B. Abdominal
   C. Retroperitoneal
   D. Pelvic

5. The proximal end of the humerus articulates with the:
   A. clavicle.
   B. glenoid fossa.
   C. scapula.
   D. acromion process.

6. The neurotransmitter that stimulates skeletal muscle to contract is called:
   A. sarcoplasmic reticulum.
   B. myosin.
   C. actin.
   D. acetylcholine.

7. The muscle group located in the anterior femur is called the:
   A. gastrocnemius.
   B. rectus abdominis.
   C. quadriceps.
   D. triceps.

8. The muscle group that points the toes away from the head is called the:
   A. gastrocnemius.
   B. rectus abdominis.
   C. tibialis anterior.
   D. pectoralis.

9. The heart valve that separates the left atrium from the left ventricle is called the _____ valve and is a _____ valve.
   A. semilunar; tricuspid
   B. pulmonic; bicuspid
   C. mitral; bicuspid
   D. aortic; tricuspid

10. The opening between the two atria of the heart in a fetus is called the:
    A. fossa ovalis.
    B. foramen ovale.
    C. interatrial septum.
    D. papillary cusp.

11. Of the vessels listed below, which is designed to withstand the highest pressures of any vessel in the body?
    A. Common carotid artery
    B. Ascending aorta
    C. Brachial artery
    D. Inferior vena cava

12. A specialized portion of the venous system that drains blood from the stomach, intestines, and spleen is called the:
    A. hepatic portal system.
    B. lymphatic system.
    C. abdominal aortic aneurism.
    D. renal residual circulation.

13. What percentage of the plasma is water?
    A. 26%
    B. 48%
    C. 72%
    D. 92%

14. Found in the plasma of the blood, which of the following is NOT considered a protein?
    A. Albumin
    B. Sodium bicarbonate
    C. Globulin
    D. Fibrinogen

15. The occipital lobe of the brain is responsible for:
    A. hearing, smell, and language.
    B. vision and storage of visual memories.
    C. basic emotions and basic reflexes, like chewing.
    D. judgment and predicting consequences of actions.

16. The portion of the brain that is responsible for emotions, temperature control, and interface with the endocrine system is called the:
    A. occipital lobe.
    B. temporal lobe.
    C. prefrontal area.
    D. diencephalon.

17. The fifth cranial nerve is called the:
    A. optic nerve.
    B. occulomotor nerve.
    C. vagus nerve.
    D. trigeminal nerve.

18. The ninth cranial nerve is called the:
    A. occulomotor nerve.
    B. glossopharyngeal nerve.
    C. facial nerve.
    D. abducens nerve.

19. The cranial nerve that is responsible for the sense of hearing and balance is the _____ cranial nerve.
    A. 3rd
    B. 8th
    C. 9th
    D. 10th

20. When a patient has been diagnosed with a history of _____, the eyes may be oriented correctly but one fails to send adequate signals to the vision center, causing a loss of depth perception and poor-quality images.
    A. strabismus
    B. amblyopia
    C. macular degeneration
    D. a blind spot

Fill-in-the-Blank

Read each item carefully, and then complete the statement by filling in the missing word(s).

1. The _liver_ is a large, solid organ that takes up most of the area immediately beneath the diaphragm. The _gallbladder_ is an outpouching from the bile ducts that serves as a reservoir and concentrating organ for _bile_ produced in the liver.

2. The _small intestine_ is the major hollow organ of the abdomen whose cells produce enzymes and mucus to aid in digestion. The _large intestine_ consists of the cecum, the _colon_, and the rectum.

3. The _endocrine_ system is made up of various glands located throughout the body. These glands release _hormones_ such as insulin into the bloodstream. The major _endocrine_ glands include the pituitary, thyroid, and adrenal glands. The major _exocrine_ glands include the sweat glands, which secrete outside the body.

4. Let's review the pituitary gland hormones. The _growth_ hormone increases the size and division rate of body cells. The _thyroid_-stimulating hormone controls the thyroid gland hormone secretion. The sex cell hormone that aids in the release of female egg cells is called the _luteinizing_ hormone. The hormone _oxytocin_ is designed to contract the uterine wall muscles as well as _contract_ milk-secreting gland muscles.

5. Now let's review the functions of the female reproductive organs. The female reproductive organ that produces oocytes and sex hormones is/are the _ovaries_. The _fallopian tubes_ transport secondary oocytes in the direction of the uterus so fertilization can normally occur. The muscular organ in which implantation, _placenta_ formation, and fetal development occur is the uterus. The uterine secretions are transported to the outside of the female's body by the _vagina_. The _labia majora_ protects and encloses the female's external reproductive organs, and the _labia minora_ protects the openings of the vagina and the urethra, which are contained in the _vestibule_.

Labeling

1. Bones of the Skull

   Label the names of the bones in the cranium.

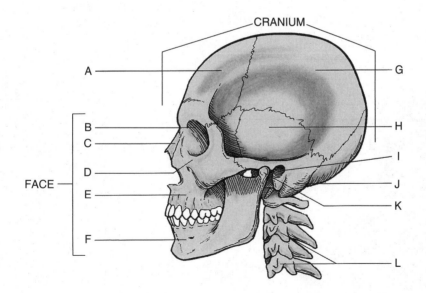

CRANIUM

A —
B —
C —
D —
E —
F —
FACE
G —
H —
I —
J —
K —
L —

A. _frontal_
B. _orbit_
C. _nasal_
D. _zygoma_
E. _maxilla_
F. _mandible_
G. _parietal_
H. _temporal_
I. _external auditory meatus_
J. _mastoid process_
K. _temporomandibular joint_
L. _cervical vertebrae_

2. The Lower Extremity

Label the names of the principal parts of the lower extremity.

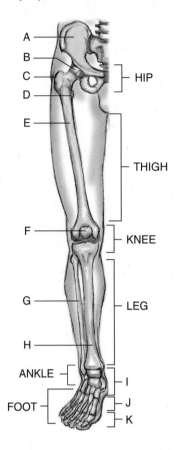

A. _pelvis_
B. _femoral head_
C. _Greater trochanter_
D. _lesser trochanter_
E. _femur_
F. _Patella_
G. _Fibulla_
H. _tibia_
I. _tarsals_
J. _metatarsals_
K. _phalanges_

3. Structures in the Respiratory System

Label the names of the structures in the respiratory system.

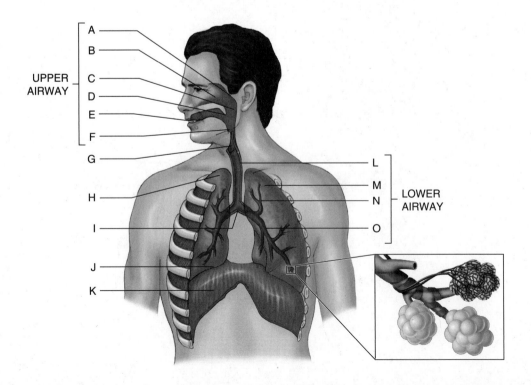

A. _nasopharynx_
B. _nasal airway passage_
C. _pharynx_
D. _oropharynx_
E. _mouth_
F. _epiglottis_
G. _larynx_
H. _apex of the lung_
I. _carina_
J. _base of the lung_
K. _diaphragm_
L. _trachea_
M. _alveoli_
N. _bronchioles_
O. _main bronchi_

True/False

If you believe the statement to be more true than false, write the letter "T" in the space provided. If you believe the statement to be more false than true, write the letter "F."

_T_ **1.** Parasympathetic stimulation can cause constriction of the pupil.

_T_ **2.** Sympathetic stimulation can cause secretion of the hormone adrenaline.

_T_ **3.** Parasympathetic stimulation can cause increased urination.

_F_ **4.** Sympathetic stimulation will cause increased emptying of the colon.

_F_ **5.** Parasympathetic stimulation will speed up the heart.

_F_ **6.** Sympathetic stimulation will constrict the bronchioles.

_T_ **7.** Parasympathetic stimulation will increase the secretion of saliva.

_T_ **8.** Sympathetic stimulation will stop the secretion of the parotid gland.

_T_ **9.** Parasympathetic stimulation will increase the motility of the small intestines.

_F_ **10.** Sympathetic division of the autonomic nervous system is referred to as the "rest and digest" reaction.

Pathophysiology

Matching

Part I

Match the adaptations in cells and tissues to the appropriate definitions.

_____ **1.** An alteration in the size, shape, and organization of cells

_____ **2.** An increase in the size of cells caused by synthesis of more subcellular components, which in turn leads to an increase in tissue and organ size

_____ **3.** A decrease in cell size caused by a loss of subcellular components, which in turn leads to a decrease in tissue and organ size

_____ **4.** Reversible, cellular adaptation in which one adult cell type is replaced by another adult cell type

_____ **5.** An increase in the actual number of cells in an organ or tissue, usually resulting in an increase in size of organ or tissue

A. Atrophy

B. Hypertrophy

C. Hyperplasia

D. Dysplasia

E. Metaplasia

Part II

Match the types of shock to the appropriate definitions.

_____ **1.** The result of widespread infection

_____ **2.** Occurs when blood flow becomes blocked in the heart or great vessels

_____ **3.** The result of spinal cord injury

_____ **4.** Occurs when histamine and other vasodilator proteins are released upon exposure to an allergen

_____ **5.** Occurs when the heart cannot circulate enough blood to maintain adequate peripheral oxygen delivery

_____ **6.** Occurs when there is widespread dilation of the resistance vessels, the capacitance vessels, or both

_____ **7.** Occurs when the circulating blood volume is unable to deliver adequate oxygen and nutrients to the body

A. Cardiogenic shock

B. Obstructive shock

C. Hypovolemic shock

D. Distributive shock

E. Anaphylactic shock

F. Septic shock

G. Neurogenic shock

Multiple Choice

Read each item carefully, and then select the best response.

1. The part of the cell that produces adenosine triphosphate (ATP), the major energy source of the body, is called:
   A. endoplasmic reticulum.
   B. golgi complex.
   C. mitochondria.
   D. lysosomes.

2. An increase in the size of cells caused by synthesis of more subcellular components, which in turn leads to an increase in tissue and organ size, is called:
   A. hypertrophy.
   B. hyperplasia.
   C. dysplasia.
   D. metaplasia.

3. The movement of a solvent from an area of low solute concentration to one of high concentration through a permeable membrane to equalize concentrations on both sides of the membrane is called:
   A. diffusion.
   B. active transport.
   C. filtration.
   D. osmosis.

4. When examining rates of disease, what term refers to the number of cases in a particular population?
   A. Incidence
   B. Prevalence
   C. Distribution
   D. Tendency

5. What percentage of the blood is made up of plasma?
   A. 0.9%
   B. 25%
   C. 45%
   D. 55%

6. Which of the following is caused by an autosomal dominant inheritance (where a person needs to inherit only one copy of the particular form of the gene to show the trait)?
   A. Sickle cell anemia
   B. Attached earlobe
   C. Tay-Sachs disease
   D. Freckles

7. Individuals who suffer from long QT syndrome are at risk of all of the following, EXCEPT:
   A. ventricular dysrhythmias.
   B. palpitations.
   C. torsades de pointes.
   D. atrial fibrillation.

8. Clinical manifestation of Alzheimer disease occurs in how many distinct stages?
   A. Four
   B. Three
   C. Two
   D. One

9. Central shock consists of what two types of shock?
   A. Hypovolemic and distributive
   B. Cardiogenic and distributive
   C. Cardiogenic and obstructive
   D. Hypovolemic and obstructive

10. The MOST abundant type of white blood cells is called:
    A. neutrophils.
    B. eosinophils.
    C. basophils.
    D. monocytes.

Fill-in-the-Blank

Read each item carefully, and then complete the statement by filling in the missing word(s).

1. The dynamic process, also called the dynamic steady state, is known as _____.

2. _____ _____ is a special type of connective tissue that contains large amounts of lipids.

3. _____ is an increase in the actual number of cells in an organ or tissue.

4. _____ are found primarily in the carotid artery, aorta, and kidneys and are sensitive to changes in blood pressure.

5. A decrease in urine output is called _____.

6. _____ is an elevated potassium level.

7. The molecules that modulate the changes in pH are called _____.

8. Normal cell death is called _____.

9. _____ _____ _____ _____ is a progressive condition usually characterized by concurrent failure of several organs, such as the lungs, liver, and kidneys.

10. _____ are lipopolysaccharides that are part of the cell walls of gram-negative bacteria. They cause inflammation, fever, and chills.

Labeling

1. Components of the Organelles of a Cell

   Label the components of the organelles of a cell.

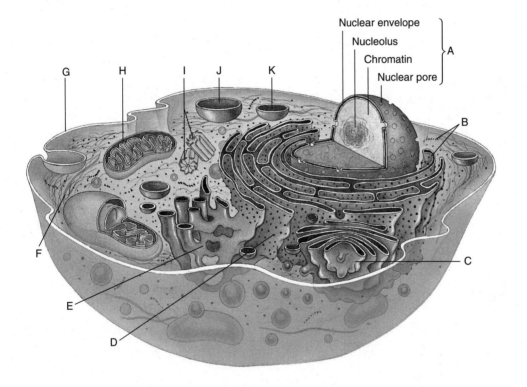

A. _____

B. _____

C. _____

D. _____

E. _____

F. _____

G. _____

H. _____

I. _____

J. _____

K. _____

2. Type I Allergic Reaction

Fill in the missing words that describe a type I allergic reaction.

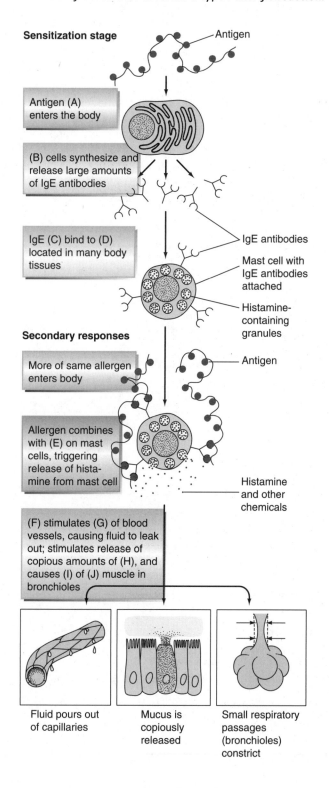

Sensitization stage

Antigen

Antigen (A) enters the body

(B) cells synthesize and release large amounts of IgE antibodies

IgE (C) bind to (D) located in many body tissues

IgE antibodies

Mast cell with IgE antibodies attached

Histamine-containing granules

Secondary responses

More of same allergen enters body

Antigen

Allergen combines with (E) on mast cells, triggering release of histamine from mast cell

Histamine and other chemicals

(F) stimulates (G) of blood vessels, causing fluid to leak out; stimulates release of copious amounts of (H), and causes (I) of (J) muscle in bronchioles

Fluid pours out of capillaries

Mucus is copiously released

Small respiratory passages (bronchioles) constrict

A. _____

B. _____

C. _____

D. _____

E. _____

F. _____

G. _____

H. _____

I. _____

J. _____

Identify

In the following case study, list the chief complaint, vital signs, and pertinent patient history.

You respond to a call to an assisted living manor for a 78-year-old man who is having difficulty breathing. Upon arrival, you find your patient sitting forward in a dining room chair with his "elbows out." He is looking rather distressed. You walk up to his table, introduce yourself, and ask what's wrong. The patient responds, with what appears to be great difficulty, "I . . . can't . . . breathe." Your partner starts to obtain vital signs as you place the patient on a nonrebreathing mask. You obtain the following history between the patient and staff for the facility. The symptoms started about 30 minutes ago with shortness of breath and coughing. The night nurse's aide tells you the patient said he was chilled, sweaty, and felt warm. His temperature was taken before your arrival and was recorded on the chart as 102.5°F. The medical record states he has chronic obstructive pulmonary disease (COPD) with a 40-year history of two packs of cigarettes a day. Your partner tells you that respirations are 28 breaths/ min and shallow, the pulse is 90 beats/min with occasional irregular beats, blood pressure is 160/90 mm Hg, and oxygen saturation is 90%. You and your partner decide to place the patient on constant positive airway pressure (CPAP) to assist. Just before placing the mask, the patient starts to cough and brings up blood-tinged sputum. You prepare the patient and transport. He is hospitalized for a week with a diagnosis of pneumonia before being placed in a nursing home.

1. Chief complaint:

_____

_____

2. Vital signs:

_____

_____

3. Pertinent patient history:

_____

_____

4. What was your presumptive diagnosis?

_____

_____

Ambulance Calls

The following case scenarios provide an opportunity to explore the concerns associated with patient management and paramedic care. Read each scenario, and then answer each question.

1. While on a chest pain call, you are taking the SAMPLE history, and the patient tells you he is taking an angiotensin-converting enzyme (ACE) inhibitor for hypertension. Your partner has placed the patient on the ECG monitor and informs you that there is a peaked T wave and a wide QRS complex with tachycardia.

a. What do you suspect is the life-threatening emergency that is being identified on the ECG?

_____

_____

b. What drug should be considered as the first-line medication for this condition?

_____

_____

2. Approximately a half million people living in the United States are believed to have Crohn disease. When a person has an acute episode, he or she may call EMS.

    a. Crohn disease is a disorder of which body system?

    _____

    _____

    b. What symptoms would you expect a patient with Crohn disease to have?

    _____

    _____

3. It is not uncommon to encounter an elderly patient who has Alzheimer disease as an underlying problem. What are some of the factors that might affect your ability to get a good SAMPLE history and provide care for an Alzheimer patient?

_____

_____

_____

True/False

If you believe the statement to be more true than false, write the letter "T" in the space provided. If you believe the statement to be more false than true, write the letter "F."

_____ **1.** Epithelium covers the external surfaces of the body.

_____ **2.** Dendrites receive electrical impulses from axons of other nerve cells and conduct the impulses toward the body cell.

_____ **3.** Metaplasia is an alteration in the size, shape, and organization of cells.

_____ **4.** Tonicity refers to the tension exerted on a cell caused by water movement across the cell membrane.

_____ **5.** A blood pH of less than 7.35 is called alkalosis.

_____ **6.** With autosomal-recessive inheritance, a person must inherit only one copy of a particular form of a gene to show that trait.

_____ **7.** Distributive shock occurs when blood flow becomes blocked in the great vessels.

_____ **8.** Acquired immunity is a highly specific, inducible, discriminatory, and unforgetting method by which armies of cells respond to an immune stimulant.

_____ **9.** Type I diabetes is considered an autoimmune disease.

_____ **10.** Rh factor is an antigen that is present in the erythrocytes of about 85% of the population and is of key importance in blood typing.

Short Answer

Complete this section with short written answers using the space provided.

1. The body loses water in a number of ways. List the four major ways.

    a. _____

    b. _____

    c. _____

    d. _____

2. What are the four forces that control the equilibrium between the capillary and the interstitial space?

    a. _____

    b. _____

c. _____

d. _____

3. Metabolic acidosis is an accumulation of abnormal acids in the blood. List four causes of this condition.

   a. _____

   b. _____

   c. _____

   d. _____

4. Cellular injury can result from various causes. List five causes.

   a. _____

   b. _____

   c. _____

   d. _____

   e. _____

5. List seven common respiratory diseases that may be caused by environmental pollutants, viruses, or bacteria.

   a. _____

   b. _____

   c. _____

   d. _____

   e. _____

   f. _____

   g. _____

6. List four conditions for which you should always consider syncope to be caused by a life-threatening dysrhythmia until proved otherwise.

   a. _____

   b. _____

   c. _____

   d. _____

7. Alzheimer disease is progressive. Describe the disease in each of the following phases:

   a. Stage 1 (early): _____

   b. Stage 2: _____

   c. Stage 3 (advanced): _____

8. List the five general types of leukocytes.

   a. _____

   b. _____

   c. _____

   d. _____

   e. _____

9. The goal of the cellular component of acute inflammatory response is for the inflammatory cells (polymorpho-nuclear neutrophils) to arrive at the site in the tissue where they are needed. The process involves two major stages: intravascular phase and extravascular phase. During the later phase, leukocytes travel to the inflammation site and kill organisms. Name the five events in this sequence.

a. _____

b. _____

c. _____

d. _____

e. _____

10. What are the three stages of general adaptation syndrome?

a. _____

b. _____

c. _____

Fill-in-the-Table

Fill in the missing parts of the table on shock.

Signs and Symptoms of Compensated and Decompensated Hypoperfusion	
Compensated	**Decompensated**
Agitation, anxiety, restlessness	Altered mental status (verbal to unresponsive)
Sense of impending doom	_____
_____	
Clammy (cool, moist) skin	Thready or absent peripheral pulses
_____	Ashen, mottled, or cyanotic skin
Shortness of breath	_____
_____	_____
Delayed capillary refill time in infants and children	Impending cardiac arrest
_____	
Normal blood pressure	

Life Span Development

Matching

Match each of the definitions in the left column to the appropriate term in the right column.

_____ **1.** Person who is 1 month to 1 year of age

_____ **2.** Person who is 0 to 1 month of age

_____ **3.** Person who is 3 to 6 years of age

_____ **4.** Person who is 18 to 40 years of age

_____ **5.** Person who is 41 to 60 years of age

_____ **6.** Life expectancy

_____ **7.** Person who is 12 to 17 years of age

_____ **8.** Person who is 61 years of age or older

_____ **9.** Person who is 6 to 12 years of age

_____ **10.** Person who is 1 to 3 years of age

A. Adolescent

B. Early adult

C. Infant

D. Late adult

E. Middle adult

F. Preschooler

G. School-age child

H. Toddler

I. Newborn

J. Average number of years one is predicted to live

Multiple Choice

Read each item carefully, and then select the best response.

1. When a newborn's cheek is touched, he or she turns toward the touch. This is called the _____ reflex.
- **A.** moro
- **B.** palmar
- **C.** sucking
- **D.** rooting

2. The tidal volume of an infant starts at _____ mL/kg.
- **A.** 4 to 6
- **B.** 6 to 8
- **C.** 8 to 12
- **D.** 12 to 14

3. Which of the infant's fontanelles can be used as a possible indicator of dehydration if sunken?
- **A.** Posterior
- **B.** Mastoid
- **C.** Sphenoidal
- **D.** Anterior

4. At approximately what age does an infant start to become afraid of strangers?
- **A.** 2 months
- **B.** 7 months
- **C.** 9 months
- **D.** 1 year

5. The filtration function of the kidneys declines by _____ between 20 and 90 years of age.
- **A.** less than 25%
- **B.** about 25%
- **C.** about 50%
- **D.** about 75%

6. Bleeding can empty into voids in the older adult brain, resulting in what type of hemorrhage?
   A. Meningeal
   B. Epidural
   C. Ventricular
   D. Subdural

7. In the 5 years preceding death, mental function is presumed to decline, a theory referred to as the:
   A. terminal drop hypothesis.
   B. organic dementia hypothesis.
   C. geriatric shrinkage syndrome.
   D. end-of-life physiopsych decline.

8. In late adults, vital capacity of the lungs decreases and residual volume increases. The effect can produce which of the following conditions?
   A. Hypercarbia
   B. Hypocarbia
   C. Hypoxia
   D. Hyperoxygenation

9. Which one of the following is NOT a usual response of the cardiovascular system with late adults?
   A. Decrease in heart rate
   B. Cardiac output matches demand
   C. Increase in systolic blood pressure
   D. Partial blockage of blood flow

10. School-age children learn various types of reasoning in their development. Which of the following is a type of reasoning they learn?
    A. Cognitive
    B. Distributive
    C. Conventional
    D. Affective

Fill-in-the-Blank

Read each item carefully, and then complete the statement by filling in the missing word(s).

1. An infant usually weighs _____ to _____ lbs at birth. After birth, infants usually lose _____ to _____ of their birth weight due to the loss of _____ in the first week.

2. A/an _____ _____ occurs when an object is placed in the infant's palm.

3. An infant's _____ allow the head to be molded when the newborn passes through the birth canal.

4. _____ _____, located on either end of the infant's bones, aid in the lengthening of a child's bones.

5. _____, or the formation of a close, personal relationship, is usually based on a secure attachment.

6. _____ and _____ refer to a stage of development from birth to about 18 months of age. Most infants desire that their world be planned, organized, and _____.

7. Atherosclerosis can contribute to the development of a/an _____, or weakening and bulging of a blood vessel wall.

8. In late adults, blood flow in the _____ (membranes that connect organs to the abdominal wall) may drop by as much as 50%.

9. In the 5 years preceding death, mental function is presumed to decline. This is a theory referred to as the _____ _____ _____.

10. In late adults, the size of the airway _____ and the surface areas of the alveoli _____.

Labeling

Label the four fontanelles of the infant's head.

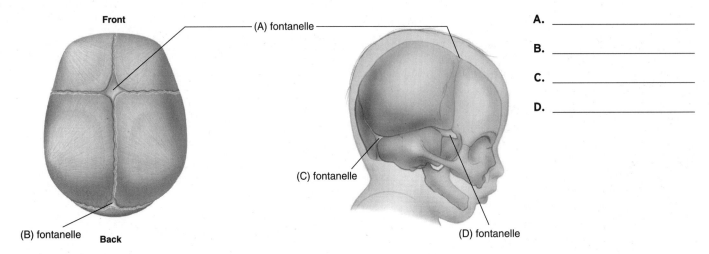

Front

(A) fontanelle

(C) fontanelle

(B) fontanelle   **Back**

(D) fontanelle

A. _____

B. _____

C. _____

D. _____

Identify

For the following case study, list the chief complaint, vital signs, and SAMPLE history.

A call to an assisted-living facility brings you to a 75-year-old woman who, while walking from the living room to the kitchen, tripped on a chair and fell. When you enter the apartment, the patient tells you she fell and has a great deal of pain in her hip. You gently palpate the injured area and the patient yells. You take a set of vital signs and find a pulse of 90 beats/min and thready, respirations of 24 breaths/min and shallow, and blood pressure of 100/70 mm Hg. The SAMPLE history identifies an externally rotated foot and discoloration of the hip on the same side. The patient reports no allergies and is on several medications for congestive heart failure. She had a heart attack last year, and she has a two-pack-a-day history of smoking for more than 30 years but stopped smoking about 5 years ago. She ate breakfast 3 hours ago. You place the patient on an ECG monitor, establish an IV, and package her for transport.

1. Chief complaint:

_____

_____

2. Vital signs:

_____

_____

3. SAMPLE history:

_____

_____

Ambulance Calls

The following case scenarios provide an opportunity to explore the concerns associated with patient management and paramedic care. Read each scenario, and then answer each question.

1. Your unit is dispatched to a call for an infant with a seizure. The response time is 5 minutes, and when you enter the residence you find a distraught mother who is very anxious. The seizure seems to have stopped, but you understand the importance of an immediate primary assessment (the MS–ABC Priority Plan). You immediately notice the child has good color except for a little cyanosis of the fingers. The child is actively breathing, and the rate is adequate. Your partner starts to administer blow-by oxygen, and you examine the child quickly from head to toe to make sure there is no external bleeding or signs of trauma. The child is starting to respond and become more active. You prepare for transport and decide the child is stable and alert enough that the neurologic status can be assessed. What reflexes would you check and how would you test them? What are considered to be the appropriate responses from the infant? Fill in the following table.

Reflex	How to Test	Appropriate Response

2. A call to an assisted living facility finds a 75-year-old woman sitting with her partner and complaining of general body weakness. You approach the patient but have trouble communicating with her, and while doing the SAMPLE history you have trouble getting necessary information from her. You decide that when asking about her past medical history you should ask about individual body systems because this might help to identify the current problem.

    a. What are some of the communication issues you might have encountered while taking the history of this patient?

_____

_____

_____

_____

    b. What are some possible concerns you are thinking of while attempting to obtain the past medical history?

_____

_____

_____

_____

3. You receive a call to the residence of a 16-year-old young woman with a chief complaint of abdominal pain. The young woman is lying on the couch in the living room and her mother and a girlfriend are also in the room. Your partner is a man who is taking the lead on the assessment and SAMPLE history. While doing the SAMPLE history, he asks the patient if there is a possibility she is pregnant. She immediately and emphatically answers no. He then decides that he should palpate the abdomen and immediately proceeds to do so with little explanation. The patient seems embarrassed. You realize that you need to package the patient and transport.

    a. What consideration should your partner have taken into account before questioning this patient about the possibility of pregnancy?

_____

_____

_____

_____

    b. Is there a more appropriate way to handle the physical exam of the abdomen?

_____

_____

_____

_____

True/False

If you believe the statement to be more true than false, write the letter "T" in the space provided. If you believe the statement to be more false than true, write the letter "F."

_____ **1.** An infant's ventilations that are too forceful can result in barotrauma.

_____ **2.** The rooting reflex occurs when an infant's lips are stroked.

_____ **3.** If the posterior fontanelle is sunken, the infant is most likely dehydrated.

_____ **4.** Anxious avoidant attachment is observed in infants who are repeatedly rejected.

_____ **5.** A toddler is at the critical age in human development to learn various types of reasoning.

_____ **6.** Cardiac function declines with age consequent to anatomic and physiologic changes largely related to atherosclerosis.

_____ **7.** In late adults, vital capacity of the lungs decreases and stagnant air remains in the alveoli and hampers gas exchange, which can produce hypercarbia.

_____ **8.** In late adults, there is a surge of increased mental functioning in the last few years of life.

_____ **9.** Age-related shrinkage creates a void between the brain and outermost layer of the meninges.

_____**10.** The number of nephrons in the kidneys increases between ages 30 and 80 years.

Short Answer

Complete this section with short written answers using the space provided.

1. Infants are born with certain reflexes and responses that can assist you in the neurologic assessment of an infant. Name four of these reflexes.

a. _____

b. _____

c. _____

d. _____

2. Cardiac function declines with age largely as a result of atherosclerosis. This disorder, which commonly affects coronary vessels, results from the formation of plaque. What two substances are responsible for the buildup of plaque?

a. _____

b. _____

3. Loss of what mechanisms in the respiratory system of the late adult makes aspiration and obstruction more likely?

a. _____

b. _____

c. _____

d. _____

e. _____

4. Late adults have sensory changes that can affect mobility and safety. What sensory changes occur in this age group?

a. _____

b. _____

c. _____

d. _____

e. _____

f. _____

g. _____

5. Colds often develop in toddlers and preschool-age children and may manifest as what types of infections?

a. _____

b. _____

6. Playing games is the way that toddlers learn. What can a child of this age learn from play?

a. _____

b. _____

c. _____

7. In the late elderly, vital capacity of the lungs decreases. Name three factors that contribute to this decline.

a. _____

b. _____

c. _____

Fill-in-the-Table

Fill in the missing parts of the tables.

1. Subtle changes occur during adolescence; one change is the development of secondary sexual characteristics. Fill in the table with these characteristics.

Male Characteristics	Female Characteristics

2. Fill in the table with the appropriate respiratory rates for the various ages listed to the left.

Vital Signs at Various Ages

Age	Pulse Rate (beats/min)	Respirations (breaths/min)	Blood Pressure (mm Hg, systolic)	Temperature (°F)
Newborn (0 to 1 mo)	_____	_____	50 to 70	98 to 100
Infant (1 month to 1 y)	_____	25 to 50	_____	96.8 to 99.6
Toddler (1 to 3 y)	90 to 150	20 to 30	_____	96.8 to 99.6
Preschool age (3 to 5 y)	80 to 140	_____	80 to 100	_____
School age _____	70 to 120	15 to 20	_____	98.6
Adolescent _____	_____	_____	_____	98.6
Early adult (18 to 40 y)	_____	12 to 20	90 to 140	98.6
Middle adult (41 to 60 y)	60 to 100	12 to 20	90 to 140	98.6
Late adult (61 y and older)	Depends on health	Depends on health	_____	98.6

CHAPTER 10

Principles of Pharmacology

Matching

Listed here are the classifications of medications considered controlled substances. Match the schedule, I to V, with the description or the example given.

_____ **1.** Hydrocodone (Vicodin)

_____ **2.** Narcotic cough medicines

_____ **3.** Heroin

_____ **4.** Fentanyl (Sublimaze)

_____ **5.** Diazepam (Valium)

_____ **6.** Lorazepam (Ativan)

_____ **7.** High abuse potential and no recognized medical purpose

_____ **8.** High abuse potential and legitimate medical purpose

_____ **9.** Cocaine

_____ **10.** Codeine

Multiple Choice

Read each item carefully, and then select the best response.

1. The nonproprietary name is a general name for a drug and is not manufacturer specific. What is another name for nonproprietary drugs?
 A. Chemical
 B. Generic
 C. Trade
 D. Official

2. What was the first US federal law, legislated in 1906, aimed at protecting the public from mislabeled and harmful drugs?
 A. Food, Drug, and Cosmetic Act
 B. Harrison Narcotic Act
 C. Pure Food and Drug Act
 D. Narcotic Control Act

3. Which US government agency has jurisdiction over approving new medications?
 A. Food and Drug Administration
 B. Centers for Disease Control and Prevention
 C. Drug Enforcement Administration
 D. Federal Trade Commission

4. The medication interaction, which is utilized when the ED physician considers administering some ethanol to a patient who has been poisoned due to drinking ethylene glycol (antifreeze), is referred to as:
 A. altered absorption.
 B. drug antagonism.
 C. altered metabolism.
 D. neutralization.

5. The form of a medication in a wax-like material that dissolves in a body cavity is called a/an:
   A. capsule.
   B. suppository.
   C. powder.
   D. inhaler.

6. Which of the following forms of medication is dissolved or suspended in liquid intended for oral consumption?
   A. Suppository
   B. Inhaler/spray
   C. Drop
   D. Liquid

7. What is the name given to the small particles of medication designed to be dissolved or mixed into a solution or liquid?
   A. Tablet
   B. Powder
   C. Pill
   D. Pulvule

8. Which receptor sites would have an agonist effect of insulin secretion, uterine relaxation, and bronchiole relaxation?
   A. Alpha-1
   B. Alpha-2
   C. Beta-1
   D. Beta-2

9. Certain medications are known to have decreased efficacy or potency when taken repeatedly by a patient, a state known as:
   A. synergy.
   B. biotransformation.
   C. tolerance.
   D. reabsorption.

10. Medications distribute into each of the following types of body substances, EXCEPT:
   A. oils.
   B. lipids.
   C. water.
   D. proteins.

Fill-in-the-Blank

Read each item carefully, and then complete the statement by filling in the missing word(s).

1. A medication's _____ are the reasons or conditions for which the medication is given.

2. Two medications can bind together in the body, creating an inactive substance. This is referred to as _____.

3. Opiate _____ medication reverses the effects of opioid drugs.

4. When the effect of one medication is greatly enhanced by the presence of another medication, which does not have the ability to produce the same effect, this is referred to as _____.

5. The agonist that produces vasoconstriction of arteries and veins is called a/an _____ receptor.

6. The agonist that stimulates bronchus and bronchiole relaxation, as well as insulin secretion and uterine relaxation, is called a/an _____ receptor.

7. _____ medications cause the kidneys to remove excess amounts of salt and water from the body.

8. Medications that reduce heart rate and blood pressure are called _____ agents.

9. _____ _____ are drugs that decrease the heart rate and improve contractility.

10. Drugs that decrease inflammation and are immunosuppressants are called _____.

Identify

For the following case study, list the chief complaint, vital signs, and pertinent negatives.

You are called to a private residence for a 65-year-old woman who has general body weakness. Upon arrival, you find a woman sitting on a couch in the living room. When you ask what the problem is, she tells you that she has heart palpitations. She appears not to be in any distress. Her husband tells you she went to the doctor's yesterday, and she seems to be doing okay because it was just a checkup. You check vital signs and find the pulse is 60 beats/min, regular and weak; respirations are slightly labored at 22 breaths/min; and blood pressure is 90/60 mm Hg. While your partner starts an IV, you listen to her lung sounds, take a 12-lead ECG, and get a SAMPLE history. You know the symptoms and observe that the patient seems pale. She tells you she has no pain or nausea and that she is on medication for high blood pressure and gastric reflux. She tells you that she was put on a new medication yesterday for her gastric reflux and an additional medication for her high blood pressure. She has had no hospitalizations and has been in relatively good health. The patient was watching TV when her symptoms started. According to her husband, it is time for the patient's afternoon medications, but you think that she should wait until she gets to the hospital, a 15-minute transport time, and discuss them with the doctor before taking. You transport and reassess the vitals en route.

1. Chief complaint:

_____

_____

2. Vital signs:

_____

_____

3. Pertinent negatives:

_____

_____

Ambulance Calls

The following case scenarios provide an opportunity to explore the concerns associated with patient management and paramedic care. Read each scenario, and then answer each question.

1. You are on the scene for a 55-year-old man who is reporting an 8 out of 10 substernal chest pain that came on while he was shoveling snow. You have placed the patient on supplemental oxygen and given aspirin, and your partner is obtaining vital signs and a 12-lead ECG. You obtain lung sounds and administer nitroglycerin, which has had no effect. The patient is now reporting 10 out of 10 for pain. His blood pressure is 160/100 mm Hg, so you decide to administer 5 mg of morphine. The six rights for medication administration run through your head as you prepare the drug for administration. What are the six rights and how do they apply?

a. _____

b. _____

c. _____

d. _____

e. _____

f. _____

2. Many medications undergo some degree of chemical change by the body, known as biotransformation. This process has four possible effects on a medication absorbed into the body, which are:

a. _____

b. _____

c. _____

d. _____

3. The young and old potentially present factors that can affect the actions of medications that are administered in the prehospital setting. What factors should the paramedic consider when providing care to the young and old, including additional factors that may need to be considered if the patient has underlying medical conditions?

a. _____

b. _____

c. _____

d. _____

e. _____

f. _____

True/False

If you believe the statement to be more true than false, write the letter "T" in the space provided. If you believe the statement to be more false than true, write the letter "F."

_____ **1.** The general, nonproprietary name for a drug is its official name.

_____ **2.** Schedule V drugs have the highest abuse potential and a propensity for severe dependency.

_____ **3.** The changes in pharmacokinetics in geriatric patients are comparable to those observed in young children.

_____ **4.** The rate of elimination of a medication is directly influenced by the plasma levels of the substance.

_____ **5.** Patients at extremes of age are disproportionately prone to paradoxical medication reactions.

_____ **6.** The medications that are diuretics can help improve the effects of sickle cell disease.

_____ **7.** In the cardiac muscle cell, during phases 0, 1, 2, and 3, no additional depolarization may occur because of external stimuli.

_____ **8.** Idiosyncrasy is an abnormal reaction by a person to a medication to which most other people do not react.

_____ **9.** The unusual tolerance to the therapeutic and adverse clinical effects of a medication or chemical is known as synergism.

_____ **10.** Promethazine (Phenergan) is an antidysrhythmic medication taken by cardiac patients.

Short Answer

Complete this section with short written answers using the space provided.

1. The medical director of your organization announces that a new medication will be introduced into the protocols. As part of an in-service to learn about this new drug, you are given the pharmaceutical company's profile. What are the three different names that will be listed on this literature?

a. _____

b. _____

c. _____

2. What are the components of a drug profile?

a. _____

b. _____

c. _____

d. _____

e. _____

f. _____

g. _____

h. _____

i. _____

j. _____

k. _____

l. _____

3. The Institute for Safe Medication Practices (ISMP) has developed a list of error-prone medication abbreviations. List five potential errors and how they can be avoided.

a. _____

b. _____

c. _____

d. _____

e. _____

4. Common adverse effects include:

a. _____

b. _____

c. _____

d. _____

e. _____

f. _____

g. _____

h. _____

5. For each of the following medication descriptions, write the medication class next to the common indications or purpose.
  a. Treat or prevent nausea and vomiting: _____
  b. Decrease gastrointestinal motility; alter GI secretion activity: _____
  c. Treat bacterial infection: _____
  d. Neutralize excess acids present in stomach: _____
  e. Block histamine receptors; dry mucous membranes; inhibit immune response in allergic reactions: _____
  f. Reduce heart rate and blood pressure: _____
  g. Treat anxiety and seizures; provide sedation: _____
  h. Decrease inflammation; immunosuppressant: _____
  i. Dissolve clots present in blood vessels or vascular access devices: _____
  j. Replace hormones; improve bone density that has decreased due to aging and hormone loss: _____
  k. Relieve pain and relieve or suppress cough: _____
  l. Increase blood pressure, heart rate, and cardiac output; constrict blood vessels: _____

Fill-in-the-Table

Fill in the missing parts of the tables.

Intraosseous Site	Veins Used During IO Infusion Vein
Proximal tibia	_____
Femur	_____
_____	Great saphenous vein
_____	Axillary vein
Manubrium (sternum)	_____

Factor	GI Medication Absorption Medication Absorption
_____	Ability of medication to pass through the GI tract into the bloodstream
_____	Perfusion of the GI system (may be decreased during systemic trauma or shock)
_____	Injury or bleeding in the GI system (both can alter GI motility, decreasing the time that oral medications can be absorbed)

Source	Sources of Medication Example
_____	Atropine, aspirin, digoxin, morphine
_____	Heparin, antivenom, thyroid preparations, insulin
_____	Streptokinase, numerous antibiotics
_____	Iron, magnesium sulfate, lithium, phosphorus, calcium

Medication Administration

Matching

Part I

In choosing a medication, selecting the route of administration relates to the medication's onset of action. For each of the following, match the onset of action with the route of administration:

_____ **1.** Intramuscular injection

_____ **2.** Nasal mucosal atomization (MAD)

_____ **3.** Endotracheal

_____ **4.** Intraosseous

_____ **5.** Sublingual

_____ **6.** Inhalation

_____ **7.** Intravenous

A. 30–60 sec

B. 2–3 min

C. 3–5 min

D. 10–20 min

Part II

Match the correct word to the definition.

_____ **1.** Carrier for red and white blood cells

_____ **2.** Inorganic molecules that do not contain carbon

_____ **3.** The fluid that dissolves components

_____ **4.** Forty-five percent of body weight; the water that is inside the cells

A. Intracellular fluid

B. Electrolytes

C. Intravascular fluid

D. Solvent

Multiple Choice

Read each item carefully, and then select the best response.

1. Interstitial fluid is:
   A. fluid that is contained inside the cells.
   B. the water within the blood.
   C. the water that bathes the cells.
   D. all the water in the body.

2. When hypocalcemia occurs in your patient, which of the following signs and symptoms would you expect to see?
   A. Muscle cramps, hypotension, and vasoconstriction
   B. Muscle spasms, lethargy, and hot, flushed skin
   C. Cardiac arrest, hyperstimulation of the nerve cells, carpopedal spasms
   D. Shortness of breath, heart dysrhythmias

3. Which of the following solutions is the BEST choice for administration, in the prehospital setting, when the patient needs to have body fluids replaced?
   A. Hypertonic
   B. Hypotonic
   C. Colloid
   D. Crystalloid

4. Which administration set will allow for 60 gtt/mL?
   A. Blood tubing
   B. Microdrip set
   C. Macrodrip set
   D. Volutrol administration set

5. When inserting an IV catheter, the bevel should be:
   A. facing down.
   B. facing up.
   C. pointed to the side.
   D. rolled as you insert it.

6. After starting an IV on a patient, which of the following is NOT necessary to document?
   A. The site of the IV
   B. The gauge of the needle you used
   C. The patient's pain scale when you started the IV
   D. The type of fluid you are using

7. There are many complications with an IV site; _____ means there is an inflammation of the vein.
   A. thrombophlebitis
   B. hematoma
   C. occlusion
   D. vein irritation

8. Which of the following is NOT a sign of an allergic reaction to IV therapy?
   A. Urticaria
   B. Shortness of breath
   C. Bradycardia
   D. Edema of the face

9. When taking a blood sample in the field, what is the green top tube used for?
   A. Determining the patient's blood type
   B. Checking glucose and electrolyte levels
   C. Determining how long it takes for the patient's blood to clot
   D. Checking for alcohol and drugs in the blood system

10. Which of the following is an example of an antiseptic?
   A. Virex
   B. Iodine
   C. Cidex
   D. Microcide

11. Which medication route is usually the fastest and most commonly used in the prehospital setting?
   A. Intradermal
   B. Subcutaneous
   C. Intramuscular
   D. Intravenous

12. A/an _____ is a breakable sterile glass container that carries a single dose of medication.
   A. vial
   B. ampule
   C. mix-o-vial
   D. prefill

13. A/an _____ injection is given at a 90° angle.
   A. subcutaneous
   B. intravascular
   C. intramuscular
   D. bolus

14. Which of the following medications is NOT given by the intranasal route?
   A. Naloxone
   B. Fentanyl
   C. Nitroglycerin
   D. Glucagon

15. How much normal saline should you use as a flush after administering a medication through a gastric tube?
   A. 15 to 30 mL
   B. 30 to 60 mL
   C. 60 to 75 mL
   D. You do not use normal saline for a flush.

Fill-in-the-Blank

Read each item carefully, and then complete the statement by filling in the missing word(s).

1. An intravenous solution that contains large molecules such as proteins is a/an _____.

2. An intravenous solution that does not contain large molecules such as proteins is a/an _____. One example of such a solution is normal _____.

3. When two solutions of different solute concentration are placed on either side of a semipermeable membrane, the more concentrated solution is said to be _____ with respect to the less concentrated solution. Conversely, the less concentrated solution is considered _____ with respect to the more concentrated solution. If the two solutions have the same concentration, they are said to be _____. Thus, for example, 4% saline is _____ with respect to serum; Ringer's solution is _____ with respect to serum; and half normal saline (0.45% NaCl) is _____ with respect to serum.

4. When two solutions of different solute concentrations are placed on either side of a semipermeable membrane, water will move from the solution of _____ (higher or lower?) solute concentration to the solution of _____ (higher or lower?) solute concentration. The process by which water migrates in that fashion is called _____.

5. The signs and symptoms of circulatory overload include _____, JVD, and _____.

Labeling

Label the common sites for intramuscular injections.

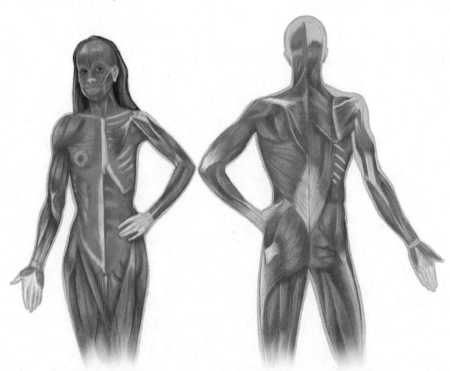

Ambulance Calls

All of the patients described in the following scenarios are experiencing a problem related to their intravenous therapy. Identify the problem in each case, and explain what you will do to manage it.

1. The patient is a 59-year-old man with severe chest pain on whom you have started a "keep-open" IV. It is a long way to the hospital, and about 10 minutes into the transport, he starts complaining of breathing difficulty. You notice that his respirations have become more rapid, and when you listen to his chest, you can hear crackling (rales) sounds. Meanwhile, you suddenly notice that the liter bag of IV fluid is empty.
    a. What is the patient's problem?

    _____

    _____

    _____

    b. What are you going to do about it?

    _____

    _____

    _____

2. You have started an IV on a frail old woman. After a few minutes, you notice that the IV is infusing more and more slowly. You open the clamp wide, but that doesn't help. You lower the IV bag below the stretcher; there is no blood return into the tubing. Then you check the IV site. There seems to be a lump in the skin, and the skin feels quite cool.
    a. What is the patient's problem?

    _____

    _____

    _____

    b. What are you going to do about it?

    _____

    _____

    _____

    c. What other problems might cause an IV to slow down or stop?

    _____

    _____

    _____

3. You are starting an IV near the wrist of a petite young woman. When the IV catheter enters the vessel, bright red blood comes spurting back onto your face shield.
    a. What is the patient's problem?

    _____

    _____

b. What are you going to do about it?

_____

_____

_____

4. You are transporting a patient between hospitals. The patient has an IV already running (it was started earlier in the day by the paramedics who brought the patient to the first hospital). The patient complains of pain at the IV site, and you notice that it is red, hot, and swollen.
   a. What is the patient's problem?

   _____

   _____

   _____

   b. What are you going to do about it?

   _____

   _____

   _____

   c. How could this problem have been prevented?
   (1) _____
   (2) _____
   (3) _____
   (4) _____

5. A driver is found conscious but very restless. He keeps asking you, "Can't you give me some water? I'm so thirsty—please give me something to drink." His skin is cold and sweaty. You do not see any external signs of serious injury.
   a. Do you think this patient has been seriously injured? Explain the reasons for your answer.

   _____

   _____

   _____

   b. You decide to start an IV with lactated Ringer's, which is a _____ (colloid or crystalloid?) solution. Your protocol calls for administering 200 mL/h in these circumstances. You have an administration set that delivers 10 gtt/mL. To set the infusion rate to deliver 200 mL/h, you will need to set the drops per minute at _____ gtt/min. (Show your calculations.)

c. A few minutes after you adjust the IV rate, you notice that the IV has slowed down to the point that it is hardly flowing at all. List the five steps you would take to try to identify and solve the problem with the IV.

(1) _____

(2) _____

(3) _____

(4) _____

(5) _____

True/False

If you believe the statement to be more true than false, write the letter "T" in the space provided. If you believe the statement to be more false than true, write the letter "F."

_____ **1.** An ion with a negative charge is called a cation.

_____ **2.** "Where sodium goes, water follows."

_____ **3.** Calcium is the primary buffer in body fluids.

_____ **4.** The normal concentration of glucose in the body is 50 to 100 mg per 100 mL.

_____ **5.** The process of moving from a higher concentration to a lower concentration is called diffusion.

_____ **6.** Tonicity is the concentration of calcium inside and outside the cell.

_____ **7.** A healthy person will lose up to 1 L of fluid a day as a result of urine output and exhalation.

_____ **8.** Lactated Ringer's or normal saline is used for patients who have lost a large amount of blood in the field.

_____ **9.** A crystalloid solution can carry oxygen to the cells.

_____ **10.** A macrodrip administration set delivers 10 or 15 gtt/mL.

_____ **11.** A good thing to do when starting an IV is to work down, in case you miss the first attempt.

_____ **12.** A butterfly catheter has a Teflon catheter over the hollow needle.

_____ **13.** You should always have the bevel to the side when starting an IV.

_____ **14.** When changing an IV bag, you must start all over with the process and restart your IV.

_____ **15.** When an IV infiltrates, you will notice edema at the catheter site.

_____ **16.** When you have cannulated an artery, you must pull the catheter out and apply direct pressure for at least 5 minutes.

_____ **17.** A healthy adult can handle only 1 to 2 extra liters of fluid.

_____ **18.** A red top tube is used to determine the blood type of a patient.

_____ **19.** An IO infusion is easier to use, so it should be used as much as possible for the pediatric patient.

_____ **20.** When placing an IO needle, you should feel two "pops."

_____ **21.** The basic unit of weight in the metric system is the gram.

_____ **22.** One lb is equal to 2.2 kg.

_____ **23.** The desired dose is what is ordered to give to the patient.

_____ **24.** Dopamine is delivered to the patient in micrograms.

_____ **25.** There are six "rights" of drug administration.

Short Answer

Complete this section with short written answers using the space provided.

1. Name three ways to make the vein "stand up" so it is easier to see.

a. _____

b. _____

c. _____

2. List the five things that are a MUST when documenting the IV.

   a. _____

   b. _____

   c. _____

   d. _____

   e. _____

3. There are seven local reactions that can happen when starting an IV. List three complications and their signs and symptoms.

   a. _____

   b. _____

   c. _____

4. List the six points of information you should document when you administer a medication to a patient.

   a. _____

   b. _____

   c. _____

   d. _____

   e. _____

   f. _____

Fill-in-the-Table

Fill in the missing parts of the table.

Route of Administration	Where on the Body the Medication Goes
Enteral	1.
Oral	2.
Intradermal	3.
Percutaneous	4.
Sublingual	5.
Endotracheal	6.
Buccal	7.
Transdermal	8.
Intramuscular	9.
Rectal	10.
Parenteral	11.
Subcutaneous	12.
Intravascular	13.
Ocular	14.
Aural	15.
Inhalation	16.
Intranasal	17.

Problem Solving

Practice your calculation skills by solving the following math problems.

1. You have started an IV on a bakery worker suffering from heat exhaustion. Your physician instructs you to run normal saline by IV at 200 mL/h. Your bag of saline is a 1,000-mL bag. Your administration set delivers 10 gtt/mL. At what rate (how many drops per minute) do you have to run the infusion to give 200 mL/h? (Show your calculations.)

2. You have started a "keep-open" IV with a microdrip infusion set (which delivers 60 gtt/mL). Your instructions are to run the IV at 30 mL/h. At what rate (how many drops per minute) should you set the flow? (Show your calculations.)

3. You are ordered to give a lidocaine drip at a rate of 2 mg/min. You have on hand:
   - A vial containing 50 mL of 4% lidocaine
   - A 500-mL bag of D_5W
   - A microdrip administration set that delivers 60 gtt/mL
   a. How many grams of lidocaine are in the vial? _____ g (Show your calculations.)

   b. When you add the contents of the vial to the IV bag, what will be the concentration of lidocaine in the IV bag? _____ mg/mL (Show your calculations.)

c. How many milliliters per minute (mL/min) will the patient have to receive to get the dosage ordered (2 mg/min)? _____ mL/min (Show your calculations.)

d. How many drops per minute (gtt/min) is that equivalent to? _____ gtt/min (Show your calculations.)

4. Convert 12 grams to milligrams: 12 g × _____ = _____ mg

5. Convert 156 pounds to kilograms: 156 lb × _____ = _____ kg (round up)

6. Now use the second method to estimate the patient's weight in kilograms.

The patient weighs 135 lb.

Step 1: Divide the patient's weight by 2: _____ ÷ 2 = _____

Step 2: Take the total from above and multiply it by 10%: _____ × .10 = _____ (round up)

*Remember to round the percentage number for easier subtraction. _____

Step 3: Take the total of step 1 and subtract the rounded percentage. _____ − _____ = _____ patient's weight in kilograms; once again you may need to round up to _____. What weight would you use for the patient? _____ kg

7. You are ordered to give a patient 6 mg of morphine. The morphine comes in 10 mg/mL. How much will you give? _____ mL

8. You are ordered to give 2 mg of Valium. Your vial contains 20 mg in 10 mL. What is the concentration on hand? _____ mg/mL

How many mL will you give? _____ mL

9. You are ordered to deliver 10 μg/kg/min of dopamine for an 80-kg patient. You have mixed 800 mg of dopamine into a 500-mL bag of normal saline. Show your calculations for the following.

a. What is your desired dose? _____ μg/min

b. Determine your dose on hand. _____ mg/mL

c. Convert the mg from answer (b) to μg. _____ μg/mL

    d. Determine the amount of volume to infuse per minute. Use your desired dose to calculate this. _____ mL/min

    e. Determine how many drops/min will deliver your desired dose, using a microdrip set (60 gtt/mL). _____ gtt/min

10. Fill in the following tables so that each row will contain different ways of representing the same values.

Microgram (µg)	Milligram (mg)	Gram (g)	Kilogram (kg)
500	0.5	0.0005	0.0000005
_____	_____	1.0	_____
_____	_____	_____	1.0
_____	1.0	_____	_____
1.0	_____	_____	_____
_____	800.0	_____	_____
15.0	_____	_____	_____

Milliliter (mL)	Deciliter (dL)	Liter (L)
5,000.0	50.0	5.0
1.0	_____	_____
10.0	_____	_____
_____	_____	1.0
250.0	_____	0.25

11. Fill in the blanks in the calculations, changing your patient's weight from pounds to kilograms using the "10% trick." Compare your answers using the formula:

patient's weight (lb) ÷ 2.2 = patient's weight (kg)

Patient's weight (lb)	Patient's weight (lb) ÷ 2	Weight (lb) ÷ 2 × 10%	Subtract your 10% from the weight ÷ 2	Patient's weight in kilograms (kg)	Patient's weight in lb ÷ 2.2 = patient's weight in kilograms (kg)
60	60 ÷ 2 = 30	30 × 10% = 3	30 − 3 = 27	27	27.27
16	_____	_____	_____	_____	_____
138	_____	_____	_____	_____	_____
8	_____	_____	_____	_____	_____
250	_____	_____	_____	_____	_____
36	_____	_____	_____	_____	_____
82	_____	_____	_____	_____	_____
180	_____	_____	_____	_____	_____
330	_____	_____	_____	_____	_____

12. Volume conversions: Fill in the blanks indicating the amount of medication found in each bag of normal saline (NS), assuming the concentration is the same in each bag. Follow the example in the first row of the table:

1,000 mL NS	500 mL NS	250 mL NS	100 mL NS	50 mL NS
100 g	50 g	25 g	10 g	5 g
_____	800 g	_____	_____	_____
_____	_____	250 g	_____	_____
_____	_____	_____	4 g	_____
_____	50 g	_____	_____	_____

13. Determine the number of milliliters of fluid infused over 1 minute to your patient by filling in the following blanks.

    a. 60 gtt admin set infused 120 gtt/min = _____ mL/min

    b. 15 gtt admin set infused 120 gtt/min = _____ mL/min

    c. 30 gtt admin set infused 120 gtt/min = _____ mL/min

14. Convert the following temperatures from Fahrenheit (F) to Celsius (C) by completing the following table. Follow the example in the third row.

This table is based on the formula $(F - 32) \times 0.555 = C$.

Temperature in degrees F	Degrees F - 32	Degrees F - 32 × 0.555	Temperature in degrees C
32			
95.0			
98.6	98.6 - 32 = 66.6	66.6 × 0.555 = 36.96	36.96 (approx 37)
101.0			
104.0			

15. Determine how much medication is prescribed for your patient by body weight by filling in the following table.

Desired dose	Patient's weight in pounds (lb)	Patient's weight in kilograms (kg)	Medication administered
1 mg/kg lidocaine	90	90 ÷ 2.2 = 40.9 kg (≈ 41 kg)	41 kg × 1 mg lidocaine = 41 mg lidocaine to administer
0.2 mg/kg atropine	30		
0.05 mg/kg lorezapam	180		
30 mg/kg methylprednisolone	220		
15 mg/kg phenobarbital	12		

16. Calculate the volume of normal saline needed to administer to the following trauma patients. Base your calculations on volumes replaced at 20 mL/kg of patient body weight.

Patient's weight in pounds (lb)	Patient's weight in kilograms: weight in lb ÷ 2.2 = wt in kg (or use the "10% trick")	Volume to be infused with first bolus at 20 mL/kg
60		
80		
100		
125		
150		
175		
190		
220		
300		

17. Find the weight of the following medications in 1 mL of solution.

    a. 100 mg/10 mL lidocaine = _____ mg/1 mL lidocaine

    b. 1 mg/10 mL epinephrine = _____ mg/1 mL epinephrine

    c. 40 mg/14 mL furosemide = _____ mg/1 mL furosemide

    d. 6 mg/2 mL adenosine = _____ mg/1 mL adenosine

    e. 20 mg/5 mL diazepam = _____ mg/1 mL diazepam

    f. 10 mg/5 mL naloxone = _____ mg/1 mL naloxone

    g. 2 mg/5 mL albuterol = _____ mg/1 mL albuterol

    h. 150 mg/3 mL amiodarone = _____ mg/1 mL amiodarone

    i. 25 g/125 mL activated charcoal = _____ g/1 mL activated charcoal = _____ mg/1 mL activated charcoal

18. Find the weight of the following medications in 1 mL of solution.

Follow this example:

50% dextrose = 50 g/100 mL = 0.5 g/1 mL

    a. 1% xylocaine

b. 10% dextrose

c. 0.5% albuterol

d. 10% calcium chloride

e. 50% magnesium sulfate

f. 5% alupent

g. 0.9% sodium chloride

19. Determine the amount of dopamine in micrograms (µg) per milliliter when 800 milligrams (mg) of dopamine is added to the following bags of normal saline (NS). (Note: 1 mg = 1,000 µg)
    a. 800 mg dopamine is added to a 500-mL bag NS = _____ µg/mL
    b. 800 mg dopamine is added to a 250-mL bag NS = _____ µg/mL
    c. 800 mg dopamine is added to a 1,000-mL bag NS = _____ µg/mL
    d. 800 mg dopamine is added to a 100-mL bag NS = _____ µg/mL

20. Medical control has directed you to administer the correct dosage of medication for your patient (desired dose). The concentration available to you is listed for each calculation. Determine the volume of medication you will administer for each order.

    Desired dose in mg ÷ concentration in mg/mL = volume to administer
    a. You are ordered to give 15 mg labetalol. You have a vial with 100 mg/20 mL solution in stock.

    b. You are ordered to give 3 mg haloperidol. You have a 1-mL ampule containing 5 mg of medication.

    c. You are directed to administer 750 mg calcium chloride. You have a bottle containing 1,000 mg of medication in 10 mL of solution.

Skill Drills

Part I

Test your knowledge of skill drills by placing the following photos in the correct order. Number the first step with a "1," the second step with a "2," and so forth.

1. Drawing Medication From an Ampule

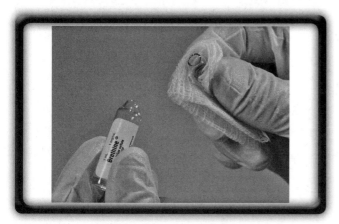

_____ Grip the neck of the ampule using a 4″ × 4″ gauze pad, and snap the neck off.

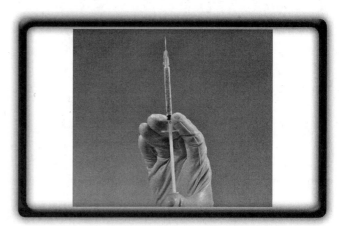

_____ Gently press on the plunger to dispel any air bubbles, and recap the needle using the one-handed method.

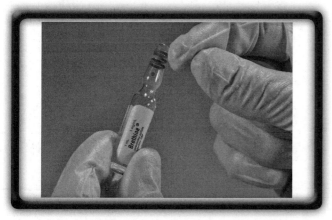

_____ Gently tap the stem of the ampule to shake medication into the base.

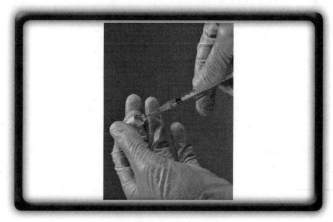

_____ Without touching the outer sides of the ampule, insert the needle into the medication in the ampule, and draw the solution into the syringe.

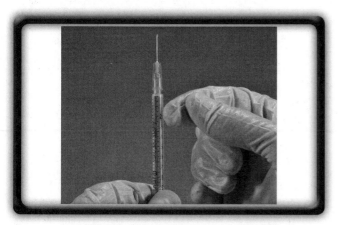

_____ Holding the syringe with the needle pointing up, gently tap the barrel to loosen air trapped inside.

2. Administering a Medication Via Small-Volume Nebulizer

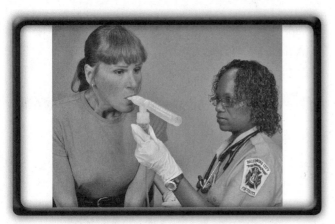

_____ Instruct the patient to breathe as deeply as possible and hold his or her breath for 3 to 5 seconds before exhaling. Monitor the patient for effects.

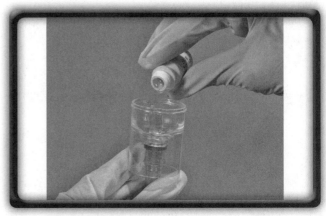

_____ Add premixed medication to the bowl of the nebulizer.

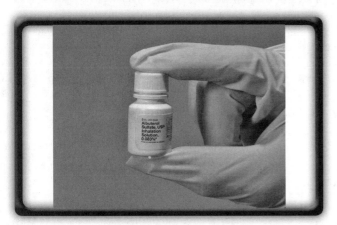

_____ Check the medication and the expiration date.

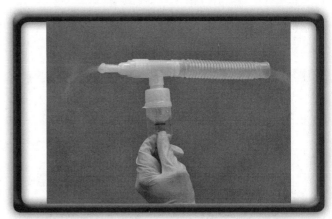

_____ Connect the T piece with the mouthpiece to the top of the bowl, connect it to the oxygen tubing, and set the flowmeter at 6 L/min.

Part II

Test your knowledge of this skill drill by filling in the correct words in the photo captions.

1. Drawing Medication From a Vial

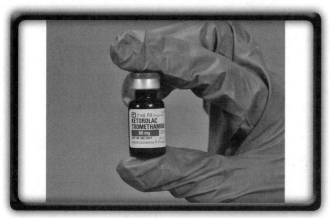

Check the medication and its _____ date.

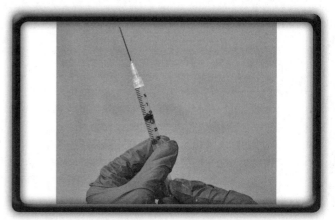

Wipe the vial rubber top with an alcohol prep before touching it with the needle. Determine the amount of medication needed, and draw that amount of _____ into the syringe.

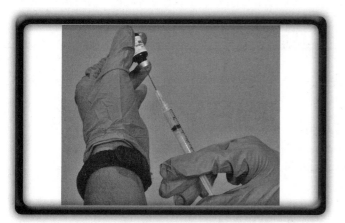

Invert the _____, and insert the needle through the rubber stopper. Expel the air in the syringe to the vial, and then withdraw the amount of medication needed.

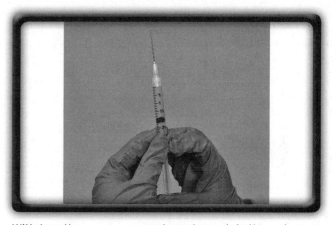

Withdraw the _____, and expel any air in the syringe.

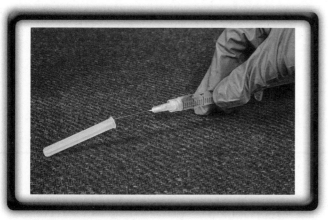

Recap the needle using the _____-_____ method. Label the syringe if the medication is not immediately given to the patient.

Emergency Medications

Matching

In choosing emergency medications, it is important for the paramedic to know the proper use of medical terminology related to pharmacology. Match the term with its definition.

_____ 1. The amount of the drug in 1 mL.

_____ 2. Any potential effect that a medication may have when administered in conjunction with or in the presence of another medication already in the patient's system.

_____ 3. A circumstance that points to the cause, pathology, treatment, or issue of an attack of disease; that which serves as a guide or warning.

_____ 4. The amount of a fluid that is present in the ampule or vial in which the medication is dissolved. This is usually expressed in milligrams, grams, or grains.

_____ 5. An abnormal or harmful effect to an organism caused by exposure to a chemical. It is indicated by some result such as death, a change in food or water consumption, altered body and organ weights, altered enzyme levels, or visible illness.

_____ 6. The quantity of a medication that is to be administered to a patient. This is usually expressed in milligrams, grams, or grains.

_____ 7. Any condition, especially any condition of disease, that renders some particular line of treatment improper or undesirable.

_____ 8. How the medication is categorized as compared to other medications. This is usually done by grouping those medications with similar characteristics, traits, or primary components.

_____ 9. The way in which a medication produces the intended response.

_____ 10. The amount of a medication that is present in the ampule or vial. This is usually expressed in milligrams, grams, or grains.

A. Adverse reaction/side effect

B. Indication

C. Yield

D. Drug interaction

E. Desired dose

F. Class

G. Volume

H. Mechanism of action

I. Contraindication

J. Concentration

Multiple Choice

Read each item carefully, and then select the best response.

1. For the duration of action of a drug, three values are generally given. Which is NOT one of those values?
   A. Peak effect
   B. Duration
   C. Adverse effects
   D. Onset

2. Using the American Heart Association (AHA) system of classifying recommendations for treatments, Class _____ would indicate that a treatment should not be administered.
   A. I
   B. Ia
   C. IIb
   D. III

3. When the scientific evidence indicates either that research is beginning on the treatment or that research is continuing, the treatment is given a Class _____ recommendation by the AHA.
   A. IIa
   B. IIb
   C. Indeterminate
   D. III

4. The FDA has categories of pregnancy safety that are used with drugs. A "category D" would indicate:
   A. studies in animals have revealed adverse effects on the fetus.
   B. there is positive evidence of human fetal risk.
   C. animal reproductive studies have not demonstrated a fetal risk, but there is no controlled study in women.
   D. controlled studies in women fail to demonstrate a risk to the fetus in the first trimester.

5. The term *antidysrhythmic* would appear in a drug profile as the medication:
   A. indication.
   B. class.
   C. mechanism of action.
   D. drug interaction.

6. When a medication is ordered to be administered by mouth, the abbreviation would be:
   A. pc.
   B. po.
   C. RL.
   D. mo.

7. When a patient is taking a medication and his prescription is written for four times a day, it should say:
   A. qid.
   B. ftd.
   C. qod.
   D. NTG.

8. The abbreviation for the form of alcohol that is served in drinks is:
   A. ET.
   B. caps.
   C. ETOH.
   D. APAP.

9. You are treating a patient who you suspect has been poisoned by ingesting a large quantity of pills. A medicine that would MOST likely be administered to the patient is:
   A. atropine.
   B. adenosine.
   C. bumetanide.
   D. activated charcoal.

10. Which of the following medicines is NOT considered an antidysrhythmic?
    A. Amiodarone
    B. Atenolol
    C. Diazepam
    D. Diltiazem

11. Of the following medications, which would be contraindicated if the patient has a history of asthma?
    A. Valium
    B. Epinephrine
    C. Dopamine
    D. Benadryl

12. Which medicine would be contraindicated in a patient who has hyperglycemia?
    A. Fentanyl
    B. Glucagon
    C. Atrovent
    D. Labetalol

13. You are treating a patient who you suspect is experiencing status epilepticus. Which medicine would MOST likely be given?
    A. Morphine sulfate
    B. Narcan
    C. Ativan
    D. Xopenex

14. Which medicine is considered when your patient is symptomatic of the ECG rhythm torsades de pointes?
    A. Magnesium sulfate
    B. Demerol
    C. Mannitol
    D. Alupent

15. Which of the following medications is MOST likely to be considered for sedation during a medical procedure?
    A. Morphine sulfate
    B. Midazolam hydrochloride
    C. Lopressor
    D. Amiodarone

Ambulance Calls

All of the patients described in the following scenarios will most likely be administered medication(s). Which medicine(s) do you suspect would be given to the patient?

1. The patient is a 50-year-old man with severe chest pain. You suspect the pain is cardiac, although his 12-lead ECG is not showing a STEMI.

   _____

2. The patient is a 22-year-old man who is having bronchoconstriction due to his asthma.

   _____

3. The patient is a 19-year-old woman who has a severely angulated right forearm from a fall on the outstretched arm. She is in severe pain and has stable vital signs.

   _____

4. The patient is a 40-year-old man who has just had his second seizure in a row without regaining consciousness.

   _____

5. The patient is a 62-year-old woman who is in cardiac arrest. CPR is in progress and her ECG shows asystole at this point.

   _____

True/False

If you believe the statement to be more true than false, write the letter "T" in the space provided. If you believe the statement to be more false than true, write the letter "F."

_____ 1. Amiodarone is an antidysrhythmic medication used to treat ventricular fibrillation.

_____ 2. The medication atropine sulfate is a platelet inhibitor used when patients complain of chest pain.

_____ 3. Bumetanide is a loop diuretic indicated for patients with pulmonary edema.

_____ 4. One indication for the corticosteroid dexamethasone is anaphylaxis.

_____ 5. Dextrose is considered an antihyperglycemic that can be used with head injuries.

_____ 6. Diazepam is a benzodiazepine that is indicated in head-injured patients and those with respiratory insufficiency.

_____ 7. Patients who have a history of glaucoma should not take diphenhydramine.

_____ **8.** If you suspect your patient has cardiogenic shock, one medication that may be considered is dobutamine hydrochloride.

_____ **9.** The typical dose of fentanyl citrate for an adult patient in severe pain is 50 to 100 mg.

_____ **10.** It would not be appropriate to give the loop diuretic furosemide to a patient with hypotension.

_____ **11.** Cerebyx is the same as fosphenytoin.

_____ **12.** Solu-Cortef is the same as hydrocortisone sodium succinate.

_____ **13.** Atarax is the same medication as ipratropium.

_____ **14.** Toradol is a nonsteroidal anti-inflammatory analgesic medication.

_____ **15.** Ativan is an antidysrhythmic medicine used for frequent premature ventricular contractions.

Short Answer

Complete this section with short written answers using the space provided.

1. Name three conditions for which lidocaine hydrochloride is contraindicated.

a. _____

b. _____

c. _____

2. Name three indications for the medication magnesium sulfate.

a. _____

b. _____

c. _____

3. Name three contraindications for the medication morphine sulfate.

a. _____

b. _____

c. _____

Fill-in-the-Table

Fill in the missing parts of the table.

Common Metric Conversions	
Weight	
1 kilogram (kg)	_____
_____	1,000 grams (g or gm)
1 gram (g or gr)	_____
_____	1,000 micrograms (µg or mcg)
Volume	
_____	1,000 milliliters or cubic centimeters (mL or cc)
Temperature	
37° Celsius (°C)	_____
Length	
_____	10 millimeters (mm)
_____	1 meter (m)

CHAPTER

13

Patient Assessment

Matching

Part I

For each of the following questions from a patient interview, indicate whether it is:

A. A well-phrased question   **B.** A poorly phrased question

_____ **1.** What seems to be the problem?

_____ **2.** When did all this start?

_____ **3.** Did the pain start when you were exerting yourself?

_____ **4.** What is the pain like?

_____ **5.** Is the pain sharp or dull?

_____ **6.** Do you get short of breath when the pain comes on?

_____ **7.** Has the pain gotten worse since it started?

_____ **8.** How has the pain changed since it started?

_____ **9.** What were you doing when the pain started?

_____ **10.** Have you ever had pain like this before?

_____ **11.** What medications do you take regularly?

_____ **12.** Are you allergic to any medications?

_____ **13.** What else is bothering you, besides the pain?

Part II

During your EMT course, you learned many assessment findings. In the paramedic program you will broaden your knowledge of assessment findings and learn their diagnostic significance so you can come to a presumptive diagnosis. Using the knowledge you already have at this point, try to match each of the signs listed to the right with the phrase that best describes its possible diagnostic significance or presumptive diagnosis. (Note: More than one sign may have the same diagnostic significance.)

_____ **1.** Narcotics overdose	**A.** Ecchymosis (discoloration) around the eyes
_____ **2.** Cardiac arrest	**B.** Fruity (acetone) odor to the breath
_____ **3.** Heart failure	**C.** Stridor on inspiration
_____ **4.** Skull fracture	**D.** Pitting edema of both ankles
_____ **5.** Stroke	**E.** Paralysis of upward gaze
_____ **6.** Hypoxemia	**F.** Muffled heart sounds
_____ **7.** Respiratory distress	**G.** Battle's sign (discoloration of mastoid area)
_____ **8.** Shock	**H.** Patient lies very still; cries out when stretcher is jarred
_____ **9.** Diabetic ketoacidosis	**I.** Pinpoint pupils
_____ **10.** Spinal cord injury	**J.** Cyanosis of the lips
_____ **11.** Increased right ventricular pressure	**K.** Capillary refill takes 5 seconds
_____ **12.** Laryngeal edema	**L.** Restlessness
_____ **13.** Pelvic fracture	**M.** Absent pulse
_____ **14.** Fluid/blood in the pericardium	**N.** Retraction of the suprasternal muscles

_____ **15.** Intra-abdominal bleeding

_____ **16.** Peritonitis

_____ **17.** Fracture of the orbit (eye socket in the skull)

_____ **18.** Pneumothorax

O. Jugular veins distended to 10 cm when the patient is sitting

P. Crackling sensation in the skin over the chest

Q. Distended, bruised abdomen in trauma victim

R. Pain on compression of the iliac crests

S. Priapism

T. No movement or sensation in the right arm or leg

U. S_3 gallop (heart sound)

V. Clear fluid draining from the ear

Part III

For each of the following patients, indicate whether their signs and/or symptoms classify them as:

S—Sick (life-threatening)   NS—Not sick

_____ **1.** 18-month-old boy who is limp and dusky blue in the face

_____ **2.** 54-year-old woman with diffuse abdominal pain

_____ **3.** 43-year-old man with confusion, sweating, and left arm pain

_____ **4.** 22-year-old woman with rapid breathing, tingling in arms and feet

_____ **5.** 4-year-old girl who is crying and has pain in her ear

_____ **6.** 75-year-old man who is unable to speak or answer questions

_____ **7.** 66-year-old woman who is unresponsive and breathing deeply and rapidly

_____ **8.** 36-year-old woman who is depressed and does not want to talk

Multiple Choice

Read each item carefully, and then select the best response.

1. When responding to a call, a paramedic's demeanor and appearance should be all of the following, EXCEPT:
   A. clean.
   B. overbearing.
   C. positive.
   D. efficient.

2. Which of the following statements/questions would be considered a facilitating communication technique?
   A. That's all the information I need.
   B. You don't have to tell me if you don't want to.
   C. Can you think of anything else about his medical history?
   D. Can you narrow down his history to just the past few months?

3. Which communication technique is NOT helpful in a stressful situation?
   A. Confrontation
   B. Facilitation
   C. Empathetic response
   D. Clarification

4. What should the thinking paramedic do when faced with a possible physical abuse situation?
   A. Document.
   B. Gather evidence in a paper bag.
   C. Accuse the abuser to try to get the real story.
   D. Call for law enforcement before leaving the scene.

5. When a patient has a period of silence during a call, it should make you:
   A. begin to ask more questions.
   B. realize the patient may not trust you and respect the silence.
   C. look for a reason the patient is not talking, such as a change in condition.
   D. look for a weapon on the patient.

6. Your patient will not quit talking! Which of the following is NOT a reason for chattiness?
   A. The patient is on meth.
   B. The patient is very nervous.
   C. The patient has had several cups of coffee.
   D. All of the above can lead to chattiness.

7. You are dealing with a very angry young man who is being arrested for DWI. He has a broken leg and arm, and you are transporting him to the hospital. What is the best way to treat this situation?
   A. Make sure you strap him down tight to the backboard so he can't get away.
   B. Tell him if he doesn't calm down you will give him some Valium and calm him down yourself.
   C. Treat him as you would any patient and keep your anger and smart comments to yourself.
   D. Yell back at him and let him know that you are the boss and will not tolerate this in the back of your squad.

8. Which statement is false when dealing with a blind person?
   A. Always put things back exactly where you picked them up from.
   B. Speak very, very slowly and clearly.
   C. Announce your identity and reason for being there.
   D. Let the person know where you are and where you are going at all times during transport.

9. Which of the following signs and symptoms is NOT a sign of depression?
   A. Feeling of high energy
   B. Irritability
   C. Eating disruptions
   D. Pain with no source

10. What is a good thing to remember when asking for history from family members?
    A. They will always know the patient's history.
    B. They will be aware of drug or alcohol use.
    C. You are not at liberty to share the patient's condition with them.
    D. You will be able to give them an update on the patient once they reach the hospital.

11. While assessing a trauma patient, you press down lightly on the abdomen. This technique is called:
    A. inspection.
    B. percussion.
    C. auscultation.
    D. palpation.

12. When using a pulse oximeter, which of the following statements is NOT true?
    A. It measures only the percentage of hemoglobin saturation.
    B. It can help determine the patient's heart rhythm.
    C. A cold person can have a false reading.
    D. A hypotensive patient can have a false reading.

13. What is essential in getting an accurate blood pressure reading?
    A. Using the right size cuff
    B. Not having any clothing on the arm
    C. Having the arm perfectly straight
    D. The age of the patient

14. When assessing a patient's mental status, P on the AVPU scale stands for which of the following?
    A. Pupil size
    B. Pallor of the skin
    C. Painful stimuli
    D. Presence

15. Clubbing of the fingertips is possibly caused by which of the following conditions?
    A. Bacterial endocarditis
    B. Systemic illness
    C. Chronic respiratory disease
    D. Cirrhosis of the liver

16. An elderly woman who was walking across the living room reports that she felt and heard a "pop" in her hip and she fell down. You think that there is a possibility she has a broken hip. What process has happened to create this injury?
    A. Pathologic fracture
    B. Physiologic fracture
    C. Psychogenic fracture
    D. Psychical fracture

17. In assessing a spine, you find an exaggerated inward curve of the lumbar area. This is known as:
    A. kyphosis.
    B. lordosis.
    C. the Cullen sign.
    D. dislocation of the lumbar spine.

18. You are auscultating the carotid arteries and hear a "whooshing." You are hearing bruit, and this indicates:
    A. a heart murmur.
    B. turbulent blood flow around a cardiac valve.
    C. turbulent blood flow in the carotid arteries.
    D. turbulent blood flow around a cardiac valve.

19. When checking the cranial nerve IV, you will be checking for which of the following?
    A. Hearing and balance
    B. Smell
    C. Visual acuity
    D. Eye movements

20. You are assessing a patient and notice cyanotic patches on the lower extremities. This is known as _____, and it is seen in severe states of shock and hypoperfusion.
    A. tenting
    B. turgor
    C. mottling
    D. crepitus

21. The scene size-up component of the patient assessment includes all of the following, EXCEPT:
    A. focused assessment.
    B. mechanism of injury (MOI).
    C. requesting additional resources.
    D. scene safety.

22. During the primary assessment, the paramedic must:
    A. treat medical and trauma patients differently.
    B. determine the SAMPLE history.
    C. identify priority patients.
    D. obtain baseline vital signs.

23. Which of the following standard precautions may be appropriate during the scene size-up and a patient examination?
    A. Gloves
    B. Gowns
    C. N-95 masks
    D. All of the above

24. When on a scene where people act aggressively, or appear to be threatening, it is best for the paramedic to:
    A. consider retreating to the rig until the scene is secure.
    B. explain that you are there to help and do not intend any harm to the patient.
    C. explain that you are not law enforcement.
    D. begin acting authoritarian and aggressive toward the instigators.

25. The most time-sensitive and important aspect of the patient assessment, where life threats are detected and quickly treated, is considered the:
    A. primary assessment.
    B. focused assessment.
    C. secondary assessment.
    D. general impression.

26. Which of the following is considered a "priority patient"?
    A. A pregnant patient involved in a minor motor vehicle crash without any complications
    B. A large multiple-casualty incident with a patient in cardiac arrest
    C. A patient who does not pass the "look test," giving a poor general impression
    D. A bystander who witnessed the event and is traumatized by what he saw

27. Evaluating an unresponsive medical patient requires you, the paramedic, to rely on:
    A. a head-to-toe physical exam.
    B. the presence of a medical identification tag.
    C. the bystander or family information.
    D. All of the above

28. The rapid trauma exam is generally completed:
    A. on all entrapped patients.
    B. on any patient who does not have a readily identifiable medical problem.
    C. before all life threats have been identified and treated.
    D. prior to conducting a secondary assessment on the patient.

29. Which of the following patients typically requires a full body exam?
    A. A man with a minor laceration obtained while cutting vegetables in the kitchen
    B. An athlete who was kicked in the shin while playing soccer
    C. An intoxicated bar patron who fell off a stool and struck his head
    D. A baseball catcher struck in the face while wearing his protective mask

30. When assessing a patient's airway status, it is often helpful to do which of the following?
    A. Think from the simple to the complex.
    B. Intubate the patient quickly to manage the airway definitively.
    C. Alter your assessment based on the patient's age.
    D. Always open an unconscious patient's airway with a head tilt–chin lift.

Labeling

Label the following diagram with the missing terms.

1. Nine Regions of the Abdomen

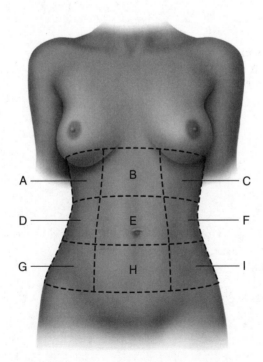

A. _____

B. _____

C. _____

D. _____

E. _____

F. _____

G. _____

H. _____

I. _____

Fill-in-the-Blank

Read each item carefully, and then complete the statement by filling in the missing word(s).

1. You will make your _____ _____ based on the patient's chief complaint, vital signs, and history.

2. The first step in making an approach to a patient is to _____ _____.

3. Once you have established the patient's chief complaint, you will want to check into the history of the _____ _____.

4. When using a translator to help interview your patient, be aware that _____ _____ and jargon often do not translate well.

5. You respond to a patient who is deaf. When communicating with the patient, you should be _____-_____-_____ with him or her.

6. _____ is described as one step further than sympathy.

7. When talking with a patient, you pause to consider something significant that you have just been told before proceeding. This technique is known as _____.

8. _____ governs the disclosure of patient information.

9. Always review transfer information before transferring a patient to a new facility so you know the patient's _____ _____.

10. During your history taking, ensure the questions you ask are _____-_____ and _____-_____.

Ambulance Calls

The following case scenarios provide an opportunity to explore the concerns associated with patient management and paramedic care. Read each scenario, and then answer each question.

1. You are called to the crash scene pictured here.

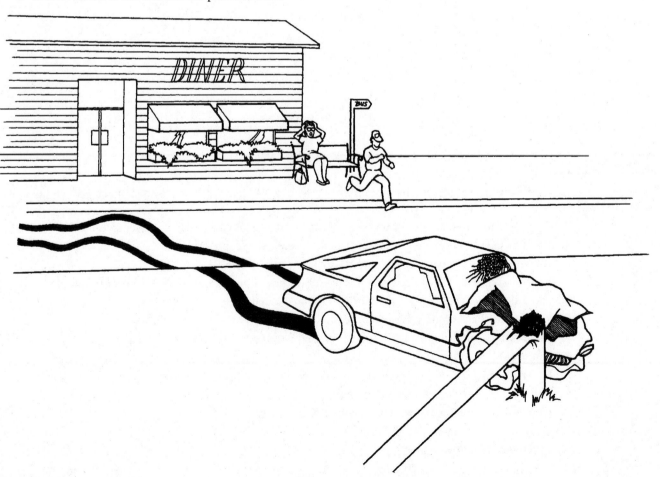

a. List four potential sources of information about what happened to the patient or about his medical background.

(1) _____

(2) _____

(3) _____

(4) _____

b. List five pieces of information you can derive simply from observing the scene.

(1) _____

(2) _____

(3) _____

(4) _____

(5) _____

c. List four reasons why it is necessary to take a history from the driver of the car.

(1) _____

(2) _____

(3) _____

(4) _____

d. Before you start taking the history, however, you need to take some preliminary steps. List them.

(1) _____

(2) _____

(3) _____

(4) _____

(5) _____

True/False

If you believe the statement to be more true than false, write the letter "T" in the space provided. If you believe the statement to be more false than true, write the letter "F."

_____ **1.** Being able to think and perform well under pressure is a big part of being a good paramedic.

_____ **2.** Patients will always be honest when it comes to their sexual history.

_____ **3.** You will always be able to tell who is a heavy user of alcohol.

_____ **4.** Patients sometimes need a few seconds to gather their thoughts and answer your questions.

_____ **5.** Law enforcement should be called for EVERY hostile patient.

_____ **6.** You should check blood glucose on every patient that has an altered mental status.

_____ **7.** Patients may suffer trauma because of a medical problem or their current health status.

_____ **8.** You should be able to make your field diagnosis based on the patient's chief complaint.

_____ **9.** Using "pet names" with a patient will put the person at ease.

_____ **10.** Clarification technique is used when trying to clear up a vague history.

_____ **11.** Children do not dehydrate as fast as adults do.

_____ **12.** Delirium is associated with an acute sudden change in mental status.

_____ **13.** Aphasia is difficulty speaking.

_____ **14.** Babinski reflex is a normal finding in an older adult.

_____ **15.** When assessing a limb for signs of venous obstruction or insufficiency, you should check for edema and wild erythema.

_____ **16.** You should always assess a pulse in three different places on the foot.

_____ **17.** To assess a shoulder dislocation, you should be in front of the patient and looking down at both shoulders.

_____ **18.** Female and male genitalia should be assessed in a limited and discreet fashion.

_____ **19.** Jugular venous distention is commonly caused by right-sided heart failure.

_____ **20.** You must have a stethoscope for evaluating blood pressure.

Short Answer

Complete this section with short written answers using the space provided.

1. A patient's chief complaint is "pain in my gut."

   a. List six questions you would ask in eliciting the history of the present illness.

   (1) _____

   (2) _____

   (3) _____

   (4) _____

   (5) _____

   (6) _____

   b. List four questions you would ask about his other medical history.

   (1) _____

   (2) _____

   (3) _____

   (4) _____

2. Taking the history of a patient with a head injury may provide important clues to the nature of the injury and its potential seriousness. List five questions that need to be answered in taking the history of a patient with a head injury:

   a. _____

   b. _____

   c. _____

   d. _____

   e. _____

3. You are called to the scene of a multi-vehicle crash on the interstate highway. As you approach the scene, you begin making your size-up of the scene. List four questions you need to answer in making your size-up of the collision scene.

   a. _____

   b. _____

   c. _____

   d. _____

4. Patient assessment consists largely of detective work—searching for and interpreting clues to form a picture of the patient's problem. At the scene of an incident or, for that matter, in the patient's home, there may be several sources of information about the patient. List four potential sources of information about the patient and what has happened to him or her.

a. _____

b. _____

c. _____

d. _____

Fill-in-the-Table

Fill in the missing parts of the tables.

1. When testing the cranial nerves, a number of simple maneuvers can be employed to determine the presence and degree of disability. Fill in the following table to indicate what to test for disability in cranial nerves.

Tests for Disability in Cranial Nerves		
Cranial Nerve		**Test**
I		
II		
III		
IV		
V		
VI		
VII		
VIII		
IX, X		
XI		
XII		

2. In the rapid trauma exam of a multisystem trauma patient, you must look for very specific clues to specific injuries. Fill in the following table to indicate what you will be looking for in particular as you examine each part of the body.

Body Region	What I Will Be Looking for in Particular (in addition to DCAP-BTLS)
Head	
Neck	
Chest	
Abdomen	
Extremities	
Back/buttocks	

Skill Drill

Test your knowledge of skill drills by placing the following photos in the correct order. Number the first step with a "1," the second step with a "2," and so forth.

1. Examining the Nervous System

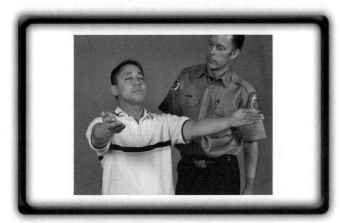

_____ Perform the pronator drift test by asking the patient to close his or her eyes and hold both arms out in front of the body.

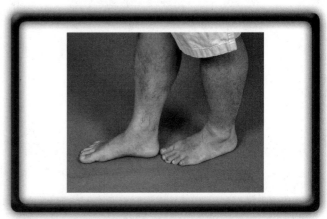

_____ If appropriate, test the patient's gait and balance by having the patient walk heel-to-toe or perform the heel-to-shin stance.

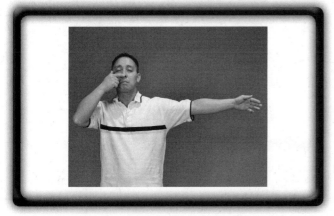

_____ Evaluate the patient's coordination by performing the finger-to-nose test using alternating hands.

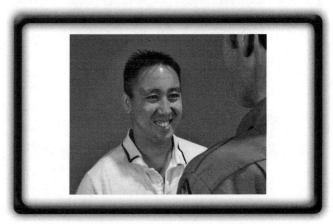

_____ Evaluate cranial nerve function.

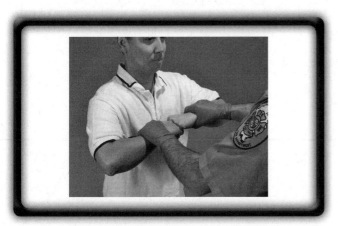

_____ Evaluate the patient's neuromuscular status by checking muscle strength against resistance.

2. Examining the Chest

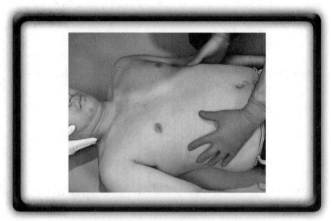

_____ Note the shape of the chest and symmetry of movement.

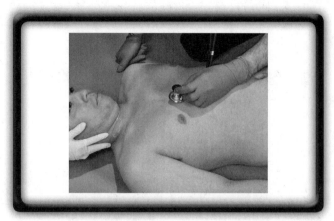

_____ Auscultate the lung fields, noting any abnormal lung sounds.

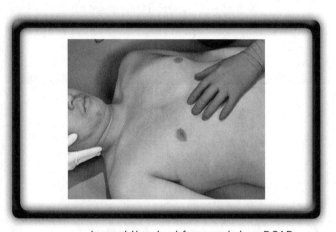

_____ Inspect the chest for any obvious DCAP-BTLS.

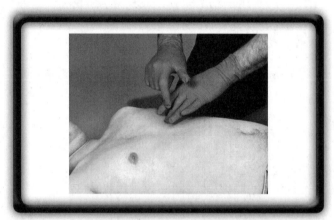

_____ Percuss the chest to detect any abnormalities.

Critical Thinking and Clinical Decision Making

Matching

For each sentence listed below, decide if you would:

A. Follow protocols   **B.** Use independent decisions

_____ **1.** An 86-year-old woman with facial droop and slurred speech

_____ **2.** A 14-year-old boy, unconscious, who is trapped in a drain pipe

_____ **3.** A diabetic woman with low blood glucose

_____ **4.** A 47-year-old man with "classic ischemic" chest pain

_____ **5.** A crop duster crash with a conscious pilot who is yelling for help

_____ **6.** A school where a person has shot several students

_____ **7.** An allergic reaction to a bee sting on a 12-year-old girl

_____ **8.** A motor vehicle crash where the car is smoking and appears to be on fire

_____ **9.** A 20-year-old basketball player in cardiac arrest during a game

_____ **10.** A man stuck inside a grain elevator, and he is being pulled under the grain

Multiple Choice

Read each item carefully, and then select the best response.

1. _____ is processing the information presented by the patient you are treating.
   A. Gathering
   B. Evaluating
   C. Synthesizing
   D. Thinking

2. Which of the following items is NOT included in the concept formation process?
   A. Smell
   B. Sample history
   C. Hearing
   D. Seeing

3. What is the second stage of critical thinking?
   A. Application of principle
   B. Reflection in action
   C. Concept formation
   D. Data interpretation

4. What does *reflection in action* mean?
   A. A call review of the run you just completed
   B. Checking your interventions as you apply them to your patient
   C. Stopping before you apply the intervention to make sure you are doing the right thing
   D. Checking the protocols prior to doing anything

5. Which of the following does NOT belong to the "Six Rs" that were discussed in the chapter?
   A. Read the scene
   B. Read the protocols
   C. Read the patient
   D. React

6. You respond to a patient's home for chest pain. You are determining the chief complaint and taking the baseline vital signs. In which of the "Six Rs" are you working right now?
   A. Reading the scene
   B. Reacting
   C. Reevaluating
   D. Reading the patient

7. When responding to a critical patient, why is it best to use a mental checklist?
   A. So you don't forget to take vital signs
   B. So you always follow your protocols
   C. To facilitate better thinking on the scene
   D. So you will never be sued

8. Which of the following is NOT used to synthesize your patient's information?
   A. Patient history
   B. Patient allergies
   C. Current complaints
   D. Previous diseases

9. Which of the following adult patients would be considered to have a serious condition?
   A. Acute presentation of a first-time event
   B. Acute presentation of a chronic event
   C. Patient with small lacerations
   D. Partial thickness burns to an extremity with less than 5% BSA

10. What is the "third" cornerstone of effective paramedic practice?
   A. Development and implementation of a patient care plan
   B. Having the ability to think and work under pressure
   C. Having the ability of judgment and making independent decisions
   D. Having the ability to gather, evaluate, and synthesize information

Fill-in-the-Blank

Read each item carefully, and then complete the statement by filling in the missing word(s).

1. By taking a sample history and baseline vital signs, you are _____ information about your patient that will be used to assess and evaluate to help form your treatment plan.

2. Your care plan for your patient is almost always defined by your _____.

3. Your final cornerstone of practicing as a paramedic is to _____ and _____ under pressure.

4. The process of gathering information by smell, sight, hearing, and touch is known as _____ _____.

5. Patients with major multisystem trauma, acute chronic conditions, and devastating single-system trauma would be examples of patients with _____ _____ _____.

6. Once you have assessed your patient and you begin treatment, you are using a/an _____ _____.

7. Some of the primary elements involved in _____ the _____ are evaluating the overall safety of the situation, the environmental conditions, the immediate surroundings, access and egress issues, and the MOI.

8. When dealing with a critical patient, you take vital signs three or more times. The readings allow you to assess _____.

Identify

In the following case study, list the chief complaint, vital signs, and any pertinent negatives.

It is 4:00 PM and you have been called to a residence for a woman who is not feeling well. When you arrive, you find a 56-year-old woman with a general feeling of malaise. You begin talking with her to gather some information while your partner takes baseline vital signs. During your SAMPLE history, you find out that she is a diabetic. Your partner tests her blood glucose level, and it is 110 mg/dL. She states she is very careful because of her illness. Her blood pressure is 160/100 mm Hg, and her pulse is 92 beats/min and regular with normal sinus rhythm showing on the ECG monitor, but she is showing a little ST-segment depression. You ask her if she has ever had a heart attack and she says no. Her oxygen saturation on room air is 97%, all lung fields are clear, and she is breathing at 18 breaths/min. She is warm and dry and her pupils are PEARRL (Pupils Equal And Round,

Regular in size, react to Light). She says she has been feeling this way for a few days and is so tired that she hasn't been able to do anything. She was afraid something major might be wrong with her, so she decided to give 9-1-1 a call. You tell the woman she might have had a cardiac event and you want to take her in. You apply oxygen by nonrebreathing mask at 15 L/min, start an IV at a TKO drip, and give her some nitroglycerin paste to bring down the blood pressure en route. You take a 12-lead ECG en route and transport her to the local ED. The nitroglycerin brings the blood pressure down to 120/70 mm Hg. All other vitals stay the same. Later you learn she has had a small MI but because of her diabetes she never had the classic signs.

1. Chief complaint:

_____

_____

_____

2. Vital signs:

_____

_____

_____

3. Pertinent negatives:

_____

_____

_____

Ambulance Calls

The following case scenario provides an opportunity to explore the concerns associated with patient management and paramedic care. Read the scenario, and then answer each question.

1. You are on a rural squad, with no regional trauma center nearby. You are dispatched to a grade school for a child who has fallen from a tree. The school is reporting that the child is still on the ground outside on the playground. When you arrive, you find a 9-year-old girl sitting up. You ask your partner to take C-spine precautions while you start your primary assessment. The teacher says she was approximately 15 feet up when she fell. You note a large broken branch about 7 feet off the ground and the teacher says she hit that branch on the way down on her left side and then landed on her head, on the hard dirt. The child is unable to tell you her name and is confused about where she is and the day of the week. After finding no obvious life threats during the primary assessment, you proceed with a rapid trauma exam because of the significant MOI. You decide she is a critical patient because of the MOI and call for Life Flight to take her to the regional trauma center. Your partner applies a C-collar and you carefully place her onto a long backboard. You apply supplemental oxygen by nonrebreathing mask at 15 L/min. Your partner takes baseline vital signs that reveal a blood pressure of 130/80 mm Hg, pulse of 52 beats/min, and respirations at 6 breaths/min. Lung sounds are clear. She responds only to painful stimuli at this point, and her oxygen saturation is at 88%. Her pupils are unequal, with the left much larger than the right pupil. The patient begins to gag and vomit. You suction all secretions, place an oral airway, and start to assist her ventilations with the bag-mask device. Your partner gets an IV started as the helicopter is landing. The patient no longer has a gag reflex, so the flight medics insert an advanced airway. The Life Flight crew loads her and takes off, heading for the regional trauma center. Later you learn the girl died as a result of massive head injury.

a. What is your first clue that this patient should be treated as a critical patient?

_____

_____

_____

b. Under what consent can you transport this child without her parents' permission?

_____

_____

_____

c. What do your baseline vital signs suggest on this patient?

_____

_____

_____

d. What is your first concern with the patient, and how can you manage that concern?

_____

_____

_____

2. You are traveling home to Grandma's house for a wonderful Thanksgiving dinner. Traffic slows and comes to a stop. Knowing what you do about traffic and collisions, you pull out your primary assessment kit and head up the road. A minivan loaded with people has crossed the centerline and hit a car with another family in it. There are people everywhere—some trying to help patients from the vehicles and others just standing around. The 9-1-1 system has already been called, but you can't hear any sirens yet because you are about 20 miles from any town. You realize there are critical patients in the van and the Jaws of Life will be needed to extricate those patients.

a. How are you going to identify yourself and gain control of this scene?

_____

_____

_____

b. What type of equipment are you going to need at this scene?

_____

_____

_____

c. Are you going to begin any type of treatment before help arrives?

_____

_____

_____

True/False

If you believe the statement to be more true than false, write the letter "T" in the space provided. If you believe the statement to be more false than true, write the letter "F."

_____ **1.** The first cornerstone of your practice is having the ability to gather, evaluate, and synthesize information on the scene.

_____ **2.** Once you have evaluated the information you obtained from the scene, the patient, or a bystander, and determined which information is valid or invalid, you need to process—or synthesize—this information.

_____ **3.** Protocols, standing orders, and patient care algorithms will address every patient for the paramedic and give a clear, defined path to treatment.

_____ **4.** The patient that presents with an acute presentation of a new medical condition is considered a patient with a critical life threat.

_____ **5.** The second stage of critical thinking is concept formation.

_____ **6.** Reflection in action is the process of reassessing your patient.

_____ **7.** When you identify a patient with medical ambiguity, it means that you have pinpointed the cause of the patient's medical problem.

_____ **8.** When reading the scene, you are looking for information that is available only at the scene.

Short Answer

Complete this section with short written answers using the space provided.

1. Discuss the use of the "Six Rs" when responding to a routine call.

   a. Read the scene:

_____

_____

_____

   b. Read the patient:

_____

_____

_____

   c. React:

_____

_____

_____

   d. Reevaluate:

_____

_____

_____

   e. Revise the plan:

_____

_____

_____

   f. Review your performance:

_____

_____

_____

2. When using the cornerstone principles of critical thinking, discuss the differences in gathering information, evaluating information, and synthesizing.

_____

_____

_____

_____

_____

_____

_____

_____

Airway Management and Ventilation

Matching

Part I

For each of the patients described here, indicate which of the following is the best method for opening the airway.

    A. Head tilt–chin lift maneuver   **B.** Jaw-thrust maneuver

_____ **1.** A construction worker found unconscious on the ground after falling 30 feet from scaffolding.

_____ **2.** A 40-year-old woman found unconscious from a drug overdose; she is breathing spontaneously.

_____ **3.** A 52-year-old man in cardiac arrest from a probable heart attack. You have arrived at his side without any ancillary equipment.

_____ **4.** A 14-year-old girl who dove into a shallow pool and struck her head on the bottom. Bystanders removed her from the pool before you arrived. She is unconscious but breathing spontaneously (and noisily) when you arrive.

Part II

Nasotracheal intubation is an excellent technique for establishing control over the airway under select circumstances. In other circumstances, it is preferable to insert the tracheal tube through the mouth; and in yet other limited circumstances, it may be necessary to establish an airway surgically, by cricothyrotomy. For each of the following patients, indicate which of the following intubation methods is preferred.

    N   Blind nasotracheal intubation is the preferred technique.

    T   Endotracheal intubation is the preferred technique.

    C   Cricothyrotomy is the preferred technique.

_____ **1.** A 65-year-old man in cardiac arrest.

_____ **2.** A 28-year-old woman with complete airway obstruction from laryngeal edema.

_____ **3.** A 26-year-old collision victim with clear fluid draining from his nose and left ear.

_____ **4.** An 18-year-old woman in a coma from a drug overdose.

_____ **5.** A 48-year-old man extricated from a wrecked car; he is unconscious and has an injury to the back of his head.

_____ **6.** A 58-year-old man with pulmonary edema; he has been taking warfarin (Coumadin; an anticoagulant drug) ever since his heart attack last year.

_____ **7.** A 6-year-old boy who choked on a piece of meat.

_____ **8.** A 52-year-old woman who was given succinylcholine (a paralyzing drug) prior to an intubation attempt; the attempt failed, and afterward it became impossible to maintain her airway by manual methods.

Part III

For each of the following patients, indicate the most appropriate device for administering supplemental oxygen. You may choose among the following. (Note: You may use any of the items once, more than once, or not at all.)

_____ **1.** A 60-year-old man in severe respiratory distress from acute pulmonary edema.

_____ **2.** A 56-year-old man complaining of crushing chest pain.

_____ **3.** A car crash victim in cardiac arrest; you are doing one-rescuer cardiopulmonary resuscitation (CPR) because your partner is busy with another casualty.

A. Nasal cannula

B. Nonrebreathing mask

C. Pocket mask (mouth to mask ventilation) with added supplemental oxygen

_____ **4.** A 78-year-old woman who suddenly stopped speaking this morning and cannot move her left arm or left leg.

_____ **5.** A 22-year-old man who has overdosed on heroin; he is unconscious and breathing shallowly at 6 breaths/min.

_____ **6.** A 32-year-old car crash victim who was thrown forward against the steering wheel; he is coughing up blood, and his lips look rather blue.

_____ **7.** A 45-year-old man who collapsed in the street; he is in cardiac arrest by the time you arrive.

_____ **8.** An unconscious 10-year-old boy who was rescued from a house fire.

D. Bag-mask device with an oxygen reservoir

E. Flow-restricted, oxygen-powered ventilation device (manually triggered ventilation device)

F. Continuous positive airway pressure (CPAP)

Multiple Choice

Read each item carefully, and then select the best response.

1. What is the leaf-shaped structure that prevents food and liquid from getting into the larynx during swallowing?
   A. Vallecula
   B. Uvula
   C. Epiglottis
   D. Pharynx

2. Which of the following is the MOST common cause of a partial airway obstruction?
   A. The tongue
   B. Food
   C. Blood
   D. Vomitus

3. What is the preferred device to deliver supplemental oxygen to the patient who is breathing?
   A. Nasal cannula
   B. Bag-mask device
   C. Simple face mask
   D. Nonrebreathing mask

4. What is the MOST definitive way to control the airway in an unconscious patient?
   A. Bag-mask device
   B. Endotracheal tube
   C. Oral airway adjunct
   D. Head tilt–chin lift

5. In what position should the patient's head be placed when preparing to intubate with a Combitube?
   A. Flexed forward
   B. Neutral position
   C. Hyperextended back
   D. Slightly to the right

6. What medication is the only depolarizing neuromuscular blocking agent that is used in the field?
   A. Vecuronium bromide
   B. Pancuronium bromide
   C. Rocuronium bromide
   D. Succinylcholine chloride

7. How much sterile saline should you have ready when you are performing a needle cricothyrotomy?
   A. 3 mL
   B. 5 mL
   C. 7 mL
   D. 10 mL

8. How much alveolar volume does the typical adult have?
   A. 150 mL
   B. 350 mL
   C. 500 mL
   D. 3,000 mL

9. The clinical finding in which the systolic BP drops more than 10 mm Hg during inhalation is called:
   A. intercostal stimulation.
   B. vagus nerve stimulation.
   C. pulsus paradoxus.
   D. asymmetric movement.

10. Which abnormal respiratory pattern do you see in the patient with ketoacidosis?
    A. Cheyne-Stokes
    B. Agonal
    C. Biots
    D. Kussmaul

11. What is the major advantage of a multilumen airway device?
    A. It fits all patients from pediatric to adult.
    B. It prevents all aspiration.
    C. It cannot be placed improperly.
    D. It always provides 100% oxygen to the patient.

12. Which of the following is NOT a complication of placing a multilumen airway device?
    A. Vomiting
    B. Unrecognized displacement of the tube
    C. Esophageal trauma
    D. Hyperventilation

13. How much air should inflate the proximal balloon on the Combitube?
    A. 15 mL
    B. 25 mL
    C. 100 mL
    D. 150 mL

14. When should you use a laryngeal mask airway (LMA) in the field?
    A. When the patient cannot be intubated, as an alternative to the bag-mask device (alone)
    B. When the patient is morbidly obese and has a difficult airway
    C. When the patient has congestive heart failure (CHF) and is unconscious
    D. When the patient is under 5 feet tall and needs attention to the airway

15. How many sizes does the LMA come in?
    A. 3
    B. 5
    C. 7
    D. 10

Fill-in-the-Blank

Read each item carefully, and then complete the statement by filling in the missing word(s).

1. The principal hazard associated with intubation is _____. That hazard can be minimized by _____.

2. For tracheal intubation to proceed smoothly, it is essential to position the patient correctly to bring the trachea into alignment with the mouth and pharynx. To do so, you need to place the patient in the _____ position.

3. An intubation attempt should take no longer than _____ seconds.

4. Breathing is normally controlled by a respiratory center in the brain stem. In a healthy person, the primary stimulus to breathe is a _____ (rise or fall) in the level of _____ (oxygen or carbon dioxide) in the blood. In some patients with chronic obstructive pulmonary disease, that mechanism is no longer fully operative, and their principal stimulus to breathe is a _____ (rise or fall) in the level of _____ (oxygen or carbon dioxide) in the blood.

5. Foreign body airway obstructions are sometimes the result of decreased airway reflexes, sometimes caused by alcohol consumption or by _____.

6. When you suction the airway, a nonrigid catheter is called a/an _____ or _____-_____ catheter, but the rigid tip is called a/an _____-_____ catheter.

7. When you insert an oral airway into a pediatric patient, the airway device is inserted with the tip facing the _____ of the _____.

8. You should always adequately _____ a patient before you intubate.

9. The King LT airway should not be used in patients with a/an _____ _____ _____, patients with known _____ _____, or patients who have ingested a/an _____ _____.

10. When examining the patient's airway with the mouth wide open, you note the posterior pharynx is _____ _____. This is considered a Class II in the _____ classification.

Labeling

Label the following diagrams with the correct terms.

1. Parts of the Larynx

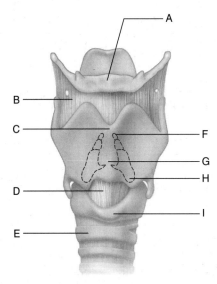

A. _____

B. _____

C. _____

D. _____

E. _____

F. _____

G. _____

H. _____

I. _____

2. The Child's Epiglottis and Surrounding Structures

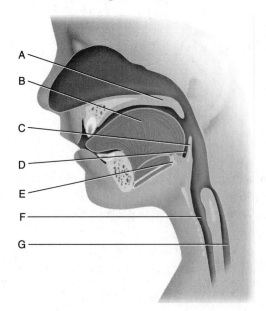

A. _____

B. _____

C. _____

D. _____

E. _____

F. _____

G. _____

Identify

In the following case study, list the chief complaint, vital signs, and pertinent negatives.

You are called to the high school for a teenager choking. When you arrive, you are directed to a 14-year-old boy who was walking down the hallway when someone scared him from behind. He was chewing on a small cap of a pen when this happened and has sucked the cap into his airway. He is seated in the tripod position and is cyanotic around the lips. You immediately assess that he is breathing because with each breath he makes a whistling noise. A teacher performed the Heimlich maneuver (abdominal thrusts) on him in the hallway initially, and he can at least draw a small breath in. Your partner applies a nonrebreathing mask at 15 L/min. The patient is breathing 28 breaths/min and shallow. He has decreased lung sounds on the right side and clear sounds on the left. His heart rate is 98 beats/min and regular and his blood pressure is 128/86 mm Hg. His skin is cyanotic in the face and fingertips and is cool. His oxygen saturation is 88%, and he is a little confused. Because the patient is conscious and you know the cap is in the lungs, and because of the sounds in the lung fields, you position the boy on the cot, sitting up, with oxygen running, and take off for the hospital. You run code 3/priority 1 (lights and siren) into the ED. Later, you learn the patient had to be taken into surgery to remove the cap.

1. Chief complaint:

   _____

   _____

2. Vital signs:

   _____

   _____

3. Pertinent negatives:

   _____

   _____

Complete the Patient Care Report (PCR)

Re-read the incident scenario in the "Identify" section above and then complete the following PCR. Feel free to create the times and numbers, as well as the date of the incident:

EMS Patient Care Report (PCR)					
Date:	**Incident No.:**	**Nature of Call:**		**Location:**	
Dispatched:	**En Route:**	**At Scene:**	**Transport:**	**At Hospital:**	**In Service:**
Patient Information					
Age: **Sex:** **Weight (in kg [lb]):**		**Allergies:** **Medications:** **Past Medical History:** **Chief Complaint:**			
Vital Signs					
Time:	**BP:**	**Pulse:**	**Respirations:**	**SpO$_2$:**	
Time:	**BP:**	**Pulse:**	**Respirations:**	**SpO$_2$:**	
Time:	**BP:**	**Pulse:**	**Respirations:**	**SpO$_2$:**	
EMS Treatment (circle all that apply)					
Oxygen @ _____ L/min via (circle one): NC NRM Bag-Mask Device		**Assisted Ventilation**	**Airway Adjunct**	**CPR**	
Defibrillation	**Bleeding Control**	**Bandaging**	**Splinting**	**Other**	
Narrative					

Ambulance Calls

The following case scenarios provide an opportunity to explore the concerns associated with patient management and paramedic care. Read each scenario, and then answer each question.

1. You finish a call and return to Joe's Steak 'n Lobster Shack where you were having dinner when a previous emergency arose. You hope that they haven't already fed your sirloin to the dog. Happily, Joe has kept your steak waiting for you, and he whips it into the microwave to rewarm it. At last, the steak is back in front of you, along with a generous order of fries. You lift your knife and fork to dig in when out of the corner of your eye you see a strange pantomime occurring two tables away. A middle-aged man in a business suit suddenly pushes himself away from the table, clutches his neck, and lurches to his feet. He staggers a few paces and then pitches to the floor—all in complete silence.

   a. The man is showing signs of:

   (1) food poisoning.

   (2) choking.

   (3) strep throat.

   (4) anaphylaxis.

   (5) hysteria.

   b. What treatment is needed?

   (1) Pump out his stomach.

   (2) Give him manual thrusts.

   (3) Have him gargle with saltwater.

   (4) Give epinephrine 1:1,000, 0.5 mL SQ.

   (5) Give diazepam (Valium), 10 mg IM.

2. You are having a barbecue in the backyard one Sunday. The beer has been flowing freely, and everyone is in a jolly mood. You tell a funny story, and everyone present starts laughing uproariously, including one of your friends who had just taken a big bite out of his hot dog. Suddenly, he starts coughing violently. His face gets very red.

   a. At that point, you should do which of the following actions?

   (1) Tilt his head back and attempt to ventilate.

   (2) Perform a quick finger sweep to remove accessible obstructing material.

   (3) Give manual thrusts.

   (4) Reach into his throat with the barbecue tongs and try to snare the hot dog.

   (5) Encourage him to keep coughing.

   b. That course of action does not seem to help. Your friend becomes completely silent, and his face turns a dusky gray as he struggles to breathe. What should you do now?

   (1) Tilt his head back and attempt to ventilate.

   (2) Perform a quick finger sweep to remove accessible obstructing material.

   (3) Do the Heimlich maneuver (abdominal thrusts).

   (4) Reach into his throat with the barbecue tongs and try to snare the hot dog.

   (5) Encourage him to keep coughing.

   c. Your friend collapses unconscious to the ground. List the next four steps you would take.

   (1) _____

   (2) _____

   (3) _____

   (4) _____

    d. Meanwhile an ambulance has arrived (someone had the sense to phone 9-1-1), and a couple of paramedics come stampeding through your flower garden carrying what looks like all the equipment from their rig. Now that you have equipment available, what steps will be taken?

        (1) _____

        (2) _____

        (3) _____

        (4) _____

3. You are struggling to intubate a 30-year-old bodybuilder who collapsed while working out at the local health club. You found him in cardiac arrest, and high-quality CPR is in progress. Despite the fact that you have positioned him just as the textbook instructs, you can't seem to bring his vocal cords into view; they remain hidden just above your laryngoscope blade.

    a. To bring the cords into view, you ask your partner to perform the _____ _____, which is _____, _____, _____ pressure on the larynx.

    b. That seems helpful in bringing the vocal cords into view. Another tool that can be useful is the _____ _____ _____, which facilitates entry into the glottis opening and enables you to feel the ridges of the tracheal wall.

    c. You manage at last to insert the endotracheal tube. After confirming proper placement, you secure it with a commercial tube restraint. List some of the specifics you should document on your patient care report (PCR) concerning this intubation.

        (1) _____

        (2) _____

        (3) _____

        (4) _____

4. You are attempting a blind nasotracheal intubation on a 60-kg 24-year-old individual who took an overdose of sleeping pills. You have succeeded in advancing the tip of the endotracheal tube just beyond the oropharynx.

    a. As you continue to advance the tube, how can you tell whether the tip is moving toward the glottis (as opposed to the esophagus)?

        (1) _____

        (2) _____

        (3) _____

    b. As you are advancing the tube, you become aware that the bleeps from the cardiac monitor are getting farther apart. What has happened?

        _____

        _____

        _____

    c. What should you do about it?

        (1) _____

        (2) _____

        (3) _____

5. You are involved in a search-and-rescue mission to find a 43-year-old male hiker lost in the woods. At last you find him, sitting down, propped against a tree. He tells you that he experienced severe chest pain and could not go on. Because there is a strong possibility that he is experiencing an acute myocardial infarction (heart attack), you and your partner will have to carry him the 40-minute walk back to the ambulance. You hook the patient to supplemental oxygen via nasal cannula at a flow rate of 5 L/min. You notice that the pressure gauge on your E cylinder is reading 800 psi.

a. How long is the oxygen in the E cylinder going to last?

_____

_____

b. Will that be long enough to get the patient back to the ambulance? (Show your calculations.)

_____

_____

6. You are sitting at the movies on your night off when you notice someone a few rows ahead of you suddenly slump over. You leap like a gazelle over several rows of seats to reach the person's side, and you discover that he has stopped breathing. You drag him into an aisle and start mouth-to-mouth ventilation with the barrier device you usually carry in your jacket. How can you tell if you are actually getting air into his lungs?

(1) _____

(2) _____

(3) _____

7. As you continue mouth-to-mouth ventilation on the patient described in question 6, you reflect that you would like to avoid causing gastric distention because you would prefer not to deal with the mess that might follow.

a. What can you do, that is noninvasive, to minimize gastric distention during artificial ventilation?

(1) _____

(2) _____

(3) _____

b. Despite your best efforts, however, you notice the man's belly is starting to get enlarged. What else should you do (that may be considered invasive)?

_____

_____

_____

8. After your experience in the movie theater, you promise yourself that you will never go anywhere without a pocket mask, or barrier shield, in your pocket, not only to make things more pleasant for yourself, but also because these devices have several advantages over other methods of giving artificial ventilation. List four specific advantages of a pocket mask.

(1) _____

(2) _____

(3) _____

(4) _____

9. A 53-year-old man calls for an ambulance because of shortness of breath. You find him in severe respiratory distress, with foam bubbling out of his mouth. Your examination reveals signs of congestive heart failure (a condition in which fluid backs up into the lungs and interferes with gas exchange).

a. The patient's pulse oximeter reading when you first arrive shows an oxygen saturation (SaO_2) of 86%. That reading is (circle the best answer):

(1) normal for the patient's age.

(2) abnormally high.

(3) abnormally low.

(4) probably an artifact.

b. What measure should you take immediately?

_____

c. You treat the patient according to your protocol for congestive heart failure, and his condition improves markedly. Now the oxygen saturation reading is 96%. You move the patient to a stretcher and bring him out to the ambulance for transport. When you have him loaded in the ambulance, you notice that the oxygen saturation is now reading 85%. The patient, however, still looks comfortable and is not in any respiratory distress, so you conclude that the reading on the pulse oximeter must be an error. List three of the possible causes of the erroneous reading in this patient:

(1) _____

(2) _____

(3) _____

10. You are attempting a blind nasotracheal intubation on an unconscious patient who took an overdose of sleeping pills. When you think you have the tracheal tube in place, you check the end-tidal carbon dioxide monitor that you've snapped onto the tracheal tube. Its color is purple, indicating that the air being exhaled through the tube contains less than 0.5% carbon dioxide.
a. What can you conclude from that reading?

_____

_____

b. What actions should you take?

_____

_____

11. A passenger riding in a car is breathing quietly at 12 breaths/min, taking in 500 mL of air with each breath.
a. What is his minute volume? _____ mL per minute
b. The car is struck by a semitrailer. The passenger receives an injury to his cervical spine, which paralyzes him from the neck down (his intercostal muscles are also affected). His respiratory rate increases to 20 breaths/min, but his tidal volume falls to 200 mL. What is his minute volume now? _____ mL/min
c. What effect do you expect that change in minute volume to have on the patient's arterial PCO_2?

_____

d. That, in turn, will cause the patient's pH to _____ (rise or fall).
e. The resulting derangement in his acid–base balance is called a _____ (respiratory or metabolic) _____ (acidosis or alkalosis).
f. What treatment is required?

_____

12. Now it's on to a cardiac arrest in a fourth-floor walk-up apartment. You grab the jump kit and the handiest D cylinder from the ambulance, while your partner takes the drug box and monitor/defibrillator, and you sprint up the four flights of stairs to the patient's apartment. While your partner starts CPR chest compressions, you "crack" the oxygen cylinder, hook up the oxygen to a bag-mask device, and open the flow control to 10 L/min. As you do so, you notice the reading on the pressure gauge is 900 psi. How much time do you have before you need to switch to a fresh cylinder? _____ minutes (The cylinder constant for a D cylinder is 0.16. Show your calculations.)

_____

_____

_____

13. A 34-year-old man has been injured in a road collision in which his head apparently struck the windshield with some force. When you first reach the scene, the patient is unconscious. He is breathing 8 breaths/min, inhaling approximately 500 mL of air with each breath.

  a. What is his minute volume? _____ per minute

  b. Is that volume greater or less than normal? _____

  c. Therefore, we can conclude that the patient's arterial PCO_2 will tend to _____ (increase or decrease), so his pH will _____ (increase or decrease). The net effect will be an acid–base disorder called a _____ (respiratory or metabolic) _____ (acidosis or alkalosis). The way you can help correct that abnormality is to _____.

14. You are doing a shift in the emergency department and the laboratory calls down with a blood gas report. You notice that the PCO_2 reported is quite high (hypercarbia)—about 55 mm Hg.

  a. Hypercarbia can be caused by:

    (1) _____

    (2) _____

    (3) _____

    (4) _____

  b. What can be done to normalize the patient's PCO_2?

    _____

    _____

15. The laboratory calls down another blood gas report. "You'd better check on this guy," the lab technician says. "His PO_2 is only 48 mm Hg." As you sprint off to alert the doctor about the blood gas results, you review in your mind the conditions that can cause hypoxemia.

  a. List six conditions that can cause respiratory distress and inadequate ventilation.

    (1) _____

    (2) _____

    (3) _____

    (4) _____

    (5) _____

    (6) _____

  b. What is the treatment for hypoxemia?

    _____

    _____

True/False

If you believe the statement to be more true than false, write the letter "T" in the space provided. If you believe the statement to be more false than true, write the letter "F."

_____ **1.** Any patient who is to be suctioned should first be preoxygenated.

_____ **2.** You should not suction while inserting the catheter.

_____ **3.** Suction for only 2 minutes at a time.

_____ **4.** A tonsil-tip catheter is a good choice for suctioning the oropharynx.

_____ **5.** Once a patient is intubated, suction through the tracheal tube every 5 to 10 minutes to keep the tube free of secretions.

_____ **6.** The physical act of moving air into and out of the lungs is oxygenation.

_____ **7.** The exchange of oxygen and carbon dioxide in the alveoli and the tissues of the body is called ventilation.

_____ **8.** A barrier to ventilation would include neuromuscular disease.

Short Answer

Complete this section with short written answers using the space provided.

1. Obstruction of the upper airway is an immediate threat to life. The upper airway may become obstructed in several ways. List four causes of upper airway obstruction, and put an asterisk beside the most common cause.

   a. _____

   b. _____

   c. _____

   d. _____

2. Endotracheal intubation has several advantages over other methods of airway control. List three advantages of endotracheal intubation.

   a. _____

   b. _____

   c. _____

3. Despite all its advantages, endotracheal intubation is not for all patients. Like every other medical procedure, it has specific indications. List three indications for endotracheal intubation.

   a. _____

   b. _____

   c. _____

4. Endotracheal intubation is not without potential complications. The most serious acute complications can, however, be avoided by meticulous attention to correct technique.
   a. List a potential complication of endotracheal intubation.

   _____

   b. How can it be avoided?

   (1) _____

   (2) _____

   (3) _____

   (4) _____

   c. How can it be detected and corrected if it does occur?

   (1) _____

   (2) _____

   (3) _____

   d. List another potential complication of endotracheal intubation.

   _____

e. How can it be avoided?

_____

f. How can it be detected and corrected if it does occur?

_____

_____

5. In some emergency medical services (EMS) systems, paramedics are authorized to use paralyzing drugs to facilitate tracheal intubation. Although such drugs undoubtedly make life easier for the paramedic, they may make life quite precarious for the patient. What is the principal hazard of administering a neuromuscular blocking agent to a patient who needs to be intubated?

_____

_____

6. A person is breathing quietly at 12 breaths/min with a tidal volume of 500 mL.
 a. Calculate his minute volume.

_____

_____

 b. List two things that could cause his minute volume to decrease.

 (1) _____

 (2) _____

 c. If the person's minute volume does decrease, what change will you see in his arterial blood gases?

_____

7. Oxygen is a drug, and like any other drug, it should be given when there are indications for its use. List six indications for administering supplemental oxygen to a patient.

 a. _____

 b. _____

 c. _____

 d. _____

 e. _____

 f. _____

8. Sometimes the patient himself will "tell" you, through his symptoms and signs, that either his oxygenation, his ventilation, or both are insufficient—that is, he is suffering from acute respiratory insufficiency. List four signs of acute respiratory insufficiency.

 a. _____

 b. _____

 c. _____

 d. _____

9. Oxygen is stored in cylinders at pressures up to 2,000 psi, which means that oxygen cylinders have to be treated with respect. List six safety precautions that should be observed when using or storing oxygen cylinders.

a. _____

b. _____

c. _____

d. _____

e. _____

f. _____

10. Respiratory arrest occurs quite a way down the pathway from life to death. List six things that can cause a person to stop breathing.

a. _____

b. _____

c. _____

d. _____

e. _____

f. _____

11. List three ways of identifying someone in respiratory arrest.

a. _____

b. _____

c. _____

12. A person who has suffered respiratory arrest will need _____ (assisted/artificial) ventilation.

13. What is the difference between artificial and assisted ventilation?

_____

_____

14. What is the objective of any form of artificial ventilation?

_____

_____

15. List three situations in which information from pulse oximetry could be helpful to you in the field.

a. _____

b. _____

c. _____

16. A car crash victim who has sustained injury to the cervical spinal cord may develop weakness or paralysis of his respiratory muscles. If so, such a patient may not have the strength to inhale as deeply as he otherwise would. Thus, his minute volume will _____ (increase or decrease), leading to a/an _____ in his arterial PCO_2.

Fill-in-the-Table

Fill in the missing parts of the table.

1. In mastering the use of any given piece of equipment, it is essential to learn not only how to use the equipment but also when to use it (and when not to use it). Artificial airways can be enormously helpful when applied in the appropriate circumstances; they can be downright dangerous when used in inappropriate circumstances. Fill in the following table to summarize the indications and contraindications for the oropharyngeal airway (OPA) and the nasopharyngeal airway (NPA).

	Oropharyngeal Airway	Nasopharyngeal Airway
Use for:		
Do not use for:		

2. Oxygen-Delivery Devices

Device	Flow Rate (L/min)	Oxygen Delivered (%)
Nasal cannula		
Nonrebreathing mask		
Bag-mask device with reservoir		

3. Airway adjuncts can be very helpful in ensuring a patent air passage, but one needs to use the right adjunct in the right situation. Fill in the following table to remind yourself what to use (and not to use) and when to use it.

Adjunct	Indicated for:	Do not use in:
Oropharyngeal airway		
Combitube		
LMA		
Endotracheal intubation		

Skill Drills

Test your knowledge of the steps in this skill drill by filling in the missing captions.

1. Nasogastric Tube Insertion in a Responsive Patient

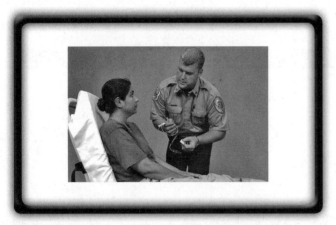

Explain the procedure to the patient, and oxygenate the patient if necessary. Ensure the patient's head is in a neutral position, and suppress the gag reflex with a topical anesthetic spray.

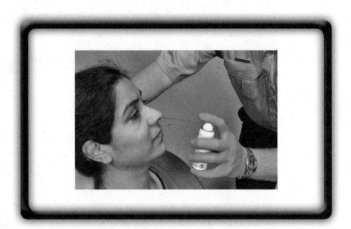

_____

_____

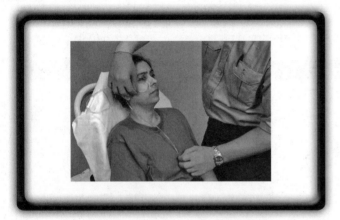

Measure the tube for the correct depth of insertion (nose to ear to xiphoid process.)

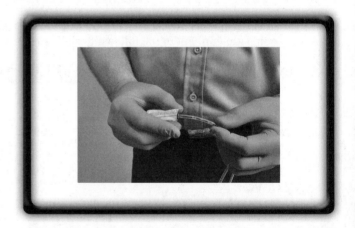

_____

_____

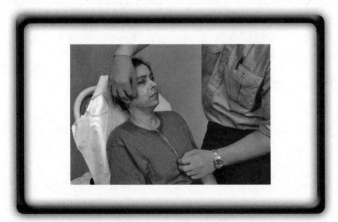

Measure the tube for the correct depth of insertion (nose to ear to xiphoid process.)

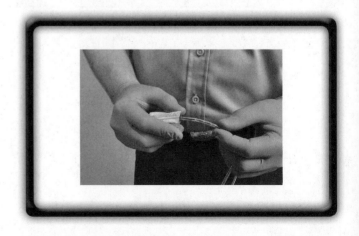

_____

_____

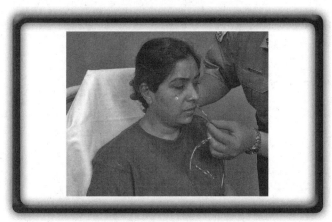

Advance the tube gently along the nasal floor.

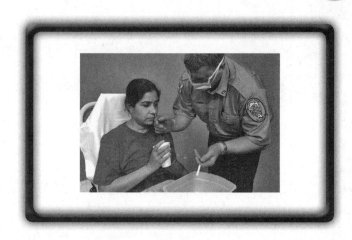

_____

_____

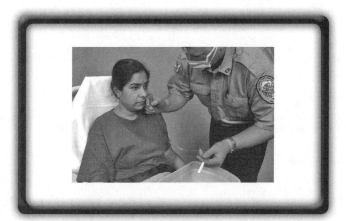

Advance the tube into the stomach.

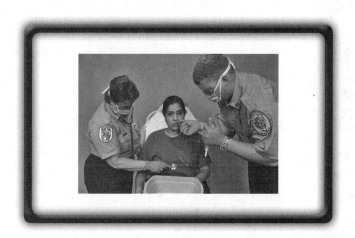

_____

_____

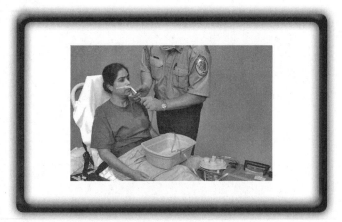

Apply suction to the tube to aspirate the gastric contents, and secure the tube in place.

CHAPTER 16

Respiratory Emergencies

Matching

Match each of the items in the left column to the appropriate term in the right column.

_____ 1. A nosebleed.

_____ 2. The mucus-producing cells found mainly in the respiratory and intestinal tracts.

_____ 3. A liquid protein substance that coats the alveoli in the lungs.

_____ 4. Weakening or loss of a palpable pulse during inhalation; characteristic of cardiac tamponade and severe asthma.

_____ 5. The infiltration of any tissue by air or gas; a chronic obstructive pulmonary disease characterized by distention of the alveoli and destructive changes in the lung parenchyma.

_____ 6. Hollow pockets on the lateral portions of the glottic opening.

_____ 7. Contorted position of the hand or foot in which the fingers or toes flex in a clawlike manner; may result from hyperventilation.

_____ 8. A vascular reaction that may have an allergic cause and may result in profound swelling of the tongue and lips.

_____ 9. The abnormal breath sounds that have a fine, crackling quality; previously called rales.

_____ 10. A ridge-like projection of tracheal cartilage located where the trachea bifurcates into the right and left mainstem bronchi.

A. Emphysema

B. Carpopedal spasm

C. Surfactant

D. Carina

E. Piriform fossae

F. Epistaxis

G. Crackles

H. Pulsus paradoxus

I. Angioedema

J. Goblet cells

Multiple Choice

Read each item carefully, and then select the best response.

1. What is the opening at the top of the trachea called?
   A. Epiglottis
   B. Glottis
   C. Larynx
   D. Piriform fossa

2. In a pneumothorax, where is air trapped?
   A. Inside the alveoli
   B. In the nasopharynx
   C. Between visceral and parietal pleurae
   D. Between the alveoli

3. Which of the following substances are thin secretions in the airway that the body can eliminate by coughing?
   A. Antitussives
   B. Corticosteroids
   C. Diuretics
   D. Expectorants

4. Right-sided heart failure that has been caused by a chronic lung disease is known as which of the following?
   A. Guillain-Barré syndrome
   B. Polycythemia
   C. Cor pulmonale
   D. Atelectasis

5. Which of the following breathing patterns is characterized by breathing that becomes faster and deeper until there is a period of apnea before the pattern begins again?
   A. Cheyne-Stokes
   B. Kussmaul
   C. Cor pulmonale
   D. Ataxic

6. What is another name for *rales*?
   A. Rhoncus
   B. Wheezing
   C. Crackles
   D. Death rattle

7. You respond to a patient who is having difficulty breathing. He is coughing up frothy sputum. What is the classic cause of frothy sputum?
   A. Rhoncus
   B. Wheezing
   C. Crackles
   D. Death rattle

8. What is the name of the response that helps regulate the depth of respiration and keeps the lungs from overinflating?
   A. Gag reflex
   B. Hering-Breuer reflex
   C. Baro-receptor reflex
   D. Atelectasis response

9. Which of the following is NOT used to treat asthma as defined in the asthma triad?
   A. Expectorants
   B. Corticosteroids
   C. Bronchodilator
   D. Hyperventilation

10. What is the correct name for a viral infection of the area around the glottis that strikes children between 6 months and 3 years of age, usually in the middle of the night?
    A. Croup
    B. Epiglottitis
    C. Diphtheria
    D. Pneumonitis

Fill-in-the-Blank

Read each item carefully, and then complete the statement by filling in the missing word(s).

1. Alveoli collapse is known as _____.

2. Hairlike structures (_____) move particulate matter up and out of the airway.

3. A surplus of red blood cells that the body makes as a result of a chronic lung disease is called _____.

4. Your patient has two or more ribs, broken in two or more places, that are inhibiting her breathing. In your radio report, you report this as a/an _____ _____.

5. The medical term for shortness of breath is _____, and the medical term for blue-tinged skin caused by lack of oxygen is _____.

6. Being awakened by difficulty breathing during the night is known as _____ _____ _____.

7. _____ _____ are vibrations felt in the chest when a patient breathes.

8. There are _____ lobes in the right lung and _____ lobes in the left lung.

9. It is helpful during ventilation through an endotracheal (ET) tube to use a/an _____-_____ carbon dioxide detector to confirm and monitor that gas exchange is happening.

10. Breathing in a way that allows patients to exhale slowly under controlled pressure is called _____-_____ _____.

Labeling

Label the following diagrams with the correct terms.

1. The Upper Airway

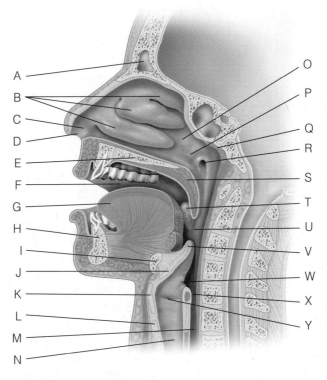

A. _____	N. _____
B. _____	O. _____
C. _____	P. _____
D. _____	Q. _____
E. _____	R. _____
F. _____	S. _____
G. _____	T. _____
H. _____	U. _____
I. _____	V. _____
J. _____	W. _____
K. _____	X. _____
L. _____	Y. _____
M. _____	

2. Anatomy of the Larynx

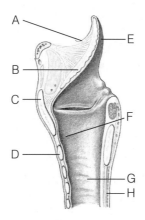

A. _____

B. _____

C. _____

D. _____

E. _____

F. _____

G. _____

H. _____

3. Respiratory Patterns

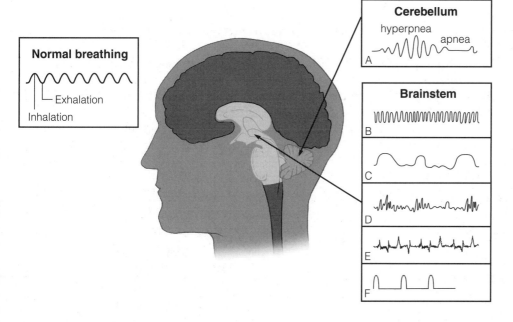

A. _____

B. _____

C. _____

D. _____

E. _____

F. _____

Identify

In the following case study, list the chief complaint, vital signs, and pertinent negatives.

You respond to a call for a baby not breathing. As you approach the home, a mother comes running out holding a 1-year-old little boy. He is limp in her arms. You immediately jump out and take the child from her, get into the back of the unit, and lay him on the cot. The child is unconscious and blue, and he has no respirations. You begin the steps of CPR by opening the airway and trying to give two breaths. Your partner has crawled into the back along with the mother and is trying to calm her down and help you at the same time. Using a pediatric bag-mask device, you give a breath and notice no chest rise and fall. You reposition the head and try again, and once again there is no rise and fall of the chest. You check the brachial artery and find a faint pulse. Your partner has pulled out the intubation kit and is ready to try to insert an advanced airway. As he looks for the trachea, he reaches for the Magill forceps and suction. After suctioning and using the forceps, he removes a small plastic game piece from the boy. You immediately start to bag the child again with 100% supplemental oxygen. The child's chest rises now. His oxygen saturation is 64%, and the pulse is bradycardic at 46 beats/min. You are unable to get a blood pressure. You manage respirations at one every 3 seconds. After a minute, the child is beginning to "pink up," his "sats" come up to 88%, and his heart rate has been on a steady climb and at the moment is 92 beats/min. The child is regaining consciousness and begins to cry and fight you. He is breathing on his own. His mother wants the child transported to be checked out. Your partner has a pediatric nonrebreathing mask ready with 100% supplemental oxygen. Mom holds the nonrebreathing mask while you strap the child into a car seat and place mom in a seat belt. By the time you reach the emergency department (ED), little Tommy's heart rate is normal and his oxygen saturation is 99%; his mom, on the other hand, begins to cry with the realization of how close Tommy was to death.

1. Chief complaint:

_____

_____

2. Vital signs:

_____

_____

3. Pertinent negatives:

_____

_____

Ambulance Calls

The following case scenarios provide an opportunity to explore the concerns associated with patient management and paramedic care. Read each scenario, and then answer each question.

1. You are called to an office building for a "possible heart attack." On arriving, you are somewhat surprised to find that the patient is a secretary who looks about 22 years old—not at all like your usual heart attack patient. The woman looks pale and anxious, however, and complains of stabbing pains in her chest that came on "out of the blue." She also complains of a "funny tingly feeling in my lips." On examination, her pulse is 110 beats/min and regular, respirations are 30 breaths/min and unlabored, and blood pressure is 140/84 mm Hg without significant variation during the respiratory cycle. There are no abnormal physical findings except that the patient's hands look a bit odd, almost like claws.

a. What is the most probable diagnosis in this case?

_____

_____

_____

b. What steps will you take in managing this case?

(1) _____

(2) _____

(3) _____

c. This woman's arterial PCO_2 is probably _____ (higher or lower) than normal. Explain why.

_____

_____

2. You are called late one night to the Koff family residence for a "man who can't breathe." The patient's wife answers the door, quite distraught, and hurries you into the bedroom, blurting, "This is the worst it's ever been. I kept telling him to leave those cigarettes alone—the doctor's been saying the same thing—but do you think he listens? Might as well be talking to a brick wall."

In the bedroom, you find a heavy-set man about 60 years old sitting up at the edge of the bed in obvious respiratory distress. In fact, his "obvious" respiratory distress is obvious only if you know the signs of respiratory distress (increased work of breathing).

a. List eight signs of respiratory distress or increased work of breathing.

(1) _____

(2) _____

(3) _____

(4) _____

(5) _____

(6) _____

(7) _____

(8) _____

b. What steps will you take at this point?

_____

_____

_____

c. In due course, you learn that the patient called for an ambulance because he wakened from sleep unable to breathe. List seven questions you need to ask in taking his history.

(1) _____

(2) _____

(3) _____

(4) _____

(5) _____

(6) _____

(7) _____

d. As you proceed systematically through the physical assessment of this man, you will be looking for some specific abnormalities at each step. In the following table, indicate what in particular you will be looking for as you examine each part of the body indicated.

Part of the Body	What I Am Looking for in Particular
General appearance	
Vital signs	
Head	
Neck	
Chest	
Abdomen	
Extremities	

e. In the course of the focused history, you learn that the patient has been a three-pack-per-day cigarette smoker for about 45 years. He "keeps a cough," but lately it has been worse than usual, and he has been bringing up a lot more sputum. His feet have also begun swelling, to the point that he can hardly get his shoes on anymore. (Most of this you learn from the patient's wife; the patient is too short of breath to provide more than two or three words at a time.)

(1) This patient most likely has which of the following conditions?

    (a) Pulmonary embolism

    (b) Chronic obstructive pulmonary disease (COPD)

   (c) Pneumonia

   (d) Pickwickian syndrome

   (e) Acute asthmatic attack

  (2) How will you manage this patient?

_____

_____

_____

_____

3. A 56-year-old man calls for an ambulance because of severe dyspnea. His wife, who greets you at the door, tells you, "My husband, he's a heart patient. Please get him to the hospital quickly. I think he's having another heart attack."

  You find the patient in the living room, sitting in an armchair in obvious distress. "Hit me like a ton of bricks," he gasps. "Not like the heart attack"—gasp—"Can't get air"—gasp—"Hurts to breathe."

  On physical examination, his skin is cool and moist. Vital signs are pulse 120 beats/min and regular, respirations 32 breaths/min and shallow, and blood pressure 174/96 mm Hg. The neck veins look a bit distended, but otherwise there are no abnormal findings.

 a. This patient is most likely suffering from which of the following conditions?

  (1) Pulmonary embolism

  (2) Decompensated COPD

  (3) Pneumonia

  (4) Pickwickian syndrome

  (5) Acute asthmatic attack

 b. What steps will you take in managing this patient?

  (1) _____

  (2) _____

  (3) _____

  (4) _____

True/False

If you believe the statement to be more true than false, write the letter "T" in the space provided. If you believe the statement to be more false than true, write the letter "F."

_____ **1.** Right-sided heart failure because of chronic lung disease is known as cor pulmonale.

_____ **2.** Typically, anatomic dead space is equal to 5 mL per pound of body weight.

_____ **3.** Gas exchange happens only in the alveoli.

_____ **4.** Hiccups, yawns, and sighs are all forms of breathing patterns.

_____ **5.** Laying a patient flat will help the patient breathe better.

_____ **6.** Stridor is a result of a partial obstruction of the upper airway.

_____ **7.** A patient who is sitting in the tripod position (elbows out) and who can speak only in two- or three-word statements is a patient in distress.

_____ **8.** Patients who suffer from severe COPD often have jugular vein distension.

_____ **9.** The diaphragm of a stethoscope is for high-pitched breath sounds.

_____ **10.** Pulse oximetry is a tool that can give false readings if the patient has a low hemoglobin level.

_____ **11.** An abnormal breathing pattern due to injury to the brainstem is central neurogenic hyperventilation.

_____ **12.** Acute pulmonary edema will sometimes present as a wheeze that sounds like an asthma attack.

_____ **13.** You should withhold high concentrations of oxygen for the patient who breathes with the hypoxic drive.

_____ **14.** An asthmatic who tells you he was previously intubated for his breathing difficulty is at increased risk of death.

_____ **15.** Anticholinergics have emerged as a central component in the management of COPD.

_____ **16.** If you use an aerosol nebulizer to deliver medication, you can expect the patient to benefit from 90% of the medication dose.

_____ **17.** Immediate fast-acting medications used for bronchodilation are beta-1 agonists.

_____ **18.** When giving a corticosteroid as an IV bolus, you will see immediate results.

_____ **19.** Morphine should be used as the first-line vasodilator in the treatment of pulmonary edema.

_____ **20.** A continuous positive airway pressure (CPAP) machine cannot be used in the field.

Short Answer

Complete this section with short written answers using the space provided.

1. List four things that can cause a pulmonary embolism.

   a. _____

   b. _____

   c. _____

   d. _____

2. Discuss the clues to diagnosing a pulmonary embolism.

   _____

   _____

   _____

3. What are the contraindications to supplemental oxygen therapy?

   _____

   _____

   _____

4. Not every patient who presents with dyspnea and wheezing has bronchial asthma. List four other conditions that can produce wheezing.

   a. _____

   b. _____

   c. _____

   d. _____

5. Asthma is common in children, so it is important to be able to distinguish a mild asthmatic attack from one that is potentially life threatening. List at least five signs that an asthmatic attack is very severe and warrants urgent transport to the hospital.

   a. _____

   b. _____

   c. _____

   d. _____

   e. _____

Fill-in-the-Table

Provide signs and symptoms of the various breathing patterns listed in the following table.

Breathing Patterns

Pattern	Comments
Agonal	_____ _____ that are widely spaced; usually represent _____ _____ _____ in a dying patient; occasional agonal gasp not unusual in patients with no pulse; not actually considered a form of breathing
Apneustic	Characterized by a _____ _____ _____ (sometimes called "_____ breathing"); follows damage to the _____ _____ in the brain; an ominous sign of severe _____ _____
Ataxic	Chaotically irregular respirations that indicate _____ brain injury or _____ _____
Biot respirations	Irregular pattern, _____, and depth of respirations, characterized by intermittent patterns of _____; indicates severe brain injury or _____ herniation
Bradypnea	Unusually _____ respirations
Central neurogenic hyperventilation	Tachypneic _____; rapid and deep respirations caused by _____ _____ _____ or direct _____ _____; drives _____ _____ level down and _____ up, resulting in respiratory _____
Cheyne-Stokes respirations	_____-_____ breathing with a period of _____ between cycles; not considered ominous unless grossly _____ or occurs in a patient with brain _____
Cough	Forced exhalation against a closed _____; an airway-clearing maneuver; also seen when _____ _____ irritate the airways; controlled by the cough center in the brain (_____ medications work on the cough center to reduce this sometimes annoying physiologic response.)
Eupnea	_____ breathing
Hiccup	Spasmodic contraction of the _____, causing short _____ with a characteristic sound; sometimes seen in cases of diaphragmatic (or _____) nerve irritation from _____ _____ _____, ulcer disease, or _____ _____
Hyperpnea	Abnormally _____ rate and depth of breathing; seen in various _____ or chemical disorders, including overdose with certain drugs
Hypopnea	Abnormally _____ rate and depth of breathing
Kussmaul respirations	The same pattern as in _____ _____ _____, but caused by the body's response to metabolic _____, attempting to rid itself of blood _____ via the lungs; seen in diabetic _____; accompanied by a _____ (acetone) breath odor and, usually, _____ and dry mouth and lips
Sighing	Periodically taking a very deep breath of about _____ the normal volume; forces open _____ that routinely close from time to time
Tachypnea	Unusually _____ breathing; does not reflect _____ of respiration and does not mean a patient is _____ (breathing too rapidly and deeply, resulting in a lowered _____ _____ level); often involves moving only small volumes of air, or _____ (much like a panting dog)
Yawning	Seems beneficial in the same manner as _____

Problem Solving

Practice your calculation skills by solving the following math problems.

1. Your patient weighs 200 lb. Typically, the dead space volume is 1 mL/lb. Also, a typical person loses 150 mL of air inside the bronchioles that are not used in the exchange of air.

a. How much dead space volume does this patient have?

b. If the patient's tidal volume is 700 mL, how many milliliters will reach the alveoli?

2. How about if your patient weighs 120 lb?
    a. How much dead space volume does this patient have?

    b. If the patient's tidal volume is 600 mL, how many milliliters will reach the alveoli?

Complete the Patient Care Report (PCR)

Read the incident scenario in the "Identify" exercise and then complete the following PCR.

EMS Patient Care Report (PCR)					
Date:	**Incident No.:**	**Nature of Call:**			**Location:**
Dispatched:	**En Route:**	**At Scene:**	**Transport:**	**At Hospital:**	**In Service:**

Patient Information	
Age:	**Allergies:**
Sex:	**Medications:**
Weight (in kg [lb]):	**Past Medical History:**
	Chief Complaint:

Vital Signs				
Time:	**BP:**	**Pulse:**	**Respirations:**	**SpO$_2$:**
Time:	**BP:**	**Pulse:**	**Respirations:**	**SpO$_2$:**
Time:	**BP:**	**Pulse:**	**Respirations:**	**SpO$_2$:**

EMS Treatment (circle all that apply)

Oxygen @ _____ L/min via (circle one): NC NRM Bag-Mask Device		Assisted Ventilation	Airway Adjunct	CPR
Defibrillation	**Bleeding Control**	**Bandaging**	**Splinting**	**Other**

Narrative

Cardiovascular Emergencies

Welcome to the cardiac chapter of the workbook. Because of the length and the amount of material covered in this chapter, we have divided the workbook chapter into three parts to facilitate your learning: Part 1: Cardiac Function, Part 2: Heart Rhythms and the ECG, and Part 3: Putting It All Together and Practice ECG Strips.

Part 1: Cardiac Function

Matching

Match each of the definitions in the left column to the appropriate term in the right column.

_____ 1. An acute elevation of blood pressure with evidence of end-organ damage.

_____ 2. A sac or bulge resulting from the weakening of the wall of a blood vessel or ventricle.

_____ 3. One of the two arteries that carry deoxygenated blood from the right ventricle to the lungs.

_____ 4. Restriction of cardiac contraction, failing cardiac output, and shock, caused by the accumulation of fluid or blood in the pericardium.

_____ 5. A condition that occurs when the heart is unable to pump powerfully enough or fast enough to empty its chambers; as a result, blood backs up into the systemic circuit, the pulmonary circuit, or both.

_____ 6. A fixed blood clot.

_____ 7. The percentage of blood that leaves the heart each time it contracts.

_____ 8. A weakening or loss of a palpable pulse during inhalation, characteristic of cardiac tamponade and severe asthma.

_____ 9. Severe shortness of breath occurring at night and after several hours of recumbency, during which fluid pools in the lungs; the person is forced to sit up to breathe; caused by left heart failure or decompensation of chronic obstructive pulmonary disease.

_____ 10. The resistance against which the ventricle contracts.

A. Thrombus

B. Congestive heart failure

C. Ejection fraction

D. Hypertensive emergency

E. Cardiac tamponade

F. Pulsus paradoxus

G. Afterload

H. Paroxysmal nocturnal dyspnea

I. Pulmonary artery

J. Aneurysm

Multiple Choice

Read each item carefully, and then select the best response.

1. The innermost smooth layer of the heart is called the:
    A. myocardium.
    B. endocardium.
    C. epicardium.
    D. pericardium.

2. The _____ separates the left atrium from the left ventricle.
    A. coronary sulcus
    B. mitral valve
    C. chordae tendineae
    D. tricuspid valve

3. The normal dominant pacemaker for the heart is the:
   A. Purkinje fibers.
   B. atrioventricular (AV) node.
   C. bundle of His.
   D. sinoatrial (SA) node.

4. The _____ component of the electrocardiogram (ECG) represents the depolarization of the ventricles.
   A. P wave
   B. QRS complex
   C. R-R interval
   D. T wave

5. The paramedic is palpating the radial pulse while listening to the apical pulse with a stethoscope. What abnormality is he or she likely to find?
   A. Pulsus paradoxus
   B. Pulse deficit
   C. Pulsus alternans
   D. Pericardial friction rub

6. Of the following, which is NOT a cause of a cardiac dysrhythmia?
   A. Myocardial ischemia
   B. Cor pulmonale
   C. Hypoglycemia
   D. Increased vagal tone

7. An area of fat in the arteries that has calcified is known as a:
   A. bruit.
   B. phlebitis.
   C. thrombophlebitis.
   D. plaque.

8. In a 65-year-old man, a systolic blood pressure of _____ would indicate hypertension.
   A. 120 mm Hg
   B. 130 mm Hg
   C. 140 mm Hg
   D. 150 mm Hg

9. What symptom is NOT associated with an acute myocardial infarction (AMI) or acute cardiac syndrome (ACS)?
   A. Bulimia
   B. Dizziness
   C. Palpitations
   D. Diaphoresis

10. The M in the mnemonic MONA stands for:
    A. myocardium.
    B. morphine.
    C. management.
    D. monitor.

Fill-in-the-Blank

Read each item carefully, and then complete the statement by filling in the missing word(s).

1. Alternative routes of blood flow around the heart are known as _____ _____. These are used in case of a blockage.

2. The _____ valve prevents blood from flowing back into the left ventricle.

3. The cardiac cycle comprises one complete phase of atrial and ventricular relaxation (_____), followed by one atrial and ventricular contraction (_____).

4. The _____ _____ comprises the blood vessels between the right ventricle and left atrium, which receive the output of the right side of the heart.

5. The smallest artery is known as a/an _____, and the largest artery in the body is the _____.

6. _____ _____ is the amount of blood pumped out by either ventricle in a single contraction.

7. The AV node serves as the _____ to the ventricles.

8. Muscle fibers _____ when they are stimulated to contract.

9. During the _____ _____ _____, the heart muscle will not contract because it is drained of all its energy.

10. Repolarization of the ventricles and atria will produce a/an _____ _____ marking on an ECG.

Labeling

Label the following diagrams with the correct terms.

1. Coronary Arteries

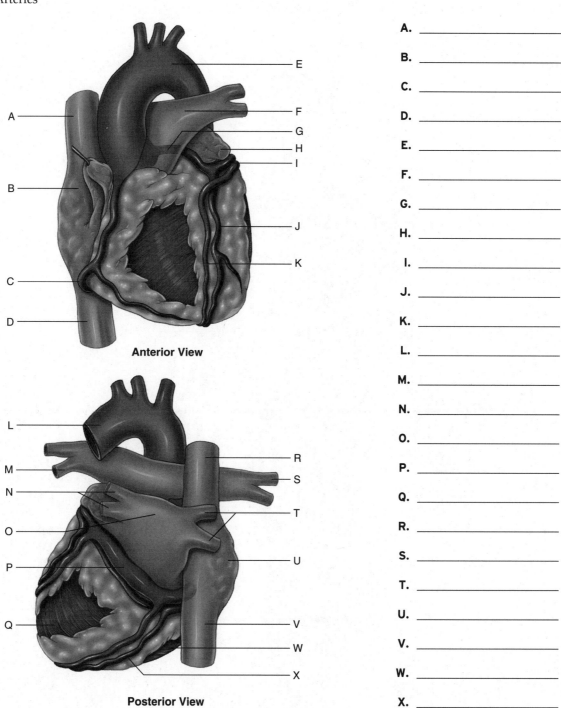

Anterior View

Posterior View

A. _____

B. _____

C. _____

D. _____

E. _____

F. _____

G. _____

H. _____

I. _____

J. _____

K. _____

L. _____

M. _____

N. _____

O. _____

P. _____

Q. _____

R. _____

S. _____

T. _____

U. _____

V. _____

W. _____

X. _____

2. Structure of a Blood Vessel

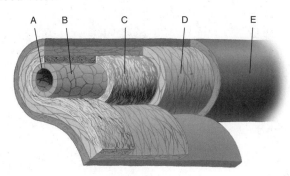

A. _____

B. _____

C. _____

D. _____

E. _____

3. Major Arteries and Veins

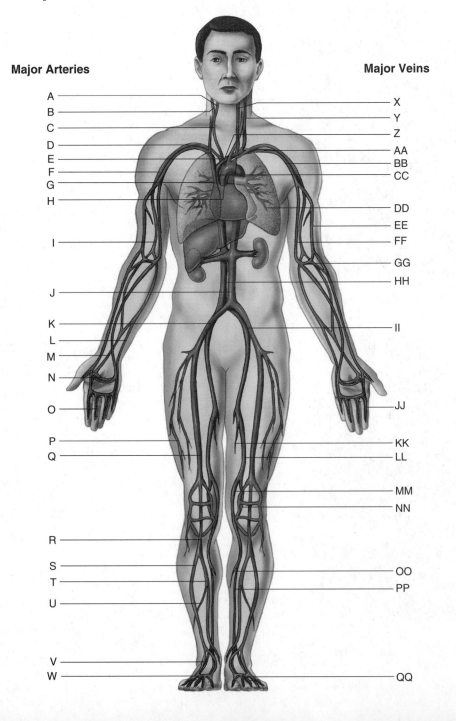

A. _____
B. _____
C. _____
D. _____
E. _____
F. _____
G. _____
H. _____
I. _____
J. _____
K. _____
L. _____
M. _____
N. _____
O. _____
P. _____
Q. _____
R. _____
S. _____
T. _____
U. _____
V. _____
W. _____
X. _____
Y. _____
Z. _____
AA. _____
BB. _____
CC. _____
DD. _____
EE. _____
FF. _____
GG. _____
HH. _____
II. _____
JJ. _____
KK. _____
LL. _____
MM. _____
NN. _____
OO. _____
PP. _____
QQ. _____

True/False

If you believe the statement to be more true than false, write the letter "T" in the space provided. If you believe the statement to be more false than true, write the letter "F."

_____ **1.** Labetalol and nitroglycerin are drugs that can lower blood pressure.

_____ **2.** The most characteristic physical finding in an abdominal aortic aneurysm (AAA) is decreased pedal pulse.

_____ **3.** An ECG will be very helpful in diagnosing cardiac tamponade.

_____ **4.** Management of left-sided heart failure should be to decrease preload.

_____ **5.** Furosemide (Lasix) is a diuretic that will help with left heart failure.

_____ **6.** Percutaneous intervention can be used for a patient who does not qualify for fibrinolytic therapy.

_____ **7.** Fibrinolytic therapy should begin 2 hours after the AMI has occurred.

_____ **8.** Diabetic patients have incredible pain when suffering from an AMI.

_____ **9.** The most common symptom of AMI is chest pain.

_____ **10.** Stable angina follows a recurrent pattern, usually after exertion.

Fill-in-the-Table

Fill in the missing parts of the table.

1. Role of Electrolytes in Cardiac Function

Role of Electrolytes in Cardiac Function	
Electrolyte	**Role in Cardiac Function**
_____	Flows into the cell to initiate depolarization
_____	Flows out of the cell to initiate _____ Decreased or increased levels of potassium result in the following: • _____ → increased myocardial irritability • _____ → decreased automaticity/conduction
_____	Has a major role in the depolarization of _____ cells (maintains depolarization) and in myocardial contractility (involved in contraction of heart muscle tissue) Decreased or increased levels of calcium result in the following: • _____ → decreased contractility and increased myocardial irritability • _____ → increased contractility
_____	Stabilizes the cell membrane; acts in concert with _____, and opposes the actions of calcium Decreased or increased levels of magnesium result in the following: • _____ → decreased conduction • _____ → increased myocardial irritability

2. Components of the ECG

Components of the ECG	
ECG Representation	**Cardiac Event**
_____	Depolarization of the atria
_____	Depolarization of the atria and delay at the AV junction
_____	Depolarization of the ventricles
_____	Period between ventricular depolarization and beginning of repolarization
_____	Repolarization of the ventricles
_____	Time between two ventricular depolarizations

Part 2: Heart Rhythms and the ECG
Matching

Match each of the items in the left column to the appropriate term in the right column.

_____ **1.** Where the "RA" or "RL" lead is traditionally placed by paramedics

_____ **2.** Where the "LL" lead is traditionally placed by paramedics

_____ **3.** The point where the QRS complex ends and the ST segment begins

_____ **4.** Represents ventricular repolarization on an ECG

_____ **5.** A regular rhythm, 60 to 100 beats/min

_____ **6.** SA node pacemaker with a rate of 100 beats/min or more

_____ **7.** A rhythm in which the atria are contracting at a rate that is too fast for the ventricles to match

_____ **8.** When an impulse reaching the AV node is delayed and results in a PR interval longer than 0.20 seconds

_____ **9.** Rhythm that occurs when the ventricles take over at a rate of 20 to 40 beats/min

_____ **10.** A delta wave is an indication of this

A. First-degree heart block
B. Heart rate
C. Left lower chest
D. T wave
E. Atrial flutter
F. Tachycardia
G. Right upper shoulder
H. Wolff-Parkinson-White syndrome
I. J point
J. Idioventricular rhythm

Multiple Choice

Read each item carefully, and then select the best response.

1. _____ is an electrolyte imbalance that causes very tall and pointed T waves.
A. Hypokalemia
B. Hyperkalemia
C. Hyperglycemia
D. Hypocalcemia

2. Lead _____ is NOT a limb lead.
A. I
B. aVR
C. aVF
D. V_2

3. During an AMI, the stage of injury appears as a/an _____ on the ECG.
A. T-wave inversion
B. ST-segment depression
C. ST-segment elevation
D. spiked P wave

4. Lead V_5 is placed on the patient on the:
A. anterior axillary line.
B. midaxillary line.
C. fourth intercostal space.
D. left arm.

5. _____ is NOT a possible cause of pulseless electrical activity (PEA).
A. Hypovolemia
B. Hyperthermia
C. Cardiac tamponade
D. Pulmonary embolism

6. The signs and symptoms of sick sinus syndrome include all of the following, EXCEPT:
A. dizziness.
B. palpitation.
C. bounding pulse.
D. near-syncope.

7. When using paddles to shock a patient, you apply _____ lb of pressure to the chest with the paddles.
   A. 10
   B. 15
   C. 20
   D. 25

8. The correct term for the use of a defibrillator to end a dysrhythmia other than V-fib or pulseless V-tach is:
   A. cardioversion.
   B. transcutaneous cardiac pacing.
   C. defibrillation.
   D. conversion.

9. A common treatment for chronic coronary heart failure or rapid atrial dysrhythmias is:
   A. atropine.
   B. digitalis.
   C. sodium bicarbonate.
   D. nitroglycerin.

10. One small box on the ECG strip represents _____ seconds.
   A. 0.04
   B. 0.40
   C. 0.02
   D. 0.20

Fill-in-the-Blank

Read each item carefully, and then complete the statement by filling in the missing word(s).

1. _____ _____ occurs when the SA node fails to fire and initiate an impulse, which in turn eliminates an entire cardiac cycle. After the missed set, a normal function returns.

2. A tachycardic rhythm that begins in the pacemaker above the ventricles is known as a/an _____ _____.

3. The SA node ceases to fire and the AV node (in the junction) takes over as the pacemaker; however, the rate is greater than 60 beats/min. This is called _____ _____ _____.

4. A/an _____-_____ _____ _____ occurs when there is no association between the AV node and the ventricles. Ventricular rate runs the heart.

5. _____ _____ occurs when the entire heart begins to quiver without any organized contractions.

6. The pattern _____ occurs when there is a normal complex followed by a premature ventricular complex. This pattern repeats itself. If every third beat is a premature ventricular complex, it is then called _____.

7. _____ occurs when the entire heart is at a standstill and there is no electrical activity.

8. A/an _____ _____ is an indication of Wolff-Parkinson-White syndrome.

9. When a premature ventricular complex comes from the same site, it is known as _____, but when the premature ventricular complexes come from different sites in the ventricles, the condition is known as _____.

10. The pacemaker is the SA node, but with a rate of less than 60 beats/min. This is called _____ _____.

True/False

If you believe the statement to be more true than false, write the letter "T" in the space provided. If you believe the statement to be more false than true, write the letter "F."

_____ **1.** The electrodes should be attached to the leads prior to placing them on the patient's skin.

_____ **2.** P waves indicate that the pacemaker for the heart is in the AV node.

_____ **3.** The "6-second method" is the simplest, but not the most accurate, method for determining the heart rate when the rhythm is slow.

_____ **4.** A heart rate of more than 100 beats/min is called tachycardia.

_____ **5.** Wandering atrial pacemaker is most commonly seen in diabetic patients.

_____ **6.** Prehospital treatment of atrial fibrillation is common.

_____ **7.** Mobitz type I occurs when each successive impulse is delayed a little longer, until finally one impulse is not able to continue.

_____ **8.** The ventricles will take over as the pacemaker if the SA node fails.

_____ **9.** Polymorphic V-tach is more serious than monomorphic V-tach.

_____ **10.** An agonal rhythm will produce a pulse.

Short Answer

Complete this section with short written answers using the space provided.

1. Discuss the basic principles in placing electrodes on a patient's chest.

_____

_____

_____

2. Explain the cause for the P wave, P-R interval, QRS complex, and T wave.

_____

_____

_____

3. Describe how a 12-lead ECG helps to "look" at the heart.

_____

_____

_____

4. What should you do if you find a patient in cardiac arrest?

_____

_____

_____

5. If you are able to terminate cardiopulmonary resuscitation (CPR) in the field, what should you and your medical director do before you implement your protocols to do so?

_____

_____

_____

Part 3: Putting It All Together and Practice ECG Strips

Matching

Match the generic name with the trade name for the following drugs.

_____ **1.** Amiodarone

_____ **2.** Metoprolol

_____ **3.** Furosemide

_____ **4.** Dopamine

_____ **5.** Nifedipine

_____ **6.** Propranolol

_____ **7.** Diltiazem

A. Procardia

B. Lopressor

C. Inderol

D. Levophed

E. Lasix

F. Intropin

G. Adrenaline

_____ **8.** Norepinephrine

_____ **9.** Albuterol

_____ **10.** Epinephrine

H. Cardizem

I. Cordarone

J. Proventil

Labeling

Label the following diagrams with the correct terms.

1. Electrical Conduction System

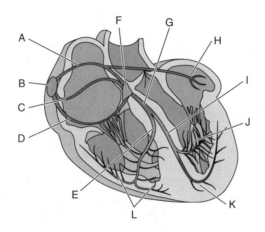

A. _____

B. _____

C. _____

D. _____

E. _____

F. _____

G. _____

H. _____

I. _____

J. _____

K. _____

L. _____

2. Schematic Representation of a 12-Lead ECG

I High lateral wall LV A_____	aVR	V₁ Interventricular septum E_____	V₄ G_____ LAD
II Inferior wall LV RCA	C_____ High lateral wall LV LCx	V₂ Interventricular septum F_____	V₅ Low lateral wall LV LCx
III B_____ RCA	D_____ Inferior wall LV RCA	V₃ Anterior wall LV LADt	H_____ Low lateral wall LV LCx

A. _____

B. _____

C. _____

D. _____

E. _____

F. _____

G. _____

H. _____

Ambulance Calls

Read each scenario, and then answer all the questions following the scenario.

1. You are called to see a 62-year-old man complaining of severe chest pain. He says that the pain came on an hour earlier and that it feels "like a thousand-pound weight on my chest." The patient is very restless and seems confused, so it is hard to get much history. On physical examination, he is obviously in marked distress. His skin is pale and cold. His pulse is 82 beats/min and thready, respirations are 32 breaths/min and shallow, and blood pressure is 90/62 mm Hg. His oxygen saturation is 91% on room air.

a. Identify the chief complaint and vital signs for this patient.

Chief complaint:

_____

_____

Vital signs:

_____

_____

b. What steps would you direct your partner to take at this time of the call?

(1) _____

(2) _____

(3) _____

(4) _____

c. After your partner hooks up the monitor, you run a 3-lead ECG strip and see this:

P wave: Typically absent. Inverted if present. Can appear after the QRS complex.
PR interval: If P wave is present prior to QRS, PR interval is typically < 120 ms.
QRS: 40 – 120 ms
Rhythm: Regular
Rate: > 100 beats/min

(1) Is the rhythm regular? _____

(2) What is the rate? _____

(3) Are the P waves present or absent? _____

(4) If present, is there a P wave before every QRS? _____

(5) P-R interval: _____ seconds

(6) QRS complex width: _____

(7) T waves present or absent? Upright? _____

(8) What is the name of this rhythm? _____

d. What field diagnosis will you give this patient and why?

_____

_____

_____

e. What treatment will you provide for this patient?

_____

_____

_____

2. You are called to see a patient whose chief complaint is dyspnea. He tells you in gasps that for several nights he has been waking up around 2:00 AM unable to breathe. He has to get up and sit on the side of the bed to catch his breath. Tonight sitting up hasn't helped. "Must be those cigarettes," he wheezes. He tells you that he "keeps a cough," but lately he's been bringing up much more sputum than usual. On physical examination, he is in obvious respiratory distress, coughing periodically. His lips look rather blue. His pulse is 102 beats/min and irregular. His respirations are 60 breaths/min and labored, and his blood pressure is 170/94 mm Hg in both arms. His neck veins are distended to the angle of the jaw. His chest is a veritable symphony of crackles and wheezes, and his oxygen saturation is 86% on room air. There is a tender fullness in the right upper quadrant of his abdomen. Both feet are swollen well above the ankles.

a. Identify the chief complaint and vital signs for this patient.

Chief complaint:

_____

Vital signs:

_____

_____

b. What steps would you take at this point in the call?

(1) _____

(2) _____

(3) _____

(4) _____

c. What do you think the patient is experiencing?

_____

_____

d. What can you do to help your patient?

_____

_____

3. The family of a 76-year-old woman calls for an ambulance after the woman fainted while preparing Sunday dinner. She is lying on the sofa when you arrive. She is conscious but somewhat confused. She was unharmed in the fall. Your partner begins with vital signs as you try to get a history. Her pulse is 44 beats/min and regular, respirations are 22 breaths/min and full, and oxygen saturation is 94%. She says that she is having some pain in her chest, but can't seem to rate the pain because of her confusion. Her blood pressure is 82/40 mm Hg, and her skin is cool. Her lungs are clear and she seems to be in good health otherwise. She takes a daily vitamin.

a. Identify the chief complaint and vital signs for this patient.

Chief complaint:

_____

_____

Vital signs:

_____

_____

b. List at least four reasons for a syncopal episode.

(1) _____

(2) _____

(3) _____

(4) _____

c. You hook up the monitor and see sinus bradycardia. What is your treatment for this patient now?

(1) _____

(2) _____

d. If pharmacologic therapies don't help, what else can you do to raise the heart rate in this patient?

_____

_____

_____

4. A 64-year-old man calls for an ambulance because he has been "feeling poorly." It's nothing he can really pin down. He has just been feeling very weak and washed out for the last few days, and so he thought maybe he ought to go to the hospital and have a doctor take a look at him. There are no striking findings on physical exam except for an irregular heartbeat. His pulse is about 76 beats/min but very irregular so that it is hard to count. His blood pressure is 110/74 mm Hg on both arms. He has no significant history and really hasn't been to a doctor except for a yearly checkup. His lungs are clear, and his oxygen saturation is 97%. His skin is a little cool. You hook up the heart monitor to take a quick peek and this is what you see.

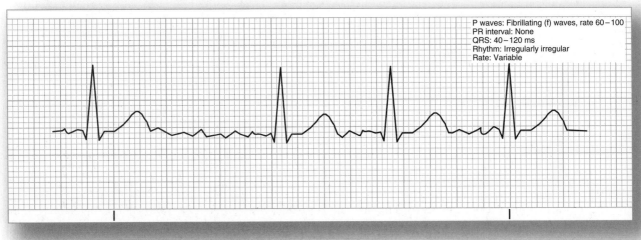

P waves: Fibrillating (f) waves, rate 60–100
PR interval: None
QRS: 40–120 ms
Rhythm: Irregularly irregular
Rate: Variable

a. Identify the chief complaint and vital signs of this patient.

Chief complaint:

_____

Vital signs:

_____

_____

b. Answer the following questions.

(1) Is the rhythm regular? _____

(2) What is the rate? _____

(3) Are the P waves present or absent? _____

(4) If present, is there a P before every QRS? _____

(5) Is there a QRS after every P? _____

(6) P-R interval: _____

(7) QRS complexes: _____ normal _____ abnormal

(8) Name of rhythm: _____

(9) Treatment: _____

5. You are taking a quick break at the emergency department (ED) after several hectic calls. You have made friends with the nurses, and they let you sit at the desk, where you can see the following heart monitors for different patients. Write the correct name of the rhythm on the line below the strip.

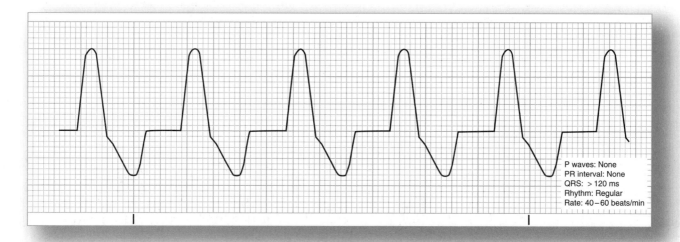

P waves: None
PR interval: None
QRS: > 120 ms
Rhythm: Regular
Rate: 40–60 beats/min

a. _____

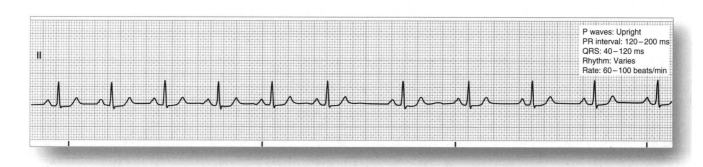

P waves: Upright
PR interval: 120–200 ms
QRS: 40–120 ms
Rhythm: Varies
Rate: 60–100 beats/min

b. _____

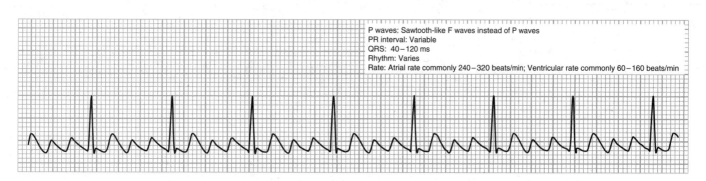

P waves: Sawtooth-like F waves instead of P waves
PR interval: Variable
QRS: 40–120 ms
Rhythm: Varies
Rate: Atrial rate commonly 240–320 beats/min; Ventricular rate commonly 60–160 beats/min

c. _____

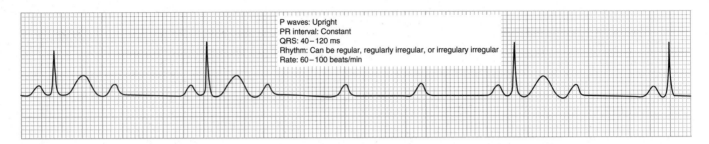

P waves: Upright
PR interval: Constant
QRS: 40–120 ms
Rhythm: Can be regular, regularly irregular, or irregulary irregular
Rate: 60–100 beats/min

d. _____

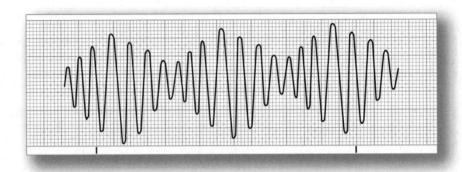

e. _____

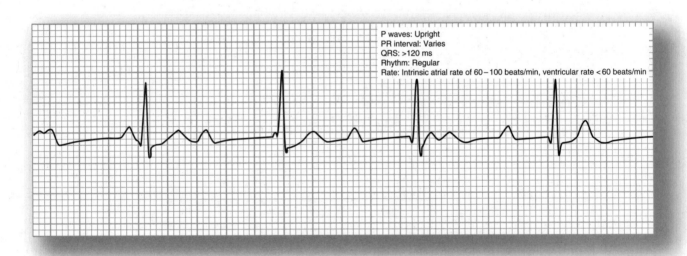

P waves: Upright
PR interval: Varies
QRS: >120 ms
Rhythm: Regular
Rate: Intrinsic atrial rate of 60–100 beats/min, ventricular rate <60 beats/min

f. _____

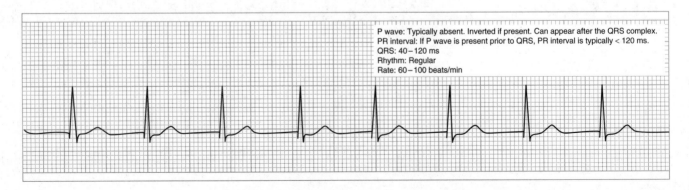

P wave: Typically absent. Inverted if present. Can appear after the QRS complex.
PR interval: If P wave is present prior to QRS, PR interval is typically < 120 ms.
QRS: 40–120 ms
Rhythm: Regular
Rate: 60–100 beats/min

g. _____

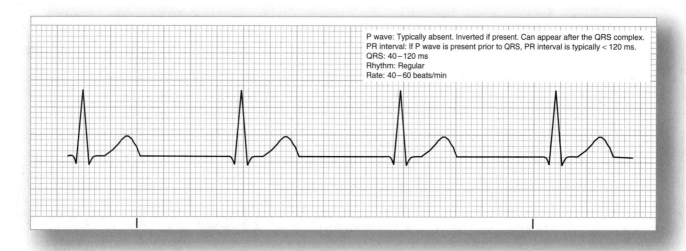

P wave: Typically absent. Inverted if present. Can appear after the QRS complex.
PR interval: If P wave is present prior to QRS, PR interval is typically < 120 ms.
QRS: 40–120 ms
Rhythm: Regular
Rate: 40–60 beats/min

h. _____

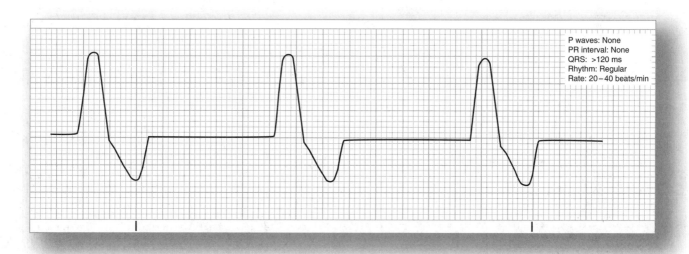

P waves: None
PR interval: None
QRS: >120 ms
Rhythm: Regular
Rate: 20–40 beats/min

i. _____

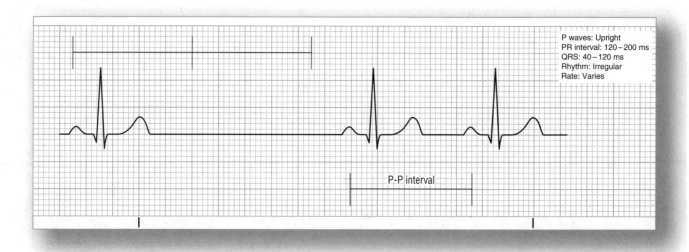

P waves: Upright
PR interval: 120–200 ms
QRS: 40–120 ms
Rhythm: Irregular
Rate: Varies

P-P interval

j. _____

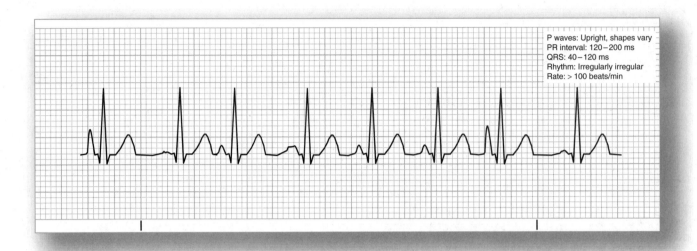

P waves: Upright, shapes vary
PR interval: 120–200 ms
QRS: 40–120 ms
Rhythm: Irregularly irregular
Rate: > 100 beats/min

k. _____

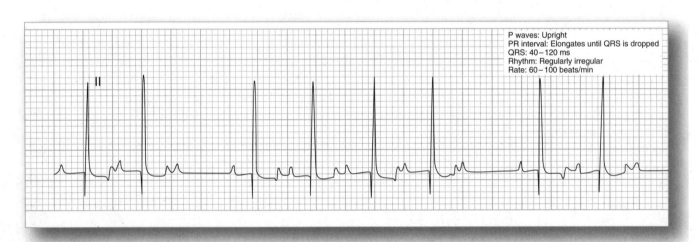

P waves: Upright
PR interval: Elongates until QRS is dropped
QRS: 40–120 ms
Rhythm: Regularly irregular
Rate: 60–100 beats/min

l. _____

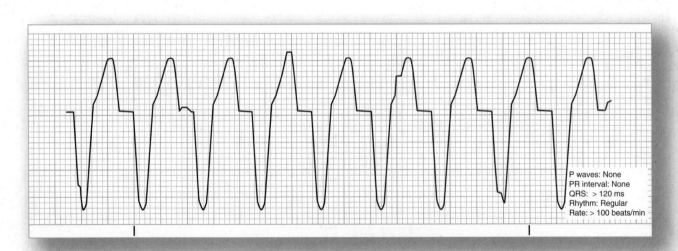

P waves: None
PR interval: None
QRS: > 120 ms
Rhythm: Regular
Rate: > 100 beats/min

m. _____

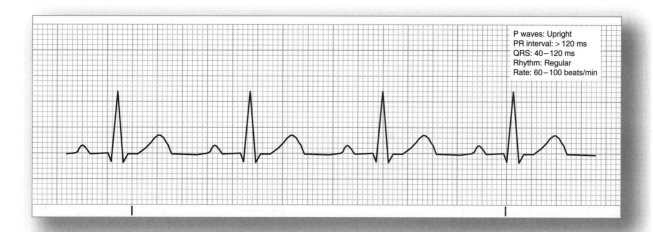

P waves: Upright
PR interval: > 120 ms
QRS: 40 – 120 ms
Rhythm: Regular
Rate: 60 – 100 beats/min

n. _____

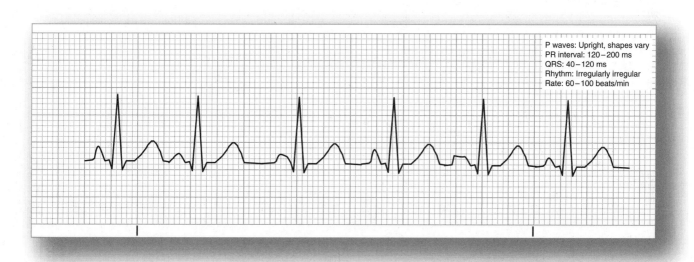

P waves: Upright, shapes vary
PR interval: 120 – 200 ms
QRS: 40 – 120 ms
Rhythm: Irregularly irregular
Rate: 60 – 100 beats/min

o. _____

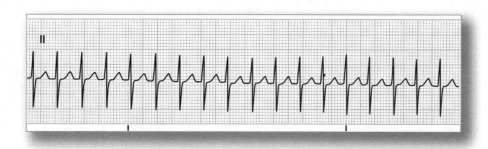

p. _____

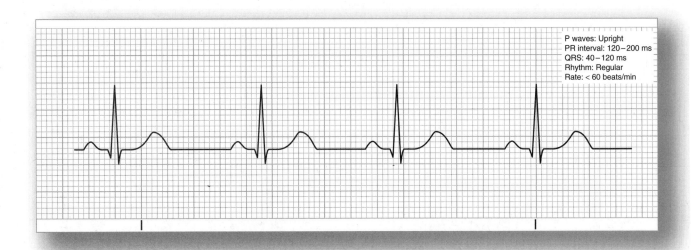

P waves: Upright
PR interval: 120–200 ms
QRS: 40–120 ms
Rhythm: Regular
Rate: < 60 beats/min

q. _____

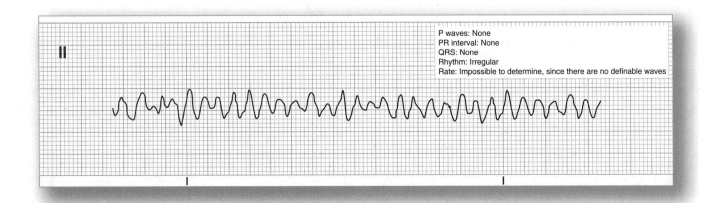

P waves: None
PR interval: None
QRS: None
Rhythm: Irregular
Rate: Impossible to determine, since there are no definable waves

r. _____

6. The nurse hands you the following three strips and asks you if you can figure out what type of ectopic beat is present in each strip.

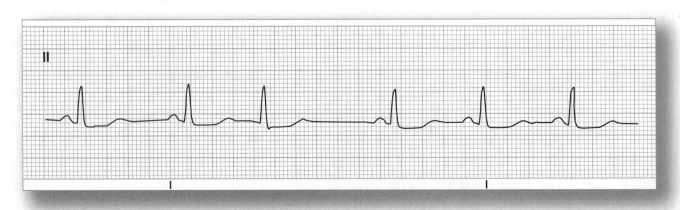

a. _____

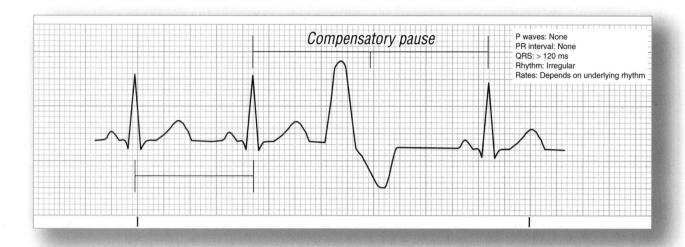

P waves: None
PR interval: None
QRS: > 120 ms
Rhythm: Irregular
Rates: Depends on underlying rhythm

Compensatory pause

b. _____

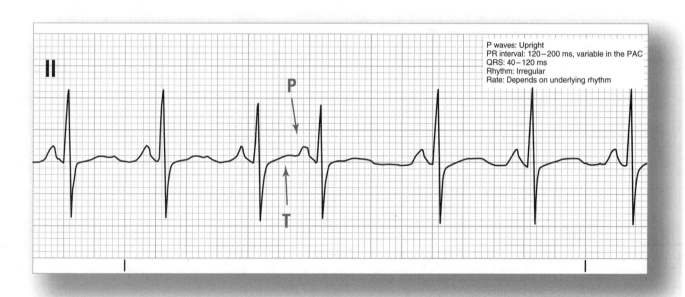

P waves: Upright
PR interval: 120–200 ms, variable in the PAC
QRS: 40–120 ms
Rhythm: Irregular
Rate: Depends on underlying rhythm

c. _____

Short Answer

1. How many seconds, or portions of a second, does a small box on an ECG graph paper represent? _____

2. How many small boxes does it take to make a large box on the ECG graph paper? _____

3. List the signs and symptoms that are present during a tachycardia that would make the patient "symptomatic" and a candidate for electric cardioversion.

   a. _____

   b. _____

   c. _____

d. _____

e. _____

4. What is the initial drug of choice when dealing with a stable tachycardia with a regular rhythm that is not breaking with a trial of vagal maneuvers?

_____

5. What drug would be a consideration with a wide complex stable tachycardia (ie, possible V-tac)? _____

_____

6. You are faced with a third-degree heart block and a rate of 48 beats/min. Your patient is showing signs of poor perfusion. After starting an IV, what would you do next?

_____

7. List the initial correct dosage of medication for the following.
   a. Epinephrine in the care of cardiac arrest: _____
   b. Vasopressin in the care of cardiac arrest: _____
   c. Dopamine as a second-line drug for a perfusing bradycardia: _____
   d. Atropine in the care of cardiac arrest: _____
   e. Epinephrine for a conscious patient with a bradycardia and poor perfusion: _____
   f. Adenosine for a stable, narrow, regular QRS tachycardia with pulses: _____
   g. Amiodarone for a stable, wide complex tachycardia or premature ventricular complexes (PVCs) in salvos:
   _____

8. List the Hs and Ts that you should be thinking about during a cardiac arrest.

   H _____   T _____
   H _____   T _____
   H _____   T _____
   H _____   T _____
   H _____   T _____
   H _____

Problem Solving

Practice your calculation skills by solving the following math problems.

1. Suppose a person at rest has a heart rate of 72 beats/min and a stroke volume of 75 mL/beat. What is his cardiac output? _____ mL/min.

2. Now that same person is running to catch a bus. His heart speeds up to 100 beats/min, and his stroke volume increases to 90 mL/beat. What is his cardiac output now? _____ mL/min

3. You often need to use your knowledge of anatomy, physiology, and pathophysiology to problem solve situations you are presented with and arrive at a working field diagnosis. In this case, take the given signs or symptoms and quickly decide if the patient could have left- or right-sided heart failure. Place an L for left-sided and an R for right-sided heart failure before the following signs and symptoms.
   a. _____ Dyspnea
   b. _____ Jugular vein distention
   c. _____ Swelling of the feet
   d. _____ Crackles on auscultation
   e. _____ Hepatomegaly
   f. _____ Sacral edema
   g. _____ Pink, frothy sputum

4. Find the mean arterial pressure (MAP) for the following blood pressures.
   a. 160/94 mm Hg _____
   b. 200/126 mm Hg _____
   c. 148/86 mm Hg _____

Practice ECG Strips

Examine each of the following ECG strips and state the rate, the rhythm, and the significant findings for each.

1.

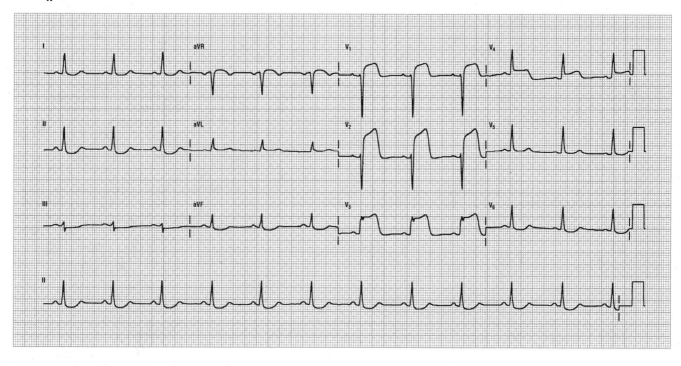

Rate: _____

Rhythm: _____

Significant findings: _____

2.

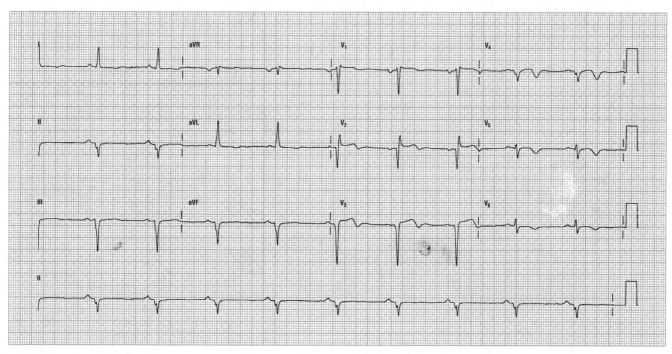

Rate: _____

Rhythm: _____

Significant findings: _____

3.

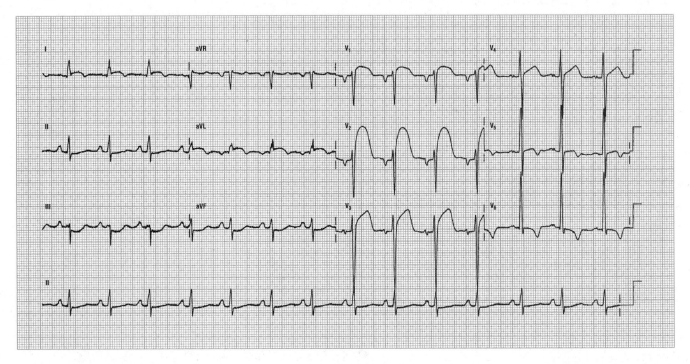

Rate: _____

Rhythm: _____

Significant findings: _____

4.

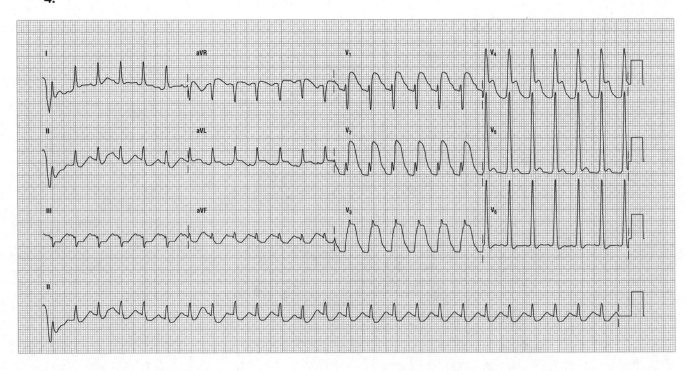

Rate: _____

Rhythm: _____

Significant findings: _____

5.

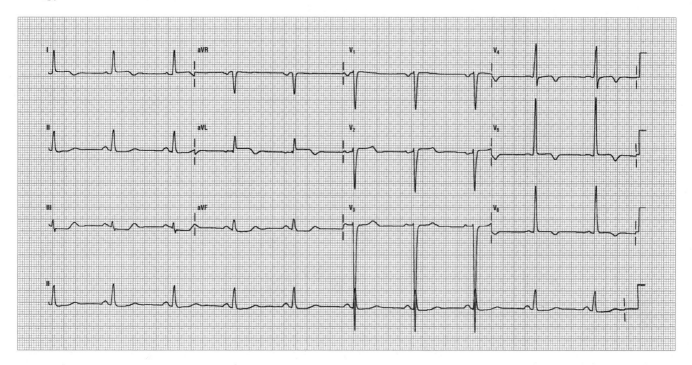

Rate: _____
Rhythm: _____
Significant findings: _____

6.

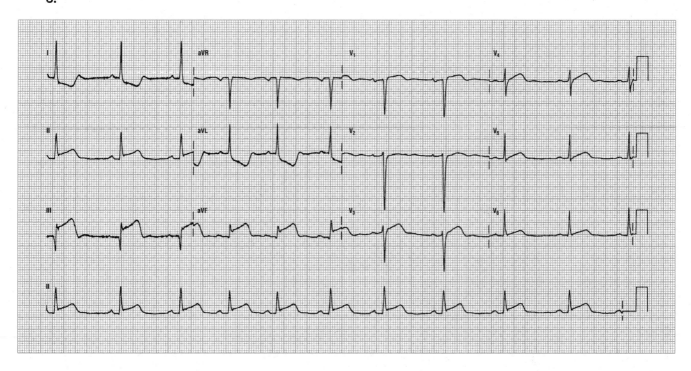

Rate: _____
Rhythm: _____
Significant findings: _____

7.

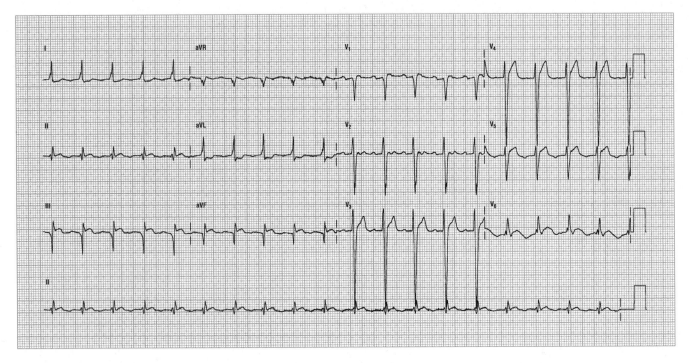

Rate: _____
Rhythm: _____
Significant findings: _____

8.

Rate: _____
Rhythm: _____
Significant findings: _____

9.

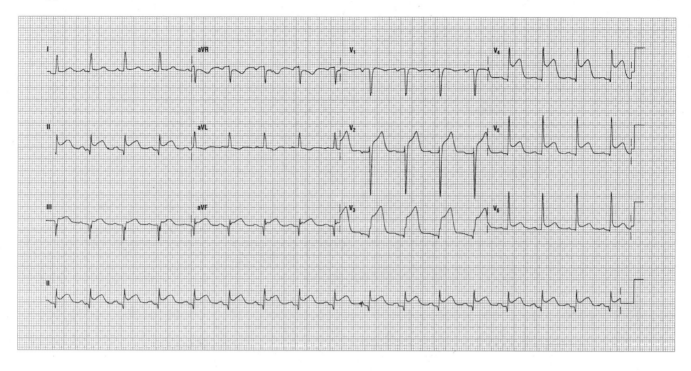

Rate: _____

Rhythm: _____

Significant findings: _____

10.

Rate: _____

Rhythm: _____

Significant findings: _____

11.

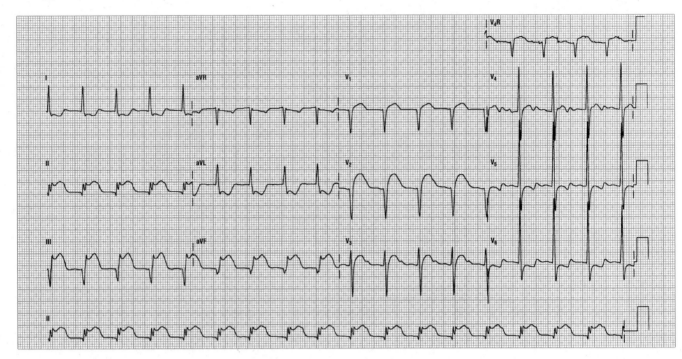

Rate: _____

Rhythm: _____

Significant findings: _____

12.

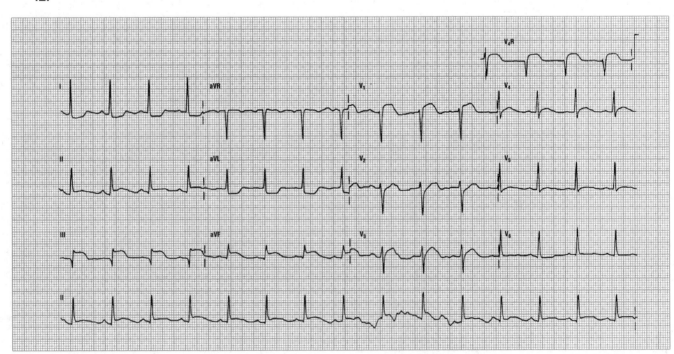

Rate: _____

Rhythm: _____

Significant findings: _____

13.

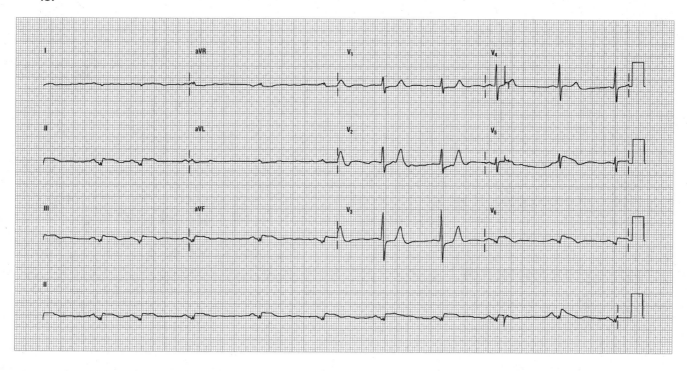

Rate: _____

Rhythm: _____

Significant findings: _____

14.

Rate: _____

Rhythm: _____

Significant findings: _____

15.

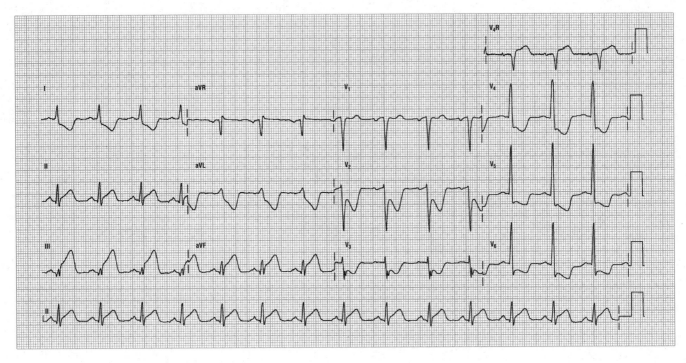

Rate: _____

Rhythm: _____

Significant findings: _____

16.

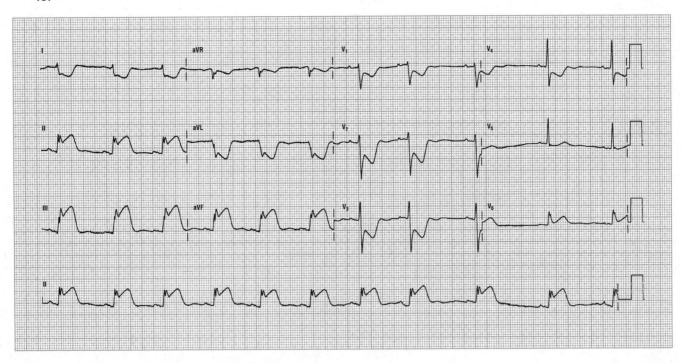

Rate: _____

Rhythm: _____

Significant findings: _____

17.

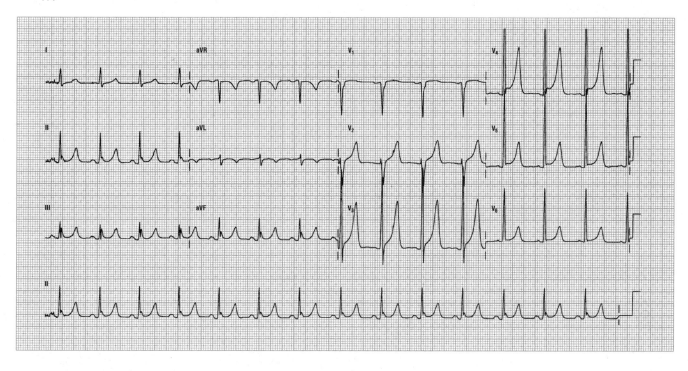

Rate: _____
Rhythm: _____
Significant findings: _____

18.

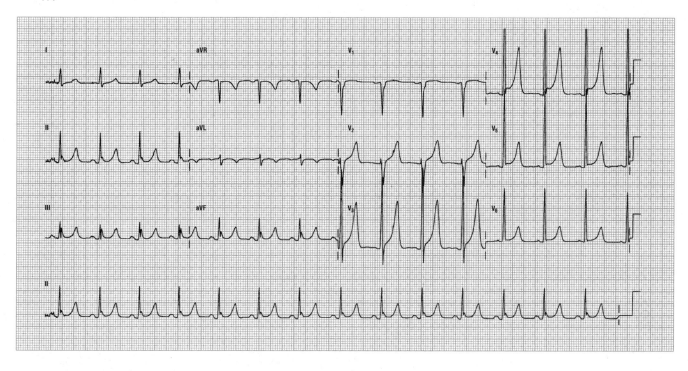

Rate: _____
Rhythm: _____
Significant findings: _____

19.

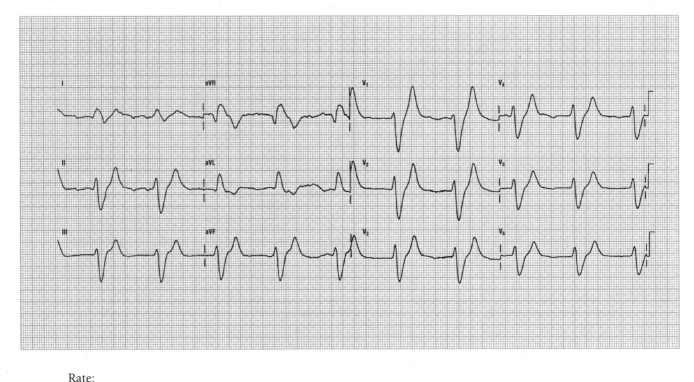

Rate: _____

Rhythm: _____

Significant findings: _____

20.

Rate: _____

Rhythm: _____

Significant findings: _____

Neurologic Emergencies

Matching

For each of the following items, indicate the letter that corresponds to each definition.

_____ **1.** Sensations experienced before an attack occurs, common in seizures and migraine headaches.

_____ **2.** Inability to connect an object with its proper use.

_____ **3.** The brain and spinal cord.

_____ **4.** Lack of feeling within a body part.

_____ **5.** The long, slender filament projecting from a nerve cell that conducts impulses to adjacent cells.

_____ **6.** A progressive organic condition in which neurons in the brain die, causing dementia.

_____ **7.** The slowing down of voluntary body movements. Found in Parkinson disease.

_____ **8.** Nerves that send information to the brain.

_____ **9.** A developmental condition in which damage is done to the brain. It presents in infancy as a delay in walking or crawling, and can take on a spastic form in which muscles are in a nearly constant state of contraction.

_____ **10.** An area in the brain or spinal cord in which cells have been attacked, typically by an infectious agent.

A. Abscess

B. Afferent nerves

C. Alzheimer disease

D. Anesthesia

E. Apraxia

F. Aura

G. Axon

H. Bradykinesia

I. Central nervous system (CNS)

J. Cerebral palsy (CP)

Multiple Choice

Read each item carefully, and then select the best response.

1. The nervous system is responsible for all of the following functions, EXCEPT:
A. heart rate.
B. blood pressure.
C. breathing.
D. heart rhythm.

2. What area of the brain acts as a relay center to filter and prioritize the information that you need for conscious thought?
A. Pons
B. Medulla oblongata
C. Diencephalon
D. Mid stem

3. Which of the following acts as an "insulation" around the axon?
   A. Myelin
   B. Neuron
   C. Diencephalon
   D. Neurotransmitter

4. When the brain receives too much oxygen, it can cause increased intracranial pressure (ICP). What happens to the cerebral arteries during this time?
   A. They vasodilate.
   B. They vasoconstrict.
   C. They leak blood.
   D. They remain normal.

5. You respond to a collision in which a woman has been thrown from a vehicle. She is unconscious; her arms are curled to her chest and her toes are pointed. How would you describe her position?
   A. Trismus posture
   B. Decerebrate posture
   C. Decorticate posture
   D. Pronation posture

6. Pupils may be changed by many different things. Which of the following does NOT change the shape of a patient's pupils?
   A. Drugs
   B. Trauma
   C. Seizure
   D. Increased ICP

7. You are treating a 17-year-old boy who is having a seizure. At this time, he is still except for his left arm, which is rocking back and forth in a rhythmic motion. What is the correct term for this activity?
   A. Clonic activity
   B. Tonic activity
   C. Intension tremors
   D. Paresthesia

8. After using naloxone (Narcan) on a patient with a suspected narcotic overdose, which of the following patient reactions would you NOT expect?
   A. The patient could wake up quickly.
   B. The patient could become aggressive.
   C. The patient could act very fearful.
   D. The patient will be sleepy but easily awakened.

9. Your patient suffers from an autoimmune disorder in which the body attacks the myelin sheath. What is this called?
   A. Dystonia
   B. Parkinson disease
   C. Trigeminal neuralgia
   D. Multiple sclerosis

10. What is the correct term for a temporary paralysis of the seventh cranial nerve?
    A. Guillain-Barré syndrome
    B. Bell palsy
    C. Poliomyelitis
    D. Myasthenia gravis

Labeling

Label the following diagrams with the correct terms.

1. Areas of the Brain

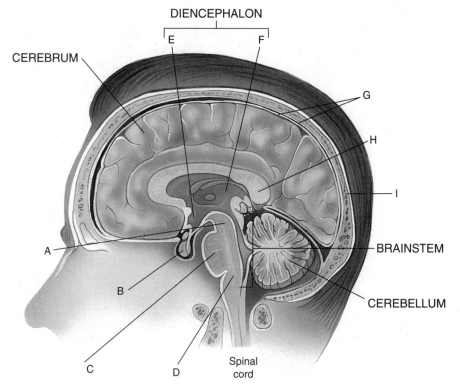

A. _____

B. _____

C. _____

D. _____

E. _____

F. _____

G. _____

H. _____

I. _____

2. Parts of a Neuron

A. _____

B. _____

C. _____

D. _____

E. _____

F. _____

3. Pupil Responses

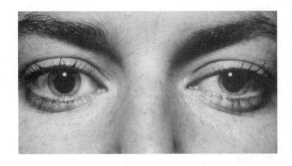

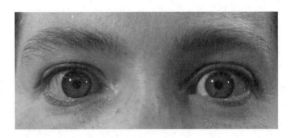

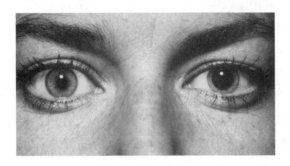

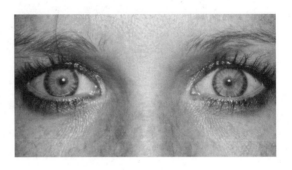

A. Normal
B. Constricted (pinpoint)
C. Dilated
D. Unequal

Fill-in-the-Blank

Read each item carefully, and then complete the statement by filling in the missing word(s).

1. The _____, located just inferior to the midbrain, regulates how deeply you breathe and your respiratory rate.

2. Dopamine and epinephrine are two types of _____.

3. When gram-negative bacteria die inside our body, they release a protein that is called a/an _____.

4. The skull is filled with three substances; they are the _____, _____, and _____ _____.

5. When a patient has increased ICP, the heart rate and respiratory rate will _____, and the blood pressure will _____.

6. The highest score on the Glasgow Coma Scale is _____, and the lowest score is _____.

7. You think your 80-year-old patient may be having a stroke. The patient can understand you, but is unable to speak clearly. This is called _____ _____.

8. _____ is the fuel for our brain. A normal reading is _____ mg/dL.

9. There are two types of strokes: _____ and _____.

10. An infant is more likely to suffer from a/an _____ seizure. There are two types of generalized seizures: _____ and _____.

Identify

In the following case study, list the chief complaint, vital signs, and pertinent negatives.

You are called to a middle-class home for a 32-year-old man. He is alert and can answer all your questions. His main complaint is general weakness because he is unable to stand or squeeze your hands. His symptoms started this morning around 9:00 AM and have intensified over the last 6 hours. He is having visual disturbances and doesn't want to open his eyes because the double vision he is experiencing is making him nauseous. You begin your assessment with vital signs and a SAMPLE history. Blood pressure is 128/76 mm Hg, and his pulse is 84 beats/min and regular. He has no allergies and takes no medications. His lungs are clear and his oxygen saturation is 98% on room air. Because you still have no clue what is going on, you place him on a nasal cannula at 4 L/min. Blood glucose check is 112 mg/dL, and he had a light lunch of a sandwich and soup around noon. He has no history of any illness and appears to be a very healthy individual. You question him about sustaining any trauma and he denies that he has suffered any in the last year. He does not have a headache or any pain anywhere in his body. He has no signs of any infections. You and your partner have spent a lot of time on scene looking for clues as to what is happening to him. One thing you are both sure of is that he needs to be seen at the emergency department. You provide supportive care and start an IV as a medication line in case the patient happens to get worse. Later you check in on the patient and find out they are leaning toward a diagnosis of multiple sclerosis (MS).

1. Chief complaint:

_____

_____

2. Vital signs:

_____

_____

3. Pertinent negatives:

_____

_____

Complete the Patient Care Report (PCR)

Read the incident scenario in the Identify exercise and then complete the following PCR.

EMS Patient Care Report (PCR)					
Date:	Incident No.:		Nature of Call:		Location:
Dispatched:	En Route:	At Scene:	Transport:	At Hospital:	In Service:
Patient Information					
Age: Sex: Weight (in kg [lb]):			Allergies: Medications: Past Medical History: Chief Complaint:		
Vital Signs					
Time:	BP:	Pulse:	Respirations:		SpO₂:
Time:	BP:	Pulse:	Respirations:		SpO₂:
Time:	BP:	Pulse:	Respirations:		SpO₂:
EMS Treatment (circle all that apply)					
Oxygen @ _____ L/min via (circle one): NC NRM Bag-Mask Device		Assisted Ventilation	Airway Adjunct		CPR
Defibrillation	Bleeding Control	Bandaging	Splinting		Other
Narrative					

Ambulance Calls

The following case scenarios provide an opportunity to explore the concerns associated with patient management and paramedic care. Read each scenario, and then answer each question.

1. You receive a call for a patient having seizures. This time it is one of the city's homeless whom the police found lying in an alley. He is having a generalized motor seizure when you arrive. It lasts about 3 minutes and then subsides. You quickly open the airway by jaw lift, start supplemental oxygen, and prepare to start an IV, but before you can do so, the patient has another generalized motor seizure that lasts about 3 minutes.

   a. Urgent treatment measures will take priority over the rapid medical assessment. When you do get around to examining this patient, what will you look for in particular?

   (1) _____

   (2) _____

   (3) _____

   (4) _____

   (5) _____

   (6) _____

   (7) _____

   (8) _____

   (9) _____

   (10) _____

   b. List the steps in the prehospital management of this patient.

   (1) _____

   (2) _____

   (3) _____

   (4) _____

   c. What medication is given in the field for repeated seizures? (You may need to refer to the pharmacology chapter.)

   _____

   _____

   (1) What are the contraindications to this medication?

   _____

   _____

   (2) What is the correct dosage in the present situation, and how is it administered?

   _____

   _____

   (3) What possible adverse side effects might occur when administering this medicine?

   _____

   _____

2. You are called to the home of a 68-year-old woman for a "possible stroke." Arriving at the scene, you are greeted at the door by the woman's daughter. "I phoned and phoned all morning," she says, "and when no one answered, I figured I'd better come and check. I found Mother lying in the bathroom." You proceed to the bathroom, where you find the patient lying on the floor. She is conscious but does not seem to be able to answer your questions—she just makes garbled noises. Her skin is warm and dry. Her vital signs are a pulse of 70 beats/min and slightly irregular, respirations of 20 breaths/min and unlabored, and a blood pressure of 190/120 mm Hg. During the physical exam, you find no evidence of head injury, but the woman's face looks a bit lopsided, and tears are streaming down. The pupils are 4 mm, equal, and reactive. The gag reflex is absent. The right arm and right leg are flaccid. There is no evidence of injury.

a. Do you think the patient is right-handed or left-handed? _____

How did you reach that conclusion?

_____

_____

b. List the steps in treating this patient.

(1) _____

(2) _____

(3) _____

(4) _____

(5) _____

(6) _____

3. You are called to a department store where a woman who appears to be about 60 years old has been found unconscious in the ladies' restroom.

a. List nine possible causes of coma.

(1) _____

(2) _____

(3) _____

(4) _____

(5) _____

(6) _____

(7) _____

(8) _____

(9) _____

b. Now list eight things you would do to manage this comatose woman.

(1) _____

(2) _____

(3) _____

(4) _____

(5) _____

(6) _____

(7) _____

(8) _____

True/False

If you believe the statement to be more true than false, write the letter "T" in the space provided. If you believe the statement to be more false than true, write the letter "F."

_____ 1. The peripheral nervous system is responsible for conducting nerve impulses between the brain and the body.

_____ 2. The function of the midbrain is to regulate heart and respiratory functions.

_____ 3. The respiratory pattern that involves extreme tachypnea and hyperpnea is called Cheyne-Stokes.

_____ 4. The medical term for cancer is neoplasms.

_____ 5. The respiratory pattern that involves rapid, regular, deep respirations is called hyperpnea.

_____ 6. The average pressure (MAP) is 100 to 120 mm Hg.

_____ 7. Trismus may result from head trauma, cerebral hypoxia, and seizures.

_____ 8. When you assess a stroke patient, you can ask the person to smile. This will show if the patient has ptosis.

_____ 9. Patients with apraxia will be unable to name a common object.

_____ 10. By stimulating the cough or gag reflex in a patient, you can decrease ICP.

_____ 11. At times you may need to give thiamine before D_{50} in chronic alcoholics or people who are malnourished.

_____ 12. Hyperglycemic patients do not need any fluid, so you must make sure to give less than 100 mL of fluid.

_____ 13. The Cincinnati Prehospital Stroke Scale uses a six-part criteria scale to assess for a stroke.

_____ 14. A little over one third of the patients who have a transient ischemic attack (TIA) will have a stroke soon after the initial event.

_____ 15. Usually an aura will precede a generalized (grand mal) seizure.

Short Answer

Complete this section with short written answers using the space provided.

1. Define the following vocabulary words:
   a. Hemiparesis

   _____

   _____

   b. Neuropathy

   _____

   _____

2. Over the course of a week of ambulance runs, you have found three patients in a coma. You don't have any information about any of them except for the medications found at the scene or on the patient's person. Nonetheless, based on those medications and assessment, you can make an educated guess at least as to each patient's underlying illnesses. For each of the comatose patients whose medications are listed here, indicate the most probable underlying illness(es).
   a. Patient 1 is carrying phenobarbital (Luminal) and phenytoin sodium (Dilantin) in her purse.

   Probable underlying illness(es): _____

   b. Patient 2 is carrying human insulin (Humulin).

   Probable underlying illness: _____

   c. Patient 3 is carrying warfarin (Coumadin).

   Probable underlying illness: _____

Fill-in-the-Table

Fill in the missing parts of the table.

1. Fill in the table with the basis for determining an adult's LOC.

Glasgow Coma Scale		
	Adult	**Pediatric (<5 y)**
Eye opening	**4.** _____ **3.** Voice **2.** Pain stimulation **1.** None	**4.** _____ **3.** _____ **2.** Pain stimulation **1.** None
Verbal	**5.** _____ **4.** Disoriented **3.** _____ **2.** _____ **1.** None	**5.** Cry, smile, coo, words correct for age **4.** _____ **3.** _____ **2.** _____ **1.** None
Motor	**6.** _____ **5.** Localizes pain **4.** _____ **3.** _____ **2.** Decerebrate **1.** None	**6.** _____ **5.** Localizes pain **4.** _____ **3.** Decorticate **2.** _____ **1.** None

2. List below all the words associated with each letter when dealing with the causes of seizures.

Common Causes of Seizures	
A	
B	
D	
F	
I	
O	
R	
S	
T	
U	

Problem Solving

Read the following scenario, and then list the portions of the scenario under the correct stroke scale or stroke screen.

You respond to a 69-year-old woman. Her daughter is waiting at the door for you when you arrive. Dispatch information said that the woman might be having a stroke. You enter the room to find "Betty" sitting in her recliner with her feet up. She acknowledges your entrance. "Hi, Mrs. Smith, my name is Jake Johnson and my partner is Julie Barnes. We are paramedics, and I am here at the request of your daughter. Can you tell me what is wrong today?" Mrs. Smith responds by telling you that her name is Betty, and she doesn't think anything is wrong with her. Her daughter is always fussing over her. You tell Betty that is because her daughter loves her and say that if Betty loves her daughter, she should be smiling about all the attention. Betty does respond with a smile, but the right side of her face doesn't respond as well as the left. Julie asks permission to do a set of vital signs, and Betty says to go right ahead. Julie gets a blood pressure of 136/82 mm Hg, a pulse of 86 beats/min and regular, oxygen saturation of 97% on room air, and respirations of 18 breaths/min. Lung sounds are clear. She checks Betty's blood glucose, which is 110 mg/dL. During this time, you ask Betty to say "You can't teach an old dog new tricks." However, Betty can't seem to get the sentence out very clearly. You proceed by having Betty squeeze both your hands at the same time. Her grip strength is about half strength in the right arm. You then ask her to close her eyes and hold both arms up straight. When she does this, her right arm drifts downward. You then ask Betty and her daughter how long she has been having these symptoms. Betty's daughter says that she had no problems this morning when she was up fixing breakfast at 8:00 AM, but she says she began to notice a few minor things around 11:00 AM, which is when she decided to call 9-1-1. You take a SAMPLE history and find that Betty has never had any medical problems at all; she takes only a vitamin every morning. Both you and Julie feel she should be seen in the ED, and Betty agrees to go with you. You prepare to take Betty in.

You and Julie did a great job using both the Cincinnati Prehospital Stroke Scale and the Los Angles Prehospital Stroke Screen Assessments. Place portions of the preceding scenario under the correct screens. Remember, they might be on both assessments.

1. Cincinnati Prehospital Stroke Scale

   a. _____

   b. _____

   c. _____

2. Los Angles Prehospital Stroke Screen

   a. _____

   b. _____

   c. _____

   d. _____

   e. _____

   f. _____

   g. _____

   h. _____

Diseases of the Eyes, Ears, Nose, and Throat

Matching

Match each of the items in the left column to the appropriate definition in the right column.

_____ **1.** A spherical structure measuring about 1 inch in diameter that is housed within the eye socket

_____ **2.** The transparent anterior portion of the eye that overlies the iris and pupil

_____ **3.** A delicate mucous membrane that covers the sclera and internal surfaces of the eyelids but not the iris

_____ **4.** The portion of the globe between the iris and the lens that is filled with vitreous humor

_____ **5.** Designed to secrete and drain tears from the eye

_____ **6.** Also called pink eye, a condition where the eye is inflamed and red

_____ **7.** A small swollen bump or pustule on the external eyelid

_____ **8.** Bleeding into the anterior chamber of the eye that obscures vision

_____ **9.** Inflammation of the iris

_____ **10.** The yellowish oily substance found in the outer ear canal

_____ **11.** The perception of sound in the inner ear with no external environmental cause

_____ **12.** The separation between the nostrils

_____ **13.** A nosebleed

_____ **14.** A nasal disorder that is most common during childhood and adolescence

_____ **15.** Commonly called thrush, a condition in which a fungus accumulates on the lining of the mouth

A. Hyphema

B. Epistaxis

C. Lacrimal apparatus

D. Anterior uveitis

E. Cornea

F. Cerumen

G. Globe

H. Chalazion

I. Posterior chamber

J. Oral candidiasis

K. Conjunctiva

L. Rhinitis

M. Nasal septum

N. Tinnitus

O. Conjunctivitis

Multiple Choice

Read each item carefully, and then select the best response.

1. The nerve that innervates the muscles that cause motion of the eyeballs and upper eyelids, as well as constriction of the pupil, is the:

   A. optic nerve.

   B. oculomotor nerve.

   C. trigeminal nerve.

   D. vagus nerve.

2. The _____ chamber of the globe is filled with _____ humor, which is a clear watery fluid.

   A. anterior; vitreous

   B. anterior; aqueous

   C. posterior; vitreous

   D. posterior; aqueous

3. There are two types of vision. The _____ vision facilitates visualization of objects directly in front of you and is processed by the _____.
   A. peripheral; macula
   B. peripheral; remaining retina
   C. central; macula
   D. central; remaining retina

4. To assess ocular function, the paramedic should assess each of the following, EXCEPT:
   A. the orbital rim.
   B. visual acuity.
   C. peripheral vision.
   D. ocular motility.

5. A group of conditions that leads to increased intraocular pressure and that is one of the leading causes of blindness is:
   A. hyphema.
   B. retinal detachment.
   C. glaucoma.
   D. papilledema.

6. An injury to the eye that is common in boxing is:
   A. retinal detachment.
   B. iritis.
   C. periorbital cellulitis.
   D. hyphema.

7. Of the following components of the ear, which is NOT in the middle ear?
   A. Tympanic membrane
   B. Ossicles
   C. Cochlea
   D. Malleus

8. The feeling of vertigo or loss of balance after an ear infection or upper respiratory infection is MOST likely:
   A. impacted cerumen.
   B. Meniere disease.
   C. otitis.
   D. labyrinthitis.

9. An inner ear disorder that usually affects adults, and in which there is ultimately damage to the organ of Corti and the semicircular canal, is:
   A. Meniere disease.
   B. labyrinthitis.
   C. perforated tympanic membrane.
   D. barotrauma.

10. You are treating a 10-year-old boy who has the chills, difficulty opening his mouth, and pain with opening of the mouth. He denies any trauma, although he appears to have facial swelling and is drooling and speaking with a muffled voice. What is MOST likely his condition?
    A. Tonsillitis
    B. Peritonsillar abscess
    C. Pharyngitis
    D. Tracheitis

Labeling

Label the following diagrams with the correct terms.

1. Structures of the Eye

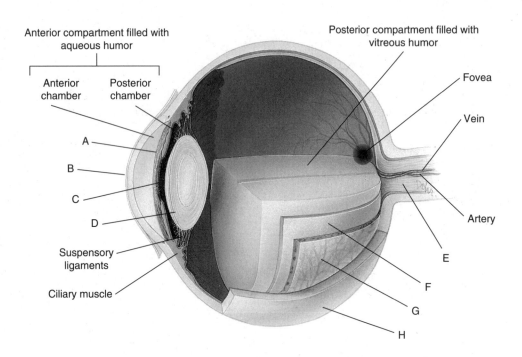

Anterior compartment filled with aqueous humor

Anterior chamber

Posterior chamber

A

B

C

D

Suspensory ligaments

Ciliary muscle

Posterior compartment filled with vitreous humor

Fovea

Vein

Artery

E

F

G

H

A. _____

B. _____

C. _____

D. _____

E. _____

F. _____

G. _____

H. _____

2. Structures of the Ear

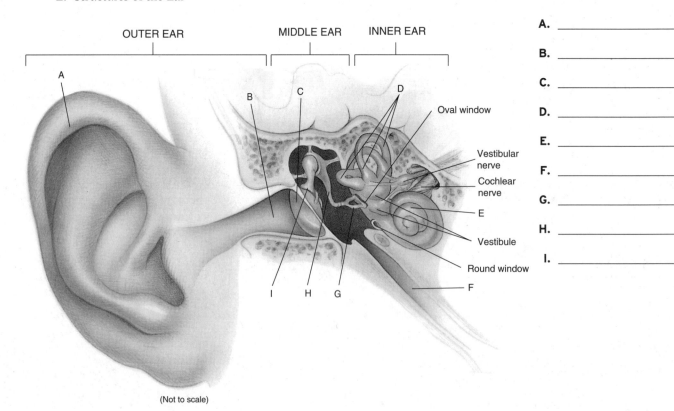

OUTER EAR

MIDDLE EAR

INNER EAR

A

B

C

D

Oval window

Vestibular nerve

Cochlear nerve

E

Vestibule

Round window

F

I H G

(Not to scale)

A. _____

B. _____

C. _____

D. _____

E. _____

F. _____

G. _____

H. _____

I. _____

Fill-in-the-Blank

Read each item carefully, and then complete the statement by filling in the missing word(s).

1. The sclera is a _____, fibrous coat that helps to _____ the shape of the eye.

2. The _____ is the transparent _____ portion of the eye that overlies the _____ and _____.

3. The _____ is a delicate mucous membrane that covers the _____ and internal surfaces of the eyelids but not the iris.

4. The _____ is the pigmented part of the eye that surrounds the _____.

5. The pupil is the _____ adjustable opening within the _____ through which light passes to the lens.

6. Sound waves enter the ear through the (A)_____, or (B)_____, the large cartilaginous external portion of the ear. They then travel through the (C)_____ _____ _____ to the (D)_____ _____. Vibration of sound waves against the tympanic membrane sets up vibration in the (E)_____, the three smaller bones on the inner side of the tympanic membrane. These vibrations are transmitted to the (F)_____ _____ at the (G)_____ _____, the opening between the middle ear and the vestibule. Movement of the oval window causes fluid within the (H)_____, a shell-shaped structure in the inner ear, to vibrate. Within the cochlea at the (I)_____ _____ _____, vibration stimulates hair movements that form nerve impulses that travel to the brain via the auditory nerve. The brain then converts these impulses to sound.

7. The top portion of the tooth, external to the gum, is the (A)_____, containing one or more (B)_____. Below the crown lie the neck and the root. The pulp cavity fills the center of the tooth and contains blood vessels, nerves, and specialized connective tissue, called (C)_____. Dentin and enamel surround the pulp cavity and protect the tooth from damage. (D)_____, which forms the principal mass of the tooth, is much denser and stronger than bone. The bony sockets for the teeth that reside in the mandible and maxilla are called (E)_____. The ridges between the teeth, the (F)_____ _____, are covered by the gingiva, or gums, which are thickened connective tissue and epithelium. Teeth are attached to the alveolar bone by periodontal membrane.

Identify

In the following case studies, list the chief complaint, vital signs, and pertinent negatives.

1. "Medic 620, respond Priority One for a 43-year-old female patient with dizziness. Patient is now conscious and alert." As you enter the apartment, you determine that the scene seems to be safe and there is only one patient so you have enough help at this point. The patient is found sitting in a chair in the kitchen. She appears pale and diaphoretic, and you notice she is drooling. You and your partner lift her off the chair and lay her on the floor, which you have covered with a blanket. Her skin color slightly improves, as does her level of consciousness (LOC). You immediately place the patient on high-flow supplemental oxygen and begin your primary assessment. You already have formed your general impression and realize that the patient is suffering from a fever. Her vital signs are a respiratory rate of 20 breaths/min, a pulse oximetry of 89%, a pulse rate (lying flat) of 118 beats/min and regular, and a blood pressure of 98/P mm Hg. She is complaining of pain when she swallows, which made her nervous so she asked her husband to call EMS. She denies any loss of consciousness or any pain to her head, chest, or abdomen.

   a. Chief complaint:

   _____

   _____

   b. Vital signs:

   _____

   _____

   c. Pertinent negatives:

   _____

   _____

2. You are dispatched to a reported "nosebleed." On arrival, you find a 78-year-old man standing in the bathroom, spitting blood into the sink. His daughter states he has been bleeding for hours and they were not able to stop the nosebleed. She said he is starting to get dizzy and has lost a lot of blood. She also mentions that he is on a "blood thinner" since he had a "mini-stroke" 5 years ago. He has not eaten all day because this nosebleed has been occupying most of his attention. His mental status is alert and you obtain the following vital signs: respirations of 20 breaths/min and regular, pulse rate of 108 beats/min and irregular, blood pressure of 170/102 mm Hg, and SpO_2 of 95%. You check his blood glucose and it is 110 mg/dL. He states he has a headache and his doctor told him he has an ECG of A-fib normally. He denies any trauma or shortness of breath. You make an attempt to control the bleeding and prepare to transport him to the hospital.

   a. Chief complaint:

   _____

   _____

   b. Vital signs:

   _____

   _____

   c. Pertinent negatives:

   _____

   _____

Ambulance Calls

The following case scenarios provide an opportunity to explore the concerns associated with patient management and paramedic care. Read each scenario, and then answer each question.

1. You are assessing and treating a conscious, alert 17-year-old boy who was playing baseball in a high school league when he was struck in the right eye with a wild pitch. He is in extreme pain and may have sustained a fracture to the orbit as well as blunt trauma to the globe of the eye. Upon examination of his eye, it appears there is bleeding into the anterior chamber.

   a. What is your initial impression of this patient's presentation?

   _____

   b. Your patient denies any other previous medical history, he is not on any medications, and he states he has an allergy to sulfa medications. His vital signs are respiratory rate of 20 breaths/min and regular, pulse of 110 beats/min and regular, blood pressure of 120/78 mm Hg, and SpO_2 of 98%. How would you treat this patient?

   _____

   _____

   _____

   c. Your patient is very nauseated and states he feels like he may vomit. What should you do?

   _____

   _____

2. You are treating a 15-year-old boy whose parent called the ambulance to their home after an accident in their back-yard. Your patient states his eye is burning up. He says he splashed concentrated chlorine into his left eye when he was pouring the chemical into their in-ground pool.
   a. What would your prehospital treatment for this patient include?

   _____

   _____

   _____

   b. What medical tool can be helpful in irrigating the eye?

   _____

   _____

   _____

   c. What medication is helpful prior to using the medical tool you just described?

   _____

True/False

If you believe the statement to be more true than false, write the letter "T" in the space provided. If you believe the state-ment to be more false than true, write the letter "F."

_____ **1.** When using the Morgan lens, you must first take out the patient's contact lens.

_____ **2.** Visual loss that does not improve when the patient blinks is an important symptom of a serious ocular condition.

_____ **3.** In front of the pupil and the iris is the lens.

_____ **4.** If vitreous humor is lost, it can easily be replaced in the operating room.

_____ **5.** The symptoms of vertigo and tinnitus are common with Meniere disease.

_____ **6.** The hollowed sections of bone, which are lined with mucous membranes and called paranasal sinuses, help to lighten the weight of the skull.

_____ **7.** The principal mass of the teeth is called the dentin.

_____ **8.** The mandibular branch of the hypoglossal nerve provides motor innervation to the muscles of mastication.

_____ **9.** Thrush is also called oral candidiasis.

_____ **10.** Epiglottitis is most commonly found in pediatric patients aged 4 to 9 years.

Abdominal and Gastrointestinal Emergencies

Matching

Match each of the items in the left column to the appropriate definition in the right column.

_____ **1.** Smelling of feces.

_____ **2.** Liquid stool.

_____ **3.** Dark, tarry, very malodorous stools caused by upper GI bleeding.

_____ **4.** An itching rash.

_____ **5.** Blood with the stool that is separate; caused by lower GI bleeds.

_____ **6.** A bowel sound characterized by increased activity in the bowel.

_____ **7.** Abdominal edema typically signaling liver failure.

_____ **8.** Foamy, fatty stools associated with liver failure or gallbladder problems.

_____ **9.** The region of the abdomen directly inferior to the xyphoid process and superior to the umbilicus.

_____ **10.** The rhythmic contractions of the intestines and esophagus that help material to move.

_____ **11.** A large vessel created by the intersection of blood vessels from the gastrointestinal (GI) system that empties into the liver.

_____ **12.** Vertical stretch marks that occur when a person loses or gains weight rapidly.

_____ **13.** Pain when pressure is applied to the right upper quadrant of the abdomen in a specific manner; helps detect gallbladder problems.

_____ **14.** The insertion of a flexible tube into the esophagus with the intent of visualizing and repairing damage or disease.

_____ **15.** A disease in which the mucous lining of the stomach and duodenum have been eroded, allowing the acid to eat into these organs.

A. Striae

B. Portal vein

C. Hematochezia

D. Peptic ulcer disease

E. Murphy sign

F. Feculent

G. Diarrhea

H. Ascites

I. Endoscopy

J. Melena

K. Urticaria

L. Borborygmi

M. Epigastric

N. Steatorrhea

O. Peristalsis

Multiple Choice

Read each item carefully, and then select the best response.

1. A 42-year-old man calls for an ambulance because of "burning" epigastric pain of several hours' duration. He says that yesterday he noticed his bowel movement was "black as pitch," and about an hour ago he vomited some "stuff that looked like coffee grounds." He also feels quite dizzy. He takes no medications except Mylanta (alumina/magnesia/simethicone) "for my heartburn." On physical examination, he looks pale and anxious, and he sits leaning forward. His skin is cold and sweaty. His pulse is 140 beats/min and regular; his respirations are 20 breaths/min and slightly labored; his blood pressure is 90/60 mm Hg. His abdomen is diffusely tender, especially over the epigastrium. There is guarding but no real rigidity. Peripheral pulses are intact. This patient's findings are most consistent with which of the following conditions?

A. Peptic ulcer disease

B. Diverticulitis

C. Mesenteric ischemia

D. A leaking abdominal aortic aneurysm

2. A 70-year-old woman calls for an ambulance because of abdominal pain of 4 hours' duration. "I just knew I shouldn't have eaten all that rich, fatty food," she says. "It never agrees with me. Oh, I hate to cause everyone so much bother." And she starts to cry. On questioning, she says she had some diarrhea, but it didn't relieve the pain. Her past medical history is notable for two previous acute myocardial infarctions. On physical examination, the woman appears to be in considerable distress. Pulse is 108 beats/min and slightly irregular; respirations are

20 breaths/min and shallow; blood pressure is 160/100 mm Hg in both arms. The chest is clear. The patient has a positive Murphy sign. This patient most likely has which of the following conditions?
- **A.** Peptic ulcer disease
- **B.** Diverticulitis
- **C.** Cholecystitis
- **D.** Leaking abdominal aortic aneurysm

3. A 52-year-old woman called for an ambulance because of severe abdominal pain. She says the pain started a couple of days ago as a kind of steady ache (she points to the left lower quadrant), and it just kept getting worse and worse. Now her whole abdomen hurts. It's been 2 days since she had a bowel movement and that one may have had some blood in it. On physical examination, the patient is in obvious distress. She lies very still on the stretcher and cries out with pain when your partner accidentally bumps the stretcher. Her pulse is 128 beats/min and regular; respirations are 28 breaths/min and shallow; blood pressure is 150/80 mm Hg. The abdomen is slightly distended, and it does not move with respiration. On palpation, it feels like a slab of concrete. The pedal pulses are equal. You are told that the patient has a history of underlying thrombotic disease. This patient's findings are most consistent with which of the following conditions?
- **A.** Peptic ulcer disease
- **B.** Diverticulitis
- **C.** Mesenteric ischemia
- **D.** A leaking abdominal aortic aneurysm

4. A 30-year-old man contacts the emergency medical dispatcher by calling 9-1-1. He states he has severe abdominal pain in the lower right quadrant. He states a history of rectal bleeding, diarrhea, arthritis, and fever. He further states episodic periods of similar symptoms. This patient's findings are most consistent with which of the following conditions?
- **A.** Peptic ulcer disease
- **B.** Diverticulitis
- **C.** Crohn disease
- **D.** A leaking abdominal aortic aneurysm

5. Pain that originates in the abdomen and causes pain in a distant location as a result of similar paths for the peripheral nerves of the abdomen and the distant location is considered _____ pain.
- **A.** referred
- **B.** parietal
- **C.** somatic
- **D.** rebound

6. On arrival, you discover that your patient is a 28-year-old woman complaining of severe vomiting. She explains that she is in the first trimester of pregnancy and has been suffering from morning sickness. Her vomiting is so severe that she is now vomiting blood. She most likely has which of the following conditions?
- **A.** Peptic ulcer disease
- **B.** Hemorrhoids
- **C.** Pancreatitis
- **D.** Mallory-Weiss syndrome

7. The proper treatment for esophageal varices includes:
- **A.** narcotic pain relief.
- **B.** treatment with 5% dextrose and water.
- **C.** fluid resuscitation.
- **D.** placement of a laryngeal mask airway (LMA) to prevent aspiration.

8. Pain that is difficult to localize, and described as a burning, cramping, gnawing, or aching, is called _____ pain.
- **A.** referred
- **B.** visceral
- **C.** somatic
- **D.** parietal

9. You receive an emergency call for a conscious, alert 26-year-old man with a sudden onset of severe abdominal pain. He is complaining of an associated fever, nausea, and vomiting. The pain appears isolated to the right lower quadrant (RLQ). Your patient most likely has which of the following conditions?
- **A.** Hypovolemia
- **B.** Inflammation of the interstitial lining

    C. Esophageal varices

    D. Appendicitis

10. Which of the following would NOT cause a bowel obstruction?

    A. Paralysis of the intestines

    B. An immune attack against the GI tract

    C. Infection

    D. Kidney disease

Fill-in-the-Blank

Read each item carefully, and then complete the statement by filling in the missing word(s).

1. When patients have _____ _____, any drug that is given may remain active within the body for _____ than anticipated.

2. Chronic consumption of _____ or _____ may increase the acidity in the stomach beyond the limits of the protective _____ layer.

3. The _____ vein transports _____ blood from the GI tract directly to the liver for processing of the nutrients that have been _____.

4. The small intestine is divided into three sections: the _____, the _____, and the _____.

5. People who are _____ are more likely to have a poor outcome from _____-_____ illness.

6. Most peptic ulcers are the result of infection of the stomach with _____ _____. Another major cause is chronic use of _____ anti-inflammatory drugs.

7. _____ _____ _____ involve inflammation of the gallbladder.

8. Ulcerative _____ is caused by inflammation of the colon.

9. _____ _____ is a disease of the young; most patients are between 15 and 30 years of age. It occurs with equal incidence in men and women. There is a strong _____ component to this disease.

10. The presentation of appendicitis can be divided into the following three stages: _____, _____, and _____.

Labeling

Label the following diagrams with the correct terms.

1. Abdominal Organs

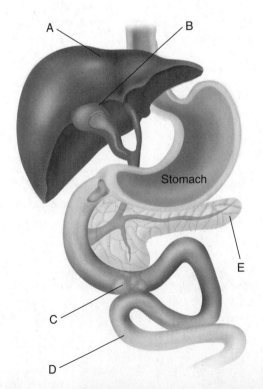

A. _____

B. _____

C. _____

D. _____

E. _____

2. The Stomach

A. _____

B. _____

C. _____

D. _____

E. _____

F. _____

G. _____

Identify

In the following case studies, list the chief complaint, vital signs, and pertinent negatives.

1. "Medic 640, respond Priority One for a 63-year-old male patient, near syncope. Patient is now conscious and alert." As you enter the apartment, you recognize the odor. It smells as though the patient has melena stools. Your paramedic instructor was right; it's an unforgettable smell even for a brand-new, inexperienced paramedic. The patient is found to be sitting on the commode in the bathroom. He appears ashen, diaphoretic, and barely able to sit up. You and your partner lift him off the commode and lay him on the floor, which you have covered with towels. His skin color slightly improves and his level of consciousness (LOC) improves as well. You immediately place the patient on high-flow supplemental oxygen and begin your primary assessment. You already have formed your general impression and realize that the patient is suffering from a GI bleed. His vital signs are a pulse oximetry of 89%, a pulse rate (lying flat) of 118 beats/min, and blood pressure of 88/P mm Hg. His abdomen is slightly distended. The patient tells you that he has an extensive history of rectal bleeding.

a. Chief complaint:

_____

_____

b. Vital signs:

_____

_____

c. Pertinent negatives:

_____

_____

2. You are dispatched to a reported "man down." On arrival, you find law enforcement standing next to a man who presents as very unkempt. He has an empty bottle of Wild Irish something in his hands. You assume that this is a street person. Regardless of your feelings, you understand the importance of remaining professional. Law enforcement explains that the patient is highly intoxicated, is a danger to himself, and needs to be transported to a detox unit. You begin to assess the patient and decide that he looks much older than his real age of 42. Assessment reveals a male patient with an odor of ethyl alcohol (ETOH) and urine. He is conscious and alert, but slurring his words. He is mostly cooperative. The patient has icteric sclera and right upper quadrant (RUQ) pain on palpation. His blood glucose is 110 mg/dL. His oxygen saturation level is 94%, pulse rate is 104 beats/min and regular, and blood pressure is 142/86 mm Hg. His skin is jaundiced, but cool and dry. He has equal bilateral motor neurologic function to all extremities. His lungs are essentially clear and equal bilaterally. The patient has slightly delayed capillary refill. He has sinus tachycardia on the monitor and appears to have had several bowel movements that appear to have been alcoholic in nature. The patient denies any recent injury or falls. He's not a very good historian.

a. Chief complaint:

_____

_____

b. Vital signs:

_____

_____

c. Pertinent negatives:

_____

_____

3. It's New Year's Eve and your patient is a 45-year-old slightly overweight woman. She is complaining of severe RUQ pain. She states that she knows better than to eat fatty foods, but after all it's New Year's Eve. She is in pain that she describes as "worse than childbirth." She is slightly nauseated and complains of gas pains. She denies any recent injury or trauma. She states a history of gallbladder disease that is usually controlled by diet. But tonight the pain is "unbearable." She further states that tonight's episode is consistent with other bouts of gallbladder attack. She says that after tonight she is going to "finally have it taken out." Her vital signs are as follows: Her pulse is 92 beats/min, strong and regular. She has equal bilateral radial pulses. The abdomen is tender in the RUQ. Her oxygen saturation is 99%. ECG reveals sinus rhythm. Capillary refill is normal. Skin color is normal, and skin is warm and slightly diaphoretic. Your patient is crying for pain relief.

a. Chief complaint:

_____

_____

b. Vital signs:

_____

_____

c. Pertinent negatives:

_____

_____

Ambulance Calls

The following case scenarios provide an opportunity to explore the concerns associated with patient management and paramedic care. Read each scenario, and then answer each question.

1. You are assessing and treating a conscious, alert 23-year-old man with a sudden severe onset of periumbilical pain that migrates to the right lower quadrant. He states that he can't find a position of comfort and feels slightly nauseated and febrile.

a. What is your initial impression of this patient's presentation?

_____

_____

b. Your patient denies any other previous medical history, he is not on any medications, and he denies allergies to medications. His vital signs would be considered within normal limits. How would you treat this patient?

(1) _____

(2) _____

(3) _____

(4) _____

(5) _____

(6) _____

c. Your patient is very nauseated and is vomiting frequently. You have a choice of the following standing order medications in your drug box: ondansetron (Zofran), diphenhydramine (Benadryl), hydroxyzine (Vistaril), and promethazine (Phenergan). List the dose and cautions of each.

(1) Ondansetron (Zofran):

_____

_____

(2) Diphenhydramine (Benadryl):

_____

_____

(3) Hydroxyzine (Vistaril):

_____

_____

(4) Promethazine (Phenergan):

_____

_____

2. Your patient presents with a history of esophageal varices. He is vomiting copious amounts of undigested blood. What would your prehospital treatment for this patient include?

a. _____

b. _____

c. _____

d. _____

3. You respond to a call for a 76-year-old woman with a possible bowel obstruction. In the prehospital setting, there might not be much you can do to treat this particular patient. List the general treatment guidelines for patients with GI disease.

a. _____

b. _____

c. _____

d. _____

e. _____

f. _____

g. _____

True/False

If you believe the statement to be more true than false, write the letter "T" in the space provided. If you believe the statement to be more false than true, write the letter "F."

_____ **1.** Promethazine is a drug for managing patients with nausea and vomiting.

_____ **2.** Ulcerative colitis presents with a chronic complaint of abdominal pain, often in the lower right area. This pain corresponds to the location of the ileum. Rectal bleeding, weight loss, and diarrhea are some symptoms of this condition.

_____ **3.** All types of severe liver damage will lead to liver failure.

_____ **4.** Patients with peptic ulcers experience a classic sequence of burning or gnawing pain in the stomach that subsides or diminishes immediately after eating, and then reemerges 2 to 3 hours later.

_____ **5.** Deep palpation can help you discern some of the organs and structures in the cavity and requires a level of technique usually employed in the prehospital setting.

_____ **6.** Pain is often an unimportant finding with GI patients. The patient's complaint of pain is something that a paramedic must learn to expect.

_____ **7.** The major presenting problems from GI diseases typically result in pain, hypovolemia, and infection.

_____ **8.** True absent bowel sounds, which are characterized by no sounds heard for 2 minutes, are typically not practical to discover in the prehospital setting.

_____ **9.** The foul-smelling stools that accompany GI emergencies are to be expected.

_____ **10.** Orthostatic vital signs are only relevant when dealing with abdominal trauma.

Short Answer

Complete this section with short written answers using the space provided.

1. Define the following vocabulary words:

a. Borborygmi:

_____

_____

b. Cholecystitis:

_____

_____

c. Scaphoid:

_____

_____

d. Mallory-Weiss syndrome:

_____

_____

2. A 15-year-old girl complains of sharp pain in the right lower quadrant. The pain is made worse by coughing or moving around. The spot she points to is the spot that is most tender to palpation. She lies very still, with her right leg flexed at the hip and knee.

a. What type of abdominal pain is this?

_____

b. What mechanism is most likely to produce this type of pain?

_____

   c. Describe the causes of this type of pain.

   _____

3. Your patient is complaining of pain localized to the right upper abdomen. The patient describes the pain as sharp and as the worst pain he's ever felt. He also states that he is nauseous and has vomited several times. Physical exam reveals fever, tachycardia, hypotension, and muscle spasms in the extremities.

   a. What type of abdominal pain is this?

   _____

   b. When does this type of pain usually occur?

   _____

Fill-in-the-Table

Fill in the missing parts of the table.

   1. In the course of a busy week (is there any other kind?), you have several calls for patients with abdominal pain. Each time you have to evaluate a different story and a different set of physical findings. Among the findings in the patients you cared for were those listed here. For each finding, explain its clinical significance.

Finding	What the Finding Tells Me
Coffee-ground vomitus	
Severe bradycardia	
Melena	
Tenting of the skin	
Patient very still	
Pulsatile abdominal mass	
Rigid abdomen	

Genitourinary and Renal Emergencies

Matching

Match each of the items in the left column to the appropriate term in the right column.

_____ 1. Progressive and irreversible inadequate kidney function caused by the permanent loss of nephrons.

_____ 2. The presence of blood in the urine.

_____ 3. Increased nitrogenous wastes in the blood.

_____ 4. Solid crystalline masses formed in the kidney, resulting from an excess of insoluble salts or uric acid crystallizing in the urine; may become trapped anywhere along the urinary tract.

_____ 5. A sudden decrease in filtration through the glomeruli.

_____ 6. Hypoperfusion of the kidneys caused by hypovolemia.

_____ 7. A condition caused by an obstruction of urine flow from the kidneys, commonly caused by a blockage of the urethra by an enlarged prostate gland, renal calculi, or structures.

_____ 8. The presence of excessive amounts of urea and other waste products in the blood.

_____ 9. Chronic inflammation of the interstitial cells around the nephrons.

_____ 10. When the urine output drops below 500 mL/day.

_____ 11. Infections, usually of the lower urinary tract, that occur when normal flora enter the urethra and multiply.

_____ 12. A powdery buildup of uric acid, especially on the skin of the face.

_____ 13. The U-shaped portion of the renal tubule that extends from the proximal to the distal convoluted tubule; concentrates the filtrate and converts it to urine.

_____ 14. A double-layered cup with the inner layer infiltrating and surrounding the capillaries of the glomerulus.

_____ 15. Inflammation of the kidney linings.

_____ 16. Solid, bean-shaped organs housed in the retroperitoneal space that filter blood and excrete body wastes in the form of urine.

A. Hematuria

B. Acute renal failure (ARF)

C. Urinary tract infection (UTI)

D. Chronic renal failure (CRF)

E. Kidney stones

F. Uremia

G. Interstitial nephritis

H. Prerenal ARF

I. Oliguria

J. Postrenal ARF

K. Azotemia

L. Pyelonephritis

M. Uremic frost

N. Loop of Henle

O. Kidneys

P. Glomerular (Bowman's) capsule

Multiple Choice

Read each item carefully, and then select the best response.

1. Which of the following is NOT considered part of the urinary system?
   A. Ureters
   B. Kidney
   C. Liver
   D. Bladder

2. How much blood does the kidney filter per day in the normal adult?
   A. 200 mL
   B. 200 L
   C. 2,000 L
   D. 200 quarts

3. Each minute _____ of the body's systemic cardiac output of blood flows through the kidneys.
   A. one tenth
   B. one quarter
   C. one half
   D. two thirds

4. What structure inside the kidney is the main filter for the blood entering the kidney?
   A. Peritubular capillaries
   B. Renal pyramids
   C. Calyces
   D. Glomerulus

5. What is the most common composition of kidney stones?
   A. Calcium
   B. Salt
   C. Glucose
   D. Fat

6. When a patient is suffering pain from a kidney stone, it is important to remember that the greater the pain:
   A. the lower the blood pressure and pulse will be.
   B. the higher the blood pressure and pulse will be.
   C. the higher the blood pressure will be and the lower the pulse will be.
   D. the lower the blood pressure will be and the higher the pulse will be.

7. What is the name of the condition when urine output stops completely?
   A. Oliguria
   B. Uremia
   C. Anuria
   D. Hematuria

8. When reading an ECG, what is a classic finding of hyperkalemia?
   A. Peaked T waves
   B. Inverted T waves
   C. Atrial flutter
   D. No T waves at all

9. Which of the following is NOT a sign of air embolism caused by a loose dialysis system?
   A. Cyanosis
   B. Hypertension
   C. Hypotension
   D. Dyspnea

10. How should pain be managed in the 25-year-old man whom you suspect has a kidney stone?
    A. Conservatively administer low doses of Valium.
    B. Aggressively administer a narcotic analgesic with medical control's permission.
    C. Administer oxygen and ASA.
    D. Withhold pain medications until arrival at the ED.

Labeling

Label the following diagrams with the correct terms.

1. The Urinary System

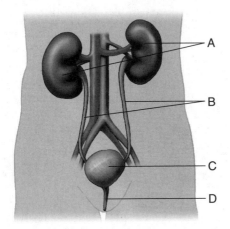

A. _____

B. _____

C. _____

D. _____

2. The Glomerulus of the Kidneys

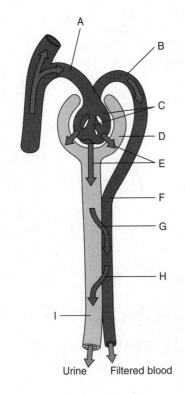

Urine   Filtered blood

A. _____

B. _____

C. _____

D. _____

E. _____

F. _____

G. _____

H. _____

I. _____

3. Male Urethra

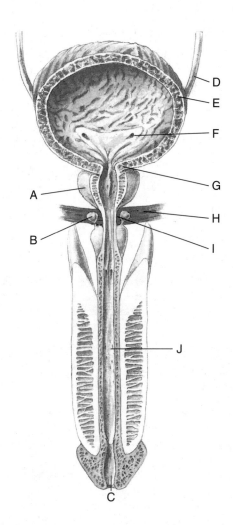

A. _____

B. _____

C. _____

D. _____

E. _____

F. _____

G. _____

H. _____

I. _____

J. _____

4. Female Urethra

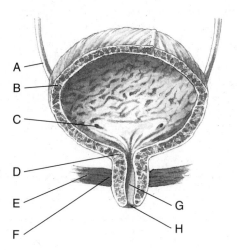

A. _____

B. _____

C. _____

D. _____

E. _____

F. _____

G. _____

H. _____

Fill-in-the-Blank

Read each item carefully, and then complete the statement by filling in the missing word(s).

1. When managing a patient whose chief complaint is renal calculi, your focus should be on _____ and _____.

2. The kidneys' internal anatomy is divided into three regions: the _____, the _____, and the _____.

3. _____ _____ is produced by the hypothalamus and is secreted when the solute concentration of the blood increases.

4. During _____, the patient's blood circulates through a dialysis machine that works the same way the patient's kidneys function.

5. _____ _____ occurs during dialysis and happens because of the water shifting from the bloodstream into the cerebrospinal fluid.

6. Leukemia and tumors, blunt penetrating trauma, cocaine abuse, and spinal cord injury can cause _____ in the male patient.

7. _____ pain is usually associated with hollow organs and presents with a crampy, aching pain deep within the body.

8. You should always monitor the patient's fluid imbalances, electrolyte abnormalities, and _____ function when dealing with an end-stage renal patient.

9. Treatment of kidney stones in the prehospital setting should revolve around _____ _____ for the patient.

10. Urinary tract infections usually occur in the _____ urinary tract.

Identify

In the following case study, list the chief complaint, vital signs, and pertinent negatives.

You're just about to hit the hay after a long day at the fire station. Unfortunately, Bill, the paramedic on duty, is not feeling very well, and so you have to fill in for him. He has had a crampy pain in his lower back all day, and he is worried he is coming down with the flu. At about 1:00 AM, Bill wakes you and tells you something is really wrong. He is having pain in his lower quadrants, and he can't take it anymore. You give him a little ribbing about all the potato chips he has been eating and the gallons of sports drink he drinks each day. You tell him to go back to sleep. It is just an upset stomach. He tells you he is about to jump through his skin because it hurts so badly and asks you to get up and haul him to the emergency department (ED). You decide that maybe Bill is having some problems, so you wake up the other EMT and start an assessment on Bill. He is 47 years old, he is alert, and his oxygen saturation is 98%. You put him on a nasal cannula at 4 L/min just for good measure. Your partner takes his pulse, which is 104 beats/min, and the heart monitor shows a sinus tachycardia with no ectopy. Blood pressure is 148/94 mm Hg, respirations are 18 breaths/min, and all lung fields are clear. His skin is warm and dry, and he has a normal temperature. Not wanting to miss anything on Bill, you measure his blood glucose, which is 96 mg/dL. His pain is a 10 on a scale of 1 to 10, and he is really hurting. Bill doesn't smoke and, other than a fast-food diet, he keeps in good shape.

Both you and Bill are now suspecting a kidney stone. You start an IV and give him a 500-mL bolus of normal saline on the way to the hospital. Medical direction agrees with you about the possibility of a stone and orders 5 mg morphine for the pain. Bill is feeling a lot better when you reach the ED. His pain is down to a 4 out of 10. You check back with him in the morning when you get off shift. He says that he passed a stone about 4 hours after you brought him in. They will run a few more tests, but he thinks he will be out of the hospital around noon. He is now swearing off sports drinks and promises water is his new buddy.

1. Chief complaint:

_____

_____

_____

2. Vital signs:

_____

_____

_____

3. Pertinent negatives:

_____

_____

_____

Ambulance Calls

The following case scenarios provide an opportunity to explore the concerns associated with patient management and paramedic care. Read each scenario, and then answer each question.

1. A 42-year-old man complains of crampy abdominal pain that builds up to a peak, subsides, and then builds again. When you ask where the pain is, he points to the general area of the umbilicus, but when you palpate his abdomen, the part that is tender is in the left lower quadrant. He tells you that he has been vomiting nearly since the pain started, about 6 hours ago.

   a. What type of abdominal pain is this?

   _____

   _____

   _____

   b. What mechanism is most likely to produce this type of pain?

   _____

   _____

   _____

   c. Describe the causes of this type of pain.

   _____

   _____

   _____

2. On the first hot day of the summer, a 35-year-old construction worker calls for an ambulance because of "excruciating" abdominal pain. He was hit in the back lower right quadrant by a steel beam that was being moved into place by a crane. It knocked him down, but he didn't want to appear hurt to his coworkers. So, after catching his breath, he went back to work. He has come home for lunch and now is hurting badly. His wife admits you to the house, where you find the patient in the bedroom, writhing about on the bed, tears rolling down his face. "I can't take it. I can't take it," he says. "Please give me something for the pain." His wife says that he came home from work complaining of back pain and then pain in his groin, and it just got worse and worse. He has been vomiting for the past hour or so. On physical examination, he is clearly in severe distress. His pulse is 124 beats/min and regular, respirations are 30 breaths/min, and blood pressure is 160/80 mm Hg. There is some guarding in the abdomen and tenderness on the left side, but no rigidity. This patient's findings are most consistent with which of the following conditions? Please explain.

   A. Peptic ulcer disease
   B. Diverticulitis
   C. Mesenteric ischemia
   D. Leaking abdominal aortic aneurysm
   E. Trauma to the kidneys
   F. None of the above

   _____

   _____

   _____

3. The following ambulance calls involve dialysis patients. For each situation described, indicate what you think is the problem and what you would do about it.

   a. A patient is due for dialysis today but says he feels "too weak and dizzy even to get out of bed." His ECG shows a rate of 40 beats/min; flattened P waves; wide QRS complexes; and tall, pointy T waves. You are 30 minutes from the hospital ED.

   (1) What do you think is the problem?

   _____

   (2) What steps will you take to manage the problem?

   (a) _____

   (b) _____

   (c) _____

   (d) _____

   (e) _____

   b. The patient calls for an ambulance because of dyspnea that wakened him from sleep. You find him sitting bolt upright, struggling for breath, and coughing up foamy, pink sputum. The lungs are full of crackles. The ECG shows sinus tachycardia (120 beats/min). His blood pressure is 190/120 mm Hg.

   (1) What do you think is the problem?

   _____

   (2) What steps will you take to manage the problem?

   (a) _____

   (b) _____

   (c) _____

   (d) _____

   c. The patient just got home from a dialysis session at the local kidney center. He complains of a severe headache and nausea. He has vomited twice since getting home. On physical examination, he seems a little confused. His pulse is 56 beats/min and regular, respirations are 16 breaths/min, and blood pressure is 180/102 mm Hg.

   (1) What do you think is the problem?

   _____

   (2) What steps will you take to manage the problem?

   (a) _____

   (b) _____

   (c) _____

   (d) _____

True/False

If you believe the statement to be more true than false, write the letter "T" in the space provided. If you believe the statement to be more false than true, write the letter "F."

_____ 1. When you suspect a patient to be in acute renal failure (ARF), you should put the patient in the shock position.

_____ 2. Hyperkalemia presents with an inverted T wave on the ECG.

_____ **3.** The "cleft" of the kidney is called the renal medulla.

_____ **4.** Nephrons are the functioning units inside the kidney that form urine.

_____ **5.** The only absorption of water and electrolytes occurs in the loop of Henle.

_____ **6.** Aldosterone is produced in the hypothalamus.

_____ **7.** When the body becomes low on water, the pituitary gland releases ADH, which causes reabsorption of water into the bloodstream.

_____ **8.** The female urethra is much shorter than the male urethra.

_____ **9.** Men are more prone to urinary tract infections than women are because of the length of their urethra.

_____ **10.** Prerenal ARF is caused by a lack of blood flow to the kidneys.

Short Answer

Complete this section with short written answers using the space provided.

1. Use a medical dictionary to look up the following words, and then write the dictionary definition beside each word:

a. Oliguria:

_____

b. Diuretics:

_____

c. Paraphimosis:

_____

d. Azotemia:

_____

e. Phimosis:

_____

f. Renal pyramids:

_____

g. Efferent arteriole:

_____

h. Uremia:

_____

2. Many patients with chronic renal failure are kept alive by periodic hemodialysis. Although dialysis does remove toxic wastes from the blood and helps restore fluid and electrolyte balance, it does not by any means solve all the patient's problems. Patients maintained on long-term dialysis for chronic renal failure are much more vulnerable than patients with normal kidneys. List five medical problems to which patients with chronic renal failure, who are taking dialysis treatments, are more vulnerable:

a. _____

b. _____

c. _____

d. _____

e. _____

Fill-in-the-Table

Fill in the missing parts of the table.

Signs and Symptoms of Acute Renal Failure	
Type of Acute Renal Failure	Signs and Symptoms
Prerenal	_____
Intrarenal	_____
Postrenal	_____

Gynecologic Emergencies

Matching

Match each of the items in the left column to the appropriate term in the right column.

_____ **1.** The area between the vaginal opening and the anus.

_____ **2.** The glands that secrete mucus for sexual lubrication.

_____ **3.** Monthly flow of blood.

_____ **4.** The beginning phase of a woman's life cycle of menstruation.

_____ **5.** Menstrual blood flow that lasts several days longer than it should or flow that is abnormally excessive.

_____ **6.** Outer fleshy "lips" covered with pubic hair that protect the vagina.

_____ **7.** A sexually transmitted disease caused by the bacterium *Chlamydia trachomatis*.

_____ **8.** A term used to describe the number of times a woman has been pregnant.

_____ **9.** Blood in the peritoneal cavity.

_____ **10.** A term used to describe the number of times a woman has delivered a viable (live) newborn.

_____ **11.** The narrowest portion (lower third of neck) of the uterus that opens into the vagina.

_____ **12.** A pregnancy in which the ovum implants somewhere other than the uterine endometrium.

_____ **13.** A situation in which the hymen completely covers the vaginal orifice.

_____ **14.** A cleft between the labia minora, where the urethral opening (orifice), the vaginal opening (orifice), and the hymen are located.

_____ **15.** A condition in which the uterus moves or drops into the vagina due to weakened pelvic muscles and connective tissues.

_____ **16.** An infection of the genitals, buttocks, or anal area caused by herpes simplex virus (HSV), which may cause sores of the genitals, mouth, or lips.

A. Hypermenorrhea

B. Para

C. Bartholin glands

D. Genital herpes

E. Menstruation

F. Gravida

G. Imperforate hymen

H. Perineum

I. Hemoperitoneum

J. Menarche

K. Labia majora

L. Prolapsed uterus

M. Vestibule

N. Ectopic pregnancy

O. Chlamydia

P. Cervix

Multiple Choice

Read each item carefully, and then select the best response.

1. How many days is the average "cycle" of a woman?
  A. 5 days
  B. 10 days
  C. 28 days
  D. 30 days

2. What is the onset of the first menses called?
  A. Menopause
  B. Premenstrual syndrome
  C. Menstruation
  D. Menarche

3. During an ectopic pregnancy, where do 97% of eggs implant?
  A. In the uterus
  B. In the fallopian tube
  C. In the ovary
  D. In the cervical opening

4. Which of the following is a symptom associated with gonorrhea?
   A. A growth in the genital area
   B. Painful urination with a foul, yellowish vaginal discharge
   C. Prolonged high fever, headache, and malaise
   D. Lower abdominal pain, and pain during intercourse

5. Which of the following is NOT one of the classic triad for diagnosing ectopic pregnancy?
   A. Vaginal bleeding
   B. Anxiety and decreased pulse pressure
   C. Amenorrhea
   D. Abdominal pain

6. Which of the following is NOT considered a life-threatening gynecologic condition?
   A. Child birth
   B. Ectopic pregnancy
   C. Tubo-ovarian abscess
   D. Ruptured ovarian cyst

7. Each of the following drugs is considered a "club drug" and has been used to facilitate a sexual rape, EXCEPT:
   A. Rohypnol.
   B. GHB.
   C. naloxone.
   D. ketamine.

8. Besides PID, which of the following is a cause of an ectopic pregnancy?
   A. Smoking
   B. IUD use
   C. Pelvic surgery
   D. All of the above

9. When dealing with a victim of sexual assault, which of the following statements is true?
   A. You should try to gain as much information as possible about the assault.
   B. You should place the patient's articles in a paper bag.
   C. You should place the patient's articles in a plastic bag to preserve DNA.
   D. You should allow the patient time to wash himself or herself.

10. Which one of the following drugs is considered a stimulant?
   A. GHB
   B. Ketalar
   C. Ecstasy (MDMA)
   D. Rohypnol

Labeling

Label the following diagrams with the correct terms.

1. Anatomy of the Female Reproductive System

FRONT VIEW   SIDE VIEW

A. _____

B. _____

C. _____

D. _____

E. _____

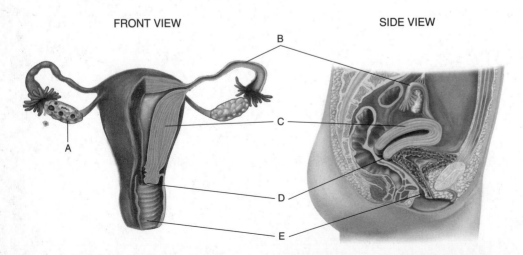

2. Reproductive System With an Ectopic Pregnancy.

A. _____

B. _____

C. _____

D. _____

Fill-in-the-Blank

Read each item carefully, and then complete the statement by filling in the missing word(s).

1. The lower portion of the birth canal is also called the _____.

2. In some cases, a/an _____ _____ will completely cover the vaginal orifice.

3. The cessation of menses is known as _____.

4. _____ is when a woman is no longer able to bear children.

5. Endometrial tissue grows outside the uterus and causes _____.

6. _____ _____ _____ is a form of septic shock.

7. _____ _____ is the first thing to ensure when called to a gynecologic emergency.

8. At all times, you should try to protect a patient's _____ when treating a gynecologic emergency.

9. _____ sign or _____ _____ sign may indicate internal bleeding.

10. _____ _____ is mainly used as a veterinary anesthetic.

Identify

In the following case study, list the chief complaint, vital signs, and pertinent negatives.

Your unit has been called to the local high school for a young woman with severe abdominal pain. When you arrive, the 16-year-old girl, Lucy, is doubled up in pain. She is crying. You begin your assessment with the MS-ABCs and apply supplemental oxygen via a nonrebreathing mask. Lucy rates her pain as 10 on a scale of 1 to 10. Your partner Abe begins with her baseline vital signs as you gather a personal history. Lucy's heart rate is 120 beats/min, her ECG rhythm is sinus tachycardia, and her blood pressure is 140/92 mm Hg. Her oxygen saturation is 99%, and respirations are 20 breaths/min. Her skin is very warm, and her temperature is 102°F. Pupils are Equal And Round, Regular in size, and reactive to Light (PEARRL). Lung sounds are clear. She has no history of illness or trauma. She denies being sexually active yet. A physical exam reveals guarding of the abdomen. She has rebound tenderness, and her abdomen is distended. She says she is going to be sick and then begins to vomit. You feel that this is a load-and-go priority patient, so your partner gets an IV started and you load the patient quickly and get to the local hospital as quickly as possible.

1. Chief complaint:

_____

_____

2. Vital signs:

_____

_____

3. Pertinent negatives:

_____

_____

Ambulance Calls

The following case scenarios provide an opportunity to explore the concerns associated with patient management and paramedic care. Read each scenario, and then answer each question.

1. A 25-year-old woman calls for an ambulance because of abdominal pain. She says the pain started yesterday and
   has just gotten worse and worse. It is a "heavy," aching pain in the lower abdomen. This afternoon, she started
   having chills as well, and she threw up once. Her last menstrual period was 5 days ago and was normal. She uses
   an intrauterine device (IUD) for contraception. On physical examination, the patient looks ill. Her skin feels hot
   and dry. Her pulse is 110 beats/min and regular while sitting, 116 beats/min while standing; her respirations are
   24 breaths/min and unlabored; and her blood pressure is 122/74 mm Hg. The abdomen is very tender to palpation
   in all quadrants.

   a. This woman is most likely experiencing which of the following conditions?
      A. A threatened abortion
      B. An inevitable abortion
      C. A septic abortion
      D. An ectopic pregnancy
      E. Pelvic inflammatory disease (PID)

   b. List the steps you would take in managing this patient.

   (1) _____

   (2) _____

2. A 24-year-old woman calls for an ambulance because she says, "I think I have appendicitis." She says she has been
   having some crampy pain in the right lower quadrant for a couple of days, but today it got much worse. She can't
   remember exactly when her last menstrual period was and says, "But I think I'm getting my period now, because
   I had some spotting this morning." She is certain, in any case, that she couldn't possibly be pregnant. On physical
   examination, she appears anxious and in moderate distress. Her skin is cool and moist. Her pulse is 100 beats/min
   and regular while sitting, 124 beats/min while standing; her respirations are 24 breaths/min and regular; and her
   blood pressure is 110/70 mm Hg. Her abdomen is very tender to palpation.

   a. What is your field diagnosis of this patient?
      A. A threatened abortion
      B. An inevitable abortion
      C. A septic abortion
      D. An ectopic pregnancy
      E. Pelvic inflammatory disease (PID)

   b. List the steps you would take in managing this patient.

   (1) _____

   (2) _____

   (3) _____

   (4) _____

   (5) _____

   (6) _____

   (7) _____

   (8) _____

True/False

If you believe the statement to be more true than false, write the letter "T" in the space provided. If you believe the statement to be more false than true, write the letter "F."

   _____ **1.** The paramedic should take a detailed history of the rape incident to enable the victim to ventilate her
feelings about what happened.

_____ **2.** All superficial wounds and abrasions suffered by a rape victim should be carefully cleaned and covered with sterile dressings before transport to prevent infection.

_____ **3.** The patient should be discouraged from cleaning up before being examined in the emergency department.

_____ **4.** The rape victim's external genitalia should be routinely inspected for injury.

_____ **5.** The diagnosis on your patient care report (PCR) for a victim of sexual assault should read "Alleged rape" rather than "Rape."

_____ **6.** Gonorrhea can cause the Bartholin glands to become cystic and abscessed.

_____ **7.** Dysmenorrhea means the patient has excessive blood flow during menses.

_____ **8.** Endometritis is hereditary and runs in families.

_____ **9.** When using the mnemonic ACHES-S, the E stands for ectopic pregnancy.

_____ **10.** If a woman has had three pregnancies and two live births, she is classified as a gravid 3, para 2.

Short Answer

Complete this section with short written answers using the space provided.

1. You are summoned to a downtown apartment for a "sick woman." On arrival, you find a 24-year-old woman complaining of severe abdominal pain.

   a. List 10 questions you would ask in taking this woman's history.

(1) _____

(2) _____

(3) _____

(4) _____

(5) _____

(6) _____

(7) _____

(8) _____

(9) _____

(10) _____

   b. List two things you would look for in particular in performing the physical examination.

(1) _____

(2) _____

2. Ectopic pregnancy is more likely in some women than in others. List two factors that predispose a woman to ectopic pregnancy.

   a. _____

   b. _____

3. Three findings in the history make up the classic diagnostic triad for ectopic pregnancy, and a woman who has those three findings must be considered to be experiencing an ectopic pregnancy until proven otherwise. What three findings make up the classic triad for ectopic pregnancy?

   a. _____

   b. _____

   c. _____

Fill-in-the-Table

Fill in the missing parts of the table.

Drug	Street Names	General Information	Symptoms	Emergency Care
	• Georgia home boy • Grievous bodily harm • Easy lay • G • Scoop • Liquid X • Soap • Salty water	• Depressant, has amnestic properties • Common in the "rave" and "club" crowds • Colorless liquid • Generally has a salty taste that is disguised when mixed in a drink	• Range from sleepiness, loss of muscle tone, and forgetfulness to seizurelike activity • Respirations and pulse rate are depressed, progressing to a comalike state that generally lasts about 2 hours	
	• Special K • Vitamin K • Cat Valium • Fort Dodge	• Predominantly marketed in the United States as a veterinary anesthetic • Blocks pain pathways • May produce frightening hallucinations • Available in liquid and powder form • Can be inhaled, injected, or mixed into a drink	• Loss of coordination • Muscle rigidity • Slurred speech • Catatonic or blank stare • General sense of numbness • Can lead to aggressive and violent behavior and an exaggerated sense of strength • Symptoms of overdose include nausea and vomiting, hypertension, and respiratory impairment leading to oxygen deprivation of the brain	
	• XTC • Adam • X • Lover's speed • Clarity	• Methamphetamine derivative with hallucinogenic properties; a stimulant • Generally sold in capsule or tablet form • Can also be found as a powder • Can be injected, inhaled, ingested, or smoked • Regular users may use paraphernalia such as rubber or candy pacifiers to ease the effects • A surgical mask smeared with Vicks VapoRub is also a clue of ecstasy use because the vapors reportedly increase the effect of the "rush" • Logos that may appear on tablets: Superman, Batman, Nike, Mercedes, Rolls Royce	• Similar to those of cocaine and speed • Rapid pulse rate • Rapid increase of body temperature, often to deadly levels • Anxiety • Hypertension • Blurred vision • Mental confusion • Nausea • Excessive sweating, leading to dangerous levels of dehydration • Rapid eye movement • Tremors • Bruxism (teeth clenching)	
	• Roofies • Roof • Roachies • Rocha • Mexican Valium	• Has sedative-hypnotic, amnestic, and anesthetic properties • Legally marketed outside the United States by Roche Pharmaceuticals as a sedative and preoperative anesthetic • White, scored tablet, with the word "Roche" appearing on one side • Tablet can be dissolved in a drink, where it is undetectable • Roche Pharmaceuticals has recently added a color base of royal blue to the tablet; if the drug is mixed with a drink, the color will appear	• Impaired judgment and motor skills • Loss of social inhibition • Decreased blood pressure • Drowsiness • Dizziness • Confusion • Memory loss (victim will have no memory of approximately the last 15 to 20 minutes before blacking out)	

Endocrine Emergencies

Matching

Match each of the definitions in the left column to the appropriate terms in the right column.

_____ **1.** A toxic condition caused by excessive levels of circulating thyroid hormone.

A. Hypothalamus

_____ **2.** Hormone that targets the adrenal cortex to secrete cortisol (a glucocorticoid).

B. Adrenocorticotropic hormone (ACTH)

_____ **3.** Hormone that stimulates the kidney to reabsorb sodium from the urine and excrete potassium by altering the osmotic gradient in the blood.

C. Hyperosmolar nonketotic coma (HONK)

_____ **4.** A form of acidosis in uncontrolled diabetes in which certain acids accumulate when insulin is not available.

D. Aldosterone

_____ **5.** A hormone secreted by the posterior pituitary lobe of the pituitary gland that constricts blood vessels and raises blood pressure; also called vasopressin.

E. Thyrotoxicosis

_____ **6.** A small region of the brain that contains several control centers for the body functions and emotions. It is the primary link between the endocrine system and the nervous system.

F. Antidiuretic hormone

_____ **7.** Also known as hyperosmolar hyperglycemic nonketotic coma.

G. Diabetic ketoacidosis (DKA)

_____ **8.** Hormones produced by the adrenal medulla that assist the body in coping with physical and emotional stress by increasing the pulse and respiratory rates and the blood pressure.

H. Myxedema coma

_____ **9.** Female gonads; they release eggs and secrete the female hormones.

I. Iodine

_____ **10.** A hormone secreted by the parathyroids that acts as an antagonist to calcitonin; secreted when calcium blood levels are low.

J. Progesterone

_____ **11.** An essential element in the diet and an important component of thyroxine. Without the proper level of intake, thyroxine cannot be produced, and physical and mental growth are diminished.

K. Ovaries

_____ **12.** A rare condition that can occur in patients who have severe, untreated hypothyroidism.

L. Calcitonin

_____ **13.** The hormone secreted by the thyroid gland that helps maintain normal calcium levels in the blood.

M. Parathyroid hormone (PTH)

_____ **14.** One of the three major female hormones.

N. Catecholamines

_____ **15.** Large gland located at the base of the neck that produces and excretes hormones that influence growth, development, and metabolism.

O. Testosterone

_____ **16.** Tissues on which hormones are directed to act.

P. Target tissues

_____ **17.** The most important androgen in men.

Q. Homeostasis

_____ **18.** A tendency to constancy or stability in the body's internal environment.

R. Thyroid

Multiple Choice

Read each item carefully, and then select the best response.

1. The endocrine system is made up of a network of glands that produce:
   - **A.** homeostasis.
   - **B.** glucose.
   - **C.** calcium.
   - **D.** hormones.

2. Agonists are molecules that bind to a cell's receptor and trigger a response by that cell; they produce some kind of action or:
   - **A.** analgesic effect.
   - **B.** fight-or-flight response.
   - **C.** biologic effect.
   - **D.** drug effect.

3. What part of the endocrine system has a role in hormone production as well as in digestion?
   - **A.** Hypothalamus
   - **B.** Pancreas
   - **C.** Thyroid
   - **D.** Parathyroid

4. The pituitary gland is often referred to as the:
   - **A.** master gland.
   - **B.** hypothalamus.
   - **C.** guardian gland.
   - **D.** None of the above

5. The thyroid secretes:
   - **A.** iodine.
   - **B.** calcitonin.
   - **C.** cardiac enzymes.
   - **D.** norepinephrine.

6. The adrenal glands consist of two parts: an outer part, called the adrenal cortex, and an inner part, called the:
   - **A.** adrenal cortex.
   - **B.** adrenal medulla.
   - **C.** posterior adrenal cortex.
   - **D.** inferior medulla.

7. Epinephrine stimulates _____ nervous system receptors throughout the body.
   - **A.** parasympathetic
   - **B.** sympathetic
   - **C.** dopamine
   - **D.** neuron

8. Type 2 diabetes mellitus used to be referred to as:
   - **A.** juvenile diabetes.
   - **B.** adult-onset diabetes.
   - **C.** diabetic hypoglycemia.
   - **D.** sweet diabetes.

9. The most common form of diabetes is type 2 diabetes, also known as:
   - **A.** insulin intolerance.
   - **B.** insulin tolerance.
   - **C.** insulin resistance.
   - **D.** insulin opposition.

10. Patients in diabetic ketoacidosis (DKA) are seldom:
    - **A.** comatose.
    - **B.** asymptomatic.
    - **C.** hyperglycemic.
    - **D.** hypoglycemic.

11. What condition is characterized by hyperglycemia, hyperosmolarity, and the absence of ketosis?
  A. Hyperosmolar nonketotic coma (HONK)
  B. Hyperosmolar hyperglycemic nonketotic coma (HHNC)
  C. Cardiometabolic syndrome
  D. Both A and B

12. Signs and symptoms of acute adrenal insufficiency may appear suddenly and are commonly referred to as:
  A. addisonian crisis.
  B. adrenal insufficiency.
  C. severe infection.
  D. None of the above

13. Cushing syndrome is caused by:
  A. an excess of cortisol production.
  B. an excess of glucocorticoid hormones.
  C. tumors of the pituitary gland or adrenal cortex.
  D. All of the above

14. An extreme manifestation of untreated hypothyroidism that is accompanied by physiologic decompensation is called:
  A. myxedema coma.
  B. thyroid storm.
  C. Cushing syndrome.
  D. diabetic ketoacidosis.

15. Thyrotoxicosis may be caused by all of the following, EXCEPT:
  A. goiters.
  B. Graves disease.
  C. thyroid cancer.
  D. ketoacidosis.

Labeling

Label the following diagrams with the correct terms.

  1. Six-Step Process of the Body's Fight-or-Flight Response to Stress

A.

B.

C.

D.

E.

F.

A. _____

B. _____

C. _____

D. _____

E. _____

F. _____

2. The Kidney

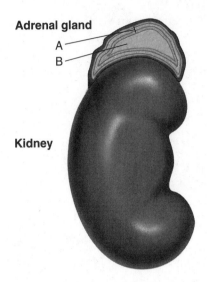

Adrenal gland

A

B

Kidney

A. _____

B. _____

3. The Endocrine System

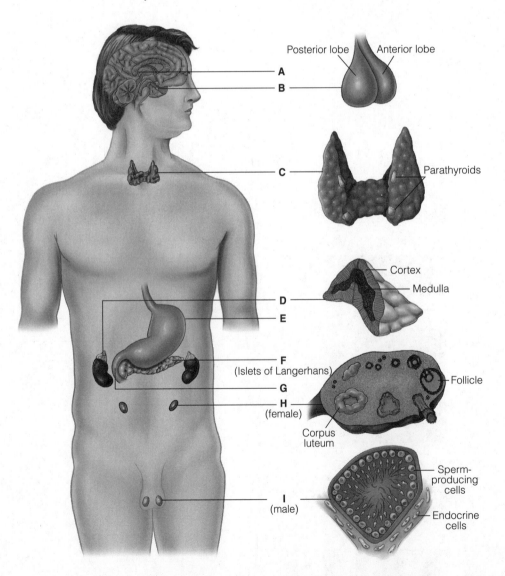

Posterior lobe   Anterior lobe

A

B

C   Parathyroids

Cortex

Medulla

D

E

F
(Islets of Langerhans)   Follicle

G

H
(female)   Corpus luteum

Sperm-producing cells

I
(male)   Endocrine cells

A. _____

B. _____

C. _____

D. _____

E. _____

F. _____

G. _____

H. _____

I. _____

4. Diabetic Emergencies

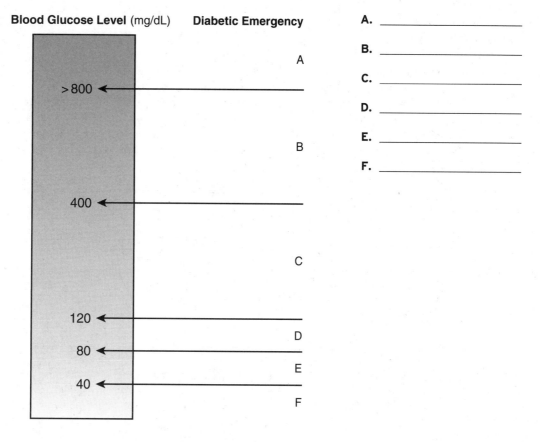

Blood Glucose Level (mg/dL)   **Diabetic Emergency**

A. _____

B. _____

C. _____

D. _____

E. _____

F. _____

>800 ←——————————— A

400 ←——————————— B

C

120 ←——————————— D

80 ←—————————————

E

40 ←————————————— F

Fill-in-the-Blank

Read each item carefully, and then complete the statement by filling in the missing word(s).

1. _____ _____ is a metabolic and cardiovascular emergency. If not diagnosed and treated immediately, the mortality rate is approximately 50%.

2. The anterior pituitary gland secretes _____-_____ _____ in response to secretion of thyrotropin-releasing hormone by the hypothalamus.

3. Aldosterone regulates and maintains the _____ and _____ balance in the blood.

4. The goals of prehospital treatment for diabetic ketoacidosis are to begin _____ and to correct the patient's _____ and acid–base abnormalities.

5. Diabetics are not immune to _____ _____, stroke, _____, meningitis, and other _____ injuries or conditions.

6. Symptoms of type 2 diabetes may include _____, _____, nausea, frequent urination, unexplained weight loss, blurred vision, unresponsiveness, and _____.

7. Two forms of diabetes exist: _____ _____ and _____ _____. Both types are serious conditions that affect many tissues and functions other than the glucose-regulating mechanism, and both require lifelong _____ _____.

8. The endocrine component is made up of the _____ _____ _____. These cell groups in the pancreas act like "an organ within an organ." The main hormones they secrete—_____ and _____—are responsible for the regulation of blood glucose levels.

9. The pituitary gland is often referred to as the _____ _____ because its secretions control, or regulate, the secretions of other _____ glands.

10. Hormones operate in _____ _____ to maintain an optimal internal operating environment in the body. Endocrine regulation, through _____ _____, is the most important method by which hormonal secretion is maintained within a physiologic range.

Identify

In the following case studies, list the chief complaint, vital signs, and pertinent negatives. Also identify the possible nature of the endocrine disorder.

1. It's a sunny but very cold and windy mid-February day. You and your partner would be content to remain inside the station practicing your advanced life support (ALS) skills. The silence is broken with a dispatch to a priority 1 call for an unconscious, unresponsive patient waiting for a prescription at the neighborhood pharmacy. On arrival, you find the 29-year-old woman being attended by the pharmacist, who states the patient was waiting for an insulin prescription. The patient is unresponsive. You note respirations are shallow and the patient is diaphoretic. Her radial pulse is 118 beats/min. Her blood pressure is 104/88 mm Hg. Her blood glucose is 48 mg/dL. As you prepare the ECG monitor and intravenous (IV) equipment, the pharmacist pulls her history.

   a. Chief complaint:

   _____

   _____

   b. Vital signs:

   _____

   _____

   c. Pertinent negatives:

   _____

   _____

   d. Nature of the endocrine disorder:

   _____

   _____

2. It's cold and flu season, and today is no exception. It seems these ailments are what everyone is calling in for. On arrival at the scene, you locate an elderly man sitting in his rocker apparently short of breath. He states that he has had the flu for a number of days and can't stop vomiting. He speaks in full, complete sentences, but has an unusual breathing pattern and fruity breath odor. You quickly place the pulse oximeter probe on his finger. Surprisingly, his oxygen saturation is 95% on room air. You immediately follow up with high-flow supplemental oxygen as you begin your assessment. The patient states a long history of diabetes. He further states that he hasn't been able to keep food down for several days, but has been taking all of his medications. His blood glucose is 405 mg/dL. He is tachycardic with a blood pressure of 108/82 mm Hg. He has poor skin turgor, and skin tenting is present. The monitor is showing a sinus tachycardia. The patient complains of thirst.

   a. Chief complaint:

   _____

   _____

   b. Vital signs:

   _____

   _____

   c. Pertinent negatives:

   _____

   _____

d. Nature of the endocrine disorder:

_____

_____

3. Once again today, you are requested to respond to a call to the local nursing home for a "routine" transport to the emergency department. You are met by family members who are concerned that Grandma's mental status has been rapidly deteriorating, and she appears to be cold. The family states that the patient has suddenly become confused and psychotic. The nursing home chart indicates a history of hypothyroidism. Her pulse rate is slightly bradycardic. She is also hypotensive. You can't get an accurate pulse oximeter reading because of poor peripheral perfusion.

a. Chief complaint:

_____

_____

b. Vital signs:

_____

_____

c. Pertinent negatives:

_____

_____

d. Nature of the endocrine disorder:

_____

_____

Ambulance Calls

The following case scenarios provide an opportunity to explore the concerns associated with patient management and paramedic care. Read each scenario, and then answer each question.

1. A 22-year-old woman is found unconscious in her apartment. Her roommate, who is nearly hysterical, tells you between sobs, "I went away for the weekend, and when I got back tonight, I found her like this. She won't die, will she?" A neighbor arrives and helps calm the roommate while you and your partner carry out the primary assessment. That accomplished, you proceed to the secondary assessment. You find that the patient wakens to a painful stimulus but rapidly returns to sleep. Her skin is warm and flushed and tents when you pinch it. Her vital signs are as follows: Pulse is 110 beats/min and regular, respirations are 30 breaths/min and deep, and blood pressure is 90/60 mm Hg. Her eyes look sunken. Pupils are 5 mm, Equal And Round, Regular in size, and reactive to Light (PEARRL). The breath smells like fruit-flavored gum (or nail polish remover). The neck is not rigid. The chest is clear. The abdomen is soft. There are multiple needle marks and skin changes over the anterior thighs. Completing your examination, you ask the patient's roommate, "Ma'am, is your friend by chance a diabetic?"

"Oh, didn't I mention that?" the roommate sniffles.

List the steps in treating this patient.

a. _____

b. _____

c. _____

d. _____

2. Over the course of a week of ambulance runs, four patients are found in a coma. You don't have any information about any of them except for the medications found at the scene or on the patient's person. Nonetheless, based on those medications, you can make an educated guess at least as to each patient's underlying illness(es). For each of the comatose patients whose medications are listed as follows, indicate the most probable underlying illness(es).

a. Patient 1 has glyburide (Micronase) on his bedside table.

Probable underlying illness(es):

_____

b. A vial of insulin is found in patient 2's refrigerator.

Probable underlying illness(es):

_____

c. Patient 3 has what appears to be an insulin pump. The patient's medical identification bracelet confirms your suspicion.

Probable underlying illness(es):

_____

d. Patient 4, a 35-year-old insulin-dependent woman, had a sudden onset of a severe headache and blurred vision before she became unconscious and fell to the floor, striking her head on a concrete surface.

Probable underlying illness(es):

_____

Complete the Patient Care Report (PCR)

Reread the first incident scenario in the preceding Ambulance Calls section, and then complete the following patient care report (PCR).

EMS Patient Care Report (PCR)					
Date:	**Incident No.:**	**Nature of Call:**		**Location:**	
Dispatched:	**En Route:**	**At Scene:**	**Transport:**	**At Hospital:**	**In Service:**
Patient Information					
Age: **Sex:** **Weight (in kg [lb]):**		**Allergies:** **Medications:** **Past Medical History:** **Chief Complaint:**			
Vital Signs					
Time:	**BP:**	**Pulse:**	**Respirations:**	**SpO$_2$:**	
Time:	**BP:**	**Pulse:**	**Respirations:**	**SpO$_2$:**	
Time:	**BP:**	**Pulse:**	**Respirations:**	**SpO$_2$:**	
EMS Treatment **(circle all that apply)**					
Oxygen @ _____ L/min via (circle one): NC NRM Bag-Mask Device		**Assisted Ventilation**	**Airway Adjunct**	**CPR**	
Defibrillation	**Bleeding Control**	**Bandaging**	**Splinting**	**Other**	
Narrative					

True/False

If you believe the statement to be more true than false, write the letter "T" in the space provided. If you believe the statement to be more false than true, write the letter "F."

_____ **1.** Cold, clammy skin is classically a sign of shock but may also signal severe hypoglycemia, as from an insulin reaction.

_____ **2.** Aldosterone stimulates the bladder to eliminate large quantities of potassium.

_____ **3.** Adult hypothyroidism is sometimes called myxedema.

_____ **4.** The anterior pituitary gland secretes thyroid-stimulating hormone (TSH) in response to the hypothalamus's secretion of thyrotropin-releasing hormone (TRH).

_____ **5.** The primary clinical manifestation of adrenal crisis is atrial fibrillation.

_____ **6.** The signs and symptoms of hypoglycemia and hyperglycemia can be quite similar.

_____ **7.** Normal blood glucose is approximately 70 to 120 mg/dL; hypoglycemia occurs when blood glucose drops to 35 mg/dL.

_____ **8.** Type 2 diabetes may be related to metabolic syndrome.

_____ **9.** Symptoms of type 2 diabetes may include fatigue; nausea; frequent urination; thirst; unexplained weight loss; blurred vision; frequent infections and slow healing of wounds; crankiness, confusion, or shakiness; unresponsiveness; and seizure.

_____ **10.** Most diabetic patients do not live a normal life span, even if they adjust their lives to the demands of the disease, especially their eating habits and activities.

_____ **11.** Endocrine disorders can be caused by either hypersecretion or insufficient secretion of a gland.

_____ **12.** The islets of Langerhans secrete glucagon and insulin, which are responsible for the regulation of blood glucose levels.

_____ **13.** When sodium is reabsorbed into the blood, water is secreted; this action decreases both blood volume and blood pressure.

_____ **14.** Iodine is an important component of thyroxine. Without the proper level of dietary iodine intake, thyroxine cannot be produced.

_____ **15.** Exocrine glands excrete chemicals for absorption.

Short Answer

Complete this section with short written answers using the space provided.

1. Define the following vocabulary words:

a. Hypoglycemia:

_____

_____

_____

b. Diabetic ketoacidosis (DKA):

_____

_____

_____

c. Thyrotoxicosis:

_____

_____

_____

d. Insulin:

_____

_____

_____

e. Cushing syndrome:

_____

_____

_____

2. Explain the treatment for the following conditions:
  a. Myxedema coma:

_____

_____

_____

_____

_____

  b. Adrenal insufficiency:

_____

_____

_____

_____

_____

  c. Hyperosmolar nonketotic coma:

_____

_____

_____

_____

_____

Fill-in-the-Table

Fill in the missing parts of the tables.

Hormones of the Adrenal Glands		
Hormone	**Class**	**Functions**
Cortisol	Glucocorticoid	
Aldosterone	Mineralocorticoid	
Epinephrine/ norepinephrine	Catecholamines	

Hormones of the Gonads	
Hormone	**Functions**
Male	
Testosterone	
Female	
Estrogen	
Progesterone	

Hematologic Emergencies

Matching

Match each of the items in the left column to the appropriate definition in the right column.

_____ 1. A disease that causes RBCs to be misshapen, resulting in poor oxygen-carrying capability and potentially resulting in lodging of the RBCs in blood vessels or the spleen.

_____ 2. A reduction in the number of WBCs.

_____ 3. Clotting of the blood.

_____ 4. Red blood cells (RBCs).

_____ 5. Another term for cancer cells.

_____ 6. The commonly used blood classification system, based on the antigens present or absent in the blood.

_____ 7. The iron-rich protein in blood that carries oxygen.

_____ 8. An overabundance or overproduction of RBCs, WBCs, and platelets.

_____ 9. Blood in the stool.

_____ 10. Unspecified itching.

_____ 11. The proportion of RBCs in total blood volume.

_____ 12. Substances (usually protein) identified as foreign to the body.

_____ 13. A lower than normal hemoglobin or erythrocyte level.

_____ 14. A temporary stop in the production of RBCs; may occur as a result of sickle cell disease.

A. Erythrocytes

B. ABO system
C. Hematocrit
D. Melena
E. Sickle cell disease
F. Pruritus

G. Hemoglobin
H. Coagulation
I. Neoplastic cells
J. Leukopenia
K. Aplastic crisis
L. Antigens
M. Anemia
N. Polycythemia

Multiple Choice

Read each item carefully, and then select the best response.

1. During the history taking and secondary assessment of a hematologic patient, it is important to do all of the following, EXCEPT:
   A. look for changes in LOC.
   B. obtain a SAMPLE history.
   C. check for skin color changes and itching.
   D. interview the family; confidentiality rules dictate that the family not be present.

2. Common findings with patients with blood disorders include which of the following?
   A. Bone fractures
   B. Mental health disorders
   C. "Clubbed" nails
   D. Epistaxis

3. Assessment and management of patients with hemophilia include which of the following procedures?
   A. Controlling bleeding
   B. Administering high-flow supplemental oxygen
   C. Administering an analgesic
   D. All of the above

4. The following organs assist in the production of RBCs, EXCEPT the:
   A. medulla.
   B. liver.
   C. spleen.
   D. bone marrow.

5. The Rh antigen was first found in:
   A. pig cells.
   B. horse serum.
   C. rhesus monkeys.
   D. cow liver.

6. Which blood type is considered the universal donor?
   A. AB
   B. A
   C. O
   D. B

7. Leukemia patients may have which of the following signs/symptoms?
   A. Frequent urinary tract infections
   B. No symptoms
   C. Unexplained bleeding
   D. Spontaneous pneumothorax

8. Disseminated intravascular coagulopathy (DIC):
   A. has a mortality rate of 75%.
   B. has a mortality rate of 10% to 15%.
   C. is rarely fatal.
   D. can be prevented with large fluid bolus.

9. Assessment and management of patients with multiple myeloma include which of the following procedures?
   A. IV therapy using a BIG device
   B. Pain management
   C. Supplemental oxygen via CPAP
   D. Transport with PASG/MAST in place

10. Blood performs which of the following functions?
   A. Transports oxygen from the lungs to the tissues
   B. Ferries waste products of metabolism
   C. Carries nutrients from the digestive tract to cells
   D. All of the above

Labeling

Label the following diagrams with the correct terms.

   1. Major Organs for Producing and Regulating the Blood

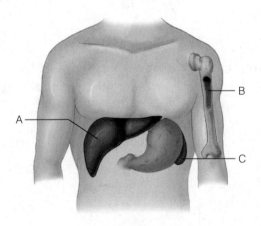

A. _____

B. _____

C. _____

2. Normal RBCs and Sickle Cells

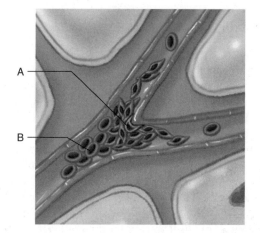

A. _____

B. _____

Fill-in-the-Blank

Read each item carefully, and then complete the statement by filling in the missing word(s).

1. Blood is the fluid of _____.

2. The _____ system includes blood components and the organs involved in their development and production.

3. The formed elements of blood include red _____ _____, white _____ _____, _____, and _____.

4. Red blood cell production occurs within _____ _____.

5. _____ _____, _____ _____, and _____ are three common blood tests done on blood samples.

6. _____ are the smallest of the formed elements and responsible for the clotting of blood.

7. _____ _____ is a painless, progressive enlargement of the lymphoid glands, most commonly affecting the spleen and the lymph nodes.

8. The leading inherited blood disorder is called _____ _____ _____.

9. Leukemia patients frequently present with _____, _____, or _____.

10. Patients with lymphoma may require _____ management.

Identify

In the following case studies, list the chief complaint, vital signs, and pertinent negatives.

1. You are called to the home of a 42-year-old woman with a history of metastatic cancer and bone marrow transplant. Her chief complaint is extreme weakness, fatigue, and exertional dyspnea. You find the patient lying in bed conscious and alert, although she appears very "withdrawn" and weighs about 90 lb. She denies chest pain or shortness of breath. She tells you that she doesn't have any energy, and the doctor's office wants her back in the hospital. Her vital signs are as follows: Pulse is 86 beats/min, slightly irregular, and difficult to palpate; blood pressure is also difficult to auscultate but appears to be 92/P mm Hg. Her skin is pale, warm, and dry. She has an oxygen saturation of 91% on ambient air. Her Pupils are Equal And Round, Regular in size, and reactive to Light (PEARRL). She has a central IV port in place.

a. Chief complaint:

_____

_____

b. Vital signs:

_____

_____

   c. Pertinent negatives:

_____

_____

2. Your unit is dispatched to a priority 1 response to Middle Road Elementary School. The dispatch information indicates a 10-year-old boy with near syncope. Once inside the nurse's office, you recognize your patient. You have transported him several times in the past. For years, he has been treated for leukemia. His mom is on the scene, and she appears comforted to see a familiar face. She explains that he was just able to return to school full time after his latest round of treatments. As you speak to the patient, it is apparent that his mental status is slightly altered. However, when you ask him about his favorite topic, baseball, he becomes quite talkative. En route to the hospital his vital signs indicate that he is now conscious and alert. He doesn't remember the near syncope. His radial pulses are equal bilaterally and regular at 86 beats/min. He currently denies any complaints as the baseball conversation continues. Blood pressure is 98/64 mm Hg. His skin is jaundiced, but cool and dry. Pupils are Equal And Round, Regular in size, and reactive to Light (PEARRL). His oxygen saturation is 98% on a nonrebreathing mask. The patient has central IV access. You contact medical control for direction and are told to continue transport while monitoring his ABCs. His IV will be activated in the ED.

   a. Chief complaint:

_____

_____

   b. Vital signs:

_____

_____

   c. Pertinent negatives:

_____

_____

3. It's been a rather busy day with mostly routine emergency calls. However, this call is a little different. A man with a history of sickle cell disease is having an acute crisis and is in extreme pain. He states that the pain is breaking through his oral morphine tablets and fentanyl transdermal patch. He states that his pain is a 9 on a scale of 1 to 10. He states that it's the worst sickle cell pain that he has ever had. His vital signs are as follows: Pulse is 112 beats/min and regular; skin is pale, warm, and moist; and blood pressure is 148/96 mm Hg. Pupils are Equal And Round, Regular in size, and reactive to Light (PEARRL). His pulse oximetry is 91%. He is anxious and keeps telling you to "get the rubber on the road."

   a. Chief complaint:

_____

_____

   b. Vital signs:

_____

_____

   c. Pertinent negatives:

_____

_____

Ambulance Calls

The following case scenarios provide an opportunity to explore the concerns associated with patient management and paramedic care. Read each scenario, and then answer each question.

1. You are transporting a patient from the local community hospital to a regional trauma center. The patient's vital signs are stable when you start the transport. He has a unit of blood running. Shortly after you set out, the patient begins complaining of severe back pain. Soon thereafter he breaks out in a cold sweat, his lips take on a bluish tinge, and his neck veins seem to bulge out. You check his pulse, and it is 60 beats/min. A few minutes later, when you check it again, it is 110 beats/min.

   a. The patient is showing signs of a/an:

   (1) allergic reaction to the transfusion.

   (2) hemolytic reaction to the transfusion.

   (3) air embolism.

   (4) pyrogenic reaction to the transfusion.

   (5) thrombophlebitis.

   b. List the steps you will take to deal with the situation.

   (1) _____

   (2) _____

   (3) _____

   (4) _____

2. Your crew receives a call for a 76-year-old man with a severe hemorrhage. On arrival you find the patient's 49-year-old daughter hysterical on the front porch. She states that her father is "bleeding to death." She is too excited and emotional to provide any additional information. You enter the house and are directed to the bathroom. You are met by a rather pleasant but obviously frustrated 76-year-old man. There is a minimal amount of blood in the sink. He is holding a tissue to his carotid region and states that he cut himself shaving. He is very apologetic for and embarrassed about his daughter's behavior. He states that he has a history of a blood disorder called polycythemia and he wears a medical identification bracelet.

   a. What is polycythemia and what are some of the symptoms?

   _____

   _____

   _____

   b. How would you treat a patient who exhibits signs and symptoms of polycythemia?

   _____

   _____

   _____

True/False

If you believe the statement to be more true than false, write the letter "T" in the space provided. If you believe the statement to be more false than true, write the letter "F."

_____ 1. White blood cells are responsible for transporting oxygenated blood.

_____ 2. Red blood cell production occurs in the pancreas.

_____ 3. "Clot busters" activate the fibrinolytic system, resulting in clot decomposition.

_____ 4. The "universal donor" is a person with AB blood type.

_____ 5. Malignant diseases that occur within the lymphoid system are called lymphomas.

_____ 6. Phlebotomy is the treatment of choice for patients with disseminated intravascular coagulopathy.

_____ **7.** In multiple myeloma, abnormal plasma cells infiltrate the bone marrow.

_____ **8.** Patients with hematologic diseases might have symptoms that include vertigo, fatigue, or syncopal episodes.

_____ **9.** Oxygen is generally contraindicated for patients with red blood cell abnormalities.

_____ **10.** Paramedics should be supportive and communicate therapeutically with the patient with a suspected blood disorder.

Short Answer

Complete this section with short written answers using the space provided.

1. Blood disorders present differently from other typical injuries and diseases encountered by paramedics. Please provide some of the common findings as they relate to the following:

a. Level of consciousness

_____

_____

_____

b. Skin

_____

_____

_____

c. Visual disturbances

_____

_____

_____

d. Gastrointestinal system

_____

_____

_____

e. Skeletal system

_____

_____

_____

f. Cardiovascular system

_____

_____

_____

g. Genitourinary system

_____

_____

2. Assessment and treatment of patients with blood disorders may differ slightly from assessment and treatment of patients with more typical diseases encountered by paramedics. Please describe how the treatment and assessment of the following diseases differ.

   a. Leukemia

   (1) _____

   (2) _____

   (3) _____

   (4) _____

   (5) _____

   b. Hemophilia

   (1) _____

   (2) _____

   (3) _____

   (4) _____

   c. Polycythemia

   (1) _____

   (2) _____

   (3) _____

   (4) _____

   (5) _____

   (6) _____

3. Define the following vocabulary words:

   a. Leukopenia:

   _____

   b. Polycythemia:

   _____

   c. ABO system:

   _____

   d. Reticuloendothelial system:

   _____

   e. Pruritus:

   _____

   f. Hematocrit:

   _____

   g. Melena:

   _____

Fill-in-the-Table

Fill in the missing parts of the table.

Blood Types			
Blood Type	ABO Antigens	ABO Antibodies	Acceptable Blood Donor Types
A	A	Anti-B	
B	B	Anti-A	
AB	A, B	None	
O	None	Anti-A Anti-B	

Immunologic Emergencies

Matching

Part I

Match each of the items in the left column to the appropriate reaction in the right column.

_____ **1.** A patient was stung by hornets while raking his lawn. He is sweaty, weak, nauseous, vomiting, pale, and diaphoretic. He is suffering from severe respiratory distress and is hypotensive.

_____ **2.** Your patient states that she is allergic to aspirin. Upon further questioning, you discover that it may cause mild nausea.

_____ **3.** While strawberry picking, your patient develops hives and urticaria.

_____ **4.** One of your partners suffers a tick bite while searching the woods for a missing person. The area is swollen and red. It is painful and itchy to touch.

_____ **5.** It is hay fever season again. With the mild winter conditions, your runny nose and swollen eyes indicate it is going to be severe.

_____ **6.** Thank goodness for credit cards. At least this bee sting wasn't as severe as the last patient you treated. Scraping away the stinger certainly minimized the pain, swelling, and redness.

_____ **7.** You are preparing the IV site. Prior to using any antiseptics, you repeatedly ask the patient if he is allergic to any medications. He explains that he is allergic to iodine. Upon further questioning, he states that he gets extremely short of breath, has chest pain, and can't swallow.

_____ **8.** After administering nitroglycerin spray to your cardiac patient, he is still complaining of chest discomfort that he describes as a 9 on a scale of 1 to 10, with 10 being the worst pain. You choose to administer morphine sulfate. The patient states that he is allergic to pain killers such as codeine. You ask him what type of reaction he typically has to those drugs. Your patient states "nausea."

_____ **9.** You have a new partner today. She is helping you complete your rig check. She notices that you are carrying latex gloves. She complains because she is allergic to latex. When you ask her what type of reaction she gets, she states that her skin cracks and itches, not to mention that messy powder.

_____ **10.** While standing by at a minor league professional baseball game, you are notified of a young child having severe respiratory distress, and he appears to be choking. As you rush toward the patient, you notice that his face is red and swollen and that he has hives all over. Nearby on a seat is a popular baseball game snack. The upset grandfather states that he didn't realize that it contained peanuts.

A. Local reaction

B. Systemic reaction

C. Hypersensitivity

D. Anaphylaxis

Part II

Match each of the items in the left column to the appropriate definition in the right column.

_____ **1.** Allergen

A. Chemicals that work to cause the immune or allergic response (eg, histamine).

_____ **2.** Anaphylactoid reaction

B. A chemical found in mast cells that, when released, causes vasodilation, capillary leaking, and bronchiole constriction.

_____ **3.** Antibody

C. An autoimmune connective tissue disease that causes fibrotic (scar tissue-like) changes to the skin, blood vessels, muscles, and internal organs.

_____ **4.** Basophils

D. The ability to recognize a foreign substance the next time it is encountered.

_____ **5.** Chemical mediators

E. A substance that produces allergic symptoms in a patient.

_____ **6.** Histamine

F. An extreme allergic response that does not involve IgE antibody mediation. The exact mechanism is unknown, but an event may occur without the patient being previously exposed to the offending agent.

_____ **7.** Hypersensitivity

G. A condition marked by exaggerated or inappropriate allergic symptoms after coming into contact with a substance the body perceives as harmful.

_____ **8.** Immunity

H. The body's ability to protect itself from acquiring a disease.

_____ **9.** Mast cells

I. Hives or reddened elevated patches on the skin.

_____ **10.** Primary response

J. A reaction that occurs throughout the body, possibly affecting multiple body systems.

_____ **11.** Scleroderma

K. A protein the body produces in response to an antigen; an immunoglobulin.

_____ **12.** Sensitivity

L. White blood cells that work to produce chemical mediators during an immune response.

_____ **13.** Systemic reaction

M. The first encounter with the foreign substance to begin the immune response.

_____ **14.** Urticaria

N. Basophils that are located in the tissues.

Multiple Choice

For the following questions, select the best response based on the scenario provided.

It's been a slow shift, so you decide to grab a quick dinner at Joe's Steak 'n Lobster. You park your rig outside and find a table near the door, in case you have to leave in a hurry on a call. You've just had your medium-rare sirloin placed in front of you when you notice a woman at the next table who does not look well. You ask her if there is anything the matter. "I don't know," she says in a very squeaky voice. "I have this lump in my throat, and I feel like I'm going to die," whereupon she collapses to the floor.

1. This woman is MOST likely suffering from:
   A. food poisoning.
   B. choking.
   C. strep throat.
   D. anaphylaxis.

2. The treatment you need to give MOST urgently is:
   A. pumping out her stomach.
   B. administering 6 to 10 manual abdominal thrusts.
   C. having her gargle with saltwater.
   D. administering epinephrine 1:1,000, 0.5 mL SQ.

3. Assuming the patient is suffering from an acute anaphylactic reaction, what other medications might be helpful?
   A. Nitroglycerin sublingual
   B. Solu-Medrol
   C. Morphine sulfate
   D. Narcan

4. You decide to administer diphenhydramine (Benadryl) to your patient as well. You determine that Benadryl may also be helpful at this time because it blocks:
   A. beta receptor sites.
   B. alpha receptor sites.
   C. neurotransmitters that cause respiratory distress.
   D. histamine receptors.

5. While assessing and treating your patient, you discover a used EpiPen next to her collapsed body. The EpiPen auto injector (if used properly) would have administered:

   A. 1 mg of 1:10,000 solution IM.

   B. 1 mg of 1:10,000 solution IV.

   C. 0.3 mg of 1:1,000 solution SQ.

   D. 0.3 mg of 1:1,000 solution IM.

6. The patient is responding slowly to the epinephrine. Which of the following medications may also be helpful if medical control concurs?

   A. Glucagon

   B. Albuterol

   C. Decadron (dexamethasone)

   D. All of the above

The patient's mother explains that the baby had been up all night tugging at her ear and crying inconsolably. She has been running a low-grade fever that appears to respond well to pediatric Tylenol (acetaminophen). Today the baby went to the pediatrician, who prescribed liquid amoxycillin for an ear infection. After the first dose of the strawberry-flavored antibiotic, the baby began to vomit and appeared to stop breathing. EMS was called. On your arrival, the child appeared conscious and alert and was acting appropriately for her age.

7. The baby was MOST likely suffering from:

   A. an anaphylactic reaction.

   B. a localized reaction.

   C. no reaction; sometimes sick children vomit and appear to hold their breath.

   D. a systemic reaction.

8. If the small child were having a reaction to the antibiotic, what would be the correct course of treatment?

   A. Check level of consciousness, open her airway, place an oral or nasal airway, ventilate with 100% supplemental oxygen, initiate IV access and pharmacologic treatment, and initiate rapid but safe transport to an appropriate facility.

   B. Initiate rapid transport and perform all assessment and treatment modalities en route.

   C. After securing the patient's ABCs, administer IM Benadryl (diphenhydramine) immediately.

   D. Contact medical control for further instructions.

9. What was the "route" of exposure?

   A. Exposure

   B. Inhalation

   C. Ingestion

   D. Injection

10. Of the following substances, which is NOT considered one of the body's chemical weapons designed to fight off the antigen?

   A. Kinins

   B. Serotonin

   C. Norepinephrine

   D. Prostaglandin

11. What would be the prehospital implication for the paramedic caring for a lupus patient exhibiting symptoms of pneumonia?

   A. You should assess for history of renal failure and electrolyte imbalance.

   B. You should assess for a fever, tachypnea, cough, and/or worsening of chest pain.

   C. You should monitor the patient for stroke and seizure precautions.

   D. Be sure to collect a history that includes bloody stools and GI distress.

12. What is the MOST common type of transplant patient in the United States?

   A. Liver

   B. Heart

   C. Skin

   D. Kidney

Labeling

Use the following figure to answer the questions regarding anaphylaxis.

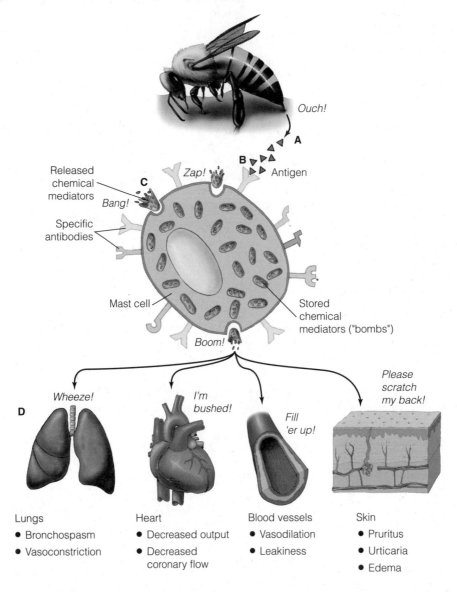

Lungs
- Bronchospasm
- Vasoconstriction

Heart
- Decreased output
- Decreased coronary flow

Blood vessels
- Vasodilation
- Leakiness

Skin
- Pruritus
- Urticaria
- Edema

1. What is the first form of attack on the human body?

_____

2. What types of cells are released?

_____

3. What signs and symptoms may be present in the respiratory system?

_____

4. What are the negative cardiovascular signs/symptoms that may be present?

_____

5. Are there any effects to the circulatory system? If so, list them.

_____

6. The skin is often the first place to show signs/symptoms; what are they?

_____

Fill-in-the-Blank

Read each item carefully, and then complete the statement by filling in the missing word(s).

1. The immunity the body develops as part of exposure to an antigen is _____ _____.
2. The immunity the body develops as part of being exposed to an antigen and developing antibodies is _____ _____.
3. A protein the body produces in response to an antibody is a/an _____.
4. _____ cells meet and greet invaders.
5. _____ is a chemical found in mast cells.
6. A/an _____ _____ airway is an early sign of impending airway occlusion due to swelling.
7. An anaphylactic reaction is a/an _____-_____ reaction and must be treated as such.
8. Patients who receive _____ must be monitored closely for adverse effects.
9. If a patient does not respond to epinephrine, _____ may be indicated.
10. High-flow _____ should be given to each anaphylactic patient.

Identify

In the following case studies, list the chief complaint, vital signs, and pertinent negatives.

1. You are treating a 16-year-old girl who was stung by a bee at her pool. She complains of hives and itching at the sting site. She denies respiratory distress or trouble swallowing. She states that she has never been stung before and doesn't carry an EpiPen. She is conscious and alert. Her skin color is normal, warm, and dry. Capillary refill is normal. Her oxygen saturation is 99%, blood pressure is 112/68 mm Hg, and Pupils are Equal And Round, Regular in size, and reactive to Light (PEARRL).

   a. Chief complaint:

   _____

   _____

   b. Vital signs:

   _____

   _____

   c. Pertinent negatives:

   _____

   _____

2. You are called to a rural location for a 23-year-old man who states that he was bitten by a tick. He appears scared but other than being "grossed-out" has no complaint. The tick is still attached to his leg. After removing the tick, you assess his vital signs. He is conscious and alert. His pulse is 110 beats/min and regular; blood pressure is 142/84 mm Hg; Pupils are Equal And Round, Regular in size, and reactive to Light (PEARRL); and skin is warm and moist. The patient has no previous medical history, no allergies, and no known drug allergies.

   a. Chief complaint:

   _____

   _____

   b. Vital signs:

   _____

   _____

c. Pertinent negatives:

_____

_____

3. A priority one response directs you to Uptown Elementary School for an eighth grader complaining of trouble breathing and swallowing after ingesting doughnuts brought by a classmate. The student is in a class that has signs posted desig- nating it as a "peanut-free" environment. The student has a medical identification bracelet indicating a severe allergy to peanuts and any by-products. The school nurse believes that the student accidentally ingested peanuts that were ingredi- ents in the doughnuts. The student is conscious and alert, anxious, and speaking in a raspy voice. He has redness around his face and neck. Vital signs are pulse of 124 beats/min, oxygen saturation of 90%, and blood pressure of 90/62 mm Hg.

a. Chief complaint:

_____

_____

b. Vital signs:

_____

_____

c. Pertinent negatives:

_____

_____

4. It's about 10:00 PM. You respond to a call for an allergic reaction to seafood. On arrival, you are met by a 32-year-old woman who states that she's allergic to shellfish and iodine. She speaks in complete full sentences and complains of nausea and vomiting. While giving her medical history, she indicates that she has never had a reaction previously to eating fish. While assessing your patient, you note the following vital signs: Her pulse is 124 beats/min and regular, oxygen saturation is 90% on ambient air, and blood pressure is easily auscultated at 112/62 mm Hg.

a. Chief complaint:

_____

_____

b. Vital signs:

_____

_____

c. Pertinent negatives:

_____

_____

5. It's late in the morning, and you are responding to a reported allergic reaction in a 10-month-old boy. Dispatch advises that the child was at the pediatrician today for a well-baby check. While there, the child received several immunizations. The child is now lethargic and gasping for breath. The child presents with urticaria all over. The baby has no other reported medical history or reported allergies. The apical pulse is 190 beats/min. The infant has delayed capillary refill and mottled skin.

a. Chief complaint:

_____

_____

b. Vital signs:

_____

_____

c. Pertinent negatives:

_____

_____

Ambulance Calls

The following case scenarios provide an opportunity to explore the concerns associated with patient management and paramedic care. Read each scenario, and then answer each question.

1. You are called to the suburban home of a 58-year-old man with "shortness of breath." You learn that while gardening, the patient was stung by numerous bees; within minutes he noticed a tight feeling in his chest and started to wheeze. Now, 10 minutes after the sting, he looks flushed and very apprehensive and has a rash on the front of his chest. His vital signs are a pulse of 124 beats/min and slightly irregular, respirations of 36 breaths/min and shallow, and blood pressure of 86/50 mm Hg. His SpO$_2$ is 93%.

   a. List the steps in managing this patient.

   (1) _____

   (2) _____

   (3) _____

   (4) _____

   (5) _____

   (6) _____

   (7) _____

   (8) _____

   b. One of the drugs that you will be giving is epinephrine. List the possible adverse effects of epinephrine if given in an excessive dosage.

   (1) _____

   (2) _____

   (3) _____

2. You are dining out on your night off at Fish Fare, a local restaurant. As you are just about to dig into your red snapper, you notice a woman at a nearby table looking distressed. "Aunt Gertrude, what's the matter?" asks another woman at the table.

   "I don't know," squeaks the distressed woman. "I feel so peculiar. Like there's a lump in my throat. And my chest feels so tight."

   Without waiting to hear another word, you bolt over to the telephone, dial 9-1-1, and ask for an ambulance posthaste. Then you go over to the woman in distress and introduce yourself as a paramedic. You notice that the woman's face is very flushed, and her eyes look puffy. Her pulse is weak and rapid.

   "Oh, dear, I think I'm going to be sick," she says.

   Just then the ambulance pulls up. List the steps in treating this patient.

   a. _____

   b. _____

   c. _____

   d. _____

   e. _____

   f. _____

3. Which of the following patients is most likely to be experiencing an anaphylactic reaction? (For those who are not, indicate what you think they are suffering from.)

    a. A 25-year-old man is dining at a fast-food joint. Suddenly he grows very pale and lurches back from the table, clutching his throat, with his eyes popping. He staggers to his feet and then collapses to the floor—all in complete silence. His problem is most likely:

    _____

    b. You are summoned for a 60-year-old man having a "bad reaction" to a medicine. Earlier in the day, the patient was prescribed erythromycin for a respiratory infection. Now he complains of severe abdominal distress and nausea. On physical examination, his skin is slightly pale and cool. His pulse is 72 beats/min and regular, his respirations are 22 breaths/min and unlabored, and his blood pressure is 160/94 mm Hg. His problem is most likely:

    _____

    c. A 22-year-old man is found sitting on the sidewalk in marked distress. He tells you hoarsely that he just got "a shot" at the VD clinic down the street, and right after he was given the shot and sent home, he started to feel "real strange." He says he got hot and itchy all over, and now he feels like he's going to die. On physical examination, his face looks quite flushed and puffy. His pulse is 140 beats/min and thready, his respirations are 32 breaths/min and shallow, and his blood pressure is 110/60 mm Hg. His problem is most likely:

    _____

4. Describe how you would manage the patient from Question 3.

    a. _____

    b. _____

    c. _____

    d. _____

    e. _____

5. After you report to medical command regarding the patient in Question 3, the physician instructs you to give diphenhydramine (Benadryl) as well. What are the contraindications to giving diphenhydramine?

    a. _____

    b. _____

    c. _____

    d. _____

    e. _____

6. What are the correct dosage and route of administration in this case?

    _____

7. What side effects of diphenhydramine (Benadryl) should you anticipate?

    a. _____

    b. _____

    c. _____

    d. _____

    e. _____

Complete the Patient Care Report (PCR)

Reread the first incident scenario in the Ambulance Calls section, and then complete the following PCR.

EMS Patient Care Report (PCR)					
Date:	**Incident No.:**	**Nature of Call:**		**Location:**	
Dispatched:	**En Route:**	**At Scene:**	**Transport:**	**At Hospital:**	**In Service:**
Patient Information					
Age: **Sex:** **Weight (in kg [lb]):**		**Allergies:** **Medications:** **Past Medical History:** **Chief Complaint:**			
Vital Signs					
Time:	**BP:**	**Pulse:**		**Respirations:**	**SpO$_2$:**
Time:	**BP:**	**Pulse:**		**Respirations:**	**SpO$_2$:**
Time:	**BP:**	**Pulse:**		**Respirations:**	**SpO$_2$:**
EMS Treatment **(circle all that apply)**					
Oxygen @ _____ L/min via (circle one): NC NRM Bag-Mask Device		**Assisted Ventilation**	**Airway Adjunct**		**CPR**
Defibrillation	**Bleeding Control**	**Bandaging**	**Splinting**		**Other**
Narrative					

True/False

If you believe the statement to be more true than false, write the letter "T" in the space provided. If you believe the statement to be more false than true, write the letter "F."

_____ 1. All patients who exhibit signs and symptoms of allergic reaction should receive epinephrine.

_____ 2. Patients should be educated to wear medical identification tags and carry their prescribed anaphylaxis kit.

_____ 3. IM epinephrine is more effective than IV.

_____ 4. Epinephrine has beta-1 properties that cause the blood vessels to constrict, reducing vasodilation.

_____ 5. Bee stings are best removed with sharp, pointy tweezers.

_____ 6. Millions of Americans are at risk for anaphylaxis.

_____ 7. Allergens can invade the body through the skin, respiratory tract, or GI tract.

_____ 8. The respiratory system usually protects the human body from substances and organisms that are considered foreign to the body.

_____ 9. Use of the polio vaccine has resulted in "herd immunity."

_____ 10. Epinephrine is generally not a first-line drug as a result of its delayed response.

Short Answer

Complete this section with short written answers using the space provided.

1. When an antigen combines with a specific antibody on the surface of a mast cell, the mast cell loses its chemical bombs ("degranulates," to use the technical term), releasing a variety of powerful mediators, such as histamine and serotonin. List seven effects produced by those mediators.

   a. _____

   b. _____

   c. _____

   d. _____

   e. _____

   f. _____

   g. _____

2. Besides bees, what other agents are commonly responsible for anaphylactic reactions? List at least four.

   a. _____

   b. _____

   c. _____

   d. _____

Fill-in-the-Table

Fill in the missing parts of the table with examples of the common substances associated with anaphylaxis.

Common Substances Associated With Anaphylaxis	
Antigen	Examples
Drugs	
Insect stings	
Foods	
Latex	
Animals	

Problem Solving

Practice your calculation skills by solving the following math problems.

1. Medical control orders you to administer 0.3 to 0.5 mg epinephrine 1:1,000 SQ to your patient. How many milliliters of fluid will you draw up?

2. Your partner was able to obtain IV access rapidly. What would be the correct dose and concentration of epinephrine?

3. Your patient is improving but still symptomatic. Medical control orders an epi drip at 2 μg/min. You are using a 250-mL bag of normal saline and a 60-gtt infusion set. You have on hand 1 mg of 1:10,000 epi (10 mL). At how many drops per minute would you run the IV?

4. Along with epinephrine, what other drug orders might you anticipate giving the patient in Question 3 and at what dose?

Infectious Diseases

Matching

Match each of the items in the left column to the appropriate term in the right column.

_____ **1.** The period during which an infected person can transmit a communicable disease to someone else.

_____ **2.** The presence or the reasonable anticipated presence of blood or other potentially infectious materials on an item or surface.

_____ **3.** Inanimate objects contaminated with microorganisms that serve as a means of transmitting an illness.

_____ **4.** A place where organisms may live and multiply.

_____ **5.** The period between exposure to an organism and the first symptoms of illness, during which the organism multiplies within the body and starts to produce symptoms.

_____ **6.** An infection acquired from a health care setting.

_____ **7.** The invasion of a host or host tissue by pathogenic organisms such as bacteria, viruses, or parasites that produces illness that may or may not have clinical manifestations.

_____ **8.** People who harbor an infectious agent and, although not personally ill, can transmit the infection to other people.

_____ **9.** Primary barrier that prevents infections.

_____ **10.** These pathogens include, but are not limited to, hepatitis B virus (HBV), human immunodeficiency virus (HIV), and hepatitis C virus (HCV).

_____ **11.** A viral disease similar to measles, best known by the distinctive red rash on the skin; not nearly as infectious or severe as measles.

_____ **12.** Having a positive blood test for an infectious agent, such as HIV or HBV.

_____ **13.** An animal or insect that carries a disease-causing organism and transmits it to a human host, without itself becoming ill.

_____ **14.** A fatal infection of the central nervous system caused by a bite from an animal that has been infected with a virus.

_____ **15.** An inflammation of the lungs caused by bacterial, viral, or fungal infections or infections with other microorganisms.

_____ **16.** The ability of an organism to invade and create disease in a host; also refers to the ability of an organism to survive outside the living host.

A. Reservoir

B. Carriers

C. Fomites

D. Incubation period
E. Communicable period

F. Nosocomial infection
G. Contaminated

H. Infection

I. Skin
J. Bloodborne pathogens

K. Vector

L. Virulence
M. Seropositive

N. Rabies

O. Pneumonia

P. Rubella

Multiple Choice

Read each item carefully, and then select the best response.

1. Agencies responsible for protecting public health include the following, EXCEPT:
   A. OSHA.
   B. CDC.
   C. state health departments.
   D. National Sanitary Foundation.

2. Communicable diseases may be transmitted by:
   A. droplets.
   B. airborne particles.
   C. vectors.
   D. All of the above

3. Host resistance refers to:
   A. drug-resistant antibiotics.
   B. your body's ability to fight off infection.
   C. virulence of the invading microorganism.
   D. the period of contagiousness.

4. Which of the following best defines the key element of the Ryan White Comprehensive AIDS Resources Emergency Act?
   A. A designated infection control officer (DICO) is required by federal law in each county.
   B. The medical facility must release source patient tests to the DICO.
   C. Emergency response personnel must be notified within 48 hours after a workplace exposure to tuberculosis.
   D. Patients' health records are protected by federal law.

5. Personal protective equipment (PPE) needs to be worn when a paramedic is working in the following situations, EXCEPT:
   A. at a collision scene.
   B. at a multiple-casualty incident.
   C. while treating contaminated patients.
   D. It needs to be worn only while working in the "clinical setting."

6. Prior to the year 2000, most exposures of health care workers in the prehospital setting occurred:
   A. by needlestick injuries.
   B. because of broken glass at crash scenes.
   C. from exposure to infected droplets.
   D. when using pocket masks without other barriers.

7. A comprehensive exposure plan for employees includes:
   A. mandatory drug and alcohol testing.
   B. anonymous blood tests.
   C. CDC-recommended work restriction guidelines.
   D. identifying "at-risk populations" in your response area.

8. Most droplets and airborne disease exposures can be prevented by:
   A. placing a mask on patients with fevers and rashes.
   B. doing nothing; confining the patient's face may exacerbate secretions.
   C. the crew wearing level III biohazard suits.
   D. notifying the hospital in advance and having the patient decontaminated prior to admission.

9. All of the following are highly communicable viral diseases, EXCEPT:
   A. measles.
   B. mumps.
   C. pertussis.
   D. meningitis.

10. Lice and scabies infections may affect:
    A. patients.
    B. families.
    C. crews.
    D. All of the above

Fill-in-the-Blank

Read each item carefully, and then complete the statement by filling in the missing word(s).

1. _____ _____ is the term used to describe infection control practices that reduce the opportunity of an exposure to occur in the daily care of patients.

2. A paramedic's major protective measure is _____.

3. Unfortunately, paramedics get exposed to communicable diseases. The third line of defense is considered _____ _____ _____-_____.

4. _____ _____ include bacteria, viruses, fungi, and parasites.

5. Mononucleosis is caused by the _____-_____ virus. Transmission occurs via direct contact with _____ secretions.

6. _____ _____ is caused when a deer tick's bite injects a bacterium into the bloodstream of the human host.

7. Gonorrhea, syphilis, herpes, and HIV are all considered _____ _____ _____.

8. An inflammation of the liver that may be produced by five distinct forms of virus is called _____ _____.

9. MRSA is believed to be transmitted from _____ to _____ via _____ hands.

10. Severe acute respiratory syndrome (SARS) arose from the merger of viruses from _____ and _____.

Identify

In the following case studies, list the chief complaint, vital signs, and pertinent negatives.

1. Your unit is called to the airport to meet an inbound flight. There is a patient reported to have flu-like symptoms that include fever, chills, and dry cough. The patient is conscious and alert but very weak. He is assisted from the aircraft when it arrives at the terminal gate. You note that the flight appears to be domestic in origin. While you are taking the patient's history, he denies any type of international travel but has been traveling extensively with very little sleep this past week. He denies other previous medical history. He denies medications and allergies to medications or prescription drugs. His skin is warm and dry. He feels febrile. After further discussion, you discover that his school-aged children were recently sick with a viral infection. His vital signs are as follows: Respiratory rate is 20 breaths/min, oxygen saturation on ambient air is 95%, pulse is 106 beats/min and regular, and blood pressure is 128/68 mm Hg.

a. Chief complaint:

_____

_____

b. Vital signs:

_____

_____

c. Pertinent negatives:

_____

_____

2. It's a hot, humid day in the mid 90s and your advanced life support (ALS) unit is dispatched to assist the police department. You arrive on scene to discover several patrol vehicles located outside an unkempt house. You are met by one of the officers, who explains that the police department received a call from an out-of-town relative to check on the welfare of the elderly resident. Once inside the house, the police officers noticed a severe lice infestation. Many of the officers are exposed to the nasty critters. Although the exposure is not life threatening, the officers appear very annoyed. They describe the conditions as squalid. You request that the exposed officers assist the elderly patient out to his front yard so that you can properly decontaminate him and minimize the lice exposure to any additional providers and equipment. Once outside, the patient appears emaciated, wearing soiled clothing, yet states he just put on the clean clothes the other morning. He has a bag of prescription medications that seem to indicate a mental health and cardiac history but says he rarely needs to take any pills. His vital signs are as follows: Pulse is 88 beats/min and irregular, blood pressure is 98/72 mm Hg, and oxygen saturation is 88%. He is tachypneic, and there is obvious skin tenting and delayed capillary refill.

a. Chief complaint:

_____

_____

b. Vital signs:

_____

_____

c. Pertinent negatives:

_____

_____

3. While preparing for an ALS interfacility transport, you are told by the nurse's station that the patient has Methicillin-resistant *Staphylococcus aureus* (MRSA). The patient has a number of drip medications, along with strict respiratory precautions. You are told that the patient is "stable" for transport. He is also on a nonrebreathing face mask and is conscious and alert. The patient is on a cardiac monitor and is in a sinus rhythm. His blood pressure as noted on the noninvasive monitor is 98/54 mm Hg, and his heart rate is 62 beats/min. He has a lengthy medical history, including kidney transplant. He is on several immunosuppressants.

   a. Chief complaint:

   _____

   _____

   b. Vital signs:

   _____

   _____

   c. Pertinent negatives:

   _____

   _____

Ambulance Calls

The following case scenarios provide an opportunity to explore the concerns associated with patient management and paramedic care. Read each scenario, and then answer each question.

1. You are called to transport a 22-year-old college student from the college infirmary to the hospital. The nurse tells you that the student has a high fever. He complains of a severe headache and stiff neck, and he seems rather confused. He vomits twice en route to the hospital.

   a. What is the patient experiencing?

   _____

   _____

   b. How can the paramedic minimize the risk of catching the illness?

   _____

   _____

2. A 54-year-old man calls for an ambulance after he coughed up some blood. He says that over the past several weeks he has been waking up in the middle of the night with his pajamas and bedclothes soaked through with sweat. He has lost about 25 pounds in the last 2 or 3 months, and today he started noticing some blood in his sputum.

   a. What is the patient experiencing?

   _____

   _____

   b. How can the paramedic minimize the risk of catching the illness?

   _____

   _____

3. A 28-year-old man calls for an ambulance because he "feels lousy." He says that for a week or so, he hasn't had any energy at all. He doesn't feel like eating or doing anything; he just feels "done in." Even cigarettes "taste like cow dung." This morning, he noticed that his urine was very dark, and he got panicky. On examination, you observe that his eyes have a yellow tinge and there are needle tracks on both his arms.

   a. What is the patient experiencing?

   _____

   _____

b. How can the paramedic minimize the risk of catching the illness?

_____

_____

4. You are called to transport an 8-year-old boy who fell and sustained a laceration to his forehead. "I told him to stay in bed," his mother says, "but no, he has to go horsing around with his brother." According to the mother, both children have been sick for a week with a fever and sore throat. On examining the 8-year-old, you find a 2-inch laceration on the left side of the forehead, and you control the bleeding with pressure. He does seem a little warm, and the angles of his jaw are indistinct, as if there is something swollen there.

a. What is the patient experiencing?

_____

_____

b. How can the paramedic minimize the risk of catching the illness?

_____

_____

5. It's back to the college infirmary for another patient with a fever—this time a 19-year-old woman. She complains of headache and says the light bothers her a lot. Her eyes are reddened, and she is coughing. She has a blotchy, red rash over her face and neck, and when you examine her throat, you notice some little white spots on the mucous membranes in her mouth.

a. What is the patient experiencing?

_____

_____

b. How can the paramedic minimize the risk of catching the illness?

_____

_____

6. You are called late one night to the scene of a two-car collision on the interstate. One of the vehicles involved in the crash skidded into a ditch and flipped upside down. The driver is unconscious inside. There is blood and broken glass everywhere. At the least, you are going to have to deal with this patient's bleeding, stabilize his spine, extricate him, and start an IV.

a. List at least four precautions you will take to protect yourself from possible infection during the care and extrication of this patient.

(1) _____

(2) _____

(3) _____

(4) _____

b. List the routine measures you will employ for cleaning the ambulance and its equipment after this call.

(1) _____

(2) _____

(3) _____

c. While you are putting fresh linens on the stretcher, your partner emerges from the "crash room" where the patient has been taken. "You oughta see that guy's eyes," he says, "they're yellow as a canary. I didn't notice it in the vehicle, but with these fluorescent lights, you can't miss it." Given that information, what further measures should you take?

_____

_____

Complete the Patient Care Report (PCR)

Reread the second scenario in the Ambulance Calls section, and then complete the following PCR.

EMS Patient Care Report (PCR)					
Date:	Incident No.:	Nature of Call:		Location:	
Dispatched:	En Route:	At Scene:	Transport:	At Hospital:	In Service:
Patient Information					
Age: Sex: Weight (in kg [lb]):			Allergies: Medications: Past Medical History: Chief Complaint:		
Vital Signs					
Time:	BP:	Pulse:		Respirations:	SpO$_2$:
Time:	BP:	Pulse:		Respirations:	SpO$_2$:
Time:	BP:	Pulse:		Respirations:	SpO$_2$:
EMS Treatment (circle all that apply)					
Oxygen @ _____ L/min via (circle one): NC NRM Bag-Mask Device		Assisted Ventilation	Airway Adjunct		CPR
Defibrillation	Bleeding Control	Bandaging	Splinting		Other
Narrative					

True/False

If you believe the statement to be more true than false, write the letter "T" in the space provided. If you believe the statement to be more false than true, write the letter "F."

_____ **1.** AIDS is a highly contagious disease.

_____ **2.** Patients with AIDS are abnormally susceptible to many infectious diseases.

_____ **3.** AIDS can be acquired through casual contact, such as shaking hands with an HIV-positive patient.

_____ **4.** AIDS is a highly communicable disease.

_____ **5.** HIV type 1 was first identified in the late 1970s.

_____ **6.** Many health care workers have acquired HIV through contact with the blood or body fluids of patients.

_____ **7.** The majority of AIDS cases that have occurred in health care workers as a result of occupational exposure have been among EMS personnel.

_____ **8.** Complications of syphilis can include cardiac, ophthalmic, auditory, and central nervous system complications.

_____ **9.** STDs require special standard precautions.

_____ **10.** The incubation period of genital herpes is 3 to 4 weeks.

Short Answer

Complete this section with short written answers using the space provided.

1. Carry out the following research project before you begin employment as a paramedic.

   a. Check off the illnesses you had as a child or up to this point:

   _____ Measles

   _____ Mumps

   _____ Chickenpox

   _____ German measles (rubella)

   _____ Polio

   _____ Hepatitis B

   b. Check off the immunizations you have had up to this point, and fill in the dates (obtain the records from your family doctor or the clinic where you received your immunizations):

   _____ Measles   Date immunized: _____

   _____ Mumps   Date immunized: _____

   _____ Rubella   Date immunized: _____

   _____ DPT (diphtheria/pertussis/tetanus)

   #1   Date immunized: _____

   #2   Date immunized: _____

   #3   Date immunized: _____

   _____ Most recent tetanus booster   Date immunized: _____

   _____ Oral polio #1   Date immunized: _____

   _____ Oral polio #2   Date immunized: _____

   _____ Oral polio #3   Date immunized: _____

   _____ Hepatitis B   Date immunized: _____

   c. Based on the preceding data you have compiled, what immunizations do you need to get before you start work?

   _____

   _____

2. With all the hysteria over AIDS, it is crucial that health professionals be as knowledgeable as possible on the subject.

    a. List three ways that AIDS can be transmitted from one person to another.

        (1) _____

        (2) _____

        (3) _____

    b. List three things you can do to minimize the risk of acquiring HIV from a patient.

        (1) _____

        (2) _____

        (3) _____

Fill-in-the-Table

Fill in the missing parts of the table.

1. Complete the following table, which outlines the PPE necessary in preventing transmission of HIV and hepatitis B. Indicate "yes" or "no" for each task or activity.

Recommended Personal Protective Equipment for Preventing Transmission of Human Immunodeficiency Virus and Hepatitis B Virus in the Prehospital Setting				
Task or Activity	**Disposable Gloves**	**Gown**	**Mask**	**Protective Eyewear**
Bleeding control with spurting blood	Yes		Yes	
Bleeding control with minimal bleeding	Yes		No	
Emergency childbirth	Yes		Yes, if splashing is likely	
Drawing blood samples	Not required by CDC, but recommended for EMS		No	
Inserting an IV line	Yes		No	
Endotracheal intubation, laryngeal mask airway, Combitube use	Yes		No, unless splashing is likely*	
Oral/nasal suctioning, manually cleaning airway	Yes		No, unless splashing is likely*	
Handling and cleaning instruments with microbial contamination	Yes		No	
Measuring blood pressure	No		No	
Measuring temperature	No		No	
Giving an injection	Not required by CDC, but recommended for EMS		No	
*Splashing is often likely, so use personal protective equipment accordingly				

2. Indicate the mode(s) of transmission and recommended protective measures for each of the diseases in the following table.

Disease	Mode(s) of Transmission	Protective Measures
AIDS		
Hepatitis type A		
Hepatitis type B		
Meningitis		
Mumps		
Syphilis		
Tuberculosis		
MRSA		
SARS		

Toxicology

Matching

Match the definitions in the left column to the appropriate terms in the right column.

_____ **1.** A synthetic narcotic not derived from opium.

_____ **2.** A common houseplant that resembles "elephant ears"; ingestion leads to burns of the mouth and tongue and, possibly, paralysis of the vocal cords and nausea and vomiting; in severe cases, may be edema of the tongue and larynx, leading to airway compromise.

_____ **3.** Chemicals that are acids or alkalis; cause direct chemical injury to the tissues they contact.

_____ **4.** A naturally occurring alkaloid found in a variety of plants (such as tea leaves).

_____ **5.** The action of two substances such as drugs, in which the total effects are greater than the sum of the independent effects of the two substances.

_____ **6.** A severe withdrawal syndrome seen in people with alcoholism who are deprived of ethyl alcohol; characterized by restlessness, fever, sweating, disorientation, agitation, and seizures; can be fatal if untreated.

_____ **7.** Psychiatric medication used primarily to treat atypical depression by increasing norepinephrine and serotonin levels in the central nervous system.

_____ **8.** A plant that contains cardiac glycosides used in making digitalis; ingestion of leaves causes nausea, vomiting, diarrhea, abdominal cramps, hyperkalemia, and a variety of dysrhythmias.

_____ **9.** A seed that contains the poison ricin; causes a variety of toxic effects, including burning of the mouth and throat; nausea, vomiting, diarrhea, and severe stomach pains; prostration; failing vision; and kidney failure, which is the usual cause of death.

_____ **10.** The emotional state of craving a drug to maintain a feeling of well-being.

_____ **11.** Compounds made up principally of hydrogen and carbon atoms mostly obtained from the distillation of petroleum.

_____ **12.** The cornerstone drug for the treatment of bipolar disorder.

_____ **13.** Class of drugs that increase alertness and excitation; includes methamphetamine, methylenedioxyamphetamine, and methylene-dioxymethamphetamine.

_____ **14.** Drugs used to treat severe depression and manage pain; minimal dosing errors can cause toxic results.

_____ **15.** Physiologic adaptation to the effects of a drug such that increasingly larger doses of the drug are required to achieve the same effect.

_____ **16.** In relation to drugs, illegal drugs such as marijuana, cocaine, and LSD.

A. Caustics

B. Monoamine oxidase inhibitors

C. Hydrocarbons

D. Castor bean

E. Tricyclic antidepressants

F. Amphetamines

G. Foxglove

H. Lithium

I. Theophylline

J. Opioid

K. Tolerance

L. Delirium tremens

M. Psychological dependence

N. Dieffenbachia

O. Synergism

P. Antagonist

_____ **17.** Something that counteracts the action of something else; in relation **Q.** Benzodiazepines
to drugs, this would be a drug with an affinity for a cell receptor
and, by binding to it, the cell is prevented from responding.

_____ **18.** Enhancement of the effect of one drug by another. **R.** Illicit

_____ **19.** An agent that produces false perceptions in any one of the five **S.** Hallucinogen
senses.

_____ **20.** The family of sedative-hypnotics most commonly used to treat **T.** Potentiation
anxiety, seizures, and alcohol withdrawal.

Multiple Choice

Read each item carefully, and then select the best response.

1. Poisoning in adults is usually a result of:
   A. improperly labeled over-the-counter medications.
   B. improperly dispensed prescribed medications.
   C. suicide attempts.
   D. workplace mishaps involving chemicals and toxic exposures.

2. All of the following are common routes of poisoning, EXCEPT:
   A. inhalation.
   B. ingestion.
   C. injection.
   D. excretion.

3. Alcoholism usually consists of two distinct phases, the first of which is _____ drinking.
   A. problem
   B. social
   C. medicinal
   D. binge

4. Alcohol abuse may cause a number of medical consequences, including:
   A. deterioration of memory and higher thinking.
   B. acute gastric distress.
   C. a higher risk of mouth and esophageal cancers.
   D. All of the above

5. Alcohol withdrawal may have life-threatening consequences, including delirium tremens. Delirium tremens, or the "DTs," are best characterized by:
   A. tremors.
   B. confusion.
   C. restlessness.
   D. All of the above

6. The general assessment approach for toxicologic emergencies includes all of the following tasks, EXCEPT:
   A. primary assessment.
   B. scene size-up.
   C. physical exam.
   D. There is no "general assessment"; these patients should receive a secondary assessment.

7. You are called to the scene of a 4-year-old who ingested a common houseplant. The best source of information regarding the accidental ingestion is:
   A. referring to the Department of Transportation (DOT) *Emergency Response Guidebook (ERG)*.
   B. contacting the Poison Center.
   C. contacting CHEMTREC.
   D. contacting medical control.

8. A chronic disorder characterized by the compulsive use of a substance resulting in physical, psychological, or social harm to the user who continues to use the substance despite the harm, is considered:
   A. tolerance.
   B. drug addiction.
   C. substance abuse.
   D. antagonist.

9. The treatment for patients abusing cocaine, amphetamine, or methamphetamine is fundamentally the same. This treatment includes the following tasks, EXCEPT:
   A. establishing and maintaining the airway. Consider an advanced airway as needed.
   B. establishing vascular access by IV or IO.
   C. administering morphine for pain relief.
   D. contacting medical control for chemical restraint when behavior is violent.

10. Signs and symptoms of overdose with cardiac drugs may include:
    A. hypotension.
    B. weakness or confusion.
    C. nausea and vomiting.
    D. All of the above

11. Salivation, lacrimation, urination, defecation, gastric upset, and emesis are symptoms associated with a toxic exposure to:
    A. psychedelics.
    B. narcotics.
    C. ketamine.
    D. organophosphates.

12. Physical examination of a patient who has been poisoned with cyanide may reveal:
    A. an altered mental state.
    B. respirations that are rapid and labored and that become slow and gasping.
    C. a rapid and thready pulse.
    D. All of the above

13. The MOST common symptom of a tricyclic antidepressant overdose is:
    A. an altered mental status.
    B. abdominal pain.
    C. internal bleeding.
    D. burning of the eyes, nose, and throat.

14. All of the following may alter the presentation of salicylate overdose, EXCEPT the:
    A. patient's age.
    B. dose ingested.
    C. duration of respiratory distress syndrome.
    D. duration of exposure.

15. Death from ingestion of large amounts of the plant foxglove usually occurs as a result of:
    A. acute respiratory distress.
    B. psychogenic shock.
    C. cardiac dysrhythmias.
    D. anaphylactic shock.

Fill-in-the-Blank

Read each item carefully, and then complete the statement by filling in the missing word(s).

1. A/an _____ is a substance that is toxic by nature, no matter how it gets into the body or in what quantities it is taken. By contrast, a/an _____ is a substance that has some therapeutic effect when given in the appropriate dose.

2. _____ _____ usually fall under one of two general headings: _____ and _____. Poisoning in adults is commonly intentional.

3. Toxins cannot exert their effects until they enter the body. The four primary methods of entry are _____, _____, _____, and _____.

4. _____ are useful for remembering the assessment and management of different substances that fall under the same _____ _____.

5. People with alcoholism tend to have chronic _____ and fall frequently, increasing the likelihood of _____ _____ injury or other trauma.

6. The most immediate danger to an acutely intoxicated person is death of _____ _____ and/or aspiration of vomitus or stomach contents secondary to a suppressed _____ _____.

7. Shortly after injecting _____, a user will appear to pass out. However, the user is typically quite _____ and remains aware of what is being done or said.

8. Signs and symptoms of overdose with cardiac drugs may include _____, weakness or confusion, nausea and vomiting, _____ _____, headache, and difficulty _____.

9. Treatment of carbon monoxide (CO) _____ in the field is aimed at providing the highest concentration of _____ possible to attempt to displace CO molecules from the _____.

10. Acids tend to be more _____-_____ than _____, and so they are often diluted relatively quickly. With _____, it is more important to keep water continually flowing because it usually takes much longer to rinse away an alkali.

11. The most dangerous drugs that increase sexual gratification include erectile dysfunction medications such as _____, which are contraindicated for patients who take _____ for cardiac problems. Their use by people taking nitrites may result in severe _____ or total cardiovascular collapse.

12. Long-term _____ abuse can lead to permanent loss of mental function as evidenced by a variety of neuropathies, such as loss of _____, loss of fine motor _____, balance and _____ disorders, and occasionally _____.

13. Hydrocarbon products cause _____ _____, which results in severe abdominal _____, diarrhea, and belching. At the other end of the spectrum, just a single hydrocarbon substance exposure may cause life-threatening _____ and on occasion, sudden _____.

14. With a serious toxic exposure of _____ _____, be alert for ventricular _____, hypotension, respiratory _____, QT prolongation on the ECG, and _____.

15. When taken in toxic levels, _____ _____ inhibitors can be lethal because they can produce _____, metabolic _____, and rhabdomyolysis.

Identify

In the following case studies, identify the appropriate toxidrome and list two drugs associated with it.

1. You arrive on scene to find a 22-year-old woman who appears confused, has a blood pressure of 88/60 mm Hg, is slurring her speech, and is somewhat sleepy.
   a. Identify the appropriate toxidrome:

   _____

   b. Name two drugs that may fit this toxidrome.
      (1) _____
      (2) _____

2. Your advanced life support (ALS) ambulance arrives on scene at the request of law enforcement for a very agitated 42-year-old man. He won't stop talking and is paranoid.
   a. Identify the appropriate toxidrome:

   _____

   b. Name two drugs that may fit this toxidrome.
      (1) _____
      (2) _____

In the following case studies, identify the possible causative agent based on the presenting symptoms.

3. On arrival, you discover a 16-year-old boy with severe nausea and vomiting. You begin assessing the patient and immediately notice an odor that appears to be alcohol.

   _____

4. You are dispatched to a "delta" response (high priority) for a patient seizing. On arrival, you discover a 56-year-old man who is actively seizing and has snoring respirations. Family members state the patient has been recently depressed and withdrawn.

   _____

Ambulance Calls

The following case scenarios provide an opportunity to explore the concerns associated with patient management and paramedic care. Read each scenario, and then answer each question.

1. You are called to a somewhat rundown apartment building where the police have forcibly entered an apartment after neighbors reported that the occupant of the apartment has not been seen for a few days and has not answered his telephone. Inside, you find a man who looks to be about 30 years old lying unconscious on a sofa in the living room. Some neighbors are milling around, giving information to the police officers.

   a. List six questions you would ask the neighbors about the patient.

   (1) _____

   (2) _____

   (3) _____

   (4) _____

   (5) _____

   (6) _____

   b. Besides the neighbors, what other sources of information might be present? What places in the apartment would you check? What would you be looking for?

   (1) _____

   (2) _____

   (3) _____

   c. When you examine the patient, you detect the following findings. For each finding listed, indicate its possible diagnostic significance.

Finding	Possible Diagnostic Significance
Cold, dry skin	
Pulse = 110 beats/min, thready	
Blood pressure = 90/60 mm Hg	
Respirations = 12 breaths/min and shallow	
Pupils dilated and not reactive to light	
Breath smells of alcohol (ETOH)	
Left arm is cold and blue	

   d. In assessing this patient's level of consciousness, you find the following:
   - He does not open his eyes.
   - His arms flex when you pinch his leg.
   - He does not make any sound in response to your calling his name or pinching him.

   In view of those findings, he is best described as which of the following?

   (1) Drowsy

   (2) Lethargic

   (3) Comatose

   (4) Stuporous

   (5) Obtunded

e. List in order the steps in managing this patient.

(1) _____

(2) _____

(3) _____

(4) _____

(5) _____

(6) _____

(7) _____

(8) _____

(9) _____

2. You are called to the home of a frantic young couple who discovered their 3-year-old happily consuming the contents of a bottle from the cleaning cupboard. List five questions you would ask in taking the history of the incident.

a. _____

b. _____

c. _____

d. _____

e. _____

3. A middle-aged man is found unconscious in his garage. He has left a suicide note on the car windshield, but the hood of the car is cold, so you are reasonably sure the engine has not been run recently. List five things to which you would give particular attention in the physical examination of this patient.

a. _____

b. _____

c. _____

d. _____

e. _____

4. A 15-year-old boy swallowed about 20 of his father's tricyclic antidepressant pills in a suicide gesture after a family argument. You arrive at the scene, some 30 minutes distant from the nearest hospital, about 15 minutes after the ingestion. In a telephone consultation, Poison Control advises you to administer activated charcoal and monitor the airway and ECG for dysrhythmias. The boy is alert, and vital signs are all within normal limits at this point.

a. What is the purpose of giving activated charcoal? That is, what is the therapeutic effect?

_____

b. List three poisonings in which activated charcoal is contraindicated.

(1) _____

(2) _____

(3) _____

c. What is the dosage of activated charcoal for this patient?

_____

    d. List in order the steps in treating this patient.

        (1) _____

        (2) _____

        (3) _____

        (4) _____

        (5) _____

5. A 35-year-old man ingested "about a tablespoon" of drain buildup remover (Drano) crystals 10 to 15 minutes before your arrival. He is fully alert and complaining of severe pain in his throat and chest. His lips and mouth are very red, and there are still crystals sticking to the mucous membranes in his mouth.

    a. List the steps in treating this patient.

        (1) _____

        (2) _____

        (3) _____

        (4) _____

6. You are summoned to a location near the railway tracks where the local "down-and-outs" gather. A police officer at the scene gestures you toward two of the group members congregated there. "They looked in pretty bad shape," he says, "so I thought I'd better call EMS."

"Been drinking real bad stuff," one of the group chimes in. "Told 'em to stay away from that rotgut—you can go blind from drinkin' stuff like that."

The first patient is in severe respiratory distress. He says he hasn't had a drink since the previous day, when he drank "some stuff they left lying around the gas station—I don't know what it was—tasted pretty good." He says he threw up a few times about 6 hours after that. On physical examination, the patient is alert. There is no alcohol odor on his breath. His vital signs are a pulse of 120 beats/min and regular, respirations of 36 breaths/min and noisy, and blood pressure of 180/105 mm Hg. The pupils are midposition, equal, and reactive to light. The gag reflex is present. The chest is full of crackles.

    a. What do you think is this patient's problem?

    _____

    b. List the steps you would take in managing this patient.

        (1) _____

        (2) _____

        (3) _____

        (4) _____

        (5) _____

        (6) _____

The second patient appears intoxicated. His speech is slurred, and he can scarcely walk. "Why ish it shnowing in Sheptember?" he mumbles. His breath smells of alcohol. His pulse is 108 beats/min and regular, his respirations are 30 breaths/min and deep, and his blood pressure is 140/86 mm Hg. There is no evidence of head injury. The pupils are about 6 mm and equal and react sluggishly to light. The gag reflex is present. The chest is clear. The abdomen is very tender and nearly rigid to palpation.

    c. What do you think is this patient's problem?

    _____

    d. List the steps you would take in managing this patient.

      (1) _____

      (2) _____

      (3) _____

      (4) _____

      (5) _____

      (6) _____

7. You are called to the home of a 46-year-old woman who swallowed an unknown quantity of silver polish in a suicide attempt. A bevy of agitated family members is hovering around her, all talking at once. As far as you can determine, the ingestion took place sometime during the past hour. While your partner telephones Poison Control for a rundown on the exact composition of that brand of silver polish, you examine the patient. You find her very confused and sleepy. There is a funny smell on her breath that you can't quite place—a little like almonds? The skin is flushed. The pulse is 132 beats/min and thready, respirations are 32 breaths/min and labored, and blood pressure is 90/64 mm Hg.

    a. What do you think is this patient's problem?

    _____

    b. What drug is indicated to treat this problem to "buy time" until you reach the emergency department?

    _____

    c. How is it given?

    _____

    d. What side effects should you anticipate?

    _____

    e. List the steps you would take in managing this patient.

      (1) _____

      (2) _____

      (3) _____

      (4) _____

      (5) _____

      (6) _____

      (7) _____

8. You are staying with friends at their cabin in the mountains for a nice ski weekend. Your host takes considerable pride in the cabin, which he built himself. "Snug as a bug in a rug," he says. "Not a draft in the place." You have to admit that he did a good insulation job and that the place is nice and cozy with the Franklin stove in the corner.

    When you get up the next morning, your friend's wife, asks, "Will you have a look at the baby? She's sick with something. She's been throwing up all morning." You don't know much about babies, and you don't feel so hot yourself, but you take a look at the baby. You find her pale and dehydrated, with a bounding pulse but no fever. As you are examining her, she has a grand mal seizure. "It must be the flu," says the baby's mother, "because I'm coming down with something, too. I feel real sick to my stomach." Meanwhile, your friend, just getting up, says, "Boy, do I have a headache; it's like Niagara Falls roaring through my skull."

    a. What do you think is the baby's problem?

    _____

b. What steps should you take in this situation?

(1) _____

(2) _____

(3) _____

(4) _____

(5) _____

(6) _____

(7) _____

9. One fine Sunday afternoon, you are called to a suburban home for a "possible heart attack." On arrival, you find a middle-aged man, clad in shorts and a T-shirt, sprawled out on the sofa in the living room. "I don't know what happened," he says. "I was just sitting outside on the lawn, and I started to feel real dizzy and sick to my stomach, and real weak. And there's this tight feeling in my chest—"

"It's that stuff Mr. Dimbledirt was spraying," his wife chimes in. "I'm sure of it. Why he has to spray his precious roses precisely when we're sitting in the garden is beyond me."

While you begin your assessment of the patient, your partner goes next door to talk with Mr. Dimbledirt. You find the patient in considerable distress. His skin is pale and diaphoretic. His vital signs are a pulse of 42 beats/min and regular, respirations are 28 breaths/min and labored, and blood pressure is 140/80 mm Hg. The pupils are very constricted. The patient is salivating profusely, and his breath smells like garlic. The neck veins are flat. The chest is full of wheezes. As you are completing the examination, your partner returns carrying a bottle labeled "parathion."

a. What do you think is this patient's problem?

_____

b. What drug is used to treat this problem?

_____

c. What is the correct dosage in this situation?

_____

d. List all the steps in treating this patient.

(1) _____

(2) _____

(3) _____

(4) _____

(5) _____

(6) _____

(7) _____

(8) _____

(9) _____

10. You are called to a local junior high school where a 12-year-old boy had a grand mal seizure. The school nurse, who is kneeling on the floor of the boys' restroom beside the boy, tells you that the boy has no known seizure history. The boy is unconscious but can be roused by painful stimuli. You cannot find any abnormalities on physical examination save for signs that he indeed just had a seizure (slight bleeding of the tongue, incontinence). A search of his pockets, however, reveals a few small bottles of typewriter correction fluid. What steps will you take in managing this patient?

a. _____

b. _____

c. _____

d. _____

e. _____

Complete the Patient Care Report (PCR)

Reread the ninth incident scenario in the Ambulance Calls section, and then complete the following PCR.

EMS Patient Care Report (PCR)				
Date:	Incident No.:	Nature of Call:		Location:
Dispatched:	En Route:	At Scene:	Transport:	At Hospital:	In Service:

Patient Information	
Age: Sex: Weight (in kg [lb]):	Allergies: Medications: Past Medical History: Chief Complaint:

Vital Signs				
Time:	BP:	Pulse:	Respirations:	SpO$_2$:
Time:	BP:	Pulse:	Respirations:	SpO$_2$:
Time:	BP:	Pulse:	Respirations:	SpO$_2$:

EMS Treatment (circle all that apply)				
Oxygen @ _____ L/min via (circle one): NC NRM Bag-Mask Device	Assisted Ventilation	Airway Adjunct		CPR
Defibrillation	Bleeding Control	Bandaging	Splinting	Other

Narrative

True/False

If you believe the statement to be more true than false, write the letter "T" in the space provided. If you believe the statement to be more false than true, write the letter "F."

_____ **1.** Your call to the Poison Control Center helps the center collect data on poisonings in your region. These data may be analyzed to help detect trends, spot developing public health problems, and evaluate current treatment protocols for different poisonings.

_____ **2.** Oxygen has a greater affinity than carbon monoxide (CO) to bind to hemoglobin on the red blood cells.

_____ **3.** There is an increasing trend of patients attempting suicide by mixing certain household chemicals while in their parked vehicle, which can be very dangerous to emergency response personnel.

_____ **4.** The major toxidromes are produced by stimulants, narcotics, cholinergics, anticholinergics, sympathomimetics, sedatives, and hypnotics.

_____ **5.** The more frequently consumption of alcohol takes place, the greater the irritation of the digestive system.

_____ **6.** The severity of alcohol withdrawal can vary according to the length and intensity of the patient's alcoholism. Minor withdrawal is characterized by restlessness, anxiousness, sleeping problems, agitation, and tremors.

_____ **7.** Prolonged heavy use of alcohol may cause ulcers, hiatal hernias, and cancers throughout the digestive tract.

_____ **8.** In a poisoning, the container and the remaining contents should never be taken with the patient to the hospital for fear of contaminating the emergency department.

_____ **9.** If the person decides to quit using stimulants, the likelihood that he or she will succeed over the long term is virtually nil. Sadly, the only way out of methamphetamine or cocaine addiction is often an early death.

_____ **10.** Patients who take lithium and nonsteroidal anti-inflammatory drugs (NSAIDs) have slowed renal clearance of the lithium, increasing the likelihood that they will inadvertently reach a toxic lithium level.

_____ **11.** Most patients who have swallowed caustic substances present with severe respiratory distress and pain in the mouth, throat, or chest.

_____ **12.** The primary goals when dealing with a patient who has inhaled hydrocarbons are to remove the patient from the noxious environment, give high-concentration supplemental oxygen, and promptly transport to the appropriate facility.

_____ **13.** When tricyclic antidepressants exert their toxic effects, the most common cause of death is cardiac dysrhythmia.

_____ **14.** Field treatment of a salicylate overdose should include the "universal antidote."

Short Answer

Complete this section with short written answers using the space provided.

1. List 10 medical problems to which alcoholics are particularly susceptible.

a. _____

b. _____

c. _____

d. _____

e. _____

f. _____

g. _____

h. _____

i. _____

j. _____

Fill-in-the-Table

Fill in the missing parts of the table.

1. Although it is advisable to consult Poison Control for definitive identification of any ingested substance, it is nonetheless worthwhile to have a general knowledge of the categories of poisons and some of the more commonly encountered examples of each category. Fill in the following table with examples of each type of poison mentioned.

Common Poisons	
Type of Poison	**Examples**
Strong acid	
Strong alkali	
Hydrocarbons	
Toxic plants	

2. Fill in the amount of time it takes for the four stages of acetaminophen toxicity.

Signs and Symptoms of Acetaminophen Toxicity		
Stage	**Time Frame**	**Signs and Symptoms**
I		Nausea, vomiting, loss of appetite, pallor, malaise
II		Right upper quadrant abdominal pain; abdomen tender to palpation
III		Metabolic acidosis, renal failure, coagulopathies, recurring GI symptoms
IV		Recovery slowly begins, or liver failure progresses and the patient dies

Psychiatric Emergencies

Matching

Part I

Match each of the descriptions in the left column to the appropriate item in the right column.

_____ 1. The basic activities a person usually accomplishes during a normal day, such as eating, dressing, and washing.

_____ 2. The outward expression of a person's inner feelings (happy, sad, angry, fearful, withdrawn).

_____ 3. An eating disorder in which a person diets by exerting extraordinary control over his or her eating, and loses weight to the point of jeopardizing his or her health or life.

_____ 4. Results of some antipsychotic medications that include side effects similar to atropine, resulting in dry mouth, blurred vision, urinary retention, and cardiac dysfunction.

_____ 5. The point at which a person's reactions to events interfere with the activities of daily living; becomes a psychiatric emergency when it cause a major life interruption, such as attempted suicide.

_____ 6. A disorder characterized by disordered images of self, impulsive and unpredictable behavior, marked shifts in mood, and instability in relationships with others.

_____ 7. Lacking expression or movement, or appearing rigid.

_____ 8. Repetitive actions carried out to relieve the anxiety of obsessive thoughts.

_____ 9. Pointing out something of interest in the patient's conversation or behavior, thereby directing the patient's attention to something he or she may have been unaware of.

_____ 10. An acute confusional state, characterized by global impairment of thinking, perception, judgment, and memory.

_____ 11. The slow onset of progressive disorientation, shortened attention span, and loss of cognitive function.

_____ 12. A condition in which a person is characterized by uncontrolled and disconnected thought, is usually incoherent or rambling in speech, and may or may not be oriented to person or place.

_____ 13. Meaningless echoing of the interviewer's words by the patient.

_____ 14. The absence of emotion; appearing to feel no emotion at all.

_____ 15. A disorder in which a person worries about everything for no particular reason, or the worrying is unproductive and the person cannot decide what to do about an upcoming situation.

_____ 16. A condition in which a person lacks the ability to resist a temptation or cannot stop acting on a drive.

A. Generalized anxiety disorder (GAD)

B. Echolalia

C. Dementia

D. Confrontation

E. Catatonic

F. Behavioral emergency

G. Anorexia nervosa

H. Activities of daily living (ADLs)

I. Affect

J. Atropine-like effects

K. Borderline personality disorder

L. Compulsions

M. Delirium

N. Disorganization

O. Flat affect

P. Impulse control disorder

Part II

For each of the following signs and symptoms, indicate whether it is:

O: More typical of organic brain syndrome

P: More typical of psychiatric illness

B: Apt to be seen in both organic and psychiatric illnesses

_____ **1.** Obsessional thinking

_____ **2.** Flat affect

_____ **3.** Delirium

_____ **4.** Distractibility

_____ **5.** Compulsions

_____ **6.** Visual hallucinations

_____ **7.** Confabulation

_____ **8.** Anxiety

_____ **9.** Coma

_____ **10.** Circumstantial thinking

Part III

For each of the psychiatric signs and symptoms listed, indicate whether it is a disturbance of:

A. Consciousness
B. Motor activity
C. Speech
D. Thinking
E. Affect or mood
F. Memory
G. Orientation
H. Perception

_____ **1.** The patient cannot name three objects that you listed out loud 5 minutes earlier.

_____ **2.** The patient is pacing back and forth.

_____ **3.** The patient smiles pleasantly as he tells you that his daughter was run over by a truck.

_____ **4.** The patient keeps shifting his attention from you to the television or to the window.

_____ **5.** The patient seems to be having a conversation with an invisible friend.

_____ **6.** The patient thinks the current year is 1931.

_____ **7.** The patient thinks he is Albert Einstein.

_____ **8.** The patient tells you, "All the world is my kingdumbell and I'm the pellmellery scullop."

_____ **9.** The patient is terrified of spiders.

_____ **10.** The patient puts two fingers to his forehead in a salute every time he finishes speaking.

_____ **11.** The patient complains of palpitations, nausea, tightness in his chest, and numbness around his lips.

_____ **12.** The patient thinks that the sound of the wind is someone calling his name.

Multiple Choice

Read each item carefully, and then select the best response.

1. In an acute behavioral emergency, which of the following causes is easiest for paramedics to treat?
   A. Hypoglycemia
   B. Severe infections
   C. Drug and alcohol intoxications
   D. Dementia

2. Pressured speech, neologisms, echolalia, and mutism are examples of:
   A. disorders of thinking.
   B. disorders of mood and affect.
   C. disorders of motor activity.
   D. disorders of speech.

3. During the primary assessment of patients with behavioral disorders, it is important for a paramedic to:
   A. hurry the call; you can't really assist the patient.
   B. assess the patient only en route to the hospital.
   C. convey that you have the time and concern.
   D. not gain consent because consent is never required.

4. The mental status exam includes:
   A. perception.
   B. affect and mood.
   C. memory.
   D. All of the above

5. Guilt, depressed appetite, sleep disturbances, lack of interest, low energy, and suicidal thoughts are diagnostic features of:
   A. depression.
   B. anxiety.
   C. mood disorders.
   D. manic-depressive illness.

6. Paramedics always need to take scene safety seriously. The following are risk factors for violence, EXCEPT:
   A. posture.
   B. speech.
   C. motor activity.
   D. prescription medication.

7. Restraining a violent patient should involve:
   A. a police presence.
   B. a Reeves stretcher.
   C. lots of duct tape.
   D. no more than two paramedics.

8. A psychiatric emergency exists when a patient:
   A. threatens to harm himself or herself.
   B. threatens to harm other people.
   C. is delusional.
   D. All of the above

9. All of the following drugs may sometimes cause a psychotic state, EXCEPT:
   A. steroids.
   B. Wellbutrin (bupropion).
   C. digitalis.
   D. LSD and PCP.

10. Which of the following is considered a disturbance of behavior?
    A. Anxiety disorder
    B. Organic brain syndrome
    C. Head injury
    D. Stroke

11. The following are appropriate guidelines for the care of any patient with a psychiatric problem, EXCEPT:
    A. being as calm and direct as possible.
    B. asking all the other disruptive family members to participate in the interview.
    C. maintaining a nonjudgmental attitude.
    D. developing a plan of action.

12. A patient who has been diagnosed as having bipolar disorder, manic behavior, and depression is categorized with what type of psychiatric disorder?
    A. Cognitive disorder
    B. Neurotic disorder
    C. Mood disorder
    D. Somatoform disorder

Fill-in-the-Blank

Read each item carefully, and then complete the statement by filling in the missing word(s).

1. The causes of abnormal behavior can be classified into four broad categories: (1) causes that are _____ or _____ in nature, (2) causes resulting from a person's _____, (3) causes resulting from acute _____ or _____, and (4) causes that are _____-_____.

2. Identify yourself _____. Tell the patient who you are and what you are trying to do. If the patient is _____ or _____, you may have to explain yourself at _____ intervals.

3. Overwhelming feelings of _____ and _____ characterize panic disorder.

4. There are two major types of eating disorders: _____ _____ and _____ _____.

5. _____, _____, and _____ are common trade names for tricyclic antidepressants.

6. One potential side effect of MAO inhibitors when taken by patients with a history of depression would be _____.

7. _____ is the third leading cause of death among 15- to 24-year-olds and the second leading cause of death among the 25- to 44-year age group.

8. One in _____ people will be affected by _____ in their lifetimes.

Identify

List the behavioral medications in the following scenarios.

1. You respond to a domestic dispute. When you arrive on scene, you are told by law enforcement that the scene is secure and safe. You and your partner proceed inside. The patient's wife is holding a bag of the patient's medications. The patient denies any complaint and simply states that he has a cardiac history and takes furosemide (Lasix) and digoxin. While you calm the patient, your partner reviews the bag of medications. He finds the furosemide and digoxin along with glyburide, fluoxetine (Prozac), and diazepam (Valium).

   _____

   _____

2. You are called to an outpatient mental health clinic for a patient requiring voluntary in-patient hospitalization. The patient has a history of hypercholesterolemia and depression. The patient is taking over-the-counter omega-3 and garlic. The patient is on the following prescription medications: phenelzine (Nardil), bupropion (Wellbutrin), simvastatin (Zocor), and atorvastatin (Lipitor).

   _____

   _____

3. You receive an emergency call for a "psychotic" patient. As you evaluate your patient, you review her medication list and discover the following prescriptions: tamoxifen, niacin (Niaspan), fluticasone/salmeterol inhaled (Advair), aripiprazole (Abilify), and famotidine (Pepcid).

   _____

   _____

Ambulance Calls

The following case scenarios provide an opportunity to explore the concerns associated with patient management and paramedic care. Read each scenario, and then answer each question.

1. The following is the transcript of an interview between an inexperienced paramedic and a disturbed patient. The interview illustrates several errors in approach. Read through the interview. Then, list the points in the interview that you think could have been handled or phrased in a better way.

   Paramedic (entering an apartment in which there is a lot of noise and confusion): Okay, which one of you is the patient?

(Someone points to a young woman crouching in a corner, crying.)

Paramedic (approaching the woman and standing in front of her): Now, dearie, what's the trouble?

(Patient continues crying.)

Paramedic: Now come on, get hold of yourself. Big girls don't cry.

Patient (sobbing): Everything's just so hopeless.

Paramedic: Things are never hopeless. You're probably just making a mountain out of a molehill, and by tomorrow you'll wonder what you were making such a big fuss about.

(Patient sits crying to herself.)

Paramedic: Well, if you don't want to tell me what's wrong, maybe one of your friends here can tell me. Is there anyone here who can tell me what's going on?

(Immediately the noise and confusion resume, as everyone starts talking at once. The patient huddles farther into the corner.)

List the things you think were done incorrectly in this interview, including errors of omission and errors of commission.

a. _____

b. _____

c. _____

d. _____

e. _____

f. _____

g. _____

h. _____

2. You are called to a downtown apartment building for a "sick man." Reaching the corridor outside the man's apartment, you are intercepted by a neighbor who had called for the ambulance. "I feel a little silly troubling you folks," she says, "but Mr. Crosby next door—he's just not himself lately—doesn't even poke his head out of that apartment. Doesn't want to see no one. He just says, 'Go away,' when I knock. So I got to worrying. I mean, I don't even think he's got himself anything to eat in there."

"Who's there?" someone finally says.

"We're paramedics, from the city ambulance service."

"Well, what do you want with me?"

"We just want to talk with you a bit," you say. "There are folks worried about you."

It takes some persuading, but finally Mr. Crosby opens the door and admits you to his apartment. The place is in complete disarray, and it appears as if no one has washed a dish or tidied up in months. Here and there you note an empty liquor bottle lying on the floor.

"So what do you want?" Mr. Crosby asks listlessly.

a. Where would you go from here? List some of the questions you would ask Mr. Crosby at this point.

_____

_____

_____

_____

b. In the course of your interview with Mr. Crosby, which seems to go very slowly, you learn that he is a 62-year-old widower. He has one son and says, "I never hear from him." He used to be a watchmaker, "but I haven't been worth anything since I got this arthritis 10 years ago." In response to your query about why he has stopped going out of the apartment, he says, "What's there to go out for? Anyway, I don't have the energy to go rambling around the city."

"Don't you have to shop for food?" you ask.

"What for? I don't feel much like eating these days anyway."

This patient is showing clear symptoms of depression. List the symptoms of depression present in this case.

(1) _____

(2) _____

(3) _____

(4) _____

c. List four other symptoms or signs of depression.

(1) _____

(2) _____

(3) _____

(4) _____

d. List the risk factors for suicide present in this patient's history.

(1) _____

(2) _____

(3) _____

(4) _____

(5) _____

e. List four other risk factors for suicide.

(1) _____

(2) _____

(3) _____

(4) _____

f. List three questions you would ask to try to evaluate the patient's risk of suicide.

(1) _____

(2) _____

(3) _____

3. You are called to a downtown office building for a "possible heart attack." When you reach the building, you are escorted into an office by a harried-looking businessman. "It's my secretary," he says. "She's having some kind of cardiac attack." In the midst of a buzzing group of people, you see a woman who looks to be about 24 years old sitting wide-eyed and pale. People are fanning her with file folders and trying to get her to drink some water. You make your way through the crowd and ask the woman what her problem is.

"Can't breathe," she gasps. "Chest all tight (gasp). Feel like I'm going to pass out (gasp). Everything is unreal (gasp), like I'm dying (gasp)."

"Quick! Quick!" squeaks one of the bystanders. "Get her to the hospital!"

Ignoring the chorus demanding that you leave immediately for the hospital, you begin taking the woman's vital signs. Her pulse is 112 beats/min and regular, her respirations are 30 breaths/min and deep, and her blood pressure is 160/88 mm Hg. You notice that her skin is cold and sweaty and her hands are shaking.

a. What do you think is this patient's problem?

_____

b. What signs and symptoms led you to that conclusion?

(1) _____

(2) _____

(3) _____

(4) _____

(5) _____

(6) _____

(7) _____

c. Are there any other diagnoses you need to take into consideration? If so, what are they?

(1) _____

(2) _____

(3) _____

(4) _____

(5) _____

d. How will you manage this patient?

(1) _____

(2) _____

(3) _____

(4) _____

(5) _____

4. You and your partner are called to a downtown bar to see a man who has apparently become disruptive there. A police officer meets you at the entrance to the bar. "Listen," he says, "the barkeeper called us to deal with an unruly customer, but personally I think the guy's a psycho case—so I thought maybe you folks ought to take a look at him."

You enter the bar and find a well-dressed but disheveled man pacing rapidly up and down. "One week from today," he is announcing, "one week from today, I'll be one of the richest men in America. I'm putting together a business empire now that will rule Wall Street." He is talking a mile a minute, cracking jokes, and gesturing extravagantly. He catches sight of you and your partner and says, "Well, hello, fellas. Bartender, give these fine young people a drink, on me. They do a great public service. This country was built on public service, yes indeed it was. So give them a public service drink."

"You haven't paid for the drinks you already ordered," says the bartender.

"Listen, fathead, I said give these nice people a drink."

"Uh, sir," you break in, "we're not allowed to drink while on duty. And we thought maybe you'd like to take a little ride with us to the hospital."

"Hospital? What do I need to go to the hospital for? Never felt better in my life. By next week, I'll be able to buy the hospital, buy this bar too, buy the whole damned town."

The police officer says, "Maybe you ought to go with them, sir, just to get a checkup."

"Any of you puts a hand on me," replies the man, "I'll sue the whole lot of you. Assault. Battery. False imprisonment. I'll sue you for the whole lot, and let me tell you, you don't want to tangle with my team of lawyers. Best legal talent in the country. You wouldn't stand a chance."

a. What do you think is this man's problem?

_____

b. What symptoms and signs led you to that conclusion?

(1) _____

(2) _____

(3) _____

(4) _____

c. How will you manage this patient?

_____

_____

5. You are called to a downtown street corner where several police officers are standing around apparently trying to talk to a somewhat wild-eyed man who could be anywhere from 55 to 75 years old. He is dressed in about six layers of tattered clothes and wearing a naval officer's cap. He clearly hasn't had a bath, shave, or haircut in weeks. "He was just walking down the middle of Main Street," says one of the police officers, "as if he didn't even notice the traffic—and all those horns blowing, people screeching on their brakes."

You introduce yourself to the man and ask whether you can be of help. He mumbles something that sounds like, "Dogs and cats."

"Sorry," you say, "I didn't quite catch what you said."

"Salt and pepper," he says. "Black and blue, I didn't, don't 'ya know, I didn't."

The police officer gives you a meaningful look.

How will you manage this case?

_____

_____

_____

_____

6. A middle-aged woman calls for an ambulance because "my son is acting real strange." When you arrive at the designated address, the woman greets you at the door. She tells you that her 20-year-old son won't come out of his room. He's been in there for 2 days now. Sometimes she hears him talking to someone, but there isn't anyone else there. "I'm sure it's all that karate stuff," she says. "It just went to his head, made him crazy, all that black belt business."

You go up to the son's room and knock on the door.

"You're not going to get me," says a voice from the other side of the door. "You won't take me alive."

"Sir, we're paramedics. We've just come to talk with you."

"You can't fool me. I know you're from the FBI. Well, you'll have to shoot me to take me."

You try the door and find it's unlocked. Inside, a young man clothed in karate garb is sitting in an armchair, gripping the armrests.

You introduce yourselves again. The patient looks away.

"You won't take me alive," he says again in a monotone. He looks suddenly toward the wall. "I know, I know," he says to the wall.

"Who are you talking to?" you ask.

He looks startled. "The voices said you would come. They killed John Lennon, and the FBI is after me. The voices said not to let you take me alive."

  a. This patient is showing signs of:

    (1) a panic attack.

    (2) psychosis.

    (3) depression.

    (4) mania.

    (5) disorganization.

  b. Are there any indications that he might become violent?

_____

  c. If so, what are four indications?

    (1) _____

    (2) _____

    (3) _____

    (4) _____

  d. How will you manage this case?

_____

_____

_____

_____

_____

_____

True/False

If you believe the statement to be more true than false, write the letter "T" in the space provided. If you believe the statement to be more false than true, write the letter "F."

_____ **1.** The most important thing a paramedic can do to help a disturbed patient is to remain calm and steady.

_____ **2.** There should be a maximum sense of urgency in evacuating a disturbed patient to the hospital because there is nothing that can be done to help the patient in the field.

_____ **3.** It is essential to correct a patient's misinterpretations of reality.

_____ **4.** The disturbed patient should be reassured that everything will turn out all right.

_____ **5.** The paramedic should remain with the disturbed patient at all times until the emergency department staff takes over the patient's care.

_____ **6.** Police intervention is usually required to transport a disturbed patient against his or her will.

Short Answer

Complete this section with short written answers using the space provided.

1. Certain situations have a higher potential for violence than others do. List three scenarios that should activate the paramedic's "nose for danger."

   a. _____

   b. _____

   c. _____

2. List four diagnostic groups that would activate the paramedic's "nose for danger."

   a. _____

   b. _____

   c. _____

   d. _____

Fill-in-the-Table

Fill in the missing parts of the table with the conditions and substances that can produce psychotic symptoms.

Selected Disease States That May Produce Psychotic Symptoms	
Disease State	**Psychotic Symptoms**
	Drug-induced psychoses, especially from: • Digitalis • Steroids • Disulfiram • Amphetamines • LSD, PCP, and other psychedelics Nutrition disorders: • Alcohol abuse • Vitamin deficiencies Poisoning with bromide or other heavy metals Kidney failure Liver failure
	Syphilis Parasites Viral encephalitis (eg, after measles) Brain abscess
	Seizure disorders (especially temporal lobe seizures) Primary and metastatic tumors of the brain Dementia Stroke Closed head injury
	Low cardiac output (eg, in heart failure)
	Thyroid hyperfunction (thyrotoxicosis) Adrenal hyperfunction (Cushing syndrome)
	Electrolyte imbalances (eg, after severe diarrhea) Hypoglycemia Diabetic ketoacidosis

Skill Drills

Test your knowledge of skill drills by placing the following photos in the correct order. Number the first step "1," the second step "2," etc.

1. Restraining a Patient

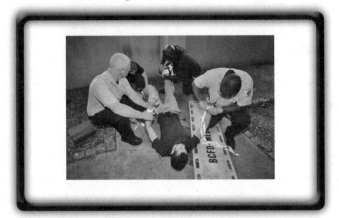

_____ On the direction of the team leader, move together toward the patient. Each team member should grasp the assigned body part and carefully, with the least amount of force, bring the patient to the ground. Carefully place the patient on the stretcher or carrying device in a face-up position.

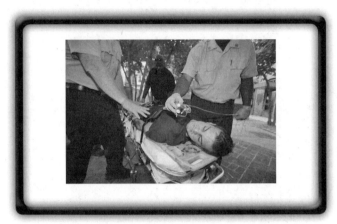

_____ If the patient is spitting, place an oxygen mask or surgical mask on his or her face.

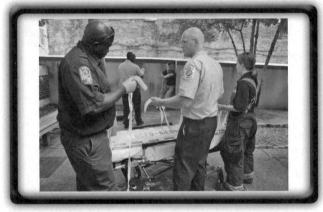

_____ Assemble four or five rescuers and have the stretcher or carrying device and soft restraints nearby. Designate a leader. Assign positions to each team member: four extremities and the head.

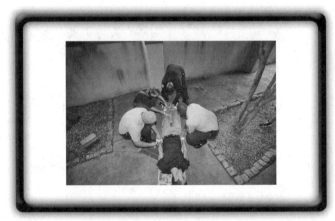

_____ Consider tying the patient with soft restraints at each wrist and ankle as well as the chest and pelvis with sheets.

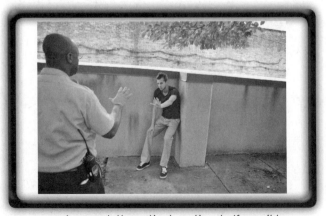

_____ Approach the patient cautiously. If possible, corner the patient in a safe area.

Trauma Systems and Mechanism of Injury

Matching

Part I

For each of the injuries listed in the left column, indicate which incident from the right column it is likely to be associated with. (*Note:* Some injuries may be associated with more than one type of mechanism.)

_____ 1. "Whiplash" injury

_____ 2. Multiple rib fractures

_____ 3. Fracture of the tibia/fibula

_____ 4. Fracture of the patella

_____ 5. Fracture of the humerus

_____ 6. Skull fracture

_____ 7. Laryngeal fracture

_____ 8. Flail chest

_____ 9. Pelvic fracture

_____ 10. Cervical spine injury

A. Head-on collision (unrestrained driver)

B. Lateral impact (unrestrained front seat passenger)

C. Rear-impact collision (unrestrained driver)

D. Pedestrian struck by an oncoming car

Part II

Match each of the terms in the left column to the appropriate definition in the right column.

_____ 1. Acceleration

_____ 2. Arterial air embolism

_____ 3. Barometric energy

_____ 4. Blast front

_____ 5. Brisance

_____ 6. Chemical energy

_____ 7. Electrical energy

_____ 8. Exit wound

_____ 9. Implosion

_____ 10. Kinetic energy

_____ 11. Law of conservation of energy

A. A score that relates to the likelihood of patient survival with the exception of a severe head injury. It is calculated on a scale from 1 to 16, with 16 being the best possible score.

B. A scoring system used for patients with head trauma.

C. The path of crushed tissue produced by a missile traversing part of the body.

D. The principle that a body at rest will remain at rest unless acted on by an outside force.

E. The way in which a traumatic injury occurs; the force that acts on the body to cause damage.

F. The energy associated with bodies in motion, expressed mathematically as half the mass times the square of the velocity.

G. The point at which a penetrating object leaves the body, which may or may not be in a straight line from the entry wound.

H. The energy released as a result of a chemical reaction.

I. The leading edge of the shock wave.

J. Air bubbles in the arterial blood vessels.

K. The rate of change in velocity; speeding up.

_____ **12.** Mechanism of injury (MOI)

_____ **13.** Multisystem trauma

_____ **14.** Newton's first law of motion

_____ **15.** Pathway expansion

_____ **16.** Permanent cavity

_____ **17.** Potential energy

_____ **18.** Revised Trauma Score (RTS)

_____ **19.** Spalling

_____ **20.** Trauma score

L. The energy that results from sudden changes in pressure as may occur in a diving accident or sudden decompression in an airplane.

M. The shattering effect of a shock wave and its ability to cause disruption of tissues and structures.

N. The energy delivered in the form of high voltage.

O. A bursting inward.

P. The principle that energy can be neither created nor destroyed; it can only change form.

Q. Trauma caused by generalized mechanisms that affect numerous body systems.

R. The tissue displacement that occurs as a result of low-displacement shock waves that travel at the speed of sound in tissue.

S. The amount of energy stored in an object—the product of mass, gravity, and height—that is converted into kinetic energy and results in injury, such as from a fall.

T. Delaminating or breaking off into chips and pieces.

Multiple Choice

Read each item carefully, and then select the best response.

1. Which of the following is NOT a criterion for referral to a regional trauma center?
   A. 45-year-old patient restrained in a low-speed auto crash
   B. Pelvic fracture
   C. Motorcycle crash > 20 mph
   D. A pregnant patient

2. The "platinum 10 minutes" refers to the:
   A. amount of time taken to extricate a patient from a motor vehicle crash.
   B. total response time to a traumatic incident.
   C. goal of the maximum time spent at a scene for a critical trauma patient.
   D. time deciding on your "transport decision."

3. Which of the following is NOT considered one of the top five causes of trauma deaths?
   A. Falls
   B. Cold injuries
   C. Motor vehicle collisions
   D. Drownings

4. Pediatric pedestrian injuries are different from adult pedestrian injuries because:
   A. the skulls of children are not fused, which allows for energy absorption.
   B. children are shorter, so they are more likely to be run over by the vehicle.
   C. children are more likely to "fly over" the vehicle.
   D. the bumper is more likely to strike the femur rather than the lower extremities.

5. The following is important information to provide to the trauma team, EXCEPT:
   A. the name of the street gang.
   B. the range at which the firearm was fired.
   C. the kind of bullet or projectile.
   D. the type of weapon used.

6. Blast injuries may also be seen in which of the following scenarios?
   A. Mining mishaps
   B. Chemical plants
   C. Terrorist activities
   D. All of the above

7. The following are factors in the seriousness of firearms injuries, EXCEPT:
   A. the type of tissue penetrated.
   B. missile velocity.
   C. fragmentation.
   D. the firearm manufacturer.

8. Which of the following is another term for mechanical energy?
   A. Kinetic energy
   B. Barometric energy
   C. Electrical energy
   D. Chemical energy

9. Criteria for transport of an adult patient to a trauma center as defined by the American College of Surgeons and Centers for Disease Control and Prevention include all of the following, EXCEPT:
   A. Glasgow Coma Scale score ≤ 13.
   B. amputation proximal to the wrist or ankle.
   C. ejection from an automobile.
   D. falls > 10 feet.

10. Facial injuries, pulmonary contusion, flail chest, ruptured aorta, and fractured sternum are examples of which of the following?
   A. "Ring" of chest injuries
   B. Lateral impacts
   C. Head-on crashes
   D. "Down and under pathway"

Labeling

Label the following diagram with the correct mechanisms of blast injuries.

A. _____

B. _____

C. _____

Fill-in-the-Blank

Read each item carefully, and then complete the statement by filling in the missing word(s).

1. The speed, duration, and pressure of the shock wave from an explosion are affected by the following:

   a. _____

   b. _____

   c. _____

   d. _____

2. The severity of a stab wound depends on the _____ area involved, depth of _____, blade length, and angle of penetration.

3. _____ _____ _____ is one of the most concerning of pulmonary blast injuries.

4. Severity of injuries in falls from heights depend on the following factors:

   a. _____

   b. _____

   c. _____

   d. _____

   e. _____

5. Specific injuries associated with seat belt use include _____ fractures and _____ sprains.

Identify

In the following case studies, list the mechanism of injury, chief complaint, vital signs, and pertinent negatives.

1. You receive a call while working in a paramedic first response vehicle for a motor vehicle crash. On arrival you find two patients who are out of the vehicle and standing along the roadside. You notice that the vehicle appears to have rolled over onto its side. No other patients are involved, and the scene is deemed safe for patient contact and treatment. One occupant denies any complaint and doesn't want anything to do with EMS. The other patient is holding his right forearm and complains of neck pain. The injured occupant states that he had his seat belt on. You notice that the air bag deployed. The injured man denies loss of consciousness, shortness of breath, or other complaints. Your physical exam indicates that the patient is slightly ashen and has an obvious bruising and deformity to his right midshaft radius/ulna. He has positive distal pulses, motor and sensory function (PMS), and the following findings: pulse is 110 beats/min and regular, respirations are 16 breaths/min and unlabored, blood pressure is 106/96 mm Hg, and SpO_2 is 98%. The patient denies significant previous medical history.

   a. Mechanism of injury:

   _____

   _____

   b. Chief complaint:

   _____

   _____

   c. Vital signs:

   _____

   _____

   d. Pertinent negatives:

   _____

   _____

2. Today you are assigned to work on an ALS ambulance. Your response area includes many high-speed interstate highways. It is toward the end of your shift and, until now, the day has been uneventful. Medcom dispatches you, priority one (a Charlie response), to a reported motorcycle crash with one critical injury. On arrival you notice a long line of stopped traffic and concerned bystanders. They are frantically waving you toward the injured patient. You notice a one-vehicle, motorcycle-versus-guardrail collision. The patient appears to be talking, but you notice a pool of blood alongside him as well as a cracked helmet. He has a badly deformed lower leg that you quickly conclude is fractured or dislocated. The patient is in obvious pain and is able to communicate that he "hurts all over." You quickly begin to assess the patient, and he appears agitated, ashen, diaphoretic, and slightly short of breath. He has delayed (> 2-second) capillary refill, and he has diminished left-side breath sounds and no tracheal deviation. His pulse is 120 beats/min, respiratory rate is 28 breaths/min, blood pressure is unobtainable, and SpO_2 is 92%. You note that the patient has a palpable femoral pulse but no radial or brachial pulse.

a. Mechanism of injury:

_____

_____

b. Chief complaint:

_____

_____

c. Vital signs:

_____

_____

d. Pertinent negatives:

_____

_____

3. You respond to a "routine" call at an adult care facility for a "fall." Your patient is an 82-year-old woman who is lying on a carpeted floor with a walker positioned beside her. She appears conscious but slightly confused. She doesn't really know why she fell or how she ended up on the ground. She asks you to help her up. You begin your primary assessment of the patient, and she denies any knowledge of the incident. During the secondary assessment, she denies any chest discomfort, shortness of breath, or neck or back pain. You note some deformity and rotation to her right lower extremity. On palpation, it is tender to the touch. The patient is confused regarding her previous medical history. The staff tells you that she has a history of transient ischemic attacks and heart problems. She is on multiple medications and is allergic to morphine sulfate. Her abdomen is soft and nontender. Her vital signs are as follows: pulse 58 beats/min and irregular; blood pressure 158/110 mm Hg; SpO_2 95%. Her skin is pale, cool, and dry.

a. Mechanism of injury:

_____

_____

b. Chief complaint:

_____

_____

c. Vital signs:

_____

_____

d. Pertinent negatives:

_____

_____

Complete the Patient Care Report (PCR)

Reread the second case study in the preceding Identify exercise and then complete the following patient care report (PCR). Feel free to create the times and numbers as well as the date of the incident.

EMS Patient Care Report (PCR)					
Date:	Incident No.:	Nature of Call:		Location:	
Dispatched:	En Route:	At Scene:	Transport:	At Hospital:	In Service:
Patient Information					
Age: Sex: Weight (in kg [lb]):		Allergies: Medications: Past Medical History: Chief Complaint:			
Vital Signs					
Time:	BP:	Pulse:		Respirations:	SpO$_2$:
Time:	BP:	Pulse:		Respirations:	SpO$_2$:
Time:	BP:	Pulse:		Respirations:	SpO$_2$:
EMS Treatment **(circle all that apply)**					
Oxygen @ _____ L/min via (circle one): NC NRM Bag-Mask Device		Assisted Ventilation	Airway Adjunct		CPR
Defibrillation	Bleeding Control	Bandaging	Splinting		Other
Narrative					

Ambulance Calls

The following case scenarios provide an opportunity to explore the concerns associated with mechanism of injury and trauma systems. Read each scenario, and then answer each question.

1. You are called to the scene of a back-road single-vehicle collision in which a car plowed into a utility pole. The driver of the car is sitting on the grass beside his wrecked vehicle looking dazed and confused. What parameters would you use to assess the mechanism of injury and suspected injuries and/or injury patterns?

   a. _____

   b. _____

   c. _____

   d. _____

   e. _____

   f. _____

2. You are summoned to the scene of a smoky apartment-house fire. When you arrive, one of the fire fighters directs you to a casualty who has been carried to a spot just beyond the fire lines. The fire fighter tells you that the man jumped from a window.

   a. What further information do you need to obtain about this patient to evaluate the potential seriousness of the injuries he might have sustained making that jump?

   _____

   _____

   _____

   _____

   _____

   _____

   b. Assuming he landed on his feet, what injuries might you expect him to have suffered?

   _____

   _____

3. On your very next call, you are summoned to a housing project where a 2-year-old child managed to crawl over the edge of a second-story balcony and fall into the playground below. What sort of injuries would this child most likely have sustained, and why?

   _____

   _____

4. You are called to a somewhat disreputable downtown area for a "man shot." You arrive on the scene to see the patient lying on the ground in the center of a small group of men, some of them apparently intoxicated and all of them talking at once.

   a. What is the *first* action you will take before entering the scene?

   _____

b. What information do you need to obtain regarding the shooting incident?

(1) _____

(2) _____

(3) _____

(4) _____

(5) _____

5. A fire at a warehouse of a large construction company ignites the stock of dynamite and produces an explosion that shatters windows for blocks around. As you respond to the scene, you review in your mind the different kinds of injuries you might soon have to deal with. List the four *mechanisms* of injuries that can be produced by an explosion, and describe each one.

a. _____

b. _____

c. _____

d. _____

6. Among the patients you treat at the scene of the explosion is a young man who had been taking a walk about half a block from the construction company when the explosion occurred. The man states that the blast "knocked me clear off my feet." He complains of a "tight feeling in my chest" and blurry vision. On physical examination, he appears somewhat confused; he cannot tell you the date or what day of the week it is. His vital signs are as follows: pulse 100 beats/min, full and regular; respirations 30 breaths/min and somewhat shallow; blood pressure 120/80 mm Hg. His skin is warm and dry. Aside from a little dried blood in the left ear canal, there are no other physical findings. What tissues are at risk? What is the evidence for you thinking so?

Tissues at Risk	Evidence
1.	
2.	
3.	

True/False

If you believe the statement to be more true than false, write the letter "T" in the space provided. If you believe the statement to be more false than true, write the letter "F."

_____ 1. One of the top five leading causes of traumatic death is drowning.

_____ 2. A Level IV trauma center provides the most comprehensive trauma care possible.

_____ 3. Transport considerations are not necessary if the patient is seriously hurt.

_____ 4. Blunt trauma typically occurs in motor vehicle crashes.

_____ 5. The "paper bag syndrome" can result in a pneumothorax.

_____ 6. Small children should be seated in the front seats of motor vehicles to benefit from the protection offered by air bags.

_____ 7. Evaluation of the patient's GCS is a component of the first step in the 2011 decision scheme for field trauma of injured patients.

_____ 8. If your patient was riding a motorcycle and was involved in a crash at about 15 mph, he should automatically be taken to a trauma center based on the 2011 decision scheme for field trauma of injured patients.

Short Answer

Complete this section with short written answers using the space provided.

1. A 2,000-lb automobile is traveling at 20 mph when it strikes a pedestrian.
   a. What happens to the kinetic energy of the vehicle at the moment of impact?

   _____

   _____

   _____

   b. If the vehicle weighed 6,000 lb instead of 2,000 lb, what difference would that make in terms of its kinetic energy?

   _____

   _____

   _____

   c. If the vehicle were traveling at 60 mph rather than 20 mph, what difference would that make in terms of its kinetic energy?

   _____

   _____

   _____

2. A car traveling at 50 mph goes out of control and slams into a concrete wall. That sequence of events in fact produces three separate collisions, each involving a transfer of kinetic energy. What objects are involved in each of the three collisions, and what happens to the kinetic energy in each case?
   a. Collision 1:

   _____

   _____

   _____

   b. Collision 2:

   _____

   _____

   _____

   c. Collision 3:

   _____

   _____

   _____

3. Careful inspection of a wrecked vehicle can enable the rescuer to detect injuries among the patients that might not otherwise be obvious. For each of the vehicular findings mentioned in the following list, list the injuries that are likely to be associated.
   a. Deformed dashboard

   (1) _____

   (2) _____

(3) _____

(4) _____

(5) _____

b. Deformed steering column

    (1) _____

    (2) _____

    (3) _____

    (4) _____

    (5) _____

    (6) _____

c. Cracked windshield

    (1) _____

    (2) _____

    (3) _____

    (4) _____

d. Door smashed in

    (1) _____

    (2) _____

    (3) _____

4. One of the most lethal objects in a motor vehicle is the steering wheel. Whenever you find structural damage to a steering wheel—indeed, whenever there is significant deformity to the front end of a car involved in a collision—you must be alert for the presence of the "ring of injuries" impact that the steering wheel may have produced in the driver of the car. List six injuries that may be associated with steering wheel trauma.

    a. _____

    b. _____

    c. _____

    d. _____

    e. _____

    f. _____

Fill-in-the-Table

Fill in the missing parts of the table.

1. Fill in the key elements for the corresponding definition.

Key Elements for Trauma Centers		
Level	Definition	Key Elements
Level I	A comprehensive regional resource that is a tertiary care facility. Capable of providing total care for every aspect of injury–from prevention through rehabilitation.	1. 2. 3. 4. 5.
Level II	Able to initiate definitive care for all injured patients.	1. 2. 3. 4. 5.
Level III	Able to provide prompt assessment, re-suscitation, and stabilization of injured patients and emergency operations.	1. 2. 3. 4. 5. 6.
Level IV	Able to provide Advanced Trauma Life Support (ATLS) before transfer of patients to a higher level trauma center.	1. 2. 3. 4.

2. List the "ring" of chest injuries from impacting the steering wheel or dashboard.

"Ring" of Chest Injuries From Impact With the Steering Wheel or Dashboard
• _____
• Soft-tissue neck trauma
• Larynx and tracheal trauma
• _____
• _____
• _____
• Pulmonary contusion
• Hemothorax, rib fractures
• _____
• _____
• Intra-abdominal injuries

Problem Solving

Use the formula for kinetic energy to answer the following questions.

$$KE = M/2 \times V^2$$

You have responded to a motor vehicle crash. This was a collision involving a car and a stationary bridge abutment. There are two patients. You note that your patient appears to be a 6-ft man who weighs approximately 200 lb. The patient is conscious and alert. While talking to him, you discover that he was not wearing a seat belt, and he was traveling at 50 mph.

1. Use the formula for calculating kinetic energy (KE) to determine the KE units involved in this crash. The second passenger in the vehicle was also unbelted, and she weighs 120 lb.

2. How many KE units are involved with the second passenger?

Bleeding

Matching

Match each of the definitions in the left column to the appropriate term in the right column.

_____ **1.** The pressure in the aorta against which the left ventricle must pump blood; increasing this can decrease cardiac output.

_____ **2.** The fluid tissue that is pumped by the heart through the arteries, veins, and capillaries and consists of plasma and formed elements or cells, such as red blood cells, white blood cells, and platelets.

_____ **3.** Amount of blood pumped by the heart per minute. Calculated by multiplying the stroke volume by the heart rate per minute.

_____ **4.** The early stage of shock, in which the body can still compensate for blood loss. The systolic blood pressure and brain perfusion are maintained.

_____ **5.** The late stage of shock, when blood pressure is falling.

_____ **6.** The percentage of blood that leaves the heart each time it contracts.

_____ **7.** Red blood cells.

_____ **8.** Vomited blood.

_____ **9.** Passage of stools containing bright red blood.

_____ **10.** A blood test that measures the portion of red blood cells in whole blood.

_____ **11.** A mass of blood in the soft tissues beneath the skin; indicates bleeding into soft tissues and may be the result of a minor or a severe injury.

_____ **12.** Blood in the urine.

_____ **13.** The oxygen-carrying pigment in red blood cells.

_____ **14.** Lacking one or more of the blood's clotting factors.

_____ **15.** Coughed-up blood.

_____ **16.** Bleeding.

_____ **17.** Volume lost as blood.

_____ **18.** Stopping hemorrhage.

_____ **19.** A condition that occurs when the level of tissue perfusion decreases below that needed to maintain normal cellular function.

_____ **20.** A condition that occurs when the circulating blood volume is inadequate to deliver adequate oxygen and nutrients to the body.

_____ **21.** The final stage of shock, prior to death.

_____ **22.** White blood cells.

_____ **23.** Passage of dark, tarry stools.

_____ **24.** The delivery of oxygen and nutrients to the cells, organs, and tissues of the body.

_____ **25.** The fluid portion of the blood from which the cells have been removed.

_____ **26.** Small cells in the blood that are essential for clot formation.

A. Erythrocytes

B. Blood

C. Afterload

D. Hemoglobin

E. Stroke volume (SV)

F. Melena

G. Hemostasis

H. Hemoptysis

I. Hematuria

J. Hematocrit

K. Ejection fraction (EF)

L. Decompensated shock (Class III)

M. Preload

N. Plasma

O. Leukocytes

P. Hypovolemic shock

Q. Hematemesis

R. Compensated shock (Class I and II)

S. Hemorrhagic shock

T. Hemorrhage

U. Irreversible shock (Class IV)

V. Perfusion

W. Cardiac output (CO)

X. Platelets

Y. Hematoma

Z. Hematochezia

_____ **27.** The precontraction pressure in the heart as the volume of blood builds up.

_____ **28.** An abnormal state associated with inadequate oxygen and nutrient delivery to the metabolic apparatus of the cell.

_____ **29.** The amount of blood that the left ventricle ejects into the aorta per contraction.

AA. Hypoperfusion

BB. Hemophilia

CC. Shock

Multiple Choice

Read each item carefully, and then select the best response.

1. _____ is a blood test that measures the portion of RBCs in the whole blood.
   A. Plasma count
   B. Hematocrit
   C. Cardiac output
   D. Ejection fraction

2. Which of the following substances accounts for more than half of the body's blood volume?
   A. Erythrocytes
   B. Leukocytes
   C. Plasma
   D. Hemoglobin

3. On average, an arterial bleed takes how many minutes to clot with direct pressure?
   A. Two
   B. Three
   C. Five
   D. Ten

4. The body cannot tolerate an acute blood loss of _____%. This loss will produce a significant change in vital signs of the adult patient, referred to as a Class III hemorrhage.
   A. < 5
   B. < 15
   C. 15–30
   D. 30–40

5. When you encounter a patient who is bleeding, the first thing you should do is:
   A. estimate the blood loss.
   B. apply direct pressure.
   C. check for breathing.
   D. don personal protective equipment.

6. A stool that has bright red blood is called:
   A. hematochezia.
   B. melena.
   C. hematuria.
   D. epistaxis.

7. Which of the following is NOT considered a significant mechanism of injury in an adult patient?
   A. Motorcycle crash
   B. Ejection from vehicle or vehicle rollover
   C. Fall of less than 12 feet without loss of consciousness
   D. Death or major injury of another occupant in the same vehicle

8. The initial stage of hemorrhagic shock is characterized by low circulating blood volume with:
   A. a respiratory rate of 30 to 40 breaths/min.
   B. minimal signs of hypoperfusion.
   C. absent capillary refill.
   D. a heart rate over 120 beats/min.

9. Which of the following statements about the use of an arterial tourniquet is correct?
   A. It is rarely used in the field today.
   B. It can be used only for arterial bleeding.
   C. It should be placed proximal to the injury on the extremity.
   D. It should be applied on and off every 20 minutes to save the limb.

10. A patient has the signs and symptoms of shock from a fracture or a burn. This is MOST likely due to which cause of shock?
   A. Poor vessel function
   B. Low fluid volume
   C. Respiratory failure
   D. Pump failure

Labeling

Label the following diagram with the correct terms.

   1. The Cardiovascular System

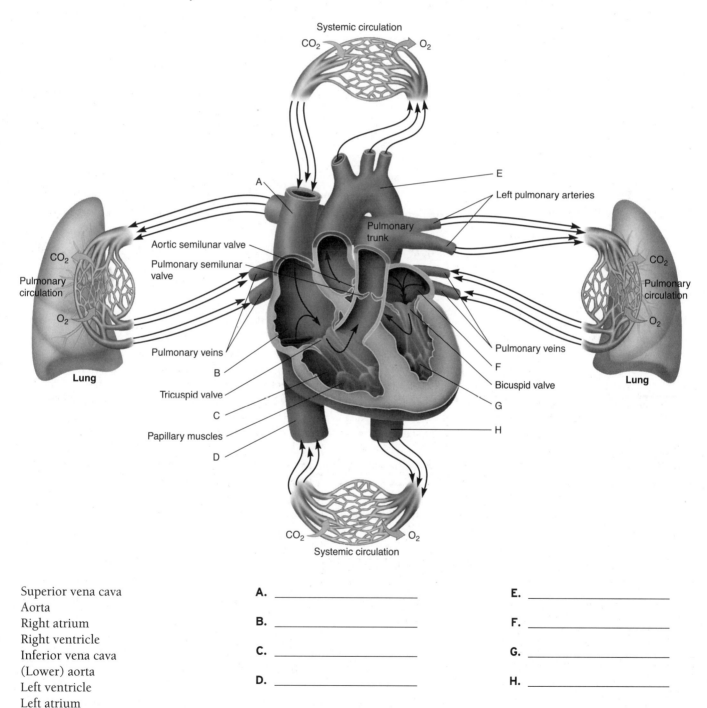

Superior vena cava
Aorta
Right atrium
Right ventricle
Inferior vena cava
(Lower) aorta
Left ventricle
Left atrium

A. _____   E. _____

B. _____   F. _____

C. _____   G. _____

D. _____   H. _____

Fill-in-the-Blank

Read each item carefully, and then complete the statement by filling in the missing word(s).

1. A now somewhat controversial treatment for shock is the military anti-shock trousers, or _____, also known as the _____.

2. Red blood cells contain _____, a protein that gives blood its reddish color.

3. Blood circulation through an organ or tissue that meets the cells' current needs for oxygen, nutrients, and waste removal is known as _____.

4. _____ is the process in which platelets aggregate at the site, plugging the hole and sealing injured portions of the vessel.

5. A lower GI bleed is indicated with the passing of _____, which is a dark, tarry-looking stool.

6. _____ is bleeding from the nose.

7. _____ happens when the level of tissue perfusion drops below normal limits.

8. When a patient is passing a bloody stool, this is referred to as _____ and can indicate hemorrhage near the external opening of the anus.

9. A small portion of the population lacks one or more of the blood's _____ factors. This condition is called _____.

10. As _____ increases and _____ drops, shock patients have cold, mottled, and pulseless extremities with _____ mental status.

11. The organs and organ systems with a _____ _____ of exsanguination from penetrating injuries include the _____, thoracic vascular system, abdominal vascular system, venous system, and _____.

12. The three phases of shock are _____, _____, and _____ shock.

13. The IV fluid of choice when replacing lost blood volume is either _____ _____ or _____ _____.

14. Shock that is caused by an allergic reaction, causing poor vessel function, is _____ shock.

15. Solutions that do not contain proteins or any other large molecules, and are typically used in shock fluid resuscitation, are known as _____.

Identify

In the following case study, list the chief complaint, vital signs, and pertinent negatives.

You are called to the scene of a local gas station where the 44-year-old man behind the counter was shot during a robbery. He is experiencing abdominal pain with a small bullet wound in the umbilical area. Upon arrival, the police determine that the perpetrator has fled the scene so the scene is safe for you to proceed with your trauma assessment. John, the patient, is clutching his belly with a towel for bleeding control. You note there is no radial pulse, yet John is still alert and oriented. Your partner quickly places John on high-flow supplemental oxygen by a nonrebreathing mask and applies an occlusive dressing to the wound. You determine that John has no obvious injury to his chest and his lung sounds are equal in both lungs. As he is being packaged to go to the trauma center, an ECG is applied and you determine that John's heart is in a sinus tachycardia with a rate of 120 beats/min and no ectopy. He is breathing at 24 breaths/min, and his room air saturation is 92%. He is very anxious but comes around with the oxygen and is able to answer all your questions. His pupils are equal and round, regular in size, and react to light (PEARRL). His blood pressure is 80/56 mm Hg, and his skin is pale, cool, and diaphoretic. You determine that there are no other injuries, although you know that an abdominal gunshot wound is significant, and it is difficult to tell how much internal bleeding he may have so far. En route to the trauma center you start two large-bore IVs of normal saline. You call ahead to prepare the ED for your arrival and then begin reassessment.

1. Chief complaint:

   _____

   _____

2. Vital signs:

   _____

   _____

3. Pertinent negatives:

   _____

   _____

Complete the Patient Care Report (PCR)

Reread the case study in the preceding Identify exercise and then complete the following patient care report (PCR) for the patient.

EMS Patient Care Report (PCR)					
Date:	Incident No.:	Nature of Call:		Location:	
Dispatched:	En Route:	At Scene:	Transport:	At Hospital:	In Service:
Patient Information					
Age: Sex: Weight (in kg [lb]):		Allergies: Medications: Past Medical History: Chief Complaint:			
Vital Signs					
Time:	BP:	Pulse:	Respirations:	SpO$_2$:	
Time:	BP:	Pulse:	Respirations:	SpO$_2$:	
Time:	BP:	Pulse:	Respirations:	SpO$_2$:	
EMS Treatment (circle all that apply)					
Oxygen @ ____ L/min via (circle one): NC NRM Bag-Mask Device		Assisted Ventilation	Airway Adjunct	CPR	
Defibrillation	Bleeding Control	Bandaging	Splinting	Other	
Narrative					

Ambulance Calls

The following case scenarios provide an opportunity to explore the concerns associated with patient management and paramedic care. Read each scenario, and then answer each question.

1. A middle-aged man was struck by a car as he was crossing the street. You find him lying by the side of the road, complaining of severe pain in his abdomen, where the car hit him. You would like to make an assessment of his state of perfusion. How will you assess the following?

   a. His *peripheral* perfusion:

   _____

   _____

   b. The perfusion to his *vital organs*:

   _____

   _____

2. You are called to a downtown bar in which firearms were used to settle a difference of opinion. You find a man lying on the floor of the bar, unconscious, his trouser leg soaked in blood. In the correct sequence, list the steps you would take in treating this patient.

   a. _____

   b. _____

   c. _____

   d. _____

   e. _____

   f. _____

3. One rainy day, a car bomb was detonated in front of a foreign consulate. A number of bystanders were injured by flying debris, including jagged pieces of metal torn from the car's body. The first patient you come upon is bleeding from multiple sites, including a deep gash on the right side of the neck and a laceration that has partially severed the right leg at the groin. The leg laceration is gushing blood; it is too proximal to benefit from a tourniquet. It is hard to evaluate skin condition in the rain. Pulse is around 100 beats/min and somewhat weak; respirations are 30 breaths/min.

   a. What steps would you take at the scene?

   (1) _____

   (2) _____

   (3) _____

   (4) _____

   b. What steps would you take during transport?

   (1) _____

   (2) _____

   (3) _____

4. A second patient from the car bombing, a young man, was sideswiped by a piece of flying debris, which made a clean 14-inch incision straight across his abdomen. He is conscious and in moderate distress. Pulse is 104 beats/min and

regular, respirations are 28 breaths/min and slightly labored, and blood pressure is 104/70 mm Hg. What looks to be a major portion of the patient's intestines is outside the abdomen.

   a. What steps would you take at the scene?

      (1) _____

      (2) _____

      (3) _____

   b. What steps would you take during transport?

      (1) _____

      (2) _____

      (3) _____

5. A third patient from the car bombing is another young man in considerable respiratory distress. There is a 2-inch-wide hole in his right chest through which you can hear air being sucked on inhalation. His skin is warm. His pulse is 108 beats/min and regular; respirations are 30 breaths/min and gasping; blood pressure is 112/64 mm Hg.

   a. What steps would you take at the scene?

      (1) _____

      (2) _____

      (3) _____

   b. What steps would you take during transport?

      (1) _____

      (2) _____

      (3) _____

6. A 59-year-old man was the driver of a car that plowed into a bridge abutment in the early hours of the morning. The patient is conscious, but very restless. He is sweating profusely. His chest is stable (it's too dark to see whether there are bruises). He can move all his extremities. His pulse is 82 beats/min, respirations are 28 breaths/min, and blood pressure is 100/70 mm Hg.

   a. What steps would you take at the scene?

      (1) _____

      (2) _____

      (3) _____

      (4) _____

      (5) _____

   b. What steps would you take during transport?

      (1) _____

      (2) _____

      (3) _____

      (4) _____

True/False

If you believe the statement to be more true than false, write the letter "T" in the space provided. If you believe the statement to be more false than true, write the letter "F."

_____ **1.** One of the earliest signs of hypovolemic shock is a fall in the blood pressure.

_____ **2.** Patients in hemorrhagic shock tend to have a normal pulse rate.

_____ **3.** The IV fluid of choice to provide volume to a patient in hypovolemic shock is 5% dextrose in water (D_5W).

_____ **4.** A patient may go into shock without losing any blood or fluid from the body.

_____ **5.** The amount of blood pumped through the circulatory system in 1 minute is known as the cardiac output.

_____ **6.** The function of plasma is to produce red blood cells (RBCs) and white blood cells (WBCs).

_____ **7.** Nontraumatic internal bleeding usually happens in the gastrointestinal tract.

_____ **8.** A 1-year-old child has a blood volume of around 800 mL.

_____ **9.** You can use a wire, rope, or any narrow material as a tourniquet.

_____ **10.** Definitive management for internal hemorrhage is in the hospital.

Short Answer

Complete this section with short written answers using the space provided.

1. Three components are required for a functioning circulatory system. If any one of those components is impaired, shock may result. List the three necessary components.

a. _____

b. _____

c. _____

2. The type of shock you will see most frequently in the prehospital setting is hemorrhagic shock. It is very important to detect hypovolemic shock early and to start treatment early. To do so, you must have a high index of suspicion in assessing patients at risk of hypovolemic shock, which means you must be aware of the situations in which hypovolemia is likely to occur. List four causes of hypovolemic shock.

a. _____

b. _____

c. _____

d. _____

3. Knowing the findings in hemorrhagic shock is important in being a paramedic. For each of the following findings, note whether the value is increased, decreased, or flat.

Findings in Hemorrhagic Shock	
Heart rate	
Blood pressure	
Central venous pressure/renal artery pressure	
Pulmonary capillary wedge pressure	
Cardiac output/cardiac index	
Systemic vascular resistance/systemic vascular resistance index	
Systemic vascular oxygen	
Urinary output	
Jugular vein distention	
Hematocrit (percentage of whole blood components versus plasma)	

4. It is not necessary in the field to make a specific diagnosis of a patient's abdominal pain, but it is necessary to be able to recognize when a potentially life-threatening situation exists. Any patient with abdominal pain showing symptoms or signs of shock must be considered to be in danger. To recognize that danger, you must be able to spot the symptoms and signs of shock. List six symptoms and signs of shock.

   a. _____

   b. _____

   c. _____

   d. _____

   e. _____

   f. _____

5. List four methods for control of external hemorrhage.

   a. _____

   b. _____

   c. _____

   d. _____

Fill-in-the-Table

Fill in the missing parts of the table.

Compensated Versus Decompensated Hypoperfusion	
Compensated Hypoperfusion	**Decompensated Hypoperfusion**
• _____	• Altered mental status (verbal to unresponsive)
• Sense of impending doom	• _____
• _____	• Labored or irregular breathing
• Clammy (cool, moist) skin	• _____
• _____	• Ashen, mottled, or cyanotic skin
• Shortness of breath	• _____
• _____	• Diminished urine output (oliguria)
• Delayed capillary refill in infants and children	• _____
• _____	
• Normal systolic blood pressure	

Skill Drills

Test your knowledge of skill drills by placing the following photos in the correct order. Number the first step with a "1," the second step with a "2," and so forth.

Managing Hemorrhagic Shock

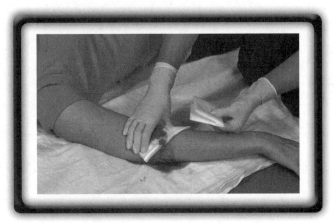

_____ Control obvious external bleeding.

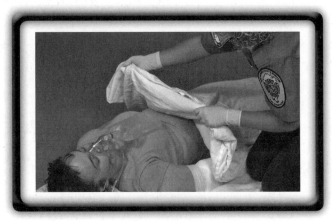

_____ Administer high-flow oxygen if you have not already done so, and keep the patient warm.

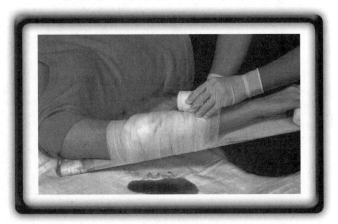

_____ Splint the patient on a backboard. Splint any broken bones or joint injuries during transport.

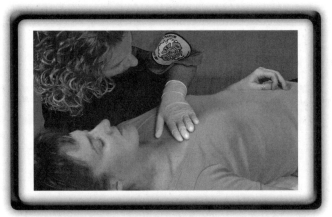

_____ Keep the patient supine, open the airway, and check breathing and pulse.

Soft-Tissue Trauma

Matching

Match each of the terms in the left column to the appropriate definition in the right column.

_____ 1. Integument

_____ 2. Collagen

_____ 3. Chemotactic factors

_____ 4. Compartment syndrome

_____ 5. Contusion

_____ 6. Pedicle

_____ 7. Deep fascia

_____ 8. Myoglobin

_____ 9. Crush syndrome

_____ 10. Rhabdomyolysis

_____ 11. Degloving

_____ 12. Keloid scar

_____ 13. Sebaceous gland

_____ 14. Adipose

_____ 15. Abrasion

_____ 16. Gangrene

_____ 17. Fasciotomy

_____ 18. Hematoma

_____ 19. Laceration

_____ 20. Epidermis

_____ 21. Elastin

_____ 22. Sebum

_____ 23. Volkmann contracture

_____ 24. Degranulation

A. Infection caused by *Clostridium perfringens*.

B. The outermost layer of the skin.

C. Superficial wound caused by scraping.

D. A wound caused by cutting or tearing tissues.

E. A protein that gives tensile strength to the connective tissues of the body.

F. The release of granules into the surrounding tissue.

G. A narrow strip by which an avulsed piece of tissue remains connected to the body.

H. A protein found in muscle that is released into the circulation after a crush injury or other muscle damage and whose presence in the circulation may produce kidney damage.

I. A traumatic injury that results in the soft tissue of a part of the body being drawn downward like a glove being removed.

J. An oily substance secreted by the sebaceous glands.

K. Significant metabolic derangement that can lead to renal failure and death. It develops when crushed extremities or other body parts remain trapped for prolonged periods.

L. The skin.

M. The factors that cause cells to migrate into an area.

N. A bruise; an injury that causes bleeding beneath the skin but does not break the skin.

O. A dense layer of fibrous tissue below the subcutaneous tissue; composed of tough bands of tissue that ensheathe muscles and other internal structures.

P. A condition that develops when edema and swelling result in increased pressure within soft tissues, causing circulation to be compromised, possibly resulting in tissue necrosis.

Q. The destruction of muscle tissue leading to a release of potassium and myoglobin.

R. Deformity of the hand, fingers, and wrist resulting from damage to forearm muscles; develops from muscle ischemia and is associated with compartment syndrome.

S. The gland located in the dermis that secretes sebum.

T. A surgical procedure that cuts away fascia to relieve pressure.

U. A localized collection of blood in the soft tissues as a result of injury or a broken blood vessel.

V. An abnormal scar commonly found in people with darkly pigmented skin. It extends over the wound margins.

W. A protein that gives the skin its elasticity.

X. Fat tissue.

Multiple Choice

Read each item carefully, and then select the best response.

1. The condition that develops when edema and swelling result in increased pressure within soft tissues is called:
   A. crush syndrome.
   B. Volkmann contracture.
   C. compartment syndrome.
   D. rhabdomyolysis.

2. Blood vessels, nerves, tendons, muscles, and internal organs can all be damaged by:
   A. compartment syndrome.
   B. improperly applied dressings.
   C. use of a wet dressing instead of a dry dressing.
   D. application of a tourniquet.

3. When should an impaled object in the abdomen be removed by the paramedic?
   A. When the object affects packaging and transport
   B. When the object does not stand up straight on its own
   C. When bleeding cannot be successfully controlled
   D. The paramedic should never remove an impaled object from that location.

4. When a foreign material is forcefully injected into soft tissue, this is called a/an:
   A. high-pressure injection injury.
   B. amputation.
   C. tympanic membrane rupture.
   D. blast injury.

5. Patients with soft-tissue injuries:
   A. rarely have life-threatening injuries.
   B. should be "signed-off" to save EMS system resources.
   C. should be treated with aggressive ALS treatment in the event of unforeseen injury.
   D. have a high incidence of morbidity and mortality.

6. Many open wounds require surgical intervention for closure to bring the wound edges together to permit optimal healing. Of the following methods, which is NOT routinely used?
   A. Medical glue
   B. Staples
   C. Rope
   D. Sutures

7. There are numerous types of soft-tissue injuries. Many of them are relatively minor, but some have potentially serious outcomes. Which of the following injuries requires transportation?
   A. Abrasion
   B. Laceration
   C. Necrotizing fasciitis
   D. Incision

8. Oftentimes soft-tissue injuries involve external hemorrhaging. All of the following would be considered appropriate bleeding management, EXCEPT:
   A. direct pressure with thick, bulky dressings.
   B. pressure with elastic bandages.
   C. "wet" dressings applied to the wound.
   D. tourniquet on a severely bleeding extremity.

9. Soft-tissue injuries to the neck may lead to which of the following complications?
   A. Air embolism
   B. Spinal injury
   C. Airway disruption
   D. All of the above

10. Which of the following can interfere with normal wound healing?
    A. An underlying cardiac history
    B. A seizure disorder
    C. Carpal tunnel syndrome
    D. A history of diabetes

Labeling

1. Label the components of the skin in the following diagram.

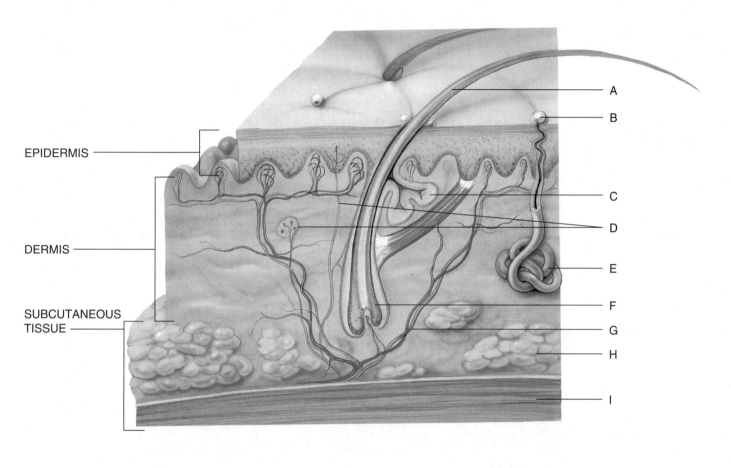

EPIDERMIS

DERMIS

SUBCUTANEOUS
TISSUE

A. _____

B. _____

C. _____

D. _____

E. _____

F. _____

G. _____

H. _____

I. _____

2. Determine which types of open wounds are shown in each of the following photos.

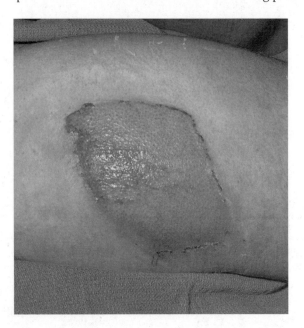

A. _____

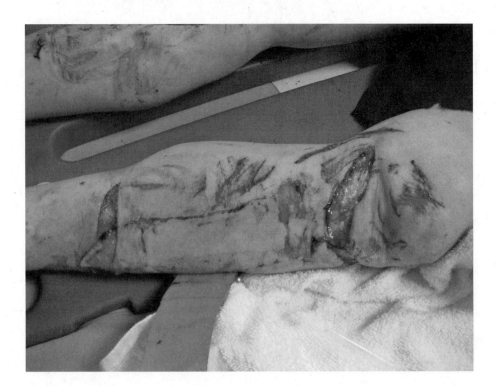

B. _____

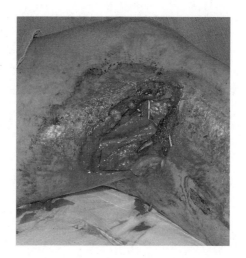

C. _____

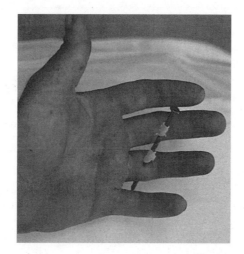

D. _____

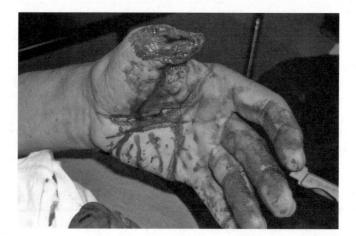

E. _____

Fill-in-the-Blank

Read each item carefully, and then complete the statement by filling in the missing word(s).

1. _____ injuries require substantial irrigation and _____ before closing by an emergency practitioner.

2. Visible clues of infection include _____, _____, _____, _____, and _____
   _____.

3. *Clostridium tetani* causes the body to produce a potent _____, which results in painful muscle _____ that are strong enough to fracture _____.

4. The darkness of a person's skin is directly proportional to the amount of _____ present.

5. Approximately 3,000 cases of _____ occur in the United States each year, of which 60% result from trauma.

6. When responding to a reported explosion, wait for _____ _____ to secure the scene and declare it _____ before you approach any victims. When a blast seems to be intentional, the paramedic should look for possible _____ devices. Responders have been injured and _____ by other explosive devices planted away from the original detonation.

7. Because wet dressings provide a medium for _____ and other pathogens to grow, their use is _____ in the field.

Identify

In the following case studies, identify the type of soft-tissue injury and the care that you would provide.

1. You are called to the scene of a local campsite where a 10-year-old boy was playing with his pocket knife, whittling some wood, when he cut himself. The injury is a jagged incision to his right forearm. There is moderate darkish-red blood oozing from the site.

   _____

   _____

   _____

2. A patient was working in his home shop when he became distracted while using a circular saw. He inadvertently cut the fingers on his left hand. When you arrive the patient is sitting in a chair, conscious and alert. He appears pale and sweaty. He has several blood-soaked towels covering his hand. You notice that his left middle and ring fingers are sitting on his wood-crafting bench.

   _____

   _____

   _____

3. It's a busy shift. On this call you are dispatched to a bar fight. On arrival, there is a crowd hovering around a woman who complains of pain in her right side and moderate shortness of breath. Her companion states that she was involved in a dispute and felt a sharp object impact her right side. The patient is somewhat angry and combative and wants to continue the dispute. As you examine the injury, you notice a minimal amount of bleeding that appears to have stopped. The patient has a quarter-inch circular opening to her chest. There appears to be a small amount of swelling and a rush of air when she breathes.

   _____

   _____

   _____

Ambulance Calls

The following case scenarios provide an opportunity to explore the concerns associated with patient management and paramedic care. Read each scenario, and then answer each question.

1. You are summoned to Bugsy's Butcher Shop to tend to the proprietor, Bugsy Butterfingers, who dropped a meat cleaver on his left leg. There is a large gash in the left calf, and it is bleeding profusely.
   a. List four methods you might use to try to control the bleeding, and put an asterisk next to the method likely to be the most effective. Please note that standard precautions are being done appropriately.

   (1) _____

   (2) _____

   (3) _____

   (4) _____

   b. Suppose Bugsy's wound had been on the forearm rather than on the leg. Which artery is most likely the cause of severe bleeding in the arm?

   _____

2. One of Bugsy's employees, Frank Fillet, becomes so distracted watching you care for his boss that he accidentally chops off two of his fingers while preparing an order of steaks.
   a. How will you treat Frank's injury?

   _____

   _____

   _____

   b. What will you do with the two fingers lying on the chopping board?

   _____

   _____

   _____

3. Yet another worker in the butcher shop, Hercules Hamburger, had been watching, slack-jawed and transfixed, as this drama was unfolding. So intent was he on the spectacle that he did not realize his right hand had entered the meat grinder—not until, that is, the hand became engaged in the grinding blades. Hearing his screams, a customer rushes over to where Hercules is standing and manages to shut off the meat grinder, but not before Hercules' hand and forearm have been badly mangled. You already have your hands full with Bugsy and Frank, so you instruct the Good Samaritan who shut off the meat grinder, "Have him lie down, and try to control the bleeding—I'll be with him in just a minute." Obligingly, the customer grabs a piece of rope that he finds behind the counter, winds it around Hercules' upper arm, and slips a ball-point pen into the knot to serve as tourniquet. He twists the rope as tight as he possibly can, secures the pen, and uses the butcher's apron to wrap the entire hand and arm.

   Although the customer was trying to be helpful, in fact he made several very serious mistakes. List the mistakes.

   a. _____

   b. _____

   c. _____

   d. _____

4. During deer-hunting season, two young backpackers were strolling through the woods when hunters, mistaking the pair for deer, discharged their crossbows at them. One arrow entered the eye of the first backpacker, while another arrow went straight through the cheek of the second backpacker.

    a. Describe the steps you would take in treating the backpacker with the arrow in his eye. Please note that standard precautions are being done appropriately.

_____

_____

_____

_____

_____

_____

    b. Describe the steps you would take in treating the backpacker who has an arrow impaled in his cheek.

_____

_____

_____

_____

_____

_____

5. You are folding up your deck chair when you happen to see a jogger running erratically down the beach toward you. His shorts are torn, and there is blood trickling down one leg. "What happened to you?" you ask.

    "Some big Doberman tackled me as I was running. I figured the best thing to do was keep running to where I left my car." You note the tooth marks and a laceration on the runner's left leg.

    How would you manage this patient? Please note that standard precautions are being done appropriately.

    a. _____

    b. _____

    c. _____

    d. _____

True/False

If you believe the statement to be more true than false, write the letter "T" in the space provided. If you believe the statement to be more false than true, write the letter "F."

    _____ **1.** Amputation is a form of avulsion.

    _____ **2.** Soft-tissue trauma is the leading form of injury.

    _____ **3.** Sweating is regulated through the parasympathetic nervous system.

    _____ **4.** Subcutaneous blood vessels have a crucial role in regulating body temperature.

    _____ **5.** The precise function of sebum secreted by the sebaceous glands is not well known.

_____ **6.** Human bites carry a higher risk of infection than animal bites do.

_____ **7.** Keloid scars typically develop in areas of high tissue stress.

_____ **8.** Tetanus infection causes the body to produce a potent toxin that results in lockjaw.

_____ **9.** One of the body's first responses to a vessel injury is localized vasoconstriction that reduces blood flow.

_____ **10.** Bleeding control is a key principle in treating open wounds.

Short Answer

Complete this section with short written answers using the space provided.

1. You can appreciate the possible consequences of injury to the skin if you understand what functions healthy, intact skin performs. List four functions performed by the skin in a healthy person.

   a. _____

   b. _____

   c. _____

   d. _____

2. Healing of wounds is a natural process that involves several overlapping stages. List the five stages of wound healing.

   a. _____

   b. _____

   c. _____

   d. _____

   e. _____

3. Wounds are characterized as either closed or open. List the characteristics of closed wounds.

   a. _____

   b. _____

   c. _____

4. Crush syndrome is a serious injury that can occur when an area of the body has been trapped for 4 hours or longer. List the progression of crush syndrome.

   a. _____

   b. _____

   c. _____

   d. _____

Skill Drills

Test your knowledge of skill drills by placing the following photos in the correct order. Number the first step with a "1," the second step with a "2," etc.

Controlling Bleeding From a Soft-Tissue Injury

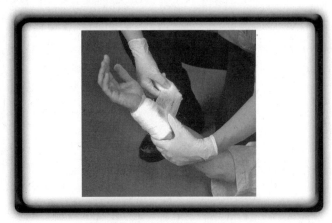

_____ Apply a pressure dressing.

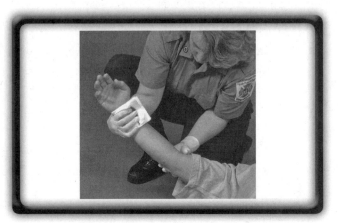

_____ Apply direct pressure over the wound with a dry, sterile dressing. Elevate the injury if no fracture is suspected.

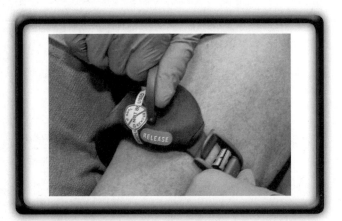

_____ If direct pressure with a pressure dressing does not rapidly control bleeding on an extremity, apply a tourniquet above the level of bleeding.

Burns

Matching

Part I

Match each of the patients with the appropriate treatment in question 1, and with the appropriate sequence in question 2.

1. In the course of a busy week, you are called on to treat eight burn victims in a variety of circumstances. In each case, you have to determine whether the patient has suffered a critical burn because, if so, he or she must be evacuated directly to the Regional Burn Center, which is 24 miles away; noncritical burns, on the other hand, can be managed by the community hospital right in town. A description of the patients you saw follows. Beside each description, indicate whether:

   A. The patient has a critical burn and should be brought to a burn center.

   B. The patient does not have a critical burn and can be managed in the community hospital.

   _____ (1) A 2-year-old boy who overturned a pot of soup from the stovetop onto himself; both legs and the anterior trunk are burned.

   _____ (2) A 57-year-old diabetic woman with a scald burn of her left lower leg.

   _____ (3) A 28-year-old woman with a scald burn of her entire right arm.

   _____ (4) A lineman who suffered an electric shock. There is a small bull's-eye entrance wound on the left hand; you cannot find the exit wound. The lineman did not fall. His left leg feels rock hard.

   _____ (5) A 22-year-old male short-order cook with partial-thickness (second-degree) burns over both anterior thighs, sustained when he spilled a pot of soup.

   _____ (6) A 34-year-old woman rescued from a burning building, where she had been trapped in her smoke-filled bedroom. She has partial-thickness burns of the right forearm. She is coughing up sooty sputum.

   _____ (7) A 25-year-old man who tripped and fell onto the hibachi on the back porch as he was preparing to barbecue some steaks. His hand went straight into the bed of red-hot charcoal, and his shirt caught fire. He has full-thickness (third-degree) burns of the left hand and forearm, and partial-thickness burns of the anterior chest.

   _____ (8) A plumber who spilled a bottle of industrial-strength liquid drain cleaner down the front of his pants.

2. You are called to treat a patient who was in a tenement fire. He is a middle-aged man who apparently fell asleep in an armchair while holding a lit cigarette. You arrive at the scene just as he is being carried unconscious from the building and note that his clothes are still smoldering. Following, in random order, are the steps you will have to take in managing this patient. Arrange the steps in the correct sequence.

   A. Administer supplemental oxygen.

   B. Start an IV.

   C. Open the airway manually.

   D. Put out the fire.

   E. Remove the patient's clothing.

   F. Pass a nasogastric tube into his stomach.

   G. Determine the extent and depth of the burn.

   H. Intubate the trachea (if a BLS airway is not adequate).

   I. Cover the burns with sterile dressings.

   J. Obtain a set of baseline vital signs.

   (1)_____   (6)_____

   (2)_____   (7)_____

   (3)_____   (8)_____

   (4)_____   (9)_____

   (5)_____   (10)_____

Part II

Match each of the terms in the left column to the appropriate definition in the right column.

_____ 1. Acute radiation syndrome

_____ 2. Burn shock

_____ 3. Circumferential burn

_____ 4. Consensus formula

_____ 5. Contact burn

_____ 6. Desquamation

_____ 7. Escharotomy

_____ 8. Flash burn

_____ 9. Lund and Browder chart

_____ 10. Partial-thickness burn

A. A detailed version of the rule of nines chart that takes into consideration the changes in body surface area brought on by growth.

B. A surgical cut through the escar or leathery covering of a burn injury to allow for swelling and to minimize the potential for development of compartment syndrome in a circumferentially burned limb or the thorax.

C. An electrothermal injury caused by arcing of electric current.

D. The continuous shedding of the dead cells on the surface of the skin.

E. A formula that recommends giving 4 mL of normal saline for each kilogram of body weight, multiplied by the percentage of body surface area burned; sometimes used to calculate fluid needs during lengthy transport times; formerly called the Parkland formula.

F. The clinical course that usually begins within hours of exposure to a radiation source. Symptoms include nausea, vomiting, diarrhea, fatigue, fever, and headache. The long-term symptoms are dose-related and are hematopoietic and gastrointestinal.

G. A burn that involves the epidermis and part of the dermis, characterized by pain and blistering; previously called a second-degree burn.

H. A burn produced by touching a hot object.

I. The shock or hypoperfusion caused by a burn injury and the tremendous loss of fluids; capillaries leak, resulting in intravascular fluid volume oozing out of the circulation and into the interstitial spaces, and cells take in increased amounts of salt and water.

J. A burn on the neck or chest that may compress the airway or on an extremity that might act like a tourniquet.

Multiple Choice

Read each item carefully, and then select the best response.

1. What is the second "rule" when in a lightning storm?
   A. Take shelter in a structure.
   B. Avoid touching a conductor.
   C. Don't be the smallest conductor.
   D. Don't stand near the tallest conductor.

2. When dealing with acute radiation syndrome, which of the following is NOT likely to happen to the patient?
   A. Central nervous system changes
   B. Urinary changes
   C. Gastrointestinal changes
   D. Hematologic changes

3. There are three methods of calculating an area of burned skin. Which method is the MOST used?
   A. Rule of nines
   B. The Lund and Browder chart
   C. Rule of palm
   D. A Broselow tape

4. You have arrived on scene to find a 12-year-old girl who has been burnt by chicken noodle soup from the stove. She has blisters and redness on her chest. How would you classify this burn?
   A. It is a full-thickness burn.
   B. It is a first-degree burn.
   C. It is a partial-thickness burn.
   D. It is a superficial burn.

5. An adult man's entire back is worth what percentage when using the rule of nines?
   A. 9%
   B. 18%
   C. 27%
   D. 36%

6. What is the *immediate management* when dealing with a 45-year-old woman who fell asleep with a cigarette in her hand?
   A. Managing the airway
   B. Starting fluid resuscitation
   C. Extinguishing the fire
   D. Keeping the patient warm

7. The Consensus (Parkland) formula determines how much fluid a burn patient should receive:
   A. during the first hour.
   B. during transport to the hospital.
   C. during the first 12 hours.
   D. during the first 24 hours.

8. What is the BEST way to give pain medication to the burn patient?
   A. IV route
   B. Subcutaneous injection
   C. By mouth
   D. Intramuscular injection

9. What should you do first when treating a patient with a chemical burn?
   A. Remove all the patient's clothing.
   B. Begin flushing with copious amounts of water.
   C. Brush the chemicals off the skin.
   D. Wait for a hazardous materials team to arrive.

10. You arrive on scene to find a child engaged in an electrical outlet. The child is "held" by the electricity. What should you do?
   A. Use a wooden pole to push the child away from the source.
   B. Throw a rope to the child and pull him away from the source.
   C. Wait until someone shuts off the power to the source.
   D. Cut the wires inside the electrical box.

Labeling

1. Label the components of the skin in the following diagram.

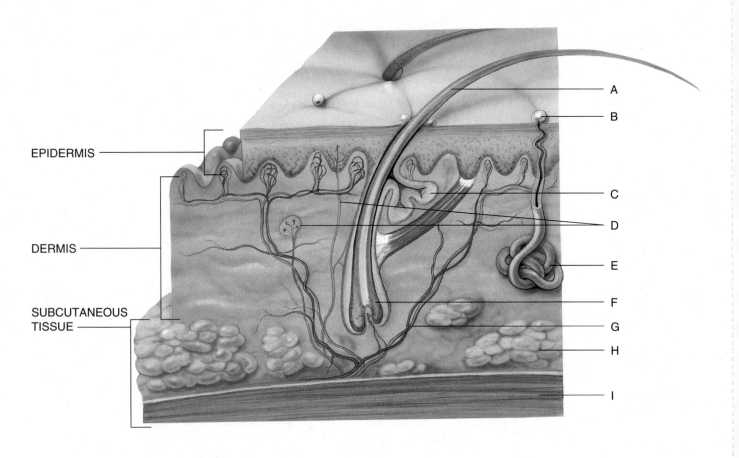

EPIDERMIS

DERMIS

SUBCUTANEOUS
TISSUE

A
B
C
D
E
F
G
H
I

A. _____   F. _____

B. _____   G. _____

C. _____   H. _____

D. _____   I. _____

E. _____

2. Classify the following images as superficial, partial-thickness, or full-thickness burns.

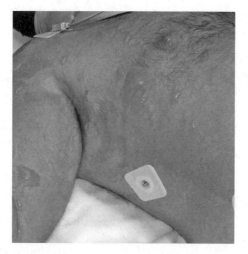

A. _____

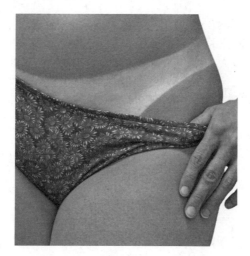

B. _____

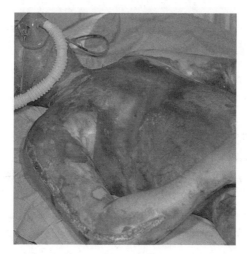

C. _____

Fill-in-the-Blank

Read each item carefully, and then complete the statement by filling in the missing word(s).

1. The _____ is the largest and one of the most complex organs in the body.
2. Sweat glands are found in the _____.
3. A _____ burn is most commonly seen in children.
4. Chemical burns can occur when the skin comes in contact with _____, _____, or _____, or other corrosive materials.
5. _____ _____ cause exothermic reaction in addition to tissue destruction.
6. You should always make sure the _____ _____ _____ before beginning any management of a patient struck by lightning.
7. There are three types of ionizing radiation: _____, _____, and _____.
8. The central area of a burn that has suffered the most damage is known as the _____ _____ _____.
9. When treating a full-thickness burn, you should apply a/an _____ _____ to the area that has been burned.
10. A patient with a radiation burn must be _____ before being transported to the emergency department.

Identify

In the following case study, list the chief complaint, vital signs, and pertinent negatives.

Around noon you are called to the local burger joint for a 56-year-old woman who has been burned by oil from a hot fryer. Upon arrival, you find her with holes in her jeans on the top of both thighs. She is crying and immediately rates her pain as unbearable. You cut the jeans away to find that there is an area covering most of the front of both thighs that is blistering and very red. She is breathing at 22 breaths/min, her oxygen saturation is 97%, and lung sounds are clear bilaterally. You apply supplemental oxygen via a nonrebreathing mask at 15 L/min. You have your partner take the rest of the vital signs as you apply a Water-Jel dressing to the burned areas. Her blood pressure is 150/100 mm Hg, her pulse is 114 beats/min, and her rhythm on the monitor is sinus tachycardia. You do catch a premature ventricular contraction on the monitor but don't see another after watching for a full minute. She is cool to the touch and you feel she might be going into shock. You cover her with a blanket and start an IV of normal saline. She is able to answer all your questions, and she has no medical history or allergies. You find no other areas of burns as you do a secondary trauma assessment. She states she slipped on the floor when carrying the hot oil to the disposal. She splashed the oil on the front of her legs. She does rate her pain 10/10, so you give her 5 mg of morphine for the pain en route to the hospital. When you arrive at the hospital, which is only 10 minutes from the burger joint, her pain has dropped to a 3/10.

1. Chief complaint:

2. Vital signs:

3. Pertinent negatives:

Complete the Patient Care Report (PCR)

Reread the case study in the preceding Identify exercise and then complete the following patient care report (PCR) for the patient.

EMS Patient Care Report (PCR)					
Date:	**Incident No.:**	**Nature of Call:**		**Location:**	
Dispatched:	**En Route:**	**At Scene:**	**Transport:**	**At Hospital:**	**In Service:**
Patient Information					
Age:		**Allergies:**			
Sex:		**Medications:**			
Weight (in kg [lb]):		**Past Medical History:**			
		Chief Complaint:			
Vital Signs					
Time:	**BP:**	**Pulse:**		**Respirations:**	**SpO$_2$:**
Time:	**BP:**	**Pulse:**		**Respirations:**	**SpO$_2$:**
Time:	**BP:**	**Pulse:**		**Respirations:**	**SpO$_2$:**
EMS Treatment (circle all that apply)					
Oxygen @ _____ L/min via (circle one): NC NRM Bag-Mask Device		**Assisted Ventilation**	**Airway Adjunct**		**CPR**
Defibrillation	**Bleeding Control**	**Bandaging**	**Splinting**		**Other**
Narrative					

Ambulance Calls

The following case scenarios provide an opportunity to explore the concerns associated with patient management and paramedic care. Read each scenario, and then answer each question.

1. You are called to the scene of a smoky apartment-house fire to treat a man who jumped from his bedroom window about 15 feet above the ground. What you observe at first glance is the following: He is now lying unconscious on the ground. His trousers are smoldering. His beard is partly burned off, and his lips are swollen. His left leg is splayed out at a peculiar angle. List in the correct sequence the steps you would take in managing this patient.

    a. _____

    b. _____

    c. _____

    d. _____

    e. _____

    f. _____

    g. _____

    h. _____

2. While you are securing the IV on the patient described in the previous question, fire fighters lead the patient's wife over to you (they just rescued her from another room). A quick check does not reveal any injuries, but you give her supplemental oxygen by nasal cannula anyway because of her exposure to smoke. Meanwhile, you take advantage of the opportunity to get some information about her husband. List five questions you would ask this woman regarding her husband and what happened to him.

    a. _____

    b. _____

    c. _____

    d. _____

    e. _____

3. Meanwhile, the fire fighters bring you yet another victim of the fire, a college student who climbed down a fire escape in the back of the building. He has burns to the right side of his body and complains of severe pain in the right arm. On examination you find the following:

    • The *right arm* is mottled red and exquisitely sensitive to the lightest touch (even the breeze blowing past it causes pain).

    • The *right flank* is fiery red and also very painful.

    • The *right lower leg* has a leathery appearance. In places, you can see thrombosed veins beneath the surface. When you touch the skin with a sterile needle, the patient does not feel the pinprick.

    a. The burn on the right arm is probably a _____ burn.

    The appropriate treatment for that burn is:

    _____

    _____

b. The burn on the flank is probably a _____ burn.
The appropriate treatment for that burn is:

_____

_____

c. The burn on the right leg is probably a _____ burn.
The appropriate treatment for that burn is:

_____

_____

4. You are called to a construction site 20 miles out of town for a "man electrocuted." According to the person who telephoned your dispatcher, one of the construction workers apparently bulldozed through a buried electric cable. He dismounted his bulldozer and picked up the cable to toss it aside, not realizing that it was live, and his hand "froze" to the cable.

    a. En route to the call, you review in your mind the types of injuries that may occur in connection with electrocution. You remember that there may be three different types of burns:

        (1) _____

        (2) _____

        (3) _____

    b. You also recall that high-voltage electricity may cause a variety of nonburn injuries. List six possible injuries or abnormal conditions that you need to be alert for in this patient.

        (1) _____

        (2) _____

        (3) _____

        (4) _____

        (5) _____

        (6) _____

    c. When you reach the construction site, you see a knot of agitated people at one end of the site. One of them is holding a long two-by-four, with which he apparently jarred the victim loose from the cable. The victim is lying very still and appears to be unconscious. The free end of the cable is now arcing along the ground like an angry snake. List the steps you will take in dealing with this situation in the sequence in which you will perform them.

        (1) _____

        (2) _____

        (3) _____

        (4) _____

        (5) _____

        (6) _____

        (7) _____

        (8) _____

        (9) _____

       (10) _____

5. You are summoned to a house fire where the fire fighters have just rescued a young man from a particularly smoky part of the building. He is unconscious, and you notice that his clothes are smoldering.

   a. Whenever a person has been unconscious in a smoky environment, you have to worry about the possibility of respiratory injury. List six signs that should lead you to suspect the presence of respiratory injury in a burned patient.

   (1) _____

   (2) _____

   (3) _____

   (4) _____

   (5) _____

   (6) _____

   b. What is the *first* step you should take in dealing with this patient?

   _____

   _____

   c. In due course, you remove his clothing and examine him from head to toe to evaluate the depth and extent of the burn. You find the following:

- Full-thickness burns of the posterior surfaces of both legs, extending well into the buttocks and groin
- Partial-thickness burns of the entire left arm and a hand-sized patch of the left flank

   (1) What percentage of the patient's body has been burned? _____%

   (2) Does the patient have a critical burn? _____ If yes, according to what criteria?

   (a) _____

   (b) _____

   (c) _____

   d. Use the Consensus formula to calculate the rate at which you should run the patient's IV. Assume that he weighs 70 kg and that your infusion set delivers 10 gtt/mL. (Show your calculations.)

   The IV should be run at _____ gtt/min.

   e. After a few minutes of oxygen therapy, the patient regains consciousness and begins complaining of excruciating pain, especially in his groin and left arm. Medical control instructs you to administer morphine.

   (1) What is the correct dosage of morphine for this patient?

   _____

   (2) By what route should it be given?

   _____

   (3) List three possible adverse side effects that you should be ready to deal with.

   (a) _____

   (b) _____

   (c) _____

6. You are standing by at a three-alarm fire when a woman is brought down a ladder by fire fighters and carried to your ambulance. "The whole apartment was full of smoke," one of the fire fighters tells you. "Everything was smoldering—carpets, mattresses, furniture." The woman is conscious but confused. She complains of a severe headache. Her vital signs are a pulse of 120 beats/min and thready, respirations of 40 breaths/min and labored, and blood pressure of 160/90 mm Hg. You find no evidence of burns or other injury.

    a. What is your major concern in this patient, given the history and her symptoms and signs?

    _____

    _____

    b. List the steps you would take in managing this patient.

        (1) _____

        (2) _____

        (3) _____

        (4) _____

        (5) _____

        (6) _____

7. In examining a patient, you find that he has mixed partial- and full-thickness burns of his entire left leg and posterior right leg, extending into his groin. There are also partial-thickness burns over most of the left forearm.

    a. What percentage of his body is burned? (Show your calculations.) _____%

    b. Does he have a critical burn? _____ Explain the reason for your answer.

        (1) _____

        (2) _____

    c. In doing the rapid trauma assessment, you are unable to detect either a dorsalis pedis or an anterior tibial pulse in the left foot. What do you think is the most likely reason?

    _____

    _____

    d. What are you going to do about it?

    _____

    _____

True/False

If you believe the statement to be more true than false, write the letter "T" in the space provided. If you believe the statement to be more false than true, write the letter "F."

    _____ **1.** If you know the identity of the chemical that caused the burn, it is preferable to start treatment with a chemical antidote (eg, applying a weak acid to an alkali burn and vice versa).

    _____ **2.** When a person has been burned by a chemical agent, the skin should be flushed for a minimum of 30 minutes with copious amounts of water.

    _____ **3.** It is important to use only sterile water to flush a chemical burn, lest you contaminate the burn wound.

_____ **4.** In burns caused by hot tar, it is crucial to remove the tar from contact with the skin as quickly as possible to prevent systemic tar poisoning.

_____ **5.** If chemicals have splashed into someone's eyes, the eyes should be continuously irrigated with a steady stream of water.

_____ **6.** Burn shock occurs because of the fluid loss across the damaged skin and the volume shifts within the rest of the body.

_____ **7.** Although fire deaths continue to decrease, children under 5 years old continue to be at a high risk of dying in a fire.

_____ **8.** Carbon monoxide binds to the hemoglobin 500 times faster than oxygen does.

_____ **9.** Currents as small as 0.1 amp may cause ventricular fibrillation if the current passes through the heart.

_____ **10.** You should peel away clothing that has "melted" into the flesh of a burn patient.

Short Answer

Complete this section with short written answers using the space provided.

   1. Discuss the four rules that can help you avoid being struck by lightning.

     a.

_____

_____

     b.

_____

_____

     c.

_____

_____

     d.

_____

_____

   2. Suspect that a patient with flame burns has a respiratory injury if any of the following signs are present:

     a. _____

     b. _____

     c. _____

     d. _____

     e. _____

     f. _____

   3. Injury from a high-voltage electric source or from lightning may produce any of the following:

     a. _____

     b. _____

     c. _____

     d. _____

e. _____

f. _____

g. _____

h. _____

i. _____

j. _____

Fill-in-the-Table

Fill in the missing columns of the table.

Approximate the amount of fluid the burned patient will need by using the Consensus formula. During the first 24 hours, the burned patient will need:

4 mL × body weight (in kg) × percentage of body surface burned

Consensus Formula Chart										
% Burn	10 kg	20 kg	30 kg	40 kg	50 kg	60 kg	70 kg	80 kg	90 kg	100 kg
10	25			100	125	150	175		225	250
20	50			200	250	300	350		450	500
30	75			300	375	450	525		675	750
40	100			400	500	600	700		900	1,000
50	125			500	625	750	875		1,125	1,250
60	150			600	750	900	1,050		1,350	1,500
70	175			700	875	1,050	1,225		1,575	1,750
80	200			800	1,000	1,200	1,400		1,800	2,000
90	225			900	1,125	1,350	1,575		2,025	2,250
20 mL/kg	200			800	1,000	1,200	1,400		1,800	2,000

This table represents the fluid recommended in the *first hour* (one eighth of the initial 8-hour dose) by the Consensus formula. The final row represents the amount of a 20-mL/kg bolus.

Problem Solving

Practice your calculation skills by solving the following math problems.

1. On examining the patient, you find burns covering the following areas:
   - The whole right leg (front and back)
   - The anterior left leg
   - The anterior trunk
   - The whole right arm
     a. Use the rule of nines to calculate what percentage of the patient's body surface area is burned: _____ %. (Show your calculations.)

b. If the patient weighs 154 lb, at what rate should you run his IV? Use the Parkland formula to calculate the rate (and don't forget to convert his weight to kilograms first!). (Show your calculations.)

IV rate = _____ mL/h

c. If you have a standard infusion set that delivers 10 gtt/mL, at how many drops per minute do you have to run the IV to deliver the volume you calculated?

IV rate = _____ gtt/min

d. What IV fluid will you use?

_____

Face and Neck Trauma

Matching

Match each of the items in the left column to the appropriate injury in the right column.

_____ **1.** Anisocoria

_____ **2.** Anterior chamber

_____ **3.** Aqueous humor

_____ **4.** Auricle

_____ **5.** Blowout fracture

_____ **6.** Central vision

_____ **7.** Cochlea

_____ **8.** Cochlear duct

_____ **9.** Conjunctiva

_____ **10.** Conjunctivitis

_____ **11.** Cornea

_____ **12.** Craniofacial disjunction

_____ **13.** Crown

_____ **14.** Cusp

_____ **15.** Dentin

_____ **16.** Diplopia

_____ **17.** Dysconjugate gaze

_____ **18.** Dysphagia

_____ **19.** Epistaxis

_____ **20.** External auditory canal

A. The area in which sound waves are received from the auricle (pinna) before they travel to the eardrum.

B. Difficulty swallowing.

C. Double vision.

D. Point at the top of a tooth.

E. A Le Fort III fracture involves a fracture of all the midface bones, thus separating the entire midface from the cranium.

F. An inflammation of the conjunctivae that usually is caused by bacteria, viruses, allergies, or foreign bodies; should be considered highly contagious if infectious in origin; also called pink eye.

G. A canal within the cochlea that receives vibrations from the ossicles.

H. The visualization of objects directly in front of oneself.

 I. The large outside portion of the ear through which sound waves enter the ear; also called the pinna.

J. The anterior area of the globe between the lens and the cornea that is filled with aqueous humor.

K. A condition in which the pupils are not equal in size.

L. The clear, watery fluid in the anterior chamber of the globe.

M. A fracture of the floor of the orbit, usually caused by a blow to the eye.

N. The shell-shaped structure within the inner ear that contains the organ of Corti.

O. A thin, transparent membrane that covers the sclera and internal surfaces of the eyelids.

P. The transparent anterior portion of the eye that overlies the iris and pupil.

Q. The part of the tooth that is external to the gum.

R. The principal mass of the tooth that is made up of a material that is much more dense and stronger than bone.

S. Paralysis of gaze or lack of coordination between the movements of the two eyes.

T. Nosebleed.

Multiple Choice

Read each item carefully, and then select the best response.

1. The sensory nerve that supplies the skin of the forehead, upper eyelid, and conjunctiva is called the:
   A. maxillary nerve.
   B. facial nerve.
   C. ophthalmic nerve.
   D. mandibular nerve.

2. There are _____ facial bones that form the structure of the face.
   A. 6
   B. 14
   C. 9
   D. 21

3. How many adult teeth does the average adult have?
   A. 32
   B. 34
   C. 30
   D. 36

4. The large cartilaginous external portion of the ear is called the:
   A. organ of Corti.
   B. auricle.
   C. tympanic membrane.
   D. cochlea.

5. What is the name of the substance that forms the principal mass of the tooth?
   A. Alveolar ridges
   B. Cusps
   C. Pulp
   D. Dentin

6. What is the function of the glossopharyngeal nerve?
   A. Motor function of the tongue
   B. Taste sensation to posterior tongue
   C. Slowing down the heart rate
   D. Motor function of mastication

7. You are treating a patient who appears to have a fracture that has affected the upper jaw and the hard palate. What is the name for this fracture?
   A. Le Fort I
   B. Le Fort II
   C. Nasal fracture
   D. Mandibular fracture

8. Which of the following is NOT advisable when covering an injured eye?
   A. Aluminum eye shield
   B. Gauze
   C. Sterile dressing
   D. Cup

9. A patient who has a maxillofacial fracture may have each of the following signs and symptoms, EXCEPT:
   A. dental malocclusion.
   B. swelling.
   C. Battle sign.
   D. blood or fluid running from the nose.

10. What is the name of the fracture resulting from blunt trauma to the face that causes the face to appear flattened?
    A. Hyoid bone fracture
    B. Zygomatic bone fracture
    C. Le Fort I fracture
    D. Orbit bone injury

11. You are treating a patient who sustained a blunt injury to his right eye from a fight. The patient reports that he is seeing flashing lights and specks. He MOST likely has a condition called:
    A. diplopia.
    B. hyphema.
    C. retinal detachment.
    D. conjunctivitis.

12. The physical examination of the eyes involves evaluating the patient for each of the following, EXCEPT:
    A. ecchymosis of the eyelids.
    B. sympathetic eye movements.
    C. redness of the globes.
    D. foreign bodies in the cornea.

13. When assessing the pupils of your patient, you note they are not equal in size. What is this condition called?
    A. Dysconjugate gaze
    B. Anisocoria
    C. Conjunctivitis
    D. Globe disruption

14. Which of the following is NOT a type of contact lens?
    A. Rigid gas permeable
    B. Soft hydrophilic
    C. Hard
    D. Chemical

15. You are treating a patient who has an injury to the anterior neck. She is complaining of difficulty swallowing, hematemesis, and hemoptysis. What is her MOST likely injury?
    A. Esophageal perforation
    B. Neurologic impairment
    C. Vascular injury
    D. Laryngeal fracture

Labeling

Label the following diagrams with the correct terms.

1. Structures of the Eye

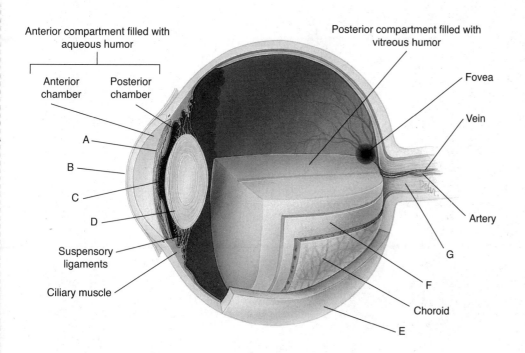

Anterior compartment filled with aqueous humor

Posterior compartment filled with vitreous humor

Anterior chamber   Posterior chamber

Fovea

Vein

A

B

C

D

Suspensory ligaments

Ciliary muscle

Artery

G

F

Choroid

E

A. _____

B. _____

C. _____

D. _____

E. _____

F. _____

G. _____

2. Structures of the Anterior Neck

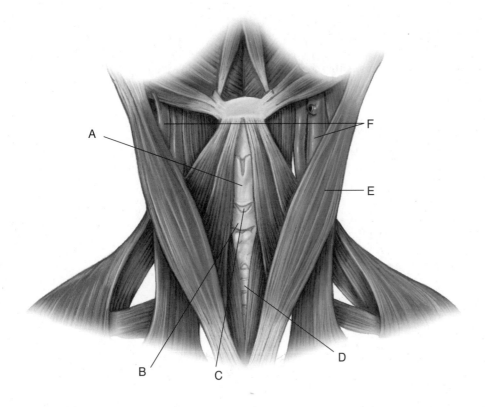

A. _____

B. _____

C. _____

D. _____

E. _____

F. _____

3. Arteries of the Neck

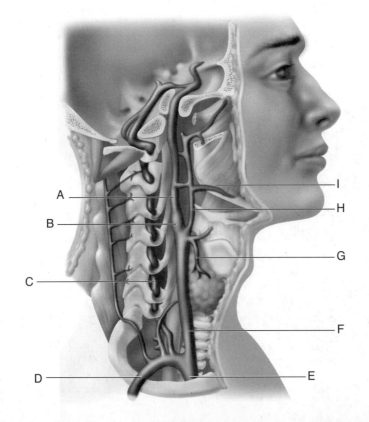

A. _____

B. _____

C. _____

D. _____

E. _____

F. _____

G. _____

H. _____

I. _____

Fill-in-the-Blank

Read each item carefully, and then complete the statement by filling in the missing word(s).

1. The most common cervical strain is often called a/an _____ injury.

2. A/an _____ is a stretching or tearing of muscle or tendon.

3. The bones around the eye are thin, and with significant trauma to the face, the eye can be dislodged. This is called a/an _____ fracture.

4. The adjustable center of the iris that allows light to pass through the eye to the lens is called the _____.

5. The _____ _____ is the portion of the globe between the iris and the lens that is filled with vitreous humor.

6. The _____ _____ secretes and drains tears from the eye.

7. There are two types of vision: _____ and _____.

8. The _____ _____ consists of the cochlea and semicircular canals.

9. When dealing with an impaled object in the face, the only time you should remove the object is when you have _____ complications.

10. Bleeding into the anterior chamber of the eye is called _____.

11. _____, _____, and _____ rays can burn the delicate tissues of the eyes.

12. If you have a burn to the eyes caused by a strong alkali or acid, you should irrigate the eye for _____ minutes.

13. The only indication for removing a contact lens in the field is a/an _____ _____.

14. Reimplantation of a tooth may be successful for up to a/an _____ after it has been avulsed from the mouth.

15. Any open neck wounds should be covered with a/an _____ dressing.

16. Performing _____ _____ in the prehospital environment is considered controversial and requires significant training.

17. When a patient has a facial injury, because _____ irritates the gastric lining, the risks of vomiting and aspiration are significant.

18. Cover the protruding eye with a moist, sterile dressing and stabilize it along with the uninjured eye to prevent further injury due to _____ _____ _____, the movement of both eyes in unison.

19. The paramedic should _____ _____ _____ _____ or manipulate the injured globe in any way.

20. The patient who has sustained a fracture of all midface bones, separating the entire midface from the cranium, has sustained a Le Fort III fracture, also called a/an _____ _____.

Identify

In the following case study, list the chief complaint, vital signs, and pertinent negatives, then answer the additional questions.

Tom and Dan arrive at the scene of a collision as additional help. It is 12:30 AM, and a carload of teenagers has rolled into a cornfield. The corn is about shoulder high, and nobody can say for sure how many kids were in the car. Tom begins a search around the crash site as Dan helps with a patient. Tom hears something to his left and finds a 17-year-old girl on the ground.

The girl is lying facedown, and when he carefully rolls her over, maintaining in-line manual stabilization with the assistance of two fire fighters, he notices that she has severe facial injuries. The primary assessment shows no life-threatening bleeding once her airway has been opened by positioning and the blood has been suctioned from her throat. The girl is "U" on the AVPU scale, and Tom suspects that she may have gone through the windshield. Her respirations are 34 breaths/min and very deep, and oxygen saturation is 95%. Pupils are sluggish, blood pressure is 160/90 mm Hg, and pulse is 72 beats/min. The girl's skin is cool, but she has been lying on the ground for at least half an hour.

Help arrives, and they apply a C-collar, secure her to a backboard, and get her in the unit.

The closest trauma center is half an hour away by helicopter, so they call for the life flight crew to meet them on scene. Because she is unresponsive, Dan and Tom decide to insert an advanced airway and administer 100% supplemental oxygen to the patient. Two large-bore IVs are placed with normal saline. They are careful not to overload this patient with fluid because of the potential for a head injury. The ECG monitor shows a sinus bradycardia now at a rate of 56 breaths/min, and the blood pressure is now 168/88 mm Hg. Life flight then takes over and flies her to the regional trauma center. They later find out that she survives. She had a Le Fort III fracture and has some neurologic defects from the closed head injury, from which it will take several months to years to recover.

1. Chief complaint:

_____

_____

2. Vital signs:

_____

_____

3. Pertinent negatives:

_____

_____

4. Why is it important to get this patient to the regional trauma center?

_____

_____

5. Why is it so important to keep this patient's airway clear of blood?

_____

_____

6. What are the patient's serial vital signs telling you?

_____

_____

Ambulance Calls

The following case scenarios provide an opportunity to explore the concerns associated with patient management and paramedic care. Read each scenario, then answer each question.

1. While enjoying a weekend off at a ski resort, you happen to see a young woman trip over the steps at the lodge and fall. As you rush to her assistance, you see blood coming from her mouth, and closer inspection reveals that she has knocked out one of her lower teeth entirely. What steps should you take?

   a. _____

   b. _____

   c. _____

   d. _____

   e. _____

2. You volunteer to accompany the young lady to the nearest hospital, some 2 hours away by road. Just as you are pulling away from the ski resort in a friend's car, the resort manager comes running after you, waving for you to stop. "I have someone else here who needs to go to the hospital," he says. Behind him, two ski instructors are

leading a young man along. The patient had been involved in a fistfight and now has two black eyes. A thorough examination of an injured eye includes assessment of which visible ocular structures and ocular functions?

a. _____

b. _____

c. _____

d. _____

e. _____

f. _____

g. _____

h. _____

3. A 12-year-old boy lost control of his bicycle as he was riding down a long, steep hill into town. At the base of the hill, his front wheel struck the curb, and he was catapulted from the bicycle straight through the show window of the local wedding dress shop. When you arrive, you find him bleeding from multiple lacerations. The most profuse bleeding seems to be coming from a large laceration on the left side of his neck.

a. What are the principal dangers associated with the laceration of the neck?

_____

b. What should be done to the wound immediately?

_____

True/False

If you believe the statement to be more true than false, write the letter "T" in the space provided. If you believe the statement to be more false than true, write the letter "F."

_____ 1. There are 22 facial bones that form the structure of the face without contributing to the cranial vault.

_____ 2. The separation between the nostrils is called the nasal septum.

_____ 3. The maxilla is the large movable bone that forms the lower jaw.

_____ 4. Hair movement at the organ of Corti forms nerve impulses that travel to the brain allowing us to "hear."

_____ 5. The glossopharyngeal nerve provides motor function to the tongue.

_____ 6. Nasal fractures are often complicated by the presence of epistaxis.

_____ 7. The Le Fort I fracture has a pyramidal shape and involves the nasal bone and inferior maxilla.

_____ 8. The patient who has sustained an orbital fracture may report symptoms of diplopia.

_____ 9. The cornea is the delicate mucous membrane that covers the sclera and internal surfaces of the eyelids, but not the iris.

_____ 10. Bruising and swelling are your first clues to a maxillofacial fracture.

_____ 11. To maintain an airway, it is okay to use blind nasotracheal intubation when there are signs of facial fractures.

_____ 12. Blunt eye trauma can lead to a retinal detachment, which is common in sports injuries.

_____ 13. It is not necessary to cover both eyes to prevent sympathetic eye movement.

_____ 14. Approximately 25% of hyphemas involve blunt trauma to the globe.

_____ 15. It may be hard to determine the extent of bleeding in the mouth as a result of the patient swallowing the blood.

_____ 16. You should always use an occlusive dressing on an open neck wound to prevent an air embolism.

_____ 17. Coughing up blood is known as dysphagia.

_____ 18. Hoarseness or voice changes may indicate laryngeal fracture.

_____ 19. A perforated tympanic membrane can occur from direct blows to the ear or pressure injuries.

_____ 20. If part of the external ear has been avulsed in a fight, you should save the piece in a container of ice.

Short Answer

Complete this section with short written answers using the space provided.

1. Injuries to the face may be quite frightening to look at, but facial injuries do not by themselves ordinarily pose an immediate threat to life. However, facial injuries may be associated with other conditions or injuries that can threaten life or limb. List two potentially serious or life-threatening conditions that may be associated with maxillofacial trauma.

   a. _____

   b. _____

2. In examining a trauma patient, what findings would lead you to suspect maxillofacial fracture? List five signs of maxillofacial fracture.

   a. _____

   b. _____

   c. _____

   d. _____

   e. _____

Fill-in-the-Table

Fill in the missing parts of the table.

1. Summary of Maxillofacial Fractures

Summary of Maxillofacial Fractures Injury	Signs and Symptoms
Multiple facial bone fractures	• Massive facial swelling • _____ • _____ • Anterior or _____ epistaxis
Zygomatic and orbital fractures	• Loss of sensation below the _____ • Flattening of the _____ • _____ of upward gaze
Nasal fractures	• Crepitus and instability • Swelling, tenderness, _____ • Anterior or _____ epistaxis
Maxillary (Le Fort) fractures	• Mobility of the _____ • Dental _____ • Facial swelling
Mandibular fractures	• Dental malocclusion • _____ instability

2. Signs and Symptoms of Injuries to the Anterior Part of the Neck

Signs and Symptoms of Injuries to the Anterior Part of the Neck	
Injury	Signs and Symptoms
Laryngeal fracture, tracheal transection	• Labored breathing or reduced _____ • Stridor • Hoarseness, voice changes • _____ (coughing up blood) • Subcutaneous emphysema • Swelling, edema • Structural irregularity
Vascular injury	• _____ bleeding • Signs of shock • Hematoma, swelling, edema • _____ deficits
Esophageal perforation	• _____ (difficulty swallowing) • _____ • _____ (suggests aspiration of blood)
Neurologic impairment	• Signs of a stroke (suggests air embolism or _____) • _____ or paresthesia • _____ nerve deficit • Signs of _____ shock

CHAPTER

34

Head and Spine Trauma

Matching

Part I

Match each of the descriptions in the left column to the appropriate term in the right column.

_____ **1.** A condition that occurs with flexion injuries or fractures, resulting in the displacement of bony fragments into the anterior portion of the spinal cord; findings include paralysis below the level of the insult and loss of pain, temperature, and touch sensation.

A. Arachnoid

_____ **2.** The middle membrane of the three meninges that enclose the brain and spinal cord.

B. Axon

_____ **3.** A potentially life-threatening late complication of spinal cord injury in which massive, uninhibited, uncompensated cardiovascular response occurs due to stimulation of the sympathetic nervous system below the level of injury.

C. Battle sign

_____ **4.** Long, slender extension of a neuron that conducts electrical impulses away from the neuronal soma.

D. Brown-Séquard syndrome

_____ **5.** Structures located deep within the cerebrum, diencephalon, and midbrain that have an important role in coordination of motor movements and posture.

E. Central nervous system (CNS)

_____ **6.** Bruising over the mastoid bone behind the ear, commonly seen following a basilar skull fracture; also called retroauricular ecchymosis.

F. Cerebral contusion

_____ **7.** Part of the central nervous system located within the cranium; contains billions of neurons that serve a variety of vital functions.

G. Cerebrospinal fluid (CSF)

_____ **8.** A condition associated with penetrating trauma with hemisection of the spinal cord and complete damage to all spinal tracts on the involved side.

H. Complete spinal cord injury

_____ **9.** A neurologic condition caused by compression of the bundle of nerve roots located at the end of the spinal cord.

I. Cribriform plate

_____ **10.** The system containing the brain and spinal cord.

J. Decerebrate (extensor) posturing

_____ **11.** The region of the brain essential in coordinating muscle movements in the body; also called the athlete's brain.

K. Herniation

_____ **12.** A focal brain injury in which brain tissue is bruised and damaged in a defined area.

L. Galea aponeurotica

_____ **13.** Cerebral water; causes or contributes to swelling of the brain.

M. Fontanelles

_____ **14.** Fluid produced in the ventricles of the brain that flows in the subarachnoid space and bathes the meninges.

N. Epidural hematoma

_____ **15.** Respirations that are fast and then become slow, with intervening periods of apnea; commonly seen following brainstem injury.

O. Diencephalon

_____ **16.** Total disruption of all tracts of the spinal cord, with all cord-mediated functions below the level of transection lost permanently.

_____ **17.** Dual impacting of the brain into the skull; the first injury occurs at the point of impact, and the second occurs on the opposite side of impact, as the brain rebounds.

_____ **18.** A horizontal bone, perforated with numerous foramina for the passage of the olfactory nerve filaments from the nasal cavity.

_____ **19.** Minimum cerebral perfusion pressure required to adequately perfuse the brain; 60 mm Hg in the adult.

_____ **20.** Abnormal posture characterized by extension of the arms and legs; indicates pressure on the brainstem.

_____ **21.** Result from high-energy direct trauma to a small surface area of the head with a blunt object (such as a baseball bat to the head); commonly result in bony fragments being driven into the brain, causing injury.

_____ **22.** The part of the brain between the brainstem and the cerebrum that includes the thalamus, subthalamus, and hypothalamus.

_____ **23.** Any injury that affects the entire brain.

_____ **24.** An accumulation of blood between the skull and the dura.

_____ **25.** A type of injury that results from forward movement of the head, typically as the result of rapid deceleration, such as in a car crash, or with a direct blow to the occiput.

_____ **26.** The soft spots in the skull of a newborn or infant where the sutures of the skull have not yet grown together.

_____ **27.** Natural openings, perforations, or orifices, such as in the bones of the cranial vault.

_____ **28.** Tough, tendinous layer of the scalp.

_____ **29.** The bony anterior part of the roof of the mouth.

_____ **30.** Process in which tissue is forced out of its normal position, such as when the brain is forced from the cranial vault, either through the foramen magnum or over the tentorium.

P. Diffuse brain injury

Q. Flexion injury

R. Foramina

S. Hard palate

T. Depressed skull fractures

U. Critical minimum threshold

V. Coup-contrecoup injury

W. Cheyne-Stokes respirations

X. Cerebral edema

Y. Cerebellum

Z. Cauda equina syndrome

AA. Brain

BB. Basal ganglia

CC. Anterior cord syndrome

DD. Autonomic dysreflexia

Part II

Match each of the items in the left column to the appropriate injury in the right column. (*Note:* Some of the injury types can be applied more than once.)

_____ **1.** A 15-year-old skateboarder has hit the side of his head after a fall. After an initial bout of unconsciousness, he regains consciousness, only to lapse again about an hour later. His mother cannot wake him up again.

A. Cerebral concussion

_____ **2.** A football player comes off the field after a helmet-to-helmet hit. He is a little disoriented and cannot remember the play. The coach says he just got his bell rung. He shows no other signs later in the evening or the next day.

B. Cerebral contusion

_____ **3.** The other football player also comes off the field. He is very confused. He loses consciousness in the locker room for about 3 minutes. He is confused for the next 2 days.

C. Epidural hematoma

____ **4.** A 40-year-old woman is scrubbing the floor. As she rises, she hits the back of her head on the sink. At the time, she gets a slight headache. Later in the evening her speech becomes slightly slurred.

D. Subdural hematoma

____ **5.** A 12-year-old girl is hit on the head with a baseball bat by her brother. She is knocked out but wakes back up to tell her mom what happened. Her mother decides to have her checked out. On the way to the doctor's office, the girl appears to go to sleep. When they arrive, the mother cannot wake her.

E. Intracerebral hematoma

____ **6.** The patient was the driver of a vehicle that was struck from the left side by another car. The door on the driver's side is dented. The patient is conscious, but witnesses say that he was "out cold" for a few minutes immediately after the collision. He complains of a headache and the feeling of pins and needles in his left hip and left leg. His skull is tender to palpation in the area just superior to the left ear. While he is under your care, his level of consciousness deteriorates until he is unconscious altogether, and his respirations become very slow.

F. Subarachnoid hemorrhage

____ **7.** The patient was a participant in a barroom brawl. This patient was "knocked out cold" for a few minutes. Now he seems alert, but he cannot remember what happened. He complains of a little dizziness. His vital signs are normal.

____ **8.** The patient was a front-seat passenger in a car that careened into a utility pole. He is confused and sleepy when you find him. His speech is slurred, and there is weakness of the right leg. He becomes more and more lethargic while under your care and vomits twice. The left pupil seems to be getting larger than the right.

____ **9.** The patient was an unrestrained front-seat passenger in a car involved in a head-on collision with another car. He apparently struck his head on the windshield because the windshield in front of the patient is cracked. The patient is found unconscious. His left pupil is larger than the right. His pulse is 56 beats/min, and his blood pressure is 190/90 mm Hg. Respirations are irregular.

____ **10.** You are called to a 70-year-old woman with a terrible headache. She hit her head on the cupboard about 2 hours ago. She initially had a severe headache at the site of the injury, but now it has moved to a larger area of her head. She is responsive only to questions and begins to vomit while you are taking care of her. She rapidly becomes unresponsive and begins to have a seizure.

Multiple Choice

Read each item carefully, and then select the best response.

1. The base of the skull has an opening that allows the spinal cord to connect to the brain. What is the opening called?
   A. Fontanelle
   B. Mastoid process
   C. Cribriform plate
   D. Foramen magnum

2. The oculomotor nerve is the _____ cranial nerve.
   A. first
   B. second
   C. third
   D. fourth

3. The brain consumes what percentage of the body's total oxygen?
   A. 10%
   B. 20%
   C. 30%
   D. 40%

4. Within the diencephalon, there are several divisions. Which division processes sensory input, influences moods, and controls general body movements?
   A. Subthalamus
   B. Thalamus
   C. Hypothalamus
   D. Epithalamus

5. What is the reticular activating system (RAS) responsible for?
   A. Blood pressure
   B. Respiration
   C. Heart rate
   D. Consciousness

6. When a patient has a basilar skull fracture, which of the following signs or symptoms would you LEAST expect to see?
   A. Raccoon eyes
   B. Battle sign
   C. Blowout fracture of the eye
   D. Draining of blood and CSF from the ear

7. What is the minimum cerebral perfusion pressure in an adult that is required to perfuse the brain adequately?
   A. 15 mm Hg
   B. 30 mm Hg
   C. 45 mm Hg
   D. 60 mm Hg

8. You are treating a patient who has starred the windshield in a car crash. The patient reports that he cannot remember what happened before the collision. This is called:
   A. anterograde amnesia.
   B. retrograde amnesia.
   C. amnesia.
   D. focal brain injury.

9. After you drop off the patient whom you treated for a fall down the stairs, the doctor tells you she had bleeding into the brain tissue. You remember the medical term for this is:
   A. epidural hematoma.
   B. intracerebral hematoma.
   C. subarachnoid hemorrhage.
   D. subdural hematoma.

10. What is the MOST important sign or symptom in evaluating a patient with a brain injury?
    A. Bleeding from the ears
    B. Pupil size and how the pupils react to light
    C. Level of consciousness
    D. Mechanism of injury

11. When using the Glasgow Coma Scale (GCS), what are the lowest and the highest scores a patient can get?
    A. 0; 15
    B. 0; 14
    C. 3; 14
    D. 3; 15

12. What is the MOST important step in managing any type of head injury?
    A. Maintaining airway and breathing
    B. Performing spinal immobilization
    C. Assessing where the bleeding is in the brain
    D. Establishing an IV

13. What portion of the spine contains the most bones of the vertebral column?
    A. Cervical
    B. Thoracic
    C. Lumbar
    D. Sacral

14. How many pairs of spinal nerves are there?
    A. 12
    B. 33
    C. 31
    D. 5

15. The _____ plexus innervates the diaphragm.
    A. cervical
    B. sacral
    C. lumbar
    D. brachial

16. Which of the following is NOT associated with high-risk mechanisms of injury for spinal injuries?
    A. Penetrating trauma near the spine
    B. Fall from two times the patient's height
    C. Unrestrained in a rollover crash
    D. Diving injury

17. What is the initial step of assessment in a suspected spinal injury?
    A. Scene safety
    B. Clearing the airway
    C. Checking for a pulse
    D. Activating the trauma system

18. What is the primary goal when immobilizing a patient with a spinal injury?
    A. Determining whether the patient will be paralyzed
    B. Determining where the exact injury is
    C. Preventing further injuries to the patient
    D. Securing the airway of the patient

19. Which of the following is NOT done prior to applying a cervical collar to a patient?
    A. Determine the need for the collar.
    B. Take manual stabilization of the head.
    C. Assess extremities for distal pulse, motor, and sensory (PMS) functions.
    D. Check the patient's ability to move the neck.

20. When should you NOT perform a rapid extrication?
    A. The patient's legs are tingling.
    B. The patient's condition requires immediate transport.
    C. The vehicle or scene is unsafe.
    D. You are unable to manage the airway.

21. How many rescuers does it take to remove a helmet from a patient?
    A. One
    B. Two
    C. Three
    D. Never remove the helmet.

22. The nerve root located at T4 is responsible for what area dermatome?
    A. Umbilicus
    B. Back of the leg
    C. Apex of axilla
    D. Nipple line

Labeling

Label the following diagrams with the correct terms.

  1. Sections of the Cervical, Thoracic, and Lumbar Spine

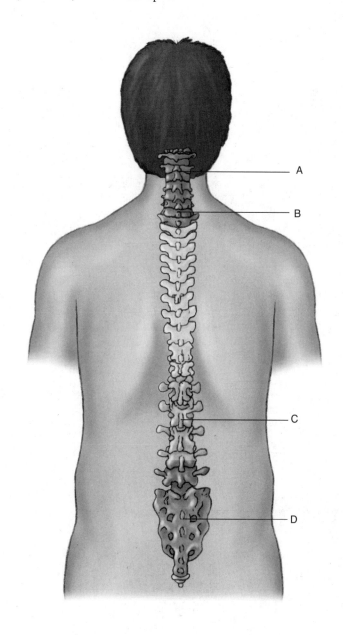

A. _____

B. _____

C. _____

D. _____

2. Layers of the Spinal Cord

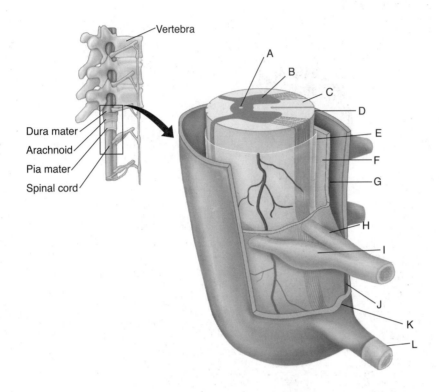

A. _____

B. _____

C. _____

D. _____

E. _____

F. _____

G. _____

H. _____

I. _____

J. _____

K. _____

L. _____

3. Major Regions of the Brain

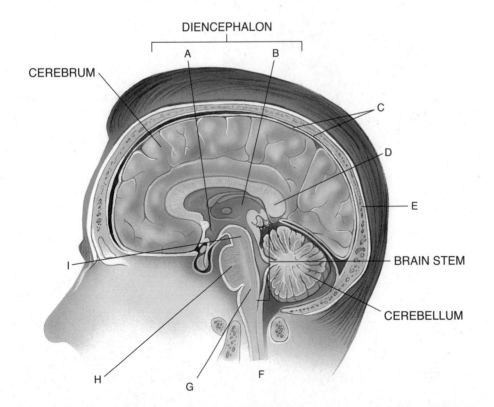

A. _____

B. _____

C. _____

D. _____

E. _____

F. _____

G. _____

H. _____

I. _____

Fill-in-the-Blank

Read each item carefully, and then complete the statement by filling in the missing word(s).

1. The skull sits atop the _____ skeleton.
2. The _____ link the sutures in the skull and are soft when a child is born.
3. The _____ is responsible for higher functions and is the largest portion of the brain.
4. The brainstem contains the midbrain, _____, and the _____.
5. The second layer of the meninges resembles a spider's web, so it is called the _____.
6. A/an _____-_____ injury happens when the brain sloshes forward and hits the front of the skull and then recoils and hits the back part of the skull.
7. Increased intracranial pressure (ICP) can produce signs of _____, bradycardia, and irregular respirations. This is known as _____ _____.
8. A/an _____ hematoma is the collection of blood between the dura mater and the skull.
9. Because of clenched teeth, the paramedic may have to perform _____ _____ _____ to intubate the head injury patient safely.
10. Unlike patients who are suffering from shock, the patient with a head injury can develop a very high _____ _____.
11. Components of the vertebral body are the spinous process, _____, and the _____.
12. The two vertebrae in the cervical area that allow for the rotational movement of the skull are _____ and _____.
13. The central nervous system consists of the _____ and the _____ _____.
14. The brainstem consists of the _____, _____, and _____.
15. The spinal cord attaches to the brain through the _____ _____, which is a hole in the base of the skull.
16. The sympathetic nervous system is controlled by the _____.
17. _____ spinal cord injury is total disruption of all tracts of the spinal cord, with all cord-mediated functions below the level of transaction lost permanently.
18. The signs and symptoms of _____ _____ are hypotension and bradycardia, accompanied by warm, dry, flushed skin.
19. The paramedic should always use the _____-_____ method for opening the airway of the patient with a suspected spinal injury.
20. During an assessment of the feet of a patient, when you stimulate the bottom of the feet, normally the toes move _____; with a positive Babinski reflex, the toes move _____.

Identify

In the following case studies, list the chief complaint, vital signs, and pertinent negatives.

Part I

Bill and Jan arrive at the scene of a motor vehicle crash as additional help. It is 2:00 AM and a van full of teenagers has rolled into an empty lot. The grass and weeds are about shoulder high and nobody can say for sure how many teens were in the vehicle. Bill begins a search around the crash site as Jan helps with a patient. Bill hears something to his left and finds a 16-year-old girl on the ground.

The girl is on her back with her arms drawn up to her chest, and her feet seem to be rigid and slightly turned in. A primary assessment shows no life-threatening bleeding. The girl is "U" on the AVPU scale, and Bill determines she is a 7 on the GCS scale. Her respirations are 34 breaths/min and very deep, and oxygen saturation is 98%. Pupils are sluggish, blood pressure is 160/90 mm Hg, and her pulse is 64 beats/min. The girl's skin is cool, but she has been lying on the ground for at least 20 minutes.

Help arrives and they apply a C-collar, secure her to a backboard, and get her in the unit.

The closest trauma center is 20 minutes away by helicopter, so they call for the life flight crew to meet them in a landing zone near the scene. Because she is unresponsive (consider intubating for a GCS less than 8), Jan and Bill decide to insert an advanced airway and administer 100% supplemental oxygen to the patient. Two large-bore IVs are placed with normal saline. They are careful not to overload this patient with fluid because of the rising ICP. The ECG monitor shows a sinus bradycardia now at a rate of 56 breaths/min, and the blood pressure is now 168/88 mm Hg. Life flight then takes over and flies her to the regional trauma center. They later find out that she makes it but has some neurologic defects, from which it will take several months to years to recover.

1. Chief complaint:

_____

_____

2. Vital signs:

_____

_____

3. Pertinent negatives:

_____

_____

4. Why is it important to get this patient to the regional trauma center?

_____

_____

5. What does the patient's position on the ground tell you?

_____

_____

6. What are the patient's serial vital signs telling you?

_____

_____

Part II

Your unit is called to a two-vehicle collision. It is a dark morning, and it is misting outside. Your patient is trapped in a vehicle that has landed on its wheels after rolling two or three times. Your patient is a young woman with long hair. Her hair is trapped between the roof of the car and the headrest, and you are unable to get inside because of the damage of the collision. You find that she responds to a few of your questions, but the only thing she can remember is her first name. You need the Jaws of Life to get her out. After the car is cut apart, you can finally get in the car to perform manual stabilization. A C-collar is applied, and you and your partners—with some help from a fire fighter—do a rapid extrication, being very careful to move her in straight lines onto the backboard.

En route you perform a rapid trauma assessment, which reveals no bleeding from anywhere. Your patient is very cold, and you learn that the crash happened about an hour before anyone found the two cars. She has a blood pressure of 100/62 mm Hg and a pulse of 124 beats/min. Her oxygen saturation is 96% before applying supplemental oxygen via nonrebreathing at 15 L/min. Her rate of breathing is 26 breaths/min and somewhat shallow. Lungs are clear. You are unable to find a pulse in either of the feet. She is unable to move her legs, and she doesn't respond to you when you touch or pinch her feet, knees, or hips. The monitor shows sinus tachycardia with no ectopy. You start two large-bore IVs with warm normal saline and use active rewarming, turning the heat on high in the squad to help bring her body temperature back up. Her serial vital signs remain largely unchanged except for the oxygen saturation, which has increased to 98%. After a 500-mL bolus of fluid, her blood pressure has come up slightly to 108/64 mm Hg. The next day you learn she had a broken L2 vertebra and is paralyzed from there down.

1. Chief complaint:

_____

_____

2. Vital signs:

_____

_____

3. Pertinent negatives:

_____

_____

Complete the Patient Care Report (PCR)

Reread the incident scenario in the preceding Identify, Part II, exercise and then complete the following PCR for the patient.

EMS Patient Care Report (PCR)			
Date:	Incident No.:	Nature of Call:	Location:
Dispatched:	En Route:	At Scene:	Transport:	At Hospital:	In Service:

Patient Information	
Age:	Allergies:
Sex:	Medications:
Weight (in kg [lb]):	Past Medical History:
	Chief Complaint:

Vital Signs				
Time:	BP:	Pulse:	Respirations:	SpO$_2$:
Time:	BP:	Pulse:	Respirations:	SpO$_2$:
Time:	BP:	Pulse:	Respirations:	SpO$_2$:

EMS Treatment (circle all that apply)			
Oxygen @ _____ L/min via (circle one): NC NRM Bag-Mask Device	Assisted Ventilation	Airway Adjunct	CPR
Defibrillation	Bleeding Control	Bandaging	Splinting	Other

Narrative

Ambulance Calls

The following case scenarios provide an opportunity to explore the concerns associated with patient management and paramedic care. Read each scenario, and then answer each question.

1. In the old cowboy movies, one of the standard ways of preventing the bad guys from making their getaway was to tie a rope securely between two trees on either side of the road, at a height about 8 or 9 feet off the ground. When the bad guys came galloping down the road, the rope would catch them across the chest or neck and throw them from their horses.

   Imagine, then, that you are the Dodge City paramedic, called to attend a bad guy who has just been thrown from his horse after riding precipitously into a rope stretched across the road. You find the bad guy lying on the road and moaning. His voice is quite hoarse as he replies to your questions about what happened, and he seems very short of breath. On examination, you find a prominent bruise over the anterior neck. The patient's face and neck appear bloated, and the skin there has a crinkly feel to it.

   a. What serious injury or injuries do you have to consider in this patient, given the mechanisms of injury and the findings on examination?

   _____

   _____

   b. List the steps you would take in treating this patient.

   (1) _____

   (2) _____

   (3) _____

2. A 15-year-old boy was shot in the abdomen during a gang dispute. You find him lying supine on the sidewalk. He is conscious, alert, and crying out, "I can't move my legs! I can't move my legs!" You find an entrance wound just to the left of the umbilicus. You cannot find an exit wound. On examination, sensation is absent from the toes up to the bottom of the ribs. The patient cannot move either leg, but he has normal strength in both hands.

   a. At approximately what level of the spinal cord has this boy probably been injured?

   _____

   b. Suppose that your examination also revealed a blood pressure of 80 mm Hg systolic. What could you conclude from that finding?

   _____

3. A 34-year-old man has been injured in a road incident in which his head apparently struck the windshield with some force. When you first reach the scene, the patient is unconscious. He is breathing 8 breaths/min, inhaling approximately 500 mL of air with each breath.

   a. What is his minute volume? _____

   b. Is that volume greater or less than normal? _____

   c. Therefore, you can conclude that the patient's arterial PCO_2 will tend to _____ (increase or decrease?), so his pH will _____ (increase or decrease?). The net effect will be an acid–base disorder called a _____ (respiratory or metabolic?) _____ (acidosis or alkalosis?). The way you can help correct that abnormality is to _____.

   d. One reason to try to correct hypoventilation in a patient with a head injury is that hypoventilation may, through its effects on acid–base balance just mentioned, worsen cerebral edema and thereby accelerate the increase in intracranial pressure (ICP). How would you know if this patient is developing an increase in ICP? List five signs of increasing ICP.

   (1) _____

   (2) _____

   (3) _____

   (4) _____

   (5) _____

e. Here are the findings of your initial neurologic assessment of the patient:

- He opens his eyes only when pinched, not when spoken to.
- He pulls his whole arm and shoulder away when you pinch his hand.
- He makes garbled sounds that you cannot understand.

(1) What is his AVPU? _____

(2) What is his score on the GCS? _____

4. Score each of the patients described in the following scenarios according to the AVPU scale and the Glasgow Coma Scale (GCS).

a. The patient is found unconscious. He opens his eyes in response to a loud voice. He does not follow commands, but he pulls his hand away when pinched and makes a few garbled noises that you cannot understand.

AVPU scale _____   GCS score _____

b. The patient is found apparently unconscious, but he opens his eyes at the sound of your voice. He can follow simple commands, but he is a bit confused and cannot tell you what month it is or what day of the week it is.

AVPU scale _____   GCS score _____

c. The patient is found unconscious. He does not open his eyes when pinched or try to pull away from the painful stimulus; instead his arms flex spasmodically across his chest while his legs go into hyperextension. He makes no sound.

AVPU scale _____   GCS score _____

d. The patient is found conscious. He gives you a coherent account of what happened to him, his name, and the day of the week, and he can follow simple commands.

AVPU scale _____   GCS score _____

5. You are called to attend to a patient injured in an altercation that took place in a downtown drinking establishment. In the course of the dispute, someone broke a whiskey bottle over the patient's head. You find the patient conscious, bleeding profusely from his scalp, and in a distinctly unfriendly frame of mind, which he manifests by hurling tables and chairs in all directions while screaming uncomplimentary names at his assailants. List the steps you would take in treating this patient.

a. _____

b. _____

c. _____

d. _____

True/False

If you believe the statement to be more true than false, write the letter "T" in the space provided. If you believe the statement to be more false than true, write the letter "F."

_____ **1.** The cranial vault consists of 10 bones.

_____ **2.** The cribriform plate allows for passage of the olfactory nerve filaments.

_____ **3.** The reticular activating system is responsible for maintenance of hearing and reading skills.

_____ **4.** The brain uses 25% of the body's glucose.

_____ **5.** The frontal lobe of the brain is responsible for personality traits.

_____ **6.** The vagus nerve originates from the pons.

_____ **7.** CSF is manufactured in the ventricles of the brain.

_____ **8.** Motor vehicle crashes are the most common cause of head injury.

_____ **9.** The body's response to a decrease of cerebral perfusion pressure is to increase mean arterial pressure.

_____ **10.** Decerebrate posturing is seen as the patient pulls the arms into the core of the body.

_____ **11.** Subarachnoid hematoma will usually present with a sudden and severe headache.

_____ **12.** The outermost of the meninges is the dura mater.

_____ **13.** There are 32 pairs of spinal nerves that emerge from the spinal cord.

_____ **14.** The vagus nerve is part of the parasympathetic nervous system.

_____ **15.** A flexion injury is usually caused by a rapid deceleration or a direct blow to the occipital region.

_____ **16.** Most fractures sustained in a vertical compression are classified as unstable.

_____ **17.** In central cord syndrome, the patient will demonstrate a greater loss of function in the lower extremities than in the upper extremities.

_____ **18.** The diaphragm is innervated by the phrenic nerve between C3 and C5.

_____ **19.** When there is an absent pulse in a patient with a spinal cord injury, it is okay not to start CPR because of the region of the injury.

_____ **20.** A normal neurologic exam can immediately rule out a spinal cord injury.

_____ **21.** The preferred method of immobilizing a person to a long backboard is the two-person log-roll method.

_____ **22.** You should assess the pulse, motor, and sensory (PMS) functions in each extremity before and after placing the patient on a long backboard.

_____ **23.** A rapid extrication technique should be used for every patient that is in a seated position in a car crash.

_____ **24.** It is okay to release manual stabilization of the neck while you are measuring for a cervical collar. Make sure, however, to let your patient know not to move the head.

_____ **25.** If the patient is standing up and walking, it is okay to have the patient lie down on the backboard for transport.

_____ **26.** Autonomic dysreflexia is typically a late complication of spinal cord injury but can occur acutely.

Short Answer

Complete this section with short written answers using the space provided.

1. In a patient who has sustained potential injury to the spinal cord, it doesn't pay to wait until there are symptoms and signs of spinal cord damage. By then it may be too late to prevent permanent disability. The only sure way to prevent such disability is to anticipate spinal injury under the appropriate circumstances and to handle the patient in a way that will protect his or her spinal cord from damage. List eight high-risk mechanisms of injury that strongly suggest spine injury:

a. _____

b. _____

c. _____

d. _____

e. _____

f. _____

g. _____

h. _____

2. When assessing a patient for traumatic injuries, you use the mnemonics DCAP-BTLS and PMS. Write the word for each letter as follows.

D _____

C _____

A _____

P _____

B _____

T _____

L _____

S _____

P _____

M _____

S _____

Fill-in-the-Table

Fill in the missing parts of the tables.

1. Signs and Symptoms of Head Injury

Signs and Symptoms of Head Injury
_____, contusions, or _____ to the scalp
Soft area or _____ noted on palpation of the scalp
Visible _____ or _____ of the skull
_____ sign or _____ eyes
CSF rhinorrhea or _____
Pupillary abnormalities • _____ pupil size • Sluggish or _____ pupils
A period of unresponsiveness
Confusion or disorientation
Repeatedly asking the same question(s) (perseveration)
Amnesia (_____ and/or _____)
Combativeness or other abnormal behavior
Numbness or tingling in the _____
Loss of sensation and/or motor function
Focal _____ deficits
Seizures
_____ triad: hypertension, _____, and irregular or erratic respirations
Dizziness
Visual disturbances, blurred vision, or double vision (_____)
Seeing "stars"
Nausea or vomiting
Posturing (_____ and/or _____)

2. Glasgow Coma Scale

Glasgow Coma Scale		
Test	**Response**	**Score**
Eye opening	Spontaneous	4
	Voice	3
	_____	2
	None	1
Verbal	_____ conversation	5
	_____ conversation	4
	_____ words	3
	_____ sounds	2
	None	1
Motor	Obeys commands	6
	Localizes pain	5
	_____	4
	Abnormal flexion (_____)	3
	Abnormal _____ (decerebrate)	2
	None	1
Score: 15 indicates no neurologic disabilities.		
Score: 13–14 may indicate mild dysfunction.		
Score: 9–12 may indicate moderate dysfunction.		
Score: 8 or less is indicative of severe dysfunction.		

3. Landmark Dermatomes

Landmark Dermatomes			
Nerve Root	**Anatomic Location**	**Nerve Root**	**Anatomic Location**
C2	_____	T10	Umbilicus
C3	_____	L1	_____ line
C5	Lateral side of _____	L2	Mid anterior thigh
C6	Thumb and medial index finger (6-shooter)	L3	Medial aspect of the _____
C7	_____ finger	L5	_____
C8	_____ finger	S1–S3	Back of _____
T2	_____	S4–S5	_____ area
T4	_____ line		

Chest Trauma

Matching

Part I

Match each of the items in the right column to the appropriate description in the left column.

_____ **1.** Prominence on the sternum that lies opposite the second intercostal space.

_____ **2.** A condition in which the atria and right ventricle are collapsed by a collection of blood and other fluid within the pericardial sac, resulting in a diminished cardiac output.

_____ **3.** An event in which an often fatal cardiac dysrhythmia is produced by a sudden blow to the thoracic cavity.

_____ **4.** Large skeletal muscle that plays a major role in breathing and separates the chest cavity from the abdominal cavity.

_____ **5.** An injury that involves two or more adjacent ribs fractured in two or more places, allowing the segment between the fractures to move independently of the rest of the thoracic cage.

_____ **6.** The collection of blood within the normally closed pleural space.

_____ **7.** A prominence of the jugular veins due to increased volume or increased pressure within the central venous system or the thoracic cavity.

_____ **8.** Space within the chest that contains the heart, major blood vessels, vagus nerve, trachea, and esophagus; located between the two lungs.

_____ **9.** An acute traumatic perforation of the ventricles, atria, intraventricular septum, intra-atrial septum, chordae, papillary muscles, or valves.

_____ **10.** A closely placed grouping of an artery, vein, and nerve that lies beneath the inferior edge of a rib.

_____ **11.** The potential space between the layers of the pericardium.

_____ **12.** Double-layered sac containing the heart and the origins of the superior vena cava, the inferior vena cava, and the pulmonary artery.

_____ **13.** The collection of air within the normally closed pleural sac.

_____ **14.** A drop in the systolic blood pressure of 10 mm Hg more than during inspiration; commonly seen in patients with cardiac tamponade or severe asthma.

_____ **15.** Also known as the breastbone, a bony structure along the midline of the thorax that provides a point of anterior attachment for the thoracic cage.

_____ **16.** A physical finding of air within the subcutaneous tissue.

_____ **17.** A life-threatening collection of air within the pleural space; the volume and pressure have both collapsed the involved lung and cause a shift of the mediastinal structures to the opposite side.

A. Xiphoid process

B. Thorax

C. Traumatic asphyxia

D. Tension pneumothorax

E. Sternum

F. Subcutaneous emphysema

G. Pneumothorax

H. Pulsus paradoxus

I. Pericardial sac

J. Pericardium

K. Angle of Louis

L. Commotio cordis

M. Cardiac tamponade

N. Flail chest

O. Diaphragm

P. Mediastinum

Q. Jugular vein distension

_____ **18.** The part of the body between the neck and the diaphragm, encased by the ribs.

_____ **19.** A pattern of injuries seen after a severe force is applied to the thorax, forcing blood from the great vessels and back into the head and neck.

_____ **20.** An inferior segment of the sternum often used as a landmark for cardiopulmonary resuscitation.

R. Hemothorax

S. Neurovascular bundle

T. Myocardial rupture

Part II
Certain signs identify specific lung injuries. Match the types of lung injuries to the signs.

_____ **1.** Hemoptysis, lack of tracheal deviation, dullness noted on the side affected during percussion.

_____ **2.** Jugular vein distention, and tracheal deviation and absence of breath sounds on affected side.

_____ **3.** Diminished breath sounds heard on auscultation, a finding that is best heard anteriorly if the patient is in the supine position or in the apices if the patient is upright.

_____ **4.** A sucking chest wound may be noted and a bubbling wound may be noted.

_____ **5.** Evidence of underlying injury may include contusions, tenderness, crepitus, or paradoxical motion. Auscultation may reveal wheezes, crackles, or rales.

A. Simple pneumothorax

B. Open pneumothorax

C. Tension pneumothorax

D. Massive hemothorax

E. Pulmonary contusion

Part III
Match the physiology terms with the definitions and descriptions.

_____ **1.** The volume of blood delivered to the body in 1 minute.

_____ **2.** The process by which CO_2 is removed from the body.

_____ **3.** This process includes the delivery of oxygen from the air to the blood.

_____ **4.** This process includes both the delivery of oxygen to the body and the elimination of carbon dioxide from the body.

_____ **5.** The amount of blood per each beat of the heart.

A. Oxygenation

B. Ventilation

C. Cardiac output

D. Stroke volume

E. Breathing

Multiple Choice
Read each item carefully, and then select the best response.

1. While riding his bicycle fast down a hill, a 16-year-old boy falls and sustains an injury to the chest. While palpating the chest during the rapid assessment of the chest, you feel what you believe to be fracture of a number of adjacent ribs and observe the patient is having paradoxical respirations. What you are feeling and observing is likely what type of injury?
   A. Flail chest
   B. Subcutaneous emphysema
   C. Commotio cordis
   D. Pulmonary contusion

2. What is it called when a knife wound to the chest wall allows air to enter the thoracic space?
   A. Pulmonary contusion
   B. Tension pneumothorax
   C. Open pneumothorax
   D. Myocardial contusion

3. While standing by with an ambulance at a college baseball game, you see a player get hit with a line drive to the chest and suddenly fall to the ground. You immediately go to the player's side and find he is in cardiac arrest. You attach the AED, and after the first defibrillation the patient gets a pulse and his eyes open. Which of the following is the condition you MOST likely observed?
   A. Myocardial rupture
   B. Commotio cordis
   C. Pulmonary contusion
   D. Diaphragmatic rupture

4. Jugular vein distention is measured when the patient is in what position?
   A. Sitting upright (Fowler's position)
   B. Lying supine
   C. Sitting at a 45° angle (semi-Fowler's position)
   D. Prone position

5. On arrival at the scene of a motor vehicle crash, you find a man who owns up to not wearing a seat belt. During your assessment, you observe significant bruising. You suspect the patient has a pericardial tamponade. Which of the following is NOT a sign of Beck triad?
   A. Hypotension
   B. Jugular vein distention
   C. Muffled heart tones
   D. Hyperresonant chest sounds

6. In what age group are the ribs MOST pliable?
   A. In children
   B. In elderly persons
   C. In young adults past puberty
   D. In the middle-aged

7. Injuries to the great vessels, as well as cardiac tamponade, are much more likely to occur with which of the following?
   A. Blunt trauma
   B. High-energy penetrating trauma
   C. Low-speed deceleration injury
   D. Posterior blunt force

8. Where are breath sounds MOST likely to diminish with an open pneumothorax?
   A. On both sides
   B. Over the unaffected side
   C. Over the affected side
   D. On neither side

9. While performing an assessment on a patient involved in a high-speed motor vehicle crash, you observe decreased breath sounds, and, upon palpation of the chest, you note hyperresonance. You immediately suspect which of the following conditions?
   A. Simple pneumothorax
   B. Tension pneumothorax
   C. Hemothorax
   D. Open pneumothorax

10. You have a critical patient who has sustained a chest injury during a fall from about 15 to 20 feet. Your assessment reveals a tension pneumothorax, and you determine an immediate needle decompression must be performed. After preparing the site, where should you insert the needle?
    A. Below the third rib midclavicular
    B. Below the third rib midaxillary
    C. Above the third rib midaxillary
    D. Above the third rib midclavicular

Labeling

Label the following diagram with the correct terms.

1. The Thorax

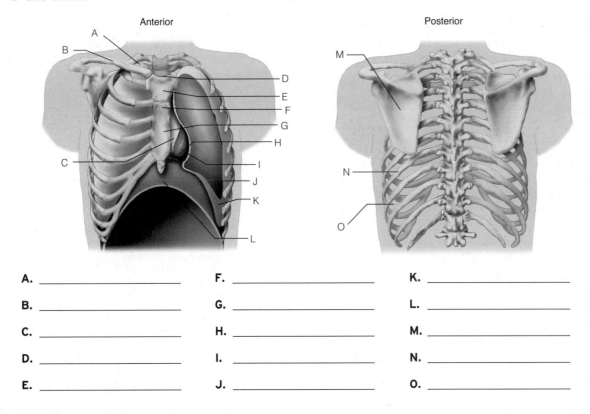

A. _____	**F.** _____	**K.** _____
B. _____	**G.** _____	**L.** _____
C. _____	**H.** _____	**M.** _____
D. _____	**I.** _____	**N.** _____
E. _____	**J.** _____	**O.** _____

Fill-in-the-Table

Fill in the possible injuries for each of the following situations.

Many, if not most, serious chest injuries cannot be specifically identified in the field. An understanding of the mechanism of injury (MOI), however, should enable you to anticipate the injuries that might be present in any given case and thereby to assess the potential urgency of the situation. For each of the following MOIs or associated injuries, indicate the serious chest injury or injuries that are likely to be present. The MOI, or easily detected injuries, may give clues to the presence of injuries that are harder to find.

If you find:	The patient may have:
1. Steering wheel imprint on anterior chest	
2. Caved-in door on driver's side	
3. Fall from a height	
4. Bullet entrance wound in fifth left intercostal space	
5. Fracture of ribs 5-7 in a young man	
6. Fracture of first and second ribs	

Identify

In the following case study, list the chief complaint, physical findings, and signs of Beck triad.

1. A 35-year-old man was involved in a motor vehicle crash. The patient is quickly extricated from the vehicle. You are the first paramedic to evaluate the patient. He is verbal and when asked about pain and other symptoms, he states, "My chest hurts." During your assessment, you observe bruising on the lower chest, diaphoresis, cyanosis, dyspnea, and jugular vein distention. While assessing the vital signs, you identify equal bilateral breath sounds, tachycardia, weak peripheral pulses, hypotension, and muffled heart tones. An ECG displays electrical alternans.

   a. Chief complaint:

   _____

   _____

   b. Physical findings:

   _____

   _____

   c. Signs of Beck triad:

   _____

   _____

   d. Do you suspect this patient has pericardial tamponade or a tension pneumothorax?

   _____

   _____

In the following trauma scenario, list the physical findings that indicate pulmonary contusion. List the description of the Spalding effect, inertial effects, and implosion.

2. You respond to an assault of a 16-year-old boy. Your patient has been struck in the chest with a baseball bat. Upon your arrival, he is conscious. You immediately perform a primary assessment. The airway is open and the patient is breathing with only mild distress. Crackles are heard upon auscultation. The pulse identifies a sinus tachycardia, and other vital signs are within normal limits. An ECG shows ischemic changes. There are no other signs of hypovolemia. You apply supplemental oxygen and initiate an IV while en route to the hospital.

   You suspect this patient has sustained a pulmonary contusion. You believe that the pressure waves generated by the blunt trauma disrupted the capillary-alveolar membrane. The pressure created by the trauma compresses the gases within the lung. The tissues accelerated and decelerated at different rates, causing a tear.

   a. Physical findings:

   _____

   _____

   b. Spalding effect:

   _____

   _____

   c. Inertial effects:

   _____

   _____

d. Implosion:

_____

_____

e. Would you run the IV wide open for this patient?

_____

_____

Ambulance Calls

The following case scenarios provide an opportunity to explore the concerns associated with patient management and paramedic care. Read each scenario, and then answer each question.

1. A 26-year-old woman was an unrestrained front-seat passenger in a car that was involved in a head-on collision. You find her lying unconscious on the front seat, her face covered with blood. The dashboard on her side is dented in, and the windshield in front of her is smashed.

  a. List four things that might jeopardize the airway in this patient.

   (1) _____

   (2) _____

   (3) _____

   (4) _____

  b. Specify precisely what you would check in assessing her breathing in the primary assessment.

   (1) LOOK for:

     (a) _____

     (b) _____

     (c) _____

     (d) _____

   (2) LISTEN for:

     (a) _____

     (b) _____

     (c) _____

   (3) FEEL for:

     (a) _____

     (b) _____

     (c) _____

  c. What steps would you take at this point to ensure adequate breathing?

   (1) _____

   (2) _____

d. Specify precisely what you would check in assessing her circulation in the primary assessment.

(1) _____

(2) _____

(3) _____

(4) _____

(5) _____

2. A 22-year-old man was shot at close range by a "friend" wielding a shotgun. You find the patient slumped in a chair in considerable respiratory distress. There is a ragged 2-inch hole in his left anterior chest, and the left chest does not seem to move with respirations.

a. This patient has a/an:

(1) simple pneumothorax.

(2) tension pneumothorax.

(3) open pneumothorax.

(4) spontaneous pneumothorax.

b. What steps would you take to manage this situation?

(1) _____

(2) _____

(3) _____

(4) _____

(5) _____

3. A 71-year-old woman was crossing the street when she was struck by a car and thrown to the ground. She is complaining of severe pain in her right chest (she points to the exact spot, over the fifth right rib in the anterior axillary line). She says the pain is much worse when she coughs or takes a deep breath. On examination, she is conscious and alert and leaning toward her right side. Her skin is warm and moist. There is no cyanosis. Her pulse is 88 beats/min and regular; respirations are 24 breaths/min and shallow. Blood pressure is 160/90 mm Hg. The neck veins are flat. There is no tracheal deviation. There is extreme tenderness over the right fifth rib in the anterior axillary line. Breath sounds are diminished over the right chest, which sounds somewhat hollow to percussion. The rest of the exam seems to be within normal limits.

a. This woman probably has:

_____

b. What is the principal danger associated with the type of injury or injuries she has suffered?

_____

c. What treatment is necessary in the field?

(1) _____

(2) _____

(3) _____

d. As you are transporting the woman to the hospital, a 20-minute drive from the collision scene, she suddenly becomes very restless and agitated and complains that she can't breathe. Her skin becomes cold and sweaty, and her pulse gets very weak. Her neck veins seem to bulge out.

(1) What do you think has happened?

_____

_____

_____

(2) What measures will you take?

_____

_____

_____

4. You are called to the scene of a two-car collision. A convertible going south on the interstate apparently jumped the median divider and plowed head-on into a station wagon traveling in the northbound lane. The driver of the convertible is lying unconscious in the road. Your primary assessment reveals gurgling respirations; broken teeth; flat neck veins; asymmetric chest movement; cold, sweaty skin; weak, rapid pulse; poor capillary refill; and brisk bleeding from wounds on the scalp and neck. You are 10 minutes from a regional trauma center. List in order the steps you would take in this case.

a. _____

b. _____

c. _____

d. _____

e. _____

f. _____

g. _____

5. A passenger was in a car that was struck from the right side by a truck running a red light. The right-hand front door of the car is rammed in, deforming the passenger compartment of the car. The patient, a middle-aged woman, is conscious and in considerable distress. Her skin is cold and moist. Her neck veins are distended. Her chest moves only minimally on respiration, and you have difficulty hearing breath sounds on the right. You can't really assess the percussion note because of all the noise at the scene. The woman's pulse is 120 beats/min and weak, and her respirations are 36 breaths/min and shallow.

a. What steps would you take at the scene?

(1) _____

(2) _____

(3) _____

(4) _____

b. What steps would you take during transport?

(1) _____

(2) _____

(3) _____

6. A passenger car has been involved in a head-on collision with a pickup truck. When you arrive at the scene, you find the driver of the passenger car propped up against a tree, where he had been placed by bystanders who pulled him from the wreckage. The patient has numerous cuts on his face and arms and is in severe respiratory distress. He seems confused. His skin is cold, cyanotic, and sweaty, and his pulse is rapid and very weak. He can barely talk, but he manages to gasp, "Can't breathe . . ." You notice that the veins of his neck are bulging out. List in order the steps you would take in assessing and managing this patient.

Assessment

a. _____

b. _____

    (1) _____

c. _____

    (1) _____

    (2) _____

    (3) _____

    (4) _____

    (5) _____

    (6) _____

d. _____

    (1) _____

    (2) _____

    (3) _____

e. _____

    (1) _____

f. _____

    (1) _____

g. _____

Management

a. _____

b. _____

c. _____

d. _____

e. _____

f. _____

g. _____

h. _____

7. For each of the following patients, indicate what the MOST likely diagnosis is, and list the steps of prehospital management.

   A. Tension pneumothorax

   B. Massive hemothorax

   C. Flail chest

   D. Cardiac tamponade

   E. Traumatic asphyxia

_____ **a.** A 20-year-old driver of a car that rammed a utility pole at high speed. He is in severe distress. His pulse is rapid and feeble, and every so often you can hardly palpate a pulse at all. His neck veins are distended. There is a steering wheel imprint on his chest. The rib cage is stable. Breath sounds are equal bilaterally. It is too noisy to hear heart sounds. You are 30 minutes from the nearest hospital. Steps of management:

(1) _____

(2) _____

(3) _____

(4) _____

_____ **b.** A 23-year-old driver of a car that rammed a utility pole at high speed. His face, neck, and chest are cyanotic and look very bloated. His eyes are bloodshot and bulging. He is vomiting blood. Breathing is labored. His pulse is rapid and very weak. The chest looks caved-in. You are 5 minutes from a regional trauma center. Steps of management:

(1) _____

(2) _____

(3) _____

(4) _____

(5) _____

_____ **c.** A 70-year-old driver of a car that rammed a utility pole at high speed. He is conscious but in severe respiratory distress. The pulse is 92 beats/min, strong, and slightly irregular. Neck veins are flat. There are bruises on the anterior chest and point tenderness along the left sternal border and over the left fifth, sixth, seventh, and eighth ribs in the anterior axillary line. The chest seems to move asymmetrically on respiration. Breath sounds seem equal. It is too noisy to hear heart sounds. You are 10 minutes from the hospital. Steps of management:

(1) _____

(2) _____

(3) _____

(4) _____

(5) _____

(6) _____

_____ **d.** A 42-year-old front-seat passenger in a car that was struck from the right side by an ambulance that ran a red light. The patient is in severe respiratory distress. Her pulse is rapid and very weak. Her skin is cold and sweaty. The neck veins are distended. Breath sounds are decreased on the right side of the chest, which is hyperresonant to palpation. It's too noisy to hear heart sounds. You are 15 minutes from the nearest hospital. Steps of management:

(1) _____

(2) _____

(3) _____

(4) _____

(5) _____

(6) _____

(7) _____

(8) _____

_____ **e.** A 22-year-old man who was stabbed in the left chest. The patient is in severe distress. His pulse is rapid and very weak. His skin is cold and sweaty. His neck veins are flat. Breath sounds are decreased in the left chest, which is dull to percussion. It's too noisy to hear heart sounds. You are 15 minutes from the nearest hospital. Steps of management:

(1) _____

(2) _____

(3) _____

True/False

If you believe the statement to be more true than false, write the letter "T" in the space provided. If you believe the statement to be more false than true, write the letter "F."

_____ **1.** Children's ribs are pliable, so underlying structures may be injured even if the ribs aren't fractured.

_____ **2.** With a sucking chest wound, a large wound opening must occur to compromise ventilations.

_____ **3.** Cardiac tamponade is defined as fluid in the myocardium causing compression of the heart and decreasing cardiac output.

_____ **4.** Commotio cordis is when the thorax receives a direct blow during the critical portion of the heart's repolarization period, resulting in cardiac arrest.

_____ **5.** Atelectasis is alveolar collapse that prevents the use of a portion of the lung.

_____ **6.** Blunt disruptions of the diaphragm are usually associated with herniation of all or part of the liver into the right side of the chest.

_____ **7.** Esophageal injuries are not usually serious injuries.

_____ **8.** Jugular vein distention is usually an early sign of tension pneumothorax.

_____ **9.** Hypotension, as a late finding, should not be considered to either confirm or exclude the possibility of a tension pneumothorax.

_____ **10.** One physical finding of tension pneumothorax is distended neck veins.

Short Answer

Complete this section with short written answers using the space provided.

A 22-year-old man was shot in the right chest with a handgun at a range of 10 feet. There is an entrance wound in the right midclavicular line about 2 fingerbreadths below the right nipple. A slightly larger exit wound is visible 3 inches (7.5 cm) to the right of the vertebral column just below the lowest rib. What organs are most likely to have been in the path of the bullet?

_____

_____

_____

Skill Drills

Test your knowledge of skill drills by placing the following photos in the correct order. Number the first step "1," the second step "2," etc.

Needle Decompression (Thoracentesis) of a Tension Pneumothorax

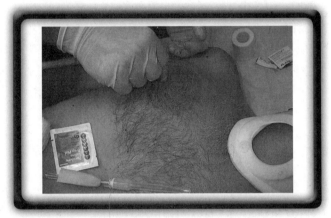

_____ Cleanse the appropriate area using aseptic technique.

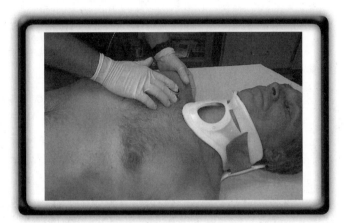

_____ Assess the patient.

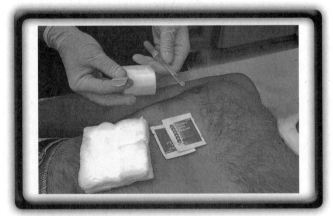

_____ Prepare and assemble all necessary equipment. Obtain orders from medical control.

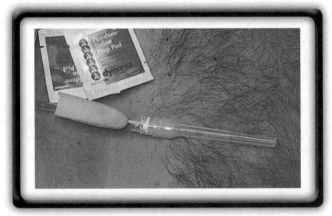

_____ Make a one-way valve or flutter valve.

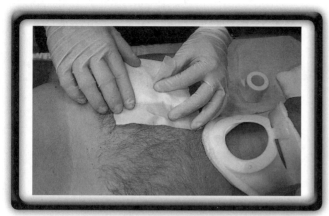

_____Secure the catheter in place. Monitor the patient closely for recurrence of the tension pneumothorax.

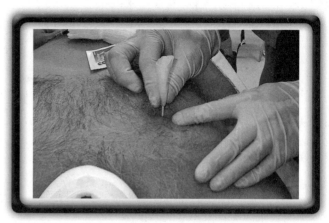

_____ Remove the needle. Properly dispose of the needle in the sharps container.

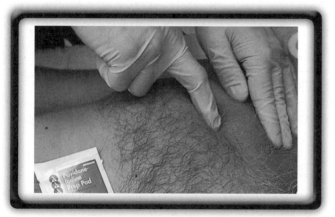

_____Locate the appropriate site between the second and third rib.

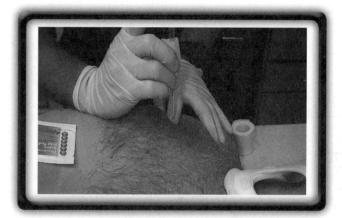

_____ Insert the needle at a 90° angle, and listen for the release of air.

Abdominal and Genitourinary Trauma

Matching

Part I

Match each of the items in the right column with the appropriate definition in the left column.

_____ **1.** Injury resulting from compression or deceleration forces, potentially crushing an organ or causing it to rupture.

_____ **2.** An injury in which there is soft-tissue damage inside the body, but the skin remains intact.

_____ **3.** The first part of the small intestine.

_____ **4.** Displacement of an organ outside the body.

_____ **5.** Blood in the urine.

_____ **6.** The presence of extravasated blood in the peritoneal cavity.

_____ **7.** Left shoulder pain that may indicate a ruptured spleen.

_____ **8.** A membranous double fold of tissue in the abdomen that attaches various organs to the body wall.

_____ **9.** An injury in which there is a break in the surface of the skin or mucous membrane, exposing deeper tissue to potential contamination.

_____ **10.** An injury in which the skin is broken; direct contact results in laceration of the structure.

_____ **11.** The area in the abdomen encased in the peritoneum, and which consists of an upper and a lower part. The upper portion contains the diaphragm, liver, spleen, stomach, gallbladder, and transverse colon. The lower portion contains the small bowel, sigmoid colon, parts of the descending and ascending colon, and, in women, the internal reproductive organs.

_____ **12.** A membrane in the abdomen encasing the liver, spleen, diaphragm, stomach, and transverse colon.

_____ **13.** Inflammation of the peritoneum that results from either blood or hollow organ contents spilling into the abdominal cavity.

_____ **14.** Pertaining to the area around the umbilicus.

_____ **15.** A circumferential muscle at the end of the stomach that acts as a valve between the stomach and duodenum.

_____ **16.** The area in the abdomen containing the aorta, vena cava, pancreas, kidneys, ureters, and portions of the duodenum and large intestine.

_____ **17.** Localized pain, usually felt deeply, which represents irritation or injury to tissue, causing activation of peripheral nerve tracts.

_____ **18.** Crampy, aching pain deep within the body, the source of which is usually difficult to pinpoint; common with genitourinary problems.

A. Visceral pain

B. Retroperitoneal space

C. Periumbilical

D. Peritoneum

E. Peritonitis

F. Pylorus

G. Somatic pain

H. Peritoneal space

I. Blunt trauma

J. Closed abdominal injury

K. Hematuria

L. Duodenum

M. Evisceration

N. Kehr sign

O. Hemoperitoneum

P. Mesentery

Q. Penetrating trauma

R. Open abdominal injury

Part II

Match each of the items in the left column to the appropriate injuries in the right column.

For each of the patients described here, given the mechanism of injury and the clinical findings, indicate which injury from the right-hand column he or she is most likely to have suffered. (Note: A patient may have sustained more than one of the injuries listed.)

_____ **1.** A 15-year-old girl was kicked in the left side by a horse. She is conscious and alert. Her pulse is rapid. She has a bruise over the left 10th rib in the anterior axillary line and has severe tenderness at that point.

A. Diaphragm injury

_____ **2.** A 50-year-old man was a passenger in a car that slammed into a wall. He was wearing a lap seat belt. He complains of shortness of breath and abdominal pain. He winces when he coughs. His vital signs are as follows: pulse 92 beats/min and regular, respirations 36 breaths/min and shallow, and blood pressure 120/80 mm Hg.

B. Ruptured spleen

_____ **3.** An 18-year-old man was shot in the right upper quadrant by his girlfriend wielding a .38 special at a distance of about 10 feet. The patient is conscious. He has cold, sweaty skin and a weak, rapid pulse. There is an entrance wound in the right upper quadrant, about 2 fingerbreadths below the costal margin in the midclavicular line. The exit wound is near the left buttock.

C. Liver laceration

_____ **4.** A 60-year-old man was struck by a car as he was crossing the street. The patient presents with gross hematuria; suprapubic pain and tenderness; difficulty voiding; and abdominal distention, guarding, and rebound tenderness.

D. Torn or ruptured bladder

_____ **5.** A 42-year-old construction worker is extricated from underneath a pile of concrete blocks that caved in on top of him. He is unconscious with cold and clammy skin. His pulse is very weak. There are no bruises on the chest, which moves symmetrically with respiration. The abdomen is not rigid, but there seems to be a fullness in the center of the lower quadrant. The pelvis is unstable.

E. Retroperitoneal injuries

_____ **6.** Your team is assessing a conscious, alert 18-year-old man who was involved in a high-speed car crash versus bridge abutment. The patient was unrestrained. The patient has an odor of ethyl alcohol; he is currently complaint free. While you are evaluating the patient, you note ecchymosis of the flanks.

F. Cullen sign

_____ **7.** It's another weekend night and another stabbing. On arrival you have a conscious, alert male patient. He is lying on the ground with what appears to be exposed abdominal contents.

G. Evisceration

_____ **8.** A patient is struck by falling debris. He was struck on the lower left quadrant and is found to be in profound shock. His lower left quadrant has point tenderness and is rigid.

_____ **9.** Your patient is a victim of blunt trauma; he is anxious and short of breath. He appears to have associated thoracic, abdominal, head, and extremity injuries.

_____ **10.** A woman fell from a height while hiking. You are assessing the patient and recognize that she has Kehr sign.

Multiple Choice

Read each item carefully, and then select the best response.

1. The physical exam conducted as a part of the secondary assessment of abdominal injuries includes all of the following, EXCEPT:
   A. inspection.
   B. palpation.
   C. percussion.
   D. determination of baseline vital signs.

2. Patients who have suffered penetrating abdominal trauma should be treated by:
   A. removing the penetrating object to facilitate immobilization and transport.
   B. avoiding direct pressure in older patients with more flaccid abdominal walls.
   C. replacing protruding abdominal contents prior to transport.
   D. stabilizing and transporting in the position found.

3. Each of the following are considered hollow organs or structures of the abdomen, except the _____, which is considered part of the genitourinary system.
   A. esophagus
   B. stomach
   C. bladder
   D. gallbladder

4. Hollow organs are less likely to be injured, unless:
   A. they are empty.
   B. the mechanism of injury is a motor vehicle crash.
   C. they are full.
   D. the patient is a pregnant woman.

5. There are numerous types of blast injuries, including:
   A. miscellaneous injury.
   B. primary blast injury.
   C. secondary blast injury.
   D. All of the above

6. Because of the nature of abdominal trauma in patients, which of the following should be required in your management plan?
   A. Obtaining a 12-lead ECG
   B. Securing the cervical spine
   C. Consulting with medical control on analgesia
   D. Establishing IV access

7. Injuries to the retroperitoneal space may include injuries to all of the following, EXCEPT the:
   A. rectum.
   B. ureters.
   C. reproductive organs.
   D. liver.

8. Crushing injuries may be caused by:
   A. crushing of abdominal contents by the abdominal wall and the spinal column.
   B. the dashboard of a car.
   C. the hood of the car.
   D. All of the above

9. In penetrating trauma, it is helpful to:
   A. identify the type of weapon used.
   B. explore the wound to detect the path of destruction.
   C. cleanse the wound site to prevent life-threatening infection.
   D. remove all exposed foreign bodies.

10. The primary assessment for abdominal injuries should include the following, EXCEPT:
    A. road rash.
    B. bruising.
    C. swelling.
    D. epistaxis.

Labeling
Label the following diagrams with the correct terms.

1. Organs in the Peritoneum

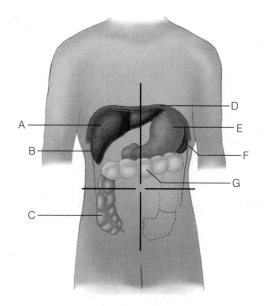

A. _____

B. _____

C. _____

D. _____

E. _____

F. _____

G. _____

2. Organs in the Retroperitoneal Space

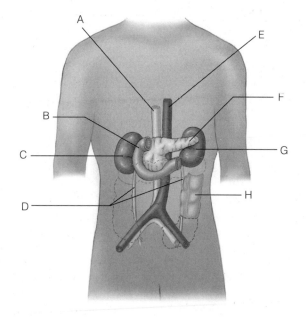

A. _____

B. _____

C. _____

D. _____

E. _____

F. _____

G. _____

H. _____

3. Organs in the Pelvis

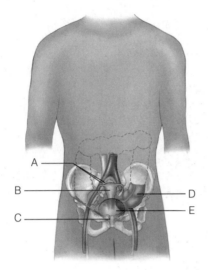

A. _____

B. _____

C. _____

D. _____

E. _____

Fill-in-the-Blank

Read each item carefully, and then complete the statement by filling in the missing word(s).

1. The first part of the small intestine, the _____, is retroperitoneal and approximately 9 to 11 inches long.
2. Retroperitoneal bleeding can lead to ecchymosis of the flanks, commonly referred to as _____ _____ _____.
3. Retroperitoneal bleeding can lead to ecchymosis around the umbilicus, commonly referred to as _____ _____.
4. Structures contained within the retroperitoneal cavity are the _____, _____, ureters, vascular structures, and part of the small intestine.
5. The _____ detoxifies blood and produces bile.
6. The stomach is an intraperitoneal _____ organ that lies in the left upper quadrant and epigastric region.
7. A hollow muscular organ situated in the pelvis is called the _____ bladder.
8. The spillage of toxins into the abdominal cavity due to trauma is called _____ and can be a potentially life-threatening infection.

Identify

In the following case studies, list the chief complaint, vital signs, and pertinent negatives.

1. You receive a priority one response for a conscious and alert 54-year-old man involved in domestic violence. When you arrive, you are advised that the scene is safe and secured by law enforcement. The patient is denying any complaint. You notice that the patient's shirt is blood soaked and the police have placed a kitchen knife in an evidence bag. The patient is not very cooperative, and he appears ashen, diaphoretic, and slightly short of breath. After several minutes of prodding, the patient agrees to remove his shirt. The patient denies any previous medical history. You observe a half-inch laceration above his umbilicus. The wound is not actively bleeding. He denies chest pain or other injuries. His vital signs are as follows: pulse is 120 beats/min and regular; skin is ashen, cool, and diaphoretic; oxygen saturation is 90%; blood pressure is 86/60 mm Hg; and sinus tachycardia is found on the ECG.

   a. Chief complaint:

   _____

   _____

b. Vital signs:

_____

_____

c. Pertinent negatives:

_____

_____

2. Your unit is standing by at your local arena for indoor motocross. This is a high-speed motorcycle racing event, with numerous elevated jumps and turns. The riders are well protected by helmets and specialized outerwear. While watching, you observe a rider crash into a retaining wall. He initially appears unconscious. As you approach, the patient is alert and speaking clearly. He is attempting to stand and get back on his motorcycle. You quickly notice that bystanders are pointing to the patient's abdomen and you see what appears to be a small protrusion of abdominal contents from his left upper quadrant. It's obvious that the patient has an evisceration. You quickly assess ABCs and immobilize the patient. He has the following vital signs: pulse is 100 beats/min and irregular; skin is pale, warm, and dry; oxygen saturation is 97% on room air; and blood pressure is 160/90 mm Hg. After quickly treating the patient and initiating rapid transport, you become suspicious because of the patient's vital signs. The patient states he has a history of atrial fibrillation and hypertension. He is currently denying chest pain.

a. Chief complaint:

_____

_____

b. Vital signs:

_____

_____

c. Pertinent negatives:

_____

_____

Ambulance Calls

The following case scenarios provide an opportunity to explore the concerns associated with patient management and paramedic care. Read each scenario, and then answer each question.

1. You are called to the scene of an interstate collision in which an apparently intoxicated 25-year-old driver plowed his car into a bridge abutment at high speed. The front end of his vehicle is accordioned against the bridge. As you approach the disabled vehicle, your keen powers of observation enable you to perceive that the patient is conscious (he is screaming obscenities at a police officer). Describe the steps in evaluating this patient for possible abdominal injuries. In particular, what issues will you be looking for?

   a. _____

   b. _____

   c. _____

   d. _____

2. A 20-year-old man was the unrestrained driver of a car that was struck on the passenger side by another vehicle. The crash caused the empty bucket seat beside him to be jammed into his right side. On your arrival at the collision, you find the patient conscious, but anxious and restless. His skin is ashen, cool, and diaphoretic. The patient

has a delayed capillary refill greater than 2 seconds. His vital signs are a pulse of 140 beats/min and thready, respirations of 40 breaths/min and shallow, and blood pressure of 72/40 mm Hg. There is a bruise over the right lower ribs. A large portion of the small bowel is eviscerated through an avulsion in the right side of the abdomen. The right elbow appears to be fractured. List the injuries and your priorities in managing this case.

Injuries:

a. _____

b. _____

c. _____

d. _____

Priorities:

a. _____

b. _____

c. _____

d. _____

e. _____

f. _____

g. _____

3. During the usual Saturday night festivities at the local Knife & Gun Club, a 16-year-old boy is stabbed with a hunting knife in the left lower quadrant of the abdomen. When you arrive, you find him lying on the ground moaning. The knife is still embedded up to its hilt in the patient's abdomen. His skin is pale, warm, and moist. Vital signs are pulse of 100 beats/min, respirations of 32 breaths/min, and blood pressure of 100/80 mm Hg. List the steps in managing this case.

a. _____

b. _____

c. _____

d. _____

e. _____

True/False

If you believe the statement to be more true than false, write the letter "T" in the space provided. If you believe the statement to be more false than true, write the letter "F."

_____ 1. Hollow organs are less likely to cause life-threatening injuries.

_____ 2. Patients who suffer ruptured spleens in a traumatic event will likely have that organ removed during lifesaving surgery.

_____ 3. Cullen sign is best described as ecchymosis around the umbilicus.

_____ 4. Treatment of impaled abdominal objects includes removal of the object to allow for proper immobilization and transport.

_____ 5. It is estimated that 80% of significant trauma involves the abdomen.

_____ **6.** The diaphragm plays a large role in the mechanical process of breathing.

_____ **7.** Visceral pain comes from organs inside the body with injury or illness.

_____ **8.** Severe injuries to the testicles are rare.

_____ **9.** Bladder injury should be suspected in any patient with trauma to the lower abdomen, lateral aspects of the middle back, or lower rib cage.

_____ **10.** A saddle-type injury is likely to cause damage to the kidneys in a female patient.

Fill-in-the-Table

Fill in the missing parts of the table.

1. Hollow and Solid Organs of the Abdominal Cavity

Hollow Organs	Solid Organs
1.	1.
2.	2.
3.	3.
4.	4.
5.	
6.	
7.	

Short Answer

Complete this section with short written answers using the space provided.

1. Which of the abdominal organs is most likely to be injured in association with:

a. Rapid deceleration in a motor vehicle crash or a fall from a height: Liver, _____, intestines, and spleen

b. Right-sided chest trauma as well as abdominal trauma: _____

c. Fracture of the pelvis: _____

d. Stab wound to the right upper quadrant: _____

CHAPTER 37

Orthopaedic Trauma

Matching

Part I

Match the orthopaedic trauma term on the right with its best definition on the left.

_____ 1. Movement away from the midline of the body.

_____ 2. Lateral extension of the scapula that forms the highest point of the shoulder.

_____ 3. Severing a part of the body.

_____ 4. The artery that travels through the anterior muscles of the leg and continues to the foot as the dorsalis pedis.

_____ 5. Inflammation of the joints.

_____ 6. Wasting away of tissue.

_____ 7. A fracture that occurs when a piece of bone is torn free at the site of attachment of a tendon or ligament.

_____ 8. The armpit.

_____ 9. An incomplete fracture, typically occurring in children, in which the bone becomes bent as the result of a compressive force.

_____ 10. The artery that runs through the arm and branches into the radial and ulnar arteries.

_____ 11. Securing an injured digit to an adjacent uninjured one to allow the intact digit to act as a splint.

_____ 12. Inflammation of a bursa.

_____ 13. Trabecular or spongy bone.

_____ 14. The eight small bones of the wrist.

_____ 15. Joints that are spanned completely by cartilage and allow for minimal motion.

_____ 16. The collarbone.

_____ 17. A fracture in which the bone is broken into three or more pieces.

_____ 18. A fracture in which the bone is broken into two or more completely separate pieces.

_____ 19. A grating sensation felt when moving the ends of a broken bone.

_____ 20. Compression of the ulnar nerve at the tunnel along the outer edge of the elbow, causing numbness, tingling, and possible partial loss of function of the little finger and medial aspect of the ring finger.

_____ 21. A fracture in which the broken region of the bone is pushed deeper into the body than the remaining intact bone.

_____ 22. The loss of blood to a part of the body.

A. Nondisplaced fracture

B. Open-book pelvic fracture

C. Osteoporosis

D. Ossification center

E. Oblique fracture

F. Cubital tunnel syndrome

G. Devascularization

H. Displaced fracture

I. Endosteum

J. Fatigue fracture

K. Fibrous joints

L. Fracture

M. Depression fracture

N. Digital arteries

O. Dorsal

P. Fascia

Q. Femoral shaft fractures

R. Flat bones

S. Glenoid fossa

T. Myalgia

U. Medullary canal

V. Malleolus

_____ 23. The arteries that supply blood to the fingers and toes.

_____ 24. A break in which the ends of the fractured bone move out of their normal positions.

_____ 25. Referring to the back or posterior side of the body or an organ.

_____ 26. The inner lining of a hollow bone.

_____ 27. A strong, fibrous membrane that covers, supports, and separates muscles.

_____ 28. Fractures that result from multiple compressive loads.

_____ 29. A break in the diaphysis of the femur.

_____ 30. The joints that contain dense fibrous tissue and allow for no motion.

_____ 31. Bones that are thin and broad, such as the scapula.

_____ 32. A break or rupture in the bone.

_____ 33. The socket in the scapula in which the head of the humerus rotates.

_____ 34. A type of fracture occurring most frequently in children in which there is incomplete breakage of the bone.

_____ 35. The bone of the upper arm.

_____ 36. High levels of uric acid in the blood.

_____ 37. A broken bone in which the end of one bone becomes wedged into another bone, as could be the case in a fall from a significant height.

_____ 38. An injury that results from a force that is applied to one region of the body but leads to an injury in another area.

_____ 39. Bones with unique shapes that allow them to perform a specific function and that do not fit into the other categories based on shape.

_____ 40. The point at which two or more bones articulate, or come together.

_____ 41. A metabolic end product of the breakdown of glucose that accumulates when metabolism proceeds in the absence of oxygen.

_____ 42. Tough bands of tissue that connect bone to bone around a joint or support internal organs within the body.

_____ 43. Bones that are longer than they are wide.

_____ 44. The large, rounded, bony protuberance on either side of the ankle joint.

_____ 45. The hollow center portion of a long bone.

_____ 46. The region of the long bone between the epiphysis and the diaphysis.

_____ 47. Muscle pain.

_____ 48. A break in which the bone remains aligned in its normal position.

_____ 49. A fracture that travels diagonally from one side of the bone to the other.

_____ 50. A life-threatening fracture of the pelvis caused by a force that displaces one or both sides of the pelvis laterally and posteriorly.

_____ 51. Areas where cartilage is transformed through calcification into a new area of bone.

_____ 52. A condition characterized by decreased bone density and increased susceptibility to fractures.

W. Ligaments

X. Joint

Y. Indirect injury

Z. Hyperuricemia

AA. Greenstick fracture

BB. Impacted fracture

CC. Irregular bones

DD. Humerus

EE. Lactic acid

FF. Long bones

GG. Metaphysis

HH. Abduction

II. Amputation

JJ. Atrophy

KK. Anterior tibial artery

LL. Acromion

MM. Crepitus

NN. Comminuted fracture

OO. Arthritis

PP. Avulsion fracture

QQ. Complete fracture

RR. Clavicle

SS. Bursitis

TT. Carpals

UU. Cartilaginous joints

VV. Buddy splinting

WW. Brachial artery

XX. Cancellous bone

YY. Axilla

ZZ. Bowing fracture

Part II

Match the musculoskeletal injury on the left with the complication or other injury that is most likely to be associated with it on the right.

_____ **1.** Pelvic fracture

_____ **2.** Calcaneal fracture

_____ **3.** Humeral shaft fracture

_____ **4.** Posterior dislocation of the clavicle

_____ **5.** Elbow fracture

_____ **6.** Posterior dislocation of the hip

_____ **7.** Open fracture

_____ **8.** Patellar fracture

A. Fracture of L1/L2 of the spine

B. Volkmann ischemic contracture

C. Fracture dislocation of the ipsilateral hip

D. Compartment syndrome

E. Deceleration injuries

F. Possible damage to underlying structures (eg, subclavian artery)

G. Infection

H. Ruptured bladder

Multiple Choice

Read each item carefully, and then select the best response.

1. Which of the following is considered one of the most common reasons that patients seek medical attention?
  A. Trauma
  B. Musculoskeletal injuries
  C. Dislocations
  D. Fractures

2. Which of the following is considered one of the functions of the musculoskeletal system?
  A. Enabling hematopoiesis
  B. Allowing the body to maintain an erect position
  C. Protecting internal organs
  D. All of the above

3. All of the following are types of joints, EXCEPT:
  A. fibrous.
  B. fused.
  C. synovial.
  D. cartilaginous.

4. Stress fractures are often referred to as _____ fractures.
  A. fatigue
  B. greenstick
  C. comminuted
  D. oblique

5. Crepitus is BEST described as a:
  A. loss of distal sensation.
  B. sure sign of dislocation.
  C. sign that occurs with fractures.
  D. grating sensation with fractures.

6. Which of the following statements MOST accurately describes an Achilles tendon rupture?
  A. It is rarely seen in adults.
  B. It often accompanies arthritis.
  C. It occurs with tendonitis.
  D. It can be identified with the Thompson test.

7. Assessing extremity injuries should include all of the following, EXCEPT:
  A. scene size-up.
  B. auscultation.
  C. inspection.
  D. examination.

8. Which of the following is the MOST common result of splinting fractured extremities?
   A. Increased pain
   B. Delay in transport
   C. Increased bleeding and nerve damage
   D. Reduced risk of further injury and less discomfort

9. Which of the following statements MOST accurately describes compartment syndrome?
   A. It can be one of the most devastating consequences of a musculoskeletal injury.
   B. It occurs as a result of loosely applied bandages.
   C. It does not occur with open fractures.
   D. It generally is not a painful injury.

10. Pelvic fractures occur infrequently; however, they are:
   A. never fatal.
   B. responsible for a relatively high percentage of deaths.
   C. not to be splinted in the prehospital setting.
   D. rarely painful, and as a result they are often misdiagnosed.

Labeling

Label the following diagrams with the correct terms.

   1. Bones of the Foot and Ankle

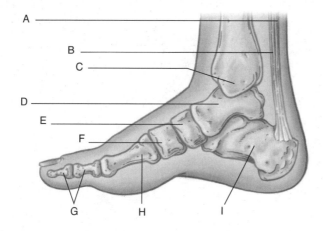

A. _____

B. _____

C. _____

D. _____

E. _____

F. _____

G. _____

H. _____

I. _____

   2. Types of Fractures

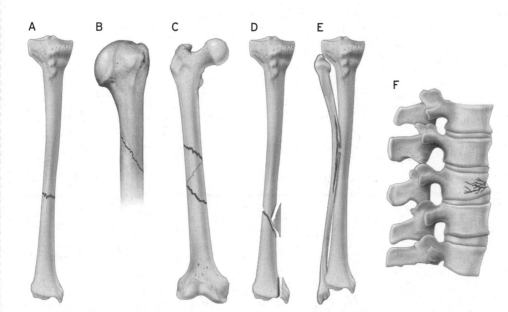

A. _____

B. _____

C. _____

D. _____

E. _____

F. _____

3. Types of Muscles

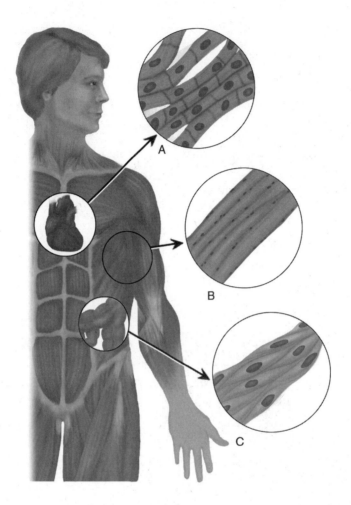

A. _____

B. _____

C. _____

Fill-in-the-Blank

Read each item carefully, and then complete the statement by filling in the missing word(s).

1. Vocabulary
   a. Wasting away of tissue is called _____.
   b. Inflammation of the joints is called _____.
   c. Location where two or more bones meet is the _____.
   d. The armpit is called the _____.
   e. The structure that acts as a strut is the _____.
   f. The shaft of a long bone is called the _____.
   g. The kneecap is also called the _____.
   h. When referring to the sole of the foot, you use the term _____.
   i. The shoulder girdle is also called the _____ _____.

2. To detect a fracture, you have to know what a fractured extremity looks and feels like. Fill in the following signs and symptoms of fractures:
   a. Unnatural shape: _____ _____ F _____ _____ _____ _____ _____ _____
   b. Reduced length: _____ _____ _____ R _____ _____ _____ _____ _____ _____

c. Fracture of the small finger: ___ ___ ___ E ___ ___ F ___ ___ ___ ___
___ ___ ___

d. Numbness or tingling: ___ ___ R ___ ___ T ___ ___ ___ ___ ___ ___

e. Grating: ___ ___ ___ ___ ___ T ___ ___

f. Devastating consequence of musculoskeletal injuries: D ___ ___ ___ ___ ___ ___ ___
___ ___

g. Protecting from movement: ___ ___ ___ R ___ ___ ___ ___

h. Hurts to touch it: ___ ___ ___ ___ ___   ___ ___ ___ ___ ___
___ E ___ ___

i. Patient with a fracture may report this: H ___ ___ ___ ___   ___ S ___ ___ ___

j. Strange moves: ___ N ___ ___ ___ ___ ___ ___   P ___ ___ ___
___ ___ ___ ___

k. Clavicle: ___ ___ ___ ___ ___ R ___ O ___ ___

l. Seen in open fracture: ___ X ___ ___ ___ ___ ___   ___ O ___ ___
___ N ___ ___

Identify

In the following case studies, list the chief complaint, vital signs, and pertinent negatives.

1. It is a snowy night in the Big Apple. Most people decided to stay indoors. You are dispatched to the scene where a 48-year-old man slipped on the ice and snow while working late on Wall Street. As you turn the corner to the scene, you notice that law enforcement is already on scene. You mentally note to yourself that the scene is safe.

Your patient states that he slipped and fell on the icy sidewalk. He complains of right ankle pain. The patient further states that he tried to catch himself and landed on his left wrist. He complains of severe wrist pain. You notice that the wrist is deformed and the patient appears to be supporting it against his chest with his right arm.

By questioning the patient, you discover that he has a previous medical history of angina, atrial fibrillation, and hypertension. He also takes one aspirin a day and an antihypertensive. He denies loss of consciousness and any head or neck pain. The patient denies any respiratory distress and denies any current chest discomfort. He denies any medical condition that may have caused him to fall. He adamantly states that he simply slipped on ice and fell. After quickly assessing the patient, you decide to move the patient into the warm ambulance for further treatment and evaluation.

His baseline vital signs reveal a pulse of 116 beats/min and irregular, respirations of 16 breaths/min and nonlabored, oxygen saturation on room air at 98%, and blood pressure of 150/90 mm Hg. His ECG shows a rapid atrial fibrillation. Pupils Equal And Round, Regular in size, and react to Light (PEARRL). Normal capillary refill < 2 seconds. Skin is, warm, dry, and a normal color.

a. Chief complaint:

_____

_____

b. Vital signs:

_____

_____

c. Pertinent negatives:

_____

_____

2. Your patient is a 48-year-old woman who was injured while waiting in line for a popular clothing store to open during the annual President's Day sale. This is the one day of the year when all the designer handbags are on sale. Unfortunately, at "crunch" time, she tripped on the curb in the parking lot and fell to the ground. Luckily, she wasn't trampled by the hordes of bargain shoppers as the doors opened. She did catch herself with her two outstretched arms. Besides her injured pride, she complains of bilateral wrist injuries and is found in extreme pain. As you approach the patient, she is sitting in a chair with ice packs already applied and mall security providing first aid. You notice that both her wrists appear bruised and deformed. Her initial mental status is conscious and alert. Her skin is slightly ashen and diaphoretic, and she has positive distal motor and neurologic sensations in both hands. She denies other injuries. Her capillary refill is > 2 seconds, and she has bilateral radial pulses that appear to be equal. Her blood pressure is obtainable only by palpation at 86 mm Hg. Her oxygen saturation is 96% on ambient air. She denies taking any medications or having allergies.

   a. Chief complaint:

   _____

   _____

   b. Vital signs:

   _____

   _____

   c. Pertinent negatives:

   _____

   _____

3. You believe that this is just another medical evacuation. As you take off from the hospital's rooftop pad and head toward the scene, you pay attention to the radio as the patient information, landing zone description, coordinates, and weather are relayed through your headset. You have a 25-minute estimated time of arrival (ETA) and request any vital signs and relevant patient information. After several minutes, you begin to realize that this call is anything but routine. The flight dispatcher describes a farm mishap where a tractor rolled on top of and is pinning a 64-year-old man. The flight dispatcher advises that the ground crew is requesting medicated facilitated intubation immediately on your arrival. Once again you request vital signs as you prepare the medications. Prior to arrival the patient is unresponsive with a Glasgow Coma Scale (GCS) score < 8, severe respiratory distress, bilateral open femoral fractures, and a possible dislocated or fractured hip or pelvis. Further transmissions indicate a delayed capillary refill, sinus tachycardia, a pulse of 128 beats/min, and a blood pressure of 64 mm Hg by palpation. The ground medics were attempting IV access while rescue crews were attempting to extricate the patient.

   a. Chief complaint:

   _____

   _____

   b. Vital signs:

   _____

   _____

   c. Pertinent negatives:

   _____

   _____

Complete the Patient Care Report (PCR)

Reread the first incident scenario in the preceding Identify exercise and then complete the following PCR for the patient.

EMS Patient Care Report (PCR)				
Date:	Incident No.:	Nature of Call:		Location:
Dispatched:	En Route:	At Scene:	Transport:	At Hospital:	In Service:

Patient Information	
Age:	Allergies:
Sex:	Medications:
Weight (in kg [lb]):	Past Medical History:
	Chief Complaint:

Vital Signs				
Time:	BP:	Pulse:	Respirations:	SpO$_2$:
Time:	BP:	Pulse:	Respirations:	SpO$_2$:
Time:	BP:	Pulse:	Respirations:	SpO$_2$:

EMS Treatment (circle all that apply)				
Oxygen @ _____ L/min via (circle one): NC NRM Bag-Mask Device	Assisted Ventilation	Airway Adjunct	CPR
Defibrillation	Bleeding Control	Bandaging	Splinting	Other

Narrative

Ambulance Calls

The following case scenarios provide an opportunity to explore the concerns associated with patient management and paramedic care. Read each scenario, and then answer each question.

1. There are injuries that frequently come in pairs because they share a common mechanism of injury. When you find one of such a pair, you should be alert for the presence of the other. For each of the following cases, indicate what other injury or injuries you would look for in particular, given the injury already detected.

    a. A young man jumped from a second-story window to escape a fire. He complains of severe pain in the left heel, which is quite bruised and swollen. What other injury or injuries might you expect to find in this patient?

_____

_____

    b. A 50-year-old woman was the front-seat passenger in a car that was hit head-on by an oncoming vehicle. Her right knee is bruised and swollen. What other injury or injuries might you expect to find in this patient?

_____

_____

    c. A 60-year-old man fell sideways onto his outstretched hand. There is ecchymosis and tenderness at the base of his thumb. What other injury or injuries might you expect to find in this patient?

_____

_____

    d. A construction worker has been extricated from under a pile of concrete blocks that fell on top of him, pinning him in a prone position, when part of a building collapsed. He has bruising over the left shoulder blade, and he cannot move the shoulder on that side. What other injury or injuries might you expect to find in this patient?

_____

_____

2. For each of the following patients, list the most likely field diagnosis, answer any questions asked about the patient, and describe how you would manage the case.

    a. A 14-year-old boy fell from his skateboard onto his extended right elbow. The elbow is massively swollen and ecchymotic. The right hand is cool and pale, and the patient cannot feel a pinprick over the dorsum of the hand in the web space between the thumb and index finger.

        (1) What is the most likely field diagnosis?

_____

_____

        (2) Is there any particular danger in this case? If so, what is the danger?

_____

_____

        (3) How would you manage this case?

_____

_____

    b. The mother of the boy just described fell over her son's skateboard as she was rushing to his assistance, and her outstretched left hand took the brunt of the impact as she hit the ground. As she walks toward the ambulance, she is gripping the dorsum of her left wrist with her right hand and holding the left wrist against her abdomen. When you inspect the left wrist from the side, it has a peculiar curve, rather like that of a dinner fork.

(1) What is the most likely field diagnosis?

_____

_____

(2) Is there any particular danger in this case? If so, what is the danger?

_____

_____

(3) How would you manage this case?

_____

_____

c. A front-seat passenger in a car that hit a tree is found with his right hip flexed, adducted, and internally rotated. The right leg looks shorter than the left leg. There are no other obvious injuries, and baseline vital signs are normal.

(1) What is the most likely field diagnosis?

_____

_____

(2) Is there any particular danger in this case? If so, what is the danger?

_____

_____

(3) How would you manage this case?

_____

_____

d. The driver of the vehicle in the preceding crash is unconscious behind the wheel. His skin is cold and sweaty. When you are extricating him from the vehicle, you notice that his hips are unstable.

(1) What is the most likely field diagnosis?

_____

_____

(2) Is there any particular danger in this case? If so, what is the danger?

_____

_____

(3) What would your primary assessment of this patient involve? How would you manage this case?

_____

_____

_____

_____

e. As your 250-lb partner leaps gracefully from the ambulance to attend to the patients of a car crash, his ankle buckles underneath him. "Ow," he says, "that is rather painful." He manages to complete his work at the scene by hopping around on one foot, but by the time he gets back to the station, his ankle is quite swollen and hurts a lot. Aside from the swelling, there is no obvious deformity and no ecchymosis.

(1) What is the most likely field diagnosis?

_____

_____

(2) Is there any particular danger in this case? If so, what is the danger?

_____

_____

(3) How would you manage this case?

_____

_____

f. You are watching the championship football game pitting your local high school team against last year's regional champions. Your quarterback, who is about 5 feet 6 inches tall and weighs perhaps 150 pounds, is looking to pass when he gets sacked and buried under a horde of 225-lb defensive linemen from the other team. When the linemen unpile, your quarterback is very slow in getting up. Of course, you race over to offer your assistance. After peeling off the boy's shirt, shoulder pads, and other gear, you notice that his chest is not symmetric. There seems to be a hollow area just to the left of the sternum, at the base of the neck, and that spot is very tender. The boy, meanwhile, is quite pale, and he gasps, "I'm choking."

(1) What is the most likely field diagnosis?

_____

_____

(2) Is there any particular danger in this case? If so, what is the danger?

_____

_____

(3) How would you manage this case?

_____

_____

g. A 25-year-old man was struck by a car while crossing the street. The bumper caught him in the middle of his shin. His lower leg is severely angulated and bleeding from an open wound. He complains of severe pain in his leg and of "pins and needles" in his foot.

(1) What is the most likely field diagnosis?

_____

_____

(2) Is there any particular danger in this case? If so, what is the danger?

_____

_____

(3) How would you manage this case?

_____

_____

h. Another 25-year-old man was shot in the thigh at close range. The left thigh is swollen compared to the right, and the left leg as a whole looks shorter than the right leg. The left dorsalis pedis pulse seems weaker than that on the right side.

(1) What is the most likely field diagnosis?

_____

_____

(2) Is there any particular danger in this case? If so, what is the danger?

_____

_____

(3) How would you manage this case?

_____

_____

(4) If your management of the case included a splint, why did you use a splint? List three reasons for splinting an injured extremity.

(a) _____

(b) _____

(c) _____

i. You are spending a weekend on the ski slopes. Sailing down a particularly challenging hill, you see a skier stopped in the middle of the slope, admiring the view. Seconds later, about five other skiers come careening down the slope and, one after another, pile into the stationary skier. When the pile is unraveled, the skier at the bottom is found to have a severely deformed right knee, which seems to be swelling before your eyes.

(1) What is the most likely field diagnosis?

_____

_____

(2) Is there any particular danger in this case? If so, what is the danger?

_____

_____

(3) How would you manage this case?

_____

_____

3. You are called to the scene of a hit-and-run collision. A 45-year-old man is lying unconscious in the street, surrounded by a crowd of highly agitated people. No one actually saw how the crash happened. At first glance, you can see that the man's right thigh is angulated, and the trouser leg on that side is soaked in blood.

a. Arrange the following steps in his management in the correct sequence. One step will be performed twice.

_____ Start an IV.

_____ Take the vital signs.

_____ Cut away the trouser leg.

_____ Determine whether he is breathing (he is).

_____ Secure the patient to a backboard.

_____ Apply the PASG/MAST (if your protocols allow), while holding the right leg in traction.

_____ Put manual pressure on the bleeding site.

_____ Open the airway.

_____ Start transport.

_____ Move the patient to a backboard.

_____ Check for a carotid pulse (pulse is present).

_____ Check for a dorsalis pedis pulse on the right side.

_____ Do the AVPU "mental status" check.

_____ Check for an open or tension pneumothorax.

_____ Put a pressure dressing over the open wound on the leg.

b. Have any steps been omitted? If so, which step(s)?

_____

4. A 56-year-old woman was struck by a car as she was crossing the street. You find her lying in the street, near the curb, her left leg severely angulated and bleeding. She is conscious. There is no tenderness to palpation over the chest or spine (you don't want to remove her shirt there in the middle of the street to inspect the chest). Her skin is warm. Pulse is 108 beats/min and regular, respirations are 28 breaths/min, and blood pressure is 132/90 mm Hg. There is an open fracture of the left tibia. The dorsalis pedis pulses are equal, and sensation to pinprick is intact in both feet.

a. What steps would you take at the scene?

(1) _____

(2) _____

(3) _____

(4) _____

b. What steps would you take during transport?

(1) _____

(2) _____

(3) _____

5. A backseat passenger, a 52-year-old woman, was wearing a lap seat belt when involved in a collision. She is shrieking, "My legs, my legs!" Her skin is warm. She has no tenderness over the chest, and the chest wall is stable. Pulse is 82 beats/min and regular, respirations are 30 breaths/min and slightly shallow, and blood pressure is 106/76 mm Hg. The patient cannot move her legs, and there is no sensation to pinprick from the toes up to around the iliac wings.

a. What steps would you take at the scene?

(1) _____

(2) _____

(3) _____

    b. What steps would you take during transport?

        (1) _____

        (2) _____

        (3) _____

True/False

If you believe the statement to be more true than false, write the letter "T" in the space provided. If you believe the statement to be more false than true, write the letter "F."

_____ **1.** Severely angulated fractures should be straightened before they are splinted.

_____ **2.** An air splint is also known as a pneumatic splint.

_____ **3.** There is no need to straighten or manipulate a fracture involving joints unless it has no distal pulse.

_____ **4.** A traction splint is contraindicated in an open femoral fracture because traction may drag broken bone ends back into the wound.

_____ **5.** Fingers or toes should be left out of the splint so that distal circulation can be monitored.

_____ **6.** A patient who sustained multitrauma is in unstable condition. One should splint the whole axial skeleton as a unit, on a long backboard, rather than take time to splint individual fractures.

_____ **7.** Vacuum splints consist of a sealed mattress that is filled with air and small plastic beads.

Fill-in-the-Table

Fill in the missing parts of the tables.

Bones in Joints	
Joint	**Bones That Make Up the Joint**
Shoulder	
Elbow	
Wrist	
Hip	
Knee	
Ankle	

Potential Blood Loss From Fracture Sites	
Fracture Site	**Potential Blood Loss (mL)**
Pelvis	
Femur	
Humerus	
Tibia or fibula	
Ankle	
Elbow	
Radius or ulna	

Short Answer

Complete this section with short written answers using the space provided.

1. Fractures of the forearm or lower leg may be complicated by a compartment syndrome when there is significant bleeding and swelling within one of the tight muscular compartments of the injured limb. A compartment syndrome, by cutting off the blood supply, can jeopardize the whole limb, so it is important to recognize the symptoms and signs that suggest that a compartment syndrome may be developing. List six symptoms and signs of compartment syndrome.

   a. _____

   b. _____

   c. _____

   d. _____

   e. _____

   f. _____

2. Review the case of the man injured on the ski slope, which is repeated here. List the steps you would take in examining him. Looking for the signs of compartment syndrome is, in fact, only part of the assessment of an injured extremity.

   You are spending a weekend on the ski slopes. Sailing down a particularly challenging hill, you see a skier stopped in the middle of the slope, admiring the view. Seconds later, about five other skiers come careening down the slope and, one after another, pile into the stationary skier. When the pile is unraveled, the skier at the bottom is found to have a severely deformed right knee, which seems to be swelling before your eyes.

   a. _____

   _____

   b. _____

   _____

   c. _____

   _____

3. The equipment you should grab and take with you when you rush to the side of a severely injured patient should include the following items:

   a. _____

   b. _____

   c. _____

   d. _____

   e. _____

   f. _____

   g. _____

Problem Solving

Practice your calculation skills by solving the following math problems.

1. Your patient has a possible fractured humerus, radius, and ulna. What is the potential blood loss from these injuries?

    _____

2. You are evaluating and treating the driver of a motorcycle involved in a high-speed crash. After assessing the patient, you believe that the patient may be suffering significant blood loss from a fractured pelvis and fractured femur. What is the potential blood loss?

    _____

3. Your intoxicated patient jumped from a height of 20 feet off a roof while attending a party. He appears to have bilateral ankle fractures. How much blood loss would you estimate from this patient's injuries?

    _____

38 Environmental Emergencies

Matching

Part I

Match each of the terms in the right column to the appropriate definition in the left column.

_____ **1.** A condition in which lung tissue is damaged, characterized by hypoxemia, low lung volume, and pulmonary edema.

_____ **2.** An altitude illness characterized by headache plus at least one of the following: fatigue or weakness, gastrointestinal symptoms, dizziness or light-headedness, or difficulty sleeping.

_____ **3.** Conditions caused by the effects from hypobaric hypoxia on the central nervous system and pulmonary systems as a result of nonacclimatized people ascending to altitude; range from acute mountain sickness to high-altitude cerebral edema and high-altitude pulmonary edema.

_____ **4.** The resultant gaseous emboli from the forcing of gas into the vasculature from barotrauma.

_____ **5.** Inability to coordinate the muscles properly; often used to describe a staggering gait.

_____ **6.** Continued fall in core temperature after a victim of hypothermia has been removed from a cold environment, due at least in part to the return of cold blood from the body surface to the body core.

_____ **7.** A measurement of ambient pressure; the weight of air at sea level, equivalent in pressure to 33 feet of seawater.

_____ **8.** Injury resulting from pressure disequilibrium across body surfaces.

_____ **9.** The heat energy produced at rest from normal body metabolic reactions, determined mostly by the liver and skeletal muscles.

_____ **10.** At a constant temperature, the volume of a gas is inversely proportional to its pressure (if you double the pressure on a gas, you halve its volume); written as $PV = K$, where P = pressure, V = volume, and K = a constant.

_____ **11.** Also called free diving, this type of diving does not require any equipment, except sometimes a snorkel.

_____ **12.** Itchy reddish and purple swollen lesions that occur primarily on the extremities, due to longer exposure to temperatures just above freezing or sudden rewarming after exposure to cold.

_____ **13.** Transfer of heat to a solid object or a liquid by direct contact.

_____ **14.** Mechanism by which body heat is picked up and carried away by moving air currents.

_____ **15.** The temperature in the part of the body comprising the heart, lungs, brain, and abdominal viscera.

_____ **16.** Each gas in a mixture exerts the same partial pressure that it would exert if it were alone in the same volume, and the total pressure of a mixture of gases is the sum of the partial pressures of all the gases in a mixture.

A. Nitrogen narcosis

B. Neuroleptic malignant syndrome

C. Malignant hyperthermia

D. Loxoscelism

E. Hypothermia

F. Wind chill factor

G. Thermoregulation

H. Thermogenesis

I. Superficial frostbite

J. Pulmonary overpressurization syndrome

K. Hypothalamus

L. Hyperthermia

M. Homeostasis

N. High-altitude pulmonary edema

O. Core body temperature

P. Convection

_____ **17.** A term for decompression sickness and air gas embolism.

_____ **18.** A broad range of signs and symptoms caused by nitrogen bubbles in blood and tissues coming out of solution on ascent.

_____ **19.** A type of frostbite in which the affected part looks white, yellow-white, or mottled blue-white and is hard, cold, and without sensation.

_____ **20.** Also called passive heatstroke, this is a serious heat illness that usually occurs during heat waves and is most likely to strike very old, very young, or bedridden people.

_____ **21.** Secretion of large amounts of urine in response to cold exposure and the consequent shunting of blood volume to the body core.

_____ **22.** The process of experiencing respiratory impairment from submersion or immersion in liquid.

_____ **23.** The injection of venom via a bite or sting.

_____ **24.** Medical conditions caused or exacerbated by the weather, terrain, or unique atmospheric conditions such as high altitude or underwater.

_____ **25.** A condition due to prolonged exertion in hot environments coupled with excessive hypotonic fluid intake that leads to nausea, vomiting, and, in severe cases, mental status changes and seizures.

_____ **26.** A serious type of heatstroke usually affecting young and fit people exercising in hot and humid conditions.

_____ **27.** An indirect measure of pressure under water, equal to one atmosphere absolute.

_____ **28.** Localized damage to tissues resulting from prolonged exposure to extreme cold.

_____ **29.** The conversion of a liquid to a gas.

_____ **30.** Early frostbite, characterized by numbness and pallor without significant tissue damage.

_____ **31.** Permanent cell death.

_____ **32.** Acute and involuntary muscle pains, usually in the lower extremities, the abdomen, or both, that occur because of profuse sweating and subsequent sodium losses in sweat.

_____ **33.** A clinical syndrome characterized by volume depletion and heat stress that is thought to be a milder form of heat illness and on a continuum leading to heatstroke.

_____ **34.** The increase in core body temperature due to inadequate thermolysis.

_____ **35.** The least common and most deadly heat illness, caused by a severe disturbance in thermoregulation, usually characterized by a core temperature of more than 104°F (40°C) and altered mental status.

_____ **36.** An altitude illness in which there is a change in mental status and/ or ataxia in a person with acute mountain sickness or the presence of mental status changes and ataxia in a person without acute mountain sickness.

_____ **37.** An altitude illness characterized by at least two of the following: dyspnea at rest, cough, weakness or decreased exercise performance, or chest tightness or congestion. Also, at least two of the following signs: central cyanosis, audible rales or wheezing in at least one lung field, tachypnea, or tachycardia.

Q. High-altitude cerebral edema

R. Henry's law

S. Heat syncope

T. Heatstroke

U. Conduction

V. Cold diuresis

W. Chilblains

X. Classic heatstroke

Y. Heat illness

Z. Heat exhaustion

AA. Breath-hold diving

BB. Boyle's law

CC. Basal metabolic rate

DD. Barotrauma

EE. Atmosphere absolute

FF. Heat cramps

GG. Gangrene

HH. Frostnip

II. Frostbite

JJ. Feet of seawater

KK. Ataxia

_____ **38.** Body processes that balance the supply and demand of the body's needs.

_____ **39.** Unusually elevated body temperature.

_____ **40.** Portion of the brain that regulates a multitude of body functions, including core temperature.

_____ **41.** Condition in which the core body temperature is significantly below normal.

_____ **42.** An orthostatic or near-syncopal episode that typically occurs in nonacclimated people who may be under heat stress.

_____ **43.** The amount of gas dissolved in a liquid is directly proportional to the partial pressure of the gas above the liquid.

_____ **44.** A condition that can result from common anesthesia medications and present with hyperthermia, muscular rigidity, altered mental status, and a hyperdynamic state.

_____ **45.** A condition caused by antipsychotic and even common antiemetic medications that presents with hyperthermia, muscular rigidity, altered mental status, and a hyperdynamic state.

_____ **46.** A state resembling alcohol intoxication produced by nitrogen gas dissolved in the blood at high ambient pressure; also called rapture of the deep.

_____ **47.** Also called "burst lung," this diving emergency can occur during rapid ascent and can cause pneumothorax, mediastinal and subcutaneous emphysema, alveolar hemorrhage, and the lethal arterial gas embolism.

_____ **48.** A potentially fatal condition resulting from a brown recluse spider bite that begins with a painful, inflamed vesicle that may progress to a gangrenous sloughing of the skin.

_____ **49.** A type of frostbite characterized by altered sensation and white, waxy skin that is firm to palpation, but the underlying tissues remain soft.

_____ **50.** The production of heat in the body.

_____ **51.** The factor that takes into account the temperature and wind velocity in calculating the effect of a given ambient temperature on living organisms.

_____ **52.** The process by which the body compensates for environmental extremes—for example, balancing between heat production and heat release.

LL. Arterial gas embolism

MM. Exertional heatstroke

NN. Exercise-associated hyponatremia

OO. Evaporation

PP. Altitude illnesses

QQ. Afterdrop

RR. Acute mountain sickness

SS. Acute lung injury

TT. Dalton's law

UU. Decompression illness

VV. Decompression sickness

WW. Deep frostbite

XX. Drowning

YY. Environmental emergencies

ZZ. Envenomation

Part II

Place the letters HP next to the factors that increase heat production and the letters HL next to the factors that interfere with heat loss (dissipation).

_____ **1.** High ambient temperature

_____ **2.** Physical exertion

_____ **3.** Heavy or tight clothing

_____ **4.** Diabetic peripheral neuropathies

_____ **5.** Hyperthyroidism

_____ **6.** Response to infection

_____ **7.** Alcoholism

_____ **8.** Overdosing on such drugs as cocaine, caffeine, or Ecstasy

_____ **9.** Impaired vasodilatation

_____ **10.** Agitated and tremulous state (such as from Parkinson disease or drug withdrawal)

Multiple Choice

Read each item carefully, and then select the best response.

1. Heat syncope is seen in nonacclimated people who may be under heat stress and typically occurs in all the following situations, EXCEPT:
   A. after standing suddenly.
   B. at mass outdoor gatherings.
   C. after prolonged standing.
   D. after swimming on a very hot day.

2. The major contributors to the basal metabolic rate (BMR), the heat energy produced at rest from normal body metabolic reactions, are the:
   A. spleen and lungs.
   B. kidneys and heart.
   C. liver and skeletal muscles.
   D. kidneys and gallbladder.

3. The loss of heat that takes place when moving air picks up heat and carries it away is:
   A. evaporation.
   B. convection.
   C. radiation.
   D. conduction.

4. A call to the scene of an outdoor high school track meet is for a 15-year-old student who was running the mile race. It is a humid day with the temperature in the 90s. The patient presents with muscle pain in the lower extremities and abdomen. Based on these symptoms, what is the MOST likely problem?
   A. Heat cramps
   B. Heat exhaustion
   C. Heatstroke
   D. Heat syncope

5. You are called to an apartment building on a hot July afternoon for a bedridden 78-year-old woman. Upon entering the apartment, you notice that it is extremely hot, and the patient is very warm with dry skin. The SAMPLE history identifies that the patient has congestive heart failure and is taking beta-blockers and diuretics. Her blood glucose is normal. You should suspect:
   A. exertional heatstroke.
   B. malignant hyperthermia.
   C. neuroleptic malignant syndrome.
   D. classic heatstroke.

6. Each of the following factors increases heat loss, EXCEPT:
   A. vasoconstriction.
   B. wet clothes.
   C. alcohol.
   D. diabetic neuropathies.

7. What unique finding might be observed on an ECG of a patient with a low core body temperature?
   A. Alternans
   B. Osborn waves
   C. Spiked waves
   D. Inverted T waves

8. You are called to a local boat dock for a patient returning from a scuba dive. His dive computer shows the maximum depth was 120 feet. The patient is reported by his buddy to have had inappropriate behavior while getting ready to ascend. The ascent was controlled with a safety stop for a few minutes at around 20 feet. Back in the dive boat, the patient complains of tingling in his lips and legs. He has no other reported symptoms. You most likely suspect that the patient may have a mild case of:
   A. arterial gas embolism.
   B. nitrogen narcosis.
   C. pulmonary overpressurization syndrome.
   D. barotitis externa.

9. You are dispatched to the pool at a private residence for an unconscious teenager. Upon arrival you are told that he was competing with a friend to see who could hold his breath underwater the longest. He was swimming underwater, and while coming to the surface, went limp and was pulled from the water. You find the patient is breathing, and you administer supplemental oxygen and continue with an assessment. What do you expect is the patient's problem?
   A. Decompression sickness
   B. Barotrauma
   C. Shallow water blackout
   D. Bends

10. Deep frostbite usually involves the hands or feet, and the extremity may initially exhibit all of the following colors, EXCEPT:
   A. white.
   B. yellow-white.
   C. mottled blue-white.
   D. gangrene.

Labeling

Label the following diagrams with the correct terms.

1. Physiologic Responses to Hot and Cold Environments

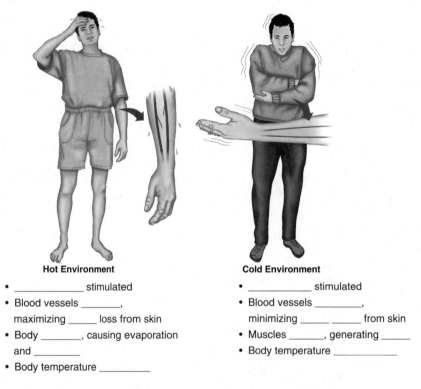

Hot Environment
- _____ stimulated
- Blood vessels _____,
  maximizing _____ loss from skin
- Body _____, causing evaporation
  and _____
- Body temperature _____

Cold Environment
- _____ stimulated
- Blood vessels _____,
  minimizing _____ _____ from skin
- Muscles _____, generating _____
- Body temperature _____

Fill-in-the-Blank

Read each item carefully, and then complete the statement by filling in the missing word(s).

1. The core temperature of the human body at any given moment represents a balance between the heat produced by the body and the heat shed by the body.
   a. List the potential sources of body heat and the mechanisms by which body heat can be dissipated.

Sources of Body Heat	Ways of Shedding Heat
1.	1.
2.	2.
3.	3.
4.	

b. The body's mechanisms for dissipating excess heat have certain limitations. First, all of the mechanisms depend on _____ _____ to shunt blood from the core to the body surface. Furthermore, to be effective, three of the body's cooling mechanisms require a temperature gradient between the body and the outside. None of these three mechanisms—_____, _____, or _____—can work if the outside temperature is not at least a few degrees cooler than the body core. Finally, one of the body's cooling mechanisms is dependent on the ambient humidity. When the humidity is high, that mechanism—namely, _____ _____ _____—is ineffective in lowering the core temperature.

c. A hatless hiker standing still on a mountaintop on a windless day loses heat from his head by _____. A breeze picks up. Now the hiker loses heat by _____ as well.

d. A white-water enthusiast who capsizes his canoe in a swift-running river loses body heat by _____.

e. A soldier on maneuvers in the desert in ambient temperatures of more than 37.7°C (100°F) can shed heat only by _____ _____ _____.

Identify

In the following case study, list the chief complaint, vital signs, and pertinent negatives.

1. You are riding on Squad 5 and are dispatched to a person who fell through the ice at a local pond. Upon arrival, you find an 18-year-old man who is shivering with a blanket wrapped around him. It is reported that a Good Samaritan threw a rope and helped the patient get to shore. When you question the patient, he says that he was trying to walk home and didn't realize he had gotten lost. There is a smell of alcohol on the patient's breath. You immediately place the patient in your squad and turn the heat on high. The wet clothes are removed and the patient is wrapped in a number of blankets. He is placed on supplemental oxygen and a cardiac monitor. The ECG rhythm is regular, with no ectopy, but you do observe Osborn waves. You establish an IV using warm crystalloid solution. The patient is transferred to the regional trauma center that is 15 minutes away. You continue to monitor the patient and perform a reassessment en route. You take serial vital signs every 5 minutes.

a. Chief complaint:

_____

_____

b. Vital signs:

_____

_____

c. Pertinent negatives:

_____

_____

d. What three pieces of information not included in this scenario would be helpful to know?

(1) _____

(2) _____

(3) _____

e. Based on this scenario, which of the following four methods of heat loss is most responsible for the greatest amount of heat lost by this patient?

A. Radiation

B. Conduction

C. Convection

D. Evaporation

f. You determine the patient is moderately hypothermic. How much IV fluid should you infuse initially?

_____

Complete the Patient Care Report (PCR)

Reread the incident scenario in the preceding Identify exercise and then complete the following PCR for the patient.

EMS Patient Care Report (PCR)					
Date:	Incident No.:	Nature of Call:		Location:	
Dispatched:	En Route:	At Scene:	Transport:	At Hospital:	In Service:
Patient Information					
Age:		Allergies:			
Sex:		Medications:			
Weight (in kg [lb]):		Past Medical History:			
		Chief Complaint:			
Vital Signs					
Time:	BP:	Pulse:	Respirations:	SpO$_2$:	
Time:	BP:	Pulse:	Respirations:	SpO$_2$:	
Time:	BP:	Pulse:	Respirations:	SpO$_2$:	
EMS Treatment (circle all that apply)					
Oxygen @ _____ L/min via (circle one): NC NRM Bag-Mask Device		Assisted Ventilation	Airway Adjunct	CPR	
Defibrillation	Bleeding Control	Bandaging	Splinting	Other	
Narrative					

Ambulance Calls

The following case scenarios provide an opportunity to explore the concerns associated with patient management and paramedic care. Read each scenario, and then answer each question.

1. At morning briefing, you are told that you will be doing a standby at an outdoor festival at a local college campus. These assignments are usually boring, but you will make the best of it. It is a very hot and humid day in late spring, and except for a few scrapes and blisters, you have little request for service. The concert has been going for about an hour when you are called to a person who has passed out. When you arrive, you find an unresponsive man about 20 years old. His friends tell you that he had been standing listening to the concert and suddenly fell. As you are assessing the patient, he starts to regain consciousness. You can tell he has been drinking. You ask how many beers he had, and he tells you he drank two. In your mind, you at least double that number. You load the patient into the ambulance and turn up the air conditioner. The assessment indicates dehydration.

   a. What is the probable cause of the syncopal episode, and what may be some contributing underlying causes?

   _____

   _____

   _____

   b. How would you manage this patient?

   _____

   _____

   _____

   c. If the patient does not recover and stabilize quickly, what may be another presenting problem to consider?

   _____

   _____

2. You are called to the local high school playing field on a hot, sticky August afternoon to deal with a "casualty" of preseason training—a 16-year-old fullback who "became crazy" during practice. You see him over near the goalposts, where several of his teammates are trying to restrain him. "None of my boys ever messed around with drugs before," the coach tells you, "and I sure never would have pegged Chuck as a junkie. But I don't know how else to explain his behavior. He's been touchy all afternoon, and he just started acting crazy."

   You find the fullback agitated and combative. He seems completely disoriented. His skin is warm and sweaty. His vital signs are as follows: Pulse is 120 beats/min and bounding, respirations are 30 breaths/min and shallow, blood pressure is 150/90 mm Hg, and oral temperature is 41.7°C (107°F). His pupils are widely dilated and react only sluggishly to light.

   a. This boy is most likely suffering from:

   _____

   _____

   b. List the steps in managing this case.

   (1) _____

   (2) _____

   (3) _____

   (4) _____

   (5) _____

   (6) _____

   (7) _____

3. The following day, it is even hotter, but mercifully the humidity has dropped considerably. You are called to the very same playing field for another casualty of preseason training, this time a 14-year-old running back. You find him lying at midfield, writhing in pain. "I swear I didn't clip him," one of the other players is insisting. "I didn't even get near him. He just fell down by himself."

"Sure, sure," says the coach, who is trying to massage the cramps out of the boy's legs. When you ask the boy what his problem is, he just moans and says, "My legs, my legs."

On examination, his skin is cool and sweaty. His pulse is 100 beats/min and regular, respirations are 30 breaths/min and shallow, blood pressure is 110/70 mm Hg, and oral temperature is 37°C (98.6°F). There are no signs of injury to the extremities.

a. This boy is most likely suffering from:

_____

_____

b. List the steps in managing this case.

(1) _____

(2) _____

(3) _____

(4) _____

4. "As long as you folks are already here," says the coach, "maybe you could take a look at our quarterback. I think he's coming down with something, and I have to decide whether to send him home."

You find the quarterback sitting on the bench looking quite miserable. He says that his girlfriend has mononucleosis, and he thinks he may be coming down with it too because he feels very tired and achy. On examination, he is sweating profusely, and his skin feels clammy. His pulse is 110 beats/min and somewhat weak, respirations are 28 breaths/min and shallow, blood pressure is 100/60 mm Hg, and oral temperature is 39.4°C (103°F).

a. This boy is most likely suffering from:

_____

_____

b. List the steps in managing this case.

(1) _____

(2) _____

(3) _____

(4) _____

(5) _____

c. What advice should you give the football coach?

_____

_____

5. On the very same day, you are called to a local supermarket for a "sick baby." You arrive to find a nearly hysterical woman who looks scarcely out of her teens holding a comatose baby. "I just left her in the car for a minute while I ran in to buy a couple of things," she says, although you note three full shopping bags in the woman's cart. The baby, a 6-month-old, is unconscious (AVPU = U). The pulse is 180 beats/min, respirations are 60 breaths/min, and blood pressure is 100/80 mm Hg. The baby's rectal temperature is 43.3°C (110°F).

a. This baby is most likely suffering from:

_____

_____

b. List the steps in managing this case.

(1) _____

(2) _____

(3) _____

(4) _____

(5) _____

(6) _____

(7) _____

6. You are enjoying a week off at a mountain ski resort. On your first morning there, the manager of the resort asks for volunteers to join a search-and-rescue party that is going out to look for three skiers who failed to return to the lodge the previous night. You, of course, volunteer, and you set off with a team on skis to comb the slopes. You are all carrying two-way radios so that you can summon a snowmobile to help transport the lost skiers if you find them. Eventually, you locate two of the skiers, about 15 miles from the ski lodge, dug into a makeshift shelter in the snow (and unaware that only about 50 meters away, beyond a stand of trees, is an empty cabin). Both skiers are alert.

a. The first skier tells you that he lost all sensation in his left leg sometime during the night. On examination the leg is white, cold, and very hard. He is most likely suffering from:

_____

_____

b. Describe how you would manage this patient.

(1) _____

(2) _____

(3) _____

(4) _____

(5) _____

c. The second skier says, "I think I've got the same problem in my left foot." On examination, the foot has a waxy, white appearance. The skin feels very stiff, but there is "give" underneath when you press down hard on the skin. He is most likely suffering from:

_____

_____

d. How would you manage this patient?

(1) _____

(2) _____

(3) _____

(4) _____

(5) _____

e. Not long after those two skiers have been evacuated on stretchers by snowmobile, you find the third skier. He is sitting up against a tree, unconscious. Apparently, he did not realize that he had come within 100 meters of the main road. His skin is very cold. You cannot detect any pulse. His pupils are dilated and unreactive. He does seem to be breathing, although only about once or twice a minute. You radio for a paramedic-staffed ambulance to meet you at the road. What is this patient suffering from?

_____

_____

f. Describe the management of this patient until the ambulance comes and en route to the hospital.

(1) _____

(2) _____

(3) _____

(4) _____

(5) _____

(6) _____

(7) _____

(8) _____

7. You and your crew are at the local lake on a chilly November afternoon, covering an annual speedboat race that invariably produces a few minor casualties (mostly from indigestion among the picnicking spectators). Making a hairpin turn at high speed, one of the speedboats capsizes. After what seems like a very long time, you see the boat's driver bob to the surface of the water (he is wearing a life jacket) and begin swimming for shore. Describe the actions you should take in this situation.

a. _____

b. _____

c. _____

d. _____

e. _____

f. _____

g. _____

h. _____

8. During the first spell of bitter cold weather of the season, you are called to the downtown bus terminal for a "man down." When you reach the scene, a police officer waves you over. "Sorry to bother you folks with this," he says. "Just a vagrant who's been sleeping in the place for a few days, and probably all he needs is a night in the lockup to sober up." You find the patient, being restrained by another police officer, over in a corner. His speech is slurred, and he staggers when he tries to walk. His breath smells of wine. His skin is pale and cold.

a. List at least three diagnoses you must consider in this case.

(1) _____

(2) _____

(3) _____

b. In view of the diagnostic possibilities, describe how you would manage this case.

(1) _____

(2) _____

(3) _____

(4) _____

(5) _____

(6) _____

(7) _____

9. You decide to take a week's vacation to do some climbing in the Canadian Rockies. Of course, you are carrying a medical kit because it's hard for you to accept the idea that you are really on vacation. On your first day out, one of your buddies starts complaining of a headache—"probably because I didn't sleep really well last night," he says. You're a little concerned that he might be suffering from the altitude, but he shrugs it off and insists that you all keep going.

a. At that point, how could you check if your friend is suffering from a serious case of acute altitude sickness?

_____

_____

b. As things turn out, you decide to continue climbing. About an hour later, you feel a tug on the rope and look back to see your friend really dragging. He seems out of breath. Now you're really concerned. List four signs or symptoms that would suggest your friend may be suffering from high-altitude pulmonary edema.

(1) _____

(2) _____

(3) _____

(4) _____

c. Assuming that you do find signs of high-altitude pulmonary edema, what steps should you take to treat your friend?

(1) _____

(2) _____

(3) _____

10. When your next vacation comes up, you decide you won't make the same mistake twice: no more mountains where emergencies will spoil your relaxation. Instead, you sign up for a cruise to the West Indies—a week of sun and sand and steel drum bands. On the ship with you is a group of scuba enthusiasts who don't miss any opportunity to explore the local coral reefs each time you anchor.

One fine afternoon, as you are sunning yourself on deck with a rum swizzle in hand, you hear a commotion off to the starboard side of the ship. You leap from your chair and peer over the rail to see some of the diving crowd in a state of agitation in the rubber raft from which they've been diving. One of their number is lying motionless in the raft, and another two are just emerging from the water and climbing into the raft to join them. The captain, meanwhile, having spotted the situation, has already lowered a winch to bring up the raft and everyone in it.

As soon as the divers are back aboard the ship, you race to the side of the diver who is unconscious. His friends tell you that he was the least experienced of their group. He had surfaced first, and a minute or so after being pulled onto the raft, he complained of chest pain and his voice had sounded funny. Then, he just blacked out.

a. What do you think has happened to this diver?

_____

_____

b. What steps should you take to manage this situation?

(1) _____

(2) _____

(3) _____

(4) _____

(5) _____

(6) _____

c. About an hour later, while you are monitoring the condition of the diver pending more definitive treatment, you hear one of his friends who was in the water with him saying to another member of the group, "Gee, my back is sure killing me. I must have pulled a muscle when I did my backflip off the raft. The hell of it is that I can't pee either." You perk up your ears when you hear that because that bit of information makes you suspect that the speaker has suffered:

_____

_____

True/False

If you believe the statement to be more true than false, write the letter "T" in the space provided. If you believe the statement to be more false than true, write the letter "F."

_____ 1. A superficial frostbitten extremity is best warmed in front of a campfire or heater.

_____ 2. In deep frostbite, the extremity feels cold and rock hard.

_____ 3. If rescue circumstances require it, a patient with deep frostbite may walk on a frostbitten leg as long as the leg is not rewarmed in the field.

_____ 4. Antibiotic ointment should be applied gently over frostbitten areas to prevent infection.

_____ 5. A frostbitten extremity will be excruciatingly painful until it is rewarmed.

_____ 6. Frostnip most often affects the tips of the ears, nose, fingers, and toes.

_____ 7. Heat exhaustion is a clinical syndrome thought to represent a milder form of heat illness on a continuum leading to heatstroke.

_____ 8. Classic heatstroke is less apt to affect older patients with chronic illnesses.

_____ 9. Patients with heatstroke usually have dilated pupils.

_____ 10. Radiation accounts for more than 65% of heat loss in a cooler setting.

Short Answer

Complete this section with short written answers using the space provided.

1. The body's normal response to entering a hot environment can place considerable stress on a person who has a limited cardiovascular reserve. Explain why.

_____

_____

_____

2. Anyone can succumb to a heat wave, but some people are more vulnerable than others. List five factors that increase a person's risk of suffering significant heat illness in response to heat stress.

a. _____

b. _____

c. _____

d. _____

e. _____

3. Paramedics, like other public safety personnel, do not have the luxury of postponing heavy exertion until weather conditions are favorable; they must do their job whatever the weather, which means they may be exposed to a significant risk of heat illness during periods of high temperature.

   a. List five measures you can take to reduce your risk of becoming ill from the heat.

   (1) _____

   (2) _____

   (3) _____

   (4) _____

   (5) _____

   b. If you do start to experience early symptoms of heat illness, you must stop your activities immediately. But to do so, you need to be able to recognize the warning symptoms of heat illness when they occur. List four warning symptoms of heat illness.

   (1) _____

   (2) _____

   (3) _____

   (4) _____

4. No one would ever suffer cold injury if they simply heeded the advice of their mother. Mothers always know, even without taking a paramedic course, how to keep warm on cold days. Following are several statements you have heard at least once from Mother. Each statement reflects an intuitive knowledge of the ways in which the body generates and loses heat. For each statement, explain why Mother was right.

   a. "Don't go out without a hat and scarf; it's freezing out there." Mother was right because:

   _____

   _____

   b. "Stop rolling around in the snow. You'll get a death of a chill." Mother was right because:

   _____

   _____

   c. "Get out of those wet clothes this minute." Mother was right because:

   _____

   _____

   d. "Those skates are much too tight. Your toes will fall off." Mother was right because:

   _____

   _____

   e. "Make sure you wear your windbreaker. It's blowing a gale out there." Mother was right because:

   _____

   _____

f. "Eat. Eat. You have to have something to keep you going in this weather." Mother was right because:

_____

_____

5. In addition to Mother's advice, the body has only a limited repertoire of defenses against the cold. List three ways the body can defend itself against a drop in core temperature.

a. _____

b. _____

c. _____

6. Although anyone can suffer cold injury, certain factors predispose a person to suffer ill effects from the cold.
a. List five factors that predispose a person to suffer frostbite when exposed to freezing conditions.

(1) _____

(2) _____

(3) _____

(4) _____

(5) _____

b. List four factors that predispose a person to suffer hypothermia.

(1) _____

(2) _____

(3) _____

(4) _____

7. The stories that many of us learned as children contain many cautionary tales about cold exposure.
a. When the three little kittens lost their mittens, they became most vulnerable to:

_____

b. Sitting on an ice-cold tuffet on a winter day, Little Miss Muffet was losing heat from her body by:

_____

c. Who is at greater risk of suffering hypothermia—Jack Sprat (who ate no fat) or his wife (who ate no lean)?

_____

d. Before venturing outside to try out his new ice skates, little Jack Horner retreated to a corner and ate his Christmas pie. Was that a good idea? Why or why not?

_____

e. Swinging about in the treetop is Baby in his cradle. When the wind blows, the cradle will rock. Furthermore, when the wind blows, Baby will lose heat from his body by the process called:

_____

Fill-in-the-Table

Fill in the missing parts of the table.

Hypothermia affects every system in the body. In the following table, list some of the effects of a drop in core temperature on each body system mentioned.

Body System	Effects of Hypothermia
Central nervous system	
Cardiovascular system	
Respiratory system	
Muscular system	
Metabolic system	

CHAPTER

39

Responding to the Field Code

Matching

Match each of the terms in the right column to the appropriate definition in the left column.

_____ **1.** In CPR, when two rescuers perform ventilations and compressions individually and not timed or waiting for the other rescuer to pause.

_____ **2.** A "smart" defibrillator that can analyze the patient's electrocardiogram (ECG) rhythm and determine whether a defibrillating shock is needed.

_____ **3.** The code team member who has the responsibility for managing the rescuers or team members during a cardiac arrest, as well as choreographing the effort of the group.

_____ **4.** A member of the resuscitation team trying to revive the patient.

_____ **5.** The use of an unsynchronized direct current electric shock to terminate ventricular fibrillation or ventricular tachycardia.

_____ **6.** A mode available on automated external defibrillators, allowing the paramedic to interpret the cardiac rhythm and determine whether defibrillation is indicated (rather than the monitor making the determination).

_____ **7.** The return of spontaneous heartbeat and blood pressure during the resuscitation of a patient in cardiac arrest.

_____ **8.** An acronym used to describe a prehospital program's objectives: Specific, Measurable, Attainable and Achievable, Realistic and Relevant, and Timely.

A. SMART

B. Manual defibrillation

C. Code team member

D. Automated external defibrillator (AED)

E. Asynchronous

F. Defibrillation

G. Return of spontaneous circulation (ROSC)

H. Code team leader

Multiple Choice
Read each item carefully, and then select the best response.

1. Which of the following is NOT considered a link in the chain of survival?
   A. Early access to 9-1-1
   B. Early high-quality CPR
   C. Early clotbuster therapy in the field
   D. State-of-the-art postresuscitative care

2. For which types of incidents does simulation training provide valuable preparation?
   A. High-frequency, low-risk
   B. Low-frequency, high-risk
   C. Low-frequency, low-risk
   D. High-frequency, high-risk

3. With the issuance of the 2005 and 2010 ECC Guidelines, there was a strong emphasis on:
   A. advanced airway procedures.
   B. choices of cardiac medications.
   C. increasing the ventilation rates.
   D. high-quality compressions.

4. When placing an advanced airway during resuscitation, the MOST important consideration would be:
   A. not to take any longer than 30 seconds.
   B. not to interrupt chest compressions for more than 10 seconds.
   C. to hyperventilate the patient as soon as possible.
   D. to insert the largest tube that will fit the patient.

5. High-quality CPR consists of each of the following, EXCEPT:
   A. compressions at a rate of at least 100 per minute.
   B. allowing complete chest recoil after each compression.
   C. avoiding excessive ventilations.
   D. compression depth of 1½ inches on the adult patient.

6. For the purposes of the ECC Guidelines, an infant is:
   A. age 1 year to adolescence.
   B. age 1 month to 1 year.
   C. within the first few hours after birth.
   D. within the first month after birth.

7. When there are two health care providers doing CPR, the infant compression-to-ventilation ratio should be:
   A. 30:2.
   B. 15:1.
   C. 15:2.
   D. 30:1.

8. When a pediatric patient needs to be defibrillated with an AED, it is acceptable to:
   A. use the pediatric dose attenuator system.
   B. use a manual defibrillator.
   C. use the standard adult pads if that is all that is available.
   D. All of the above

9. You are treating an adult patient who has overdosed from a narcotic. The patient is in respiratory arrest. What is the rate of ventilations that should be given to the patient?
   A. 1 breath every 6–8 seconds
   B. 2 breaths every 30 compressions
   C. 1 breath every 3 seconds
   D. 2 breaths every 3 seconds

10. Of the following treatments for the patient with ROSC, which would NOT be appropriate?
   A. Increase the blood pressure with dopamine (Intropin) to approximately 120 mm Hg systolic.
   B. Elevate the patient's head to 30 degrees if the blood pressure allows.
   C. Stabilize the cardiac rhythm with an antidysrhythmic.
   D. Begin hypothermia treatment if the patient is comatose.

Labeling

Label the following diagrams with the correct terms.

    1. CPR Devices

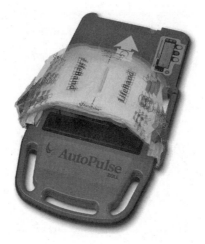

    A. _____

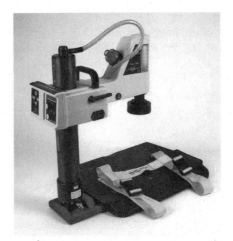

    B. _____

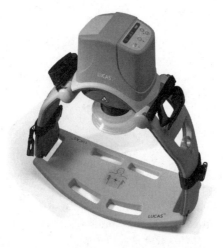

    C. _____

2. Resuscitation Pyramid

```
        A
        B
      ─────
        C

        D

        E
```

A. _____

B. _____

C. _____

D. _____

E. _____

Fill-in-the-Blank

Read each item carefully, and then complete the statement by filling in the missing word(s).

1. The _____ is an adjunct to adult CPR that provides both continuous chest compressions and ventilations.
2. If a/an _____ _____ is in place, there are no longer cycles of compressions to ventilations.
3. The _____ _____ _____ is marketed as the ResQPOD in the United States.
4. If an advanced airway is inserted, you should switch to _____ compressions of at least 100 per minute and ventilate every _____ to _____ seconds.
5. For _____ or _____, do not deliver shocks.
6. Drug therapy for pulseless electrical activity (PEA) or asystole includes a _____ (epinephrine or vasopressin).

Identify

In the following case study, list the chief complaint, vital signs, and pertinent negatives.

1. You are riding on Medic 480 and are dispatched along with a basic life support (BLS) unit to a person who is unresponsive in the shopping mall restroom. Upon arrival, you find a bystander and a security guard doing CPR on a 58-year-old man. When you question the patient's spouse, she says that he was complaining of pressure in his chest and indigestion before he went into the bathroom. She stated that he was only in there for a couple of moments when the bystander who started chest compressions had his son come out to get her and call 9-1-1. The security guard arrived soon thereafter with the AED. You immediately rotate the compressor, who is starting to get tired, and determine that the initial rhythm is not a shockable rhythm. As the other unit arrives, you begin to choreograph the resuscitation, making sure the patient is receiving high-quality chest compressions with as few interruptions as possible. Your partner is placing an intraosseous line in the leg so the first epinephrine can be administered. At this

point the EMT doing the ventilations reports that bag-valve mask ventilation is working just fine. After 2 minutes (of five cycles of compressions and ventilations), you note a rhythm change to ventricular fibrillation (V-Fib), so the defibrillator is charged and a shock is administered. After the shock is administered, the chest compressions are started immediately. Within moments you note that the monitor is now showing a "normal"-looking ECG, so you stop the compressions and note the patient has a strong carotid pulse. Since the patient is not yet breathing on his own, you decide to intubate and start the hypothermia protocol. The wife, who has been observing all of the care, is very happy when the pulse returns. Further history reveals that the patient has been having these periods of chest discomfort for the past few weeks. He has no allergies and takes only vitamins each day. He has never had previous problems with his heart, head, or lungs, although his father did die from heart problems at a young age. En route to the hospital, a 12-lead ECG is taken and medications are administered to keep the patient from shivering from the cooled saline you are administering. The patient's blood pressure is 108 mm Hg systolic, and his pulse rate is 96 beats/min and regular.

After delivering the patient right to the coronary catherization lab for post–successful resuscitative measures, you note that the success of this resuscitation was definitely due to the bystander's immediate actions!

a. Chief complaint:

_____

_____

b. Vital signs:

_____

_____

c. Pertinent negatives:

_____

_____

d. What two medications would most likely be administered to this patient?

_____

_____

e. Based on this scenario, what are the links in the Chain of Survival for this patient and all victims of sudden cardiac arrest?

(1) _____

(2) _____

(3) _____

(4) _____

(5) _____

Complete the Patient Care Report (PCR)

Reread the incident scenario in the preceding Identify exercise and then complete the following PCR for the patient.

EMS Patient Care Report (PCR)			
Date:	**Incident No.:**	**Nature of Call:**	**Location:**
Dispatched:	**En Route:**	**At Scene:** **Transport:**	**At Hospital:** **In Service:**

Patient Information	
Age:	**Allergies:**
Sex:	**Medications:**
Weight (in kg [lb]):	**Past Medical History:**
	Chief Complaint:

Vital Signs				
Time:	**BP:**	**Pulse:**	**Respirations:**	**SpO$_2$:**
Time:	**BP:**	**Pulse:**	**Respirations:**	**SpO$_2$:**
Time:	**BP:**	**Pulse:**	**Respirations:**	**SpO$_2$:**

EMS Treatment (circle all that apply)			
Oxygen @ _____ L/min via (circle one): NC NRM Bag-Mask Device	**Assisted Ventilation**	**Airway Adjunct**	**CPR**
Defibrillation	**Bleeding Control**	**Bandaging**	**Splinting**	**Other**

Narrative

Ambulance Calls

The following case scenarios provide an opportunity to explore the concerns associated with patient management and paramedic care. Read each scenario, and then answer each question.

1. At morning briefing, you are interrupted with a call for a possible cardiac arrest. The police have just arrived on the scene and the supervisor is en route to the call also. As you arrive, you are met by a neighbor who states, "Mr. Jones was out shoveling snow when he suddenly collapsed. He was told by his heart doctor to leave the heavy work for his grandson!" Apparently the grandson found him, carried him into the garage, called 9-1-1, and began hands-only CPR. As you and your partner are bringing in your equipment, you think to yourself, *The good news is CPR was started . . . The bad news is that he has a cardiac history.* Just then a backup unit pulls up, as does the supervisor's truck. That means there are two medics (including you), two EMTs, a supervisor, and a police officer, and you will need to assign tasks so this code runs with the speed and precision of a NASCAR pit stop.

   a. What is the highest priority during the entire code?

   _____

   _____

   _____

   b. If your role is that of the code team leader, what are your responsibilities?

   (1) _____

   (2) _____

   (3) _____

   (4) _____

   (5) _____

   (6) _____

   (7) _____

   (8) _____

   c. If you need to assign roles to the code team members, what do they include?

   (1) _____

   (2) _____

   (3) _____

   (4) _____

2. Based on the scenario just described, if the grandson had come home to find his grandfather on the floor in the kitchen in cardiac arrest and there was an unknown downtime before calling 9-1-1, the results could be entirely different. On your arrival at the scene this time, the grandson was not doing hands-only CPR because he missed that day in his high school when it was taught.

   a. What are the criteria for not starting resuscitation?

   _____

   _____

   _____

b. With regard to the success of this resuscitation, what is the significance of chest compressions not being started prior to your arrival on the scene?

_____

_____

_____

3. Later that day, you and your partner respond to a private home where on entering the living room you note there is a hospital bed set up in the corner of the room. The daughter has called 9-1-1 because she thinks her father, who has been suffering for a long time, has passed away. She leads you to the bathroom where you can hear the son counting 19 and 20 and 21 and . . . as he provides chest compressions to his father on the floor of the small bathroom. The daughter states, "We just didn't know what to do. Dad wouldn't have wanted all this." You and your partner quickly move the patient, who weighs about 100 pounds, out into the living room where there is more room.

   a. List the conditions (termination rules) when it would be appropriate to stop the resuscitation in consult with medical control.

   (1) _____

   (2) _____

   (3) _____

   (4) _____

   b. From the scenario described, what might lead you to ask if the patient was in a hospice program or has a do not resuscitate (DNR) order?

   (1) _____

   (2) _____

   (3) _____

   (4) _____

True/False

If you believe the statement to be more true than false, write the letter "T" in the space provided. If you believe the statement to be more false than true, write the letter "F."

_____   **1.** A possible cause of PEA is hypovolemia.

_____   **2.** A clue to the patient in cardiac arrest due to cardiac tamponade may be jugular vein distention.

_____   **3.** Beyond managing a cardiac arrest, if you suspect a tension pneumothorax, you should do a needle decompression on the affected side.

_____   **4.** Sodium bicarbonate should be considered in a cardiac arrest if the patient is in V-Fib.

_____   **5.** If the patient has torsades de pointes, the paramedic should consider administering magnesium.

_____   **6.** Once you start CPR in the field, you should not stop until 15 minutes have gone by.

_____   **7.** An impedance threshold device (ITD) selectively prevents excess air from rushing into the chest during resuscitation.

_____   **8.** Once ROSC occurs, the ITD can be used to assist in the patient's ventilations.

_____   **9.** The two-hands encircling method should be used by a single rescuer doing infant CPR.

_____   **10.** In an adult who is unconscious where you suspect a foreign body airway obstruction, CPR chest compressions are the most effective method for clearing the obstruction.

Short Answer

Complete this section with short written answers using the space provided.

1. The ECC guidelines include recommendations on tube placement confirmation and continuous monitoring of the tube's position to avoid dislodgement. List the initial techniques of verification paramedics should employ on a tube's placement.

    a. _____

    b. _____

    c. _____

    d. _____

    e. _____

    f. _____

2. The chapter describes a plan for prehospital response to a cardiac arrest with a five-person team. This is just an example of a "best practice" that could be practiced in your community, but it certainly is not the only way to manage a cardiac arrest; each community has different responders and resources. List the roles of the five-person team, and describe what they are responsible for.

    a.
    _____
    _____
    _____
    _____

    b.
    _____
    _____
    _____
    _____

    c.
    _____
    _____
    _____
    _____

    d.
    _____
    _____
    _____
    _____

    e.
    _____
    _____
    _____

Fill-in-the-Table

Fill in the missing parts of the table.

Key Elements of CPR for Adults, Children, and Infants, 2010 Guidelines			
Procedure	**Age 9 to Adult**	**Age 1 to 8 Years**	**Younger Than 1 Year[a]**
Circulation			
Recognition	Unresponsive with no breathing, or only agonal (gasping) respirations		
Pulse check	_____	_____	Brachial artery
Compression location	In the center of the chest, in between the nipples	In the center of the chest, in between the nipples	_____
Compression area	Heel of both hands	_____	Two fingers or two-thumb encircling-hands technique
Compression depth	At least 2 inches	At least one third of chest depth Approximately 2 inches	_____
Compression rate	_____		
Chest wall recoil	Allow full chest recoil in between compressions Rotate professional rescuers delivering compressions every 2 minutes		
Interruptions	Limit interruptions in delivery of chest compressions to less than 10 seconds		
Ratio of compressions to ventilations (until an advanced airway is inserted)	_____	_____ (one rescuer); _____ (two professional rescuers)	
Airway			
	Head tilt–chin lift maneuver; jaw-thrust maneuver if _____ is suspected		
Breathing			
Untrained rescuer	Compressions only		
Ventilations without advanced airway	2 breaths with a duration of _____ each, with enough volume to produce _____ [b]		
Ventilations with advanced airway	1 breath every 6 to 8 seconds (8 to 10/min) Asynchronous with chest compressions. Duration of 1 second each with enough volume to produce chest rise		
Rescue breaths	1 breath every _____ (12 breaths/min)	1 breath every _____ (20 breaths/min)	1 breath every _____ (20 breaths/min)
Defibrillation			
Device	Adult AED	Use _____ unit if available; if not available, use adult unit	Use _____ if available; if not, use unit with pediatric dose attenuator; if neither is available, use adult unit
Procedure	Attach AED as soon as it is available. If two rescuers are available, one should immediately begin CPR while the second retrieves and applies the AED. Minimize CPR interruptions. Resume CPR immediately after shock, beginning with _____.		
Airway Obstruction			
Foreign body obstruction	Conscious: _____	Conscious: _____	Conscious: _____
	Unconscious: _____ [c]		

[a]Excluding newborns, in whom arrest is usually the result of asphyxiation and requires the rescue ventilations.
[b]Pause compressions to deliver ventilations.
[c]Look in the mouth for objects before delivering breaths in a patient with a known airway obstruction.

Skill Drill

Place the skill drill steps in the correct order.

1. Performing Two-Rescuer Adult CPR

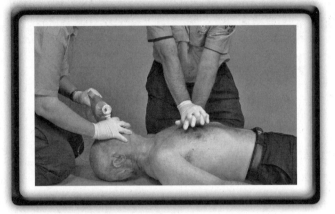

_____ If there is no pulse and an AED is not available or the elapsed time from collapse is greater than 4 to 5 minutes, begin chest compressions at a ratio of 30:2. Once an advanced airway is inserted, rescuers should switch from cycles of CPR to continuously delivered compressions at a rate of at least 100/min.

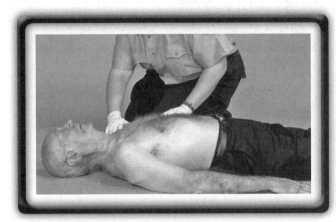

_____ Determine unresponsiveness and take positions.

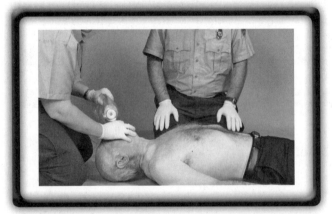

_____ If not breathing, give two breaths of 1 second each. After 2 minutes, switch rescuer positions to minimize fatigue. Keep switch time to 5 to 10 seconds. Depending on patient condition, continue CPR, continue ventilations only, or place in recovery position and monitor breathing and pulse.

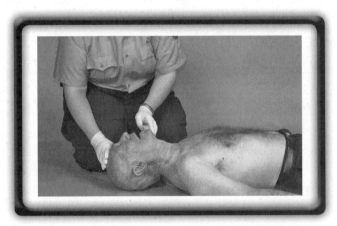

_____ Open the airway. Check for breathing. If breathing is adequate, place the patient in the recovery position and monitor.

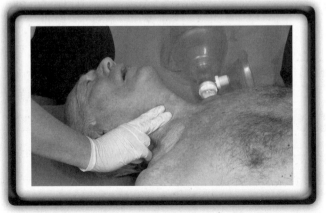

_____ Check for a carotid pulse (maximum of 10 seconds). If there is no pulse but an AED is available, apply it now.

2. Performing CPR on a Child

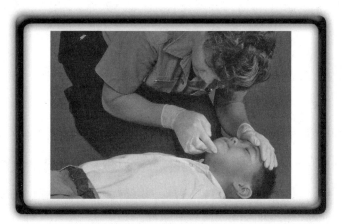

_____ Coordinate compressions with ventilations in a 30:2 ratio (one rescuer) or 15:2 (two rescuers). At the end of each cycle, pause for two ventilations.

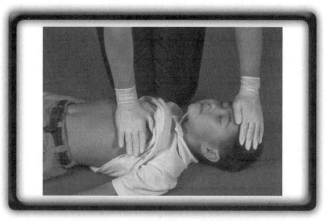

_____ Compress the chest one third the anterior-posterior diameter of the chest at a rate of 100/min.

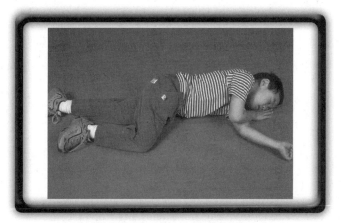

_____ Continue cycles of compressions and ventilations until an AED becomes available or the patient shows signs of spontaneous breathing. If the child resumes effective breathing, place him or her in a position that allows for frequent reassessment of the airway and vital signs during transport.

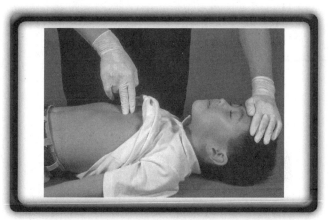

_____ Place the child on a firm surface. Prepare to place the heel of one or both hands in the center of the chest, in between the nipples, avoiding the xiphoid process.

3. Infant CPR

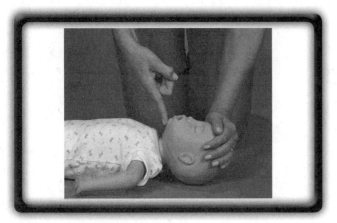

_____ Position the infant on a firm surface while maintaining the airway.

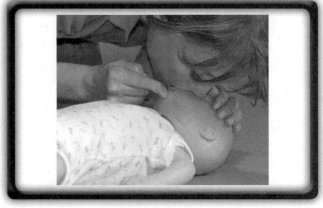

_____ Coordinate compressions with ventilations in a 30:2 ratio (one rescuer) or 15:2 (two rescuers), pausing for two ventilations at the end of each cycle. Continue cycles of compressions and ventilations until an AED becomes available or the infant shows signs of spontaneous breathing.

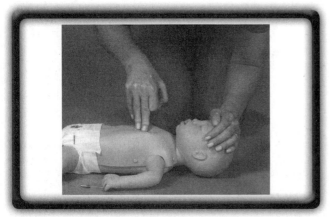

_____ Place two fingers in the middle of the sternum just below a line between the nipples. Use two fingers to compress the chest one third the anterior-posterior diameter of the chest at a rate of at least 100/min. Allow the sternum to return to its normal position between compressions.

Management and Resuscitation of the Critical Patient

40

Matching

Match each of the terms in the right column to the appropriate definition in the left column.

_____ **1.** The early stage of shock, in which the body can still compensate for blood loss. The systolic blood pressure and brain perfusion are maintained.

_____ **2.** Occurs with the tendency to gather and rely on information that confirms your existing views and to avoid or downplay information that does not conform to your preexisiting hypothesis or field differential.

_____ **3.** A progressive condition usually characterized by combined failure of several organs, such as the lungs, liver, and kidneys, along with some clotting mechanisms, which occurs after severe illness or injury.

_____ **4.** A process in which molecules move from an area of higher concentration to an area of lower concentration.

_____ **5.** A condition that occurs when there is widespread dilation of the resistance vessels, the capacitance vessels, or both.

_____ **6.** The effect on the velocity of conduction.

_____ **7.** A principle stating that the movement and use of oxygen in the body is dependent on an adequate concentration of inspired oxygen, appropriate movement of oxygen across the alveolar-capillary membrane into the arterial bloodstream, adequate number of red blood cells to carry the oxygen, proper tissue perfusion, and efficient off-loading of oxygen at the tissue level.

_____ **8.** A condition that occurs when the circulating blood volume is inadequate to deliver adequate oxygen and nutrients to the body.

_____ **9.** Affecting the contractility of muscle tissue, especially cardiac muscle.

_____ **10.** The late stage of shock, when blood pressure is falling.

_____ **11.** The short list of the potential causes of the patient's presenting condition.

_____ **12.** The final stage of shock, resulting in death.

_____ **13.** A condition that occurs when the level of tissue perfusion decreases below that needed to maintain normal cellular functions; also called shock.

_____ **14.** The blood pressure required to sustain organ perfusion; roughly 60 mm Hg in the average person.

_____ **15.** The ability of the heart to contract.

A. Chemoreceptors

B. Central shock

C. Cardiovascular collapse

D. Aerobic metabolism

E. Afterload

F. Anaerobic metabolism

G. Baroreceptors

H. Capacitance vessels

I. Cardiac output (CO)

J. Cardiogenic shock

K. Angioedema

L. Anchoring bias

M. Anaphylactic shock

N. Confirmation bias

O. Critical patients

_____ **16.** Circulatory failure caused by paralysis of the nerves that control the size of the blood vessels, leading to widespread dilation; seen in patients with spinal cord injuries.

_____ **17.** Shock that occurs as a result of fluid loss contained within the body, such as in dehydration, burn injury, crush injury, and anaphylaxis.

_____ **18.** A drop in systolic blood pressure when moving a patient from a sitting to a standing position.

_____ **19.** The resistance to blood flow within all of the blood vessels except the pulmonary vessels.

_____ **20.** The delivery of oxygen and nutrients to the cells, organs, and tissues of the body.

_____ **21.** The period either just before or just after cardiac arrest when the patient is critical and care must be taken to prevent progression or regression into cardiac arrest.

_____ **22.** Patients either in premorbid conditions, with major trauma, or in the peri-arrest period.

_____ **23.** Shock that occurs when there is a block to blood flow to the heart or great vessels, causing an insufficient blood supply to the body's tissues.

_____ **24.** A condition that consists of hypovolemic shock and distributive shock (Weil-Shubin classification).

_____ **25.** The initial stretching of the cardiac muscles prior to contraction. It is related to the chamber volume of blood just prior to the contraction.

_____ **26.** A condition preceding the onset of disease.

_____ **27.** The difference between the systolic and diastolic pressures.

_____ **28.** The smallest arterioles.

_____ **29.** Shock caused by severe infection, usually a bacterial infection.

_____ **30.** A sudden reaction of the nervous system that produces a temporary, generalized vascular dilation, resulting in syncope (vasovagal syncope).

_____ **31.** An abnormal state associated with inadequate oxygen and nutrient delivery to the metabolic apparatus of the cell; also called hypoperfusion.

_____ **32.** Developing sensitivity to a substance that initially causes no allergic reaction.

_____ **33.** Circular muscular walls of capillaries that constrict and dilate, acting as a gate to increase or decrease blood flow.

_____ **34.** The local neurologic condition that occurs after a spinal injury produces motor and sensory losses (which may not be permanent).

_____ **35.** The amount of blood that the left ventricle ejects into the aorta per contraction.

_____ **36.** Metabolism that can proceed only in the presence of oxygen.

P. Decompensated shock

Q. Differential field diagnosis

R. Dromotropic effect

S. Fick principle

T. Hypoperfusion

U. Mean arterial pressure (MAP)

V. Irreversible shock

W. Inotropic effect

X. Hypovolemic shock

Y. Distributive shock

Z. Compensated shock

AA. Multiple-organ dysfunction syndrome (MODS)

BB. Neurogenic shock

CC. Myocardial contractility

DD. Systemic vascular resistance (SVR)

EE. Stroke volume (SV)

FF. Resistance vessels

GG. Sensitization

HH. Pulse pressure

II. Non-hemorrhagic shock

JJ. Obstructive shock

_____ **37.** The pressure in the aorta against which the left ventricle must pump blood.

_____ **38.** Metabolism that takes place in the absence of oxygen.

_____ **39.** A severe hypersensitivity reaction that involves bronchoconstriction and cardiovascular collapse.

_____ **40.** Occurs when an initial reference point distorts your estimates.

_____ **41.** Recurrent large areas of subcutaneous edema of sudden onset, usually disappearing within 24 hours, which is seen mainly in young women, frequently as a result of allergy to food or drugs.

_____ **42.** Receptors in the blood vessels, kidneys, brain, and heart that respond to changes in pressure in the heart or main arteries to help maintain homeostasis.

_____ **43.** The smallest venules.

_____ **44.** The volume of blood pumped through the circulatory system in 1 minute.

_____ **45.** A condition caused by loss of 40% or more of the functioning myocardium; the heart is no longer able to circulate sufficient blood to maintain adequate oxygen delivery.

_____ **46.** Failure of the heart and blood vessels; shock.

_____ **47.** A condition that consists of cardiogenic shock and obstructive shock (Weil-Shubin classification).

_____ **48.** Sense organs that monitor the levels of oxygen and carbon dioxide and the pH of cerebrospinal fluid and blood, and provide feedback to the respiratory centers to modify the rate and depth of breathing based on the body's needs at any given time.

KK. Peripheral shock

LL. Preload

MM. Premorbid condition

NN. Orthostatic hypotension

OO. Perfusion

PP. Peri-arrest period

QQ. Septic shock

RR. Shock

SS. Sphincters

TT. Spinal shock

UU. Diffusion

VV. Psychogenic shock

Multiple Choice

Read each item carefully, and then select the best response.

1. The short list of potential causes of the patient's presenting condition is called the:
   - **A.** definitive diagnosis.
   - **B.** presenting problem.
   - **C.** differential field diagnosis.
   - **D.** disposition.

2. Conditions that come before the onset of disease are called:
   - **A.** peri-arrest conditions.
   - **B.** premorbid conditions.
   - **C.** risk factors.
   - **D.** congenital defects.

3. With a patient who has a chief complaint of altered mental status, a starting point for the differential diagnosis can be remembered using the acronym:
   - **A.** SAMPLE.
   - **B.** M-T-SHIP.
   - **C.** OPQRST.
   - **D.** AVPU.

4. Intuition has a definite role in assessment of critical patients by experienced providers. Intuition can:
   A. forewarn you of what may happen next.
   B. lead you to make treatment errors.
   C. be difficult to teach.
   D. All of the above

5. A tendency to gather and rely on information that confirms your existing assessment views is called a/an:
   A. personal bias.
   B. confirmation bias.
   C. relieved decision.
   D. anchoring bias.

6. The amount of circulation of blood within an organ or tissue in adequate amounts to meet the cells' current needs for oxygen nutrients and waste removal is referred to as:
   A. stroke volume.
   B. contractility.
   C. preload.
   D. perfusion.

7. The initial stretching of the cardiac muscle prior to contraction is called the:
   A. cardiac output.
   B. preload.
   C. afterload.
   D. stroke volume.

8. Your patient has a blood pressure of 110/70 mm Hg. What is his mean arterial pressure?
   A. 40
   B. 56
   C. 83
   D. 92

9. Stimulation of the sympathetic nervous system can cause the pupils to _____ and the heart rate to _____.
   A. dilate; increase
   B. dilate; decrease
   C. constrict; increase
   D. constrict; decrease

10. Stimulation of the parasympathetic nervous system can cause the gastrointestinal tract to:
    A. decrease motility.
    B. shut down.
    C. increase salivation.
    D. All of the above

11. Of the following, which is NOT considered an essential element of the Fick principle?
    A. Proper tissue perfusion
    B. Adequate number of white blood cells to carry oxygen
    C. Adequate concentration of inspired oxygen
    D. Efficient off-loading of oxygen at the tissue level

12. Beta-1 stimulation produces each of the following, EXCEPT:
    A. positive chronotropic effects.
    B. positive inotropic effects.
    C. inhibited insulin release.
    D. positive dromotropic effects.

13. A progressive condition characterized by combined failure of two or more organs or organ systems that were initially unharmed by the patient's initial illness, is called:

A. cardiovascular collapse.

B. compensated shock.

C. decompensated shock.

D. multiple-organ dysfunction syndrome.

14. Your patient has sustained a serious internal injury. He is agitated, anxious, and restless. He complains of nausea and thirst and has a normal blood pressure. What phase of shock is he MOST likely in?

A. Irreversible shock

B. Compensated shock

C. Decompensated shock

D. Terminal shock

15. Pediatric patients are unique, as compared to adults, in that they can often compensate even when they have lost up to _____ of their blood volume.

A. 10–15%

B. 20–25%

C. 30–35%

D. 40–45%

Labeling

Label the following diagram with the correct terms.

1. Relationship Between the Organism and the Cells

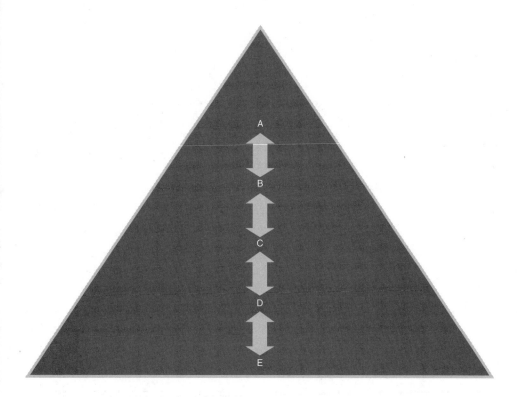

A. _____

B. _____

C. _____

D. _____

E. _____

Fill-in-the-Blank

Read each item carefully, and then complete the statement by filling in the missing word(s).

1. When the paramedic allows his/her initial reference point to distort an estimate while conducting the assessment, this is known as a/an _____ bias.

2. To protect vital organs, the body attempts to _____ by _____ blood flow from organs that are more tolerant of low flow to vital organs that cannot tolerate hypoperfusion.

3. Blood flow through capillary beds is regulated by the capillary _____, circular muscular walls that constrict and dilate to increase or decrease flow.

4. Along with the baroreceptors are _____, which measure subtle shifts in the amount of carbon dioxide in the arterial blood.

5. The switch from _____ metabolism to _____ metabolism is a critical point that begins to produce lactic acidosis from this inefficient form of metabolism.

6. Effects of norepinephrine are primarily _____ and _____ in nature and center on vasoconstriction and _____ (increasing/decreasing) peripheral vascular resistance.

7. A reduction in _____ blood flow produces acute tubular _____, which in turn leads to _____ (urine output of less than 20 mL/h).

8. The last phase of shock, when this condition has progressed to a terminal stage, is _____ shock.

9. In cases of suspected _____ _____, you must recognize the need for expeditious transport for pericardiocentesis at the ED.

10. _____ shock occurs when the heart is unable to circulate sufficient blood to maintain adequate peripheral oxygen delivery.

Identify

In the following case study, list the chief complaint, vital signs, and pertinent negatives.

You are called to the home of a 74-year-old man who is experiencing chest pain. Upon arrival, you begin your chest pain protocol. John, the patient, is experiencing tightness in his chest and left arm. You place John on high-flow supplemental oxygen and obtain a 12-lead electrocardiogram (ECG). You determine that John's heart is in a sinus bradycardia with a rate of 52 beats/min. Both his lungs have some crackles at their bases, he is breathing 24 breaths/min, and his room air saturation is SpO_2 92%. He is slightly confused, but comes around with the oxygen and is able to answer all your questions. His pupils are equal and round, regular in size, and react to light (PEARRL). You are unable to feel a pulse in his wrist. His blood pressure is 80/56 mm Hg, and he is diaphoretic. You determine that the rate and strength of John's heart are causing the problem. You realize that John could be in cardiogenic shock. You start an IV and a low-dose dopamine (Intropin) drip. You feel that John is a top priority and head to the most appropriate hospital as quickly as possible.

1. Chief complaint:

_____

_____

2. Vital signs:

_____

_____

3. Pertinent negatives:

_____

_____

Complete the Patient Care Report (PCR)

Reread the case study in the preceding Identify exercise and then complete the following PCR for the patient.

EMS Patient Care Report (PCR)					
Date:	**Incident No.:**	**Nature of Call:**		**Location:**	
Dispatched:	**En Route:**	**At Scene:**	**Transport:**	**At Hospital:**	**In Service:**

Patient Information	
Age:	**Allergies:**
Sex:	**Medications:**
Weight (in kg [lb]):	**Past Medical History:**
	Chief Complaint:

Vital Signs				
Time:	**BP:**	**Pulse:**	**Respirations:**	**SpO$_2$:**
Time:	**BP:**	**Pulse:**	**Respirations:**	**SpO$_2$:**
Time:	**BP:**	**Pulse:**	**Respirations:**	**SpO$_2$:**

EMS Treatment (circle all that apply)				
Oxygen @ _____ L/min via (circle one): NC NRM Bag-Mask Device		**Assisted Ventilation**	**Airway Adjunct**	**CPR**
Defibrillation	**Bleeding Control**	**Bandaging**	**Splinting**	**Other**

Narrative

Ambulance Calls

The following case scenarios provide an opportunity to explore the concerns associated with patient management and paramedic care. Read each scenario, and then answer each question.

1. A middle-aged man was struck by a car as he was crossing the street. You find him lying by the side of the road, complaining of severe pain in his abdomen, where the car hit him. You would like to make an assessment of his state of perfusion. How will you assess the following?

   a. His peripheral perfusion:

   _____

   b. The perfusion to his vital organs:

   _____

2. You are called to a downtown bar in which firearms were deployed to settle a difference of opinion. You find a man lying on the floor of the bar, unconscious, his trouser leg soaked in blood. In the correct sequence, list the steps you will take in treating this patient.

   a. _____

   b. _____

   c. _____

   d. _____

   e. _____

   f. _____

3. One rainy day, a car bomb was detonated in front of a foreign consulate, and a number of bystanders were injured by flying debris, including jagged pieces of metal torn from the car's body. The first patient you come upon is bleeding from multiple sites, including a deep gash on the right side of the neck and a laceration that has partially severed the right leg at the groin. The leg laceration is gushing blood; it is too proximal to benefit from a tourniquet. It is hard to evaluate skin condition in the rain. Pulse is around 100 beats/min and somewhat weak; respirations are 30 breaths/min.

   a. What steps would you take at the scene?

   (1) _____

   (2) _____

   (3) _____

   (4) _____

   b. What steps would you take during transport?

   (1) _____

   (2) _____

   (3) _____

4. A second patient from the car bombing, a young man, was sideswiped by a piece of flying debris, which made a clean 14-inch incision straight across his abdomen. He is conscious and in moderate distress. Pulse is 104 beats/min and regular, respirations are 28 breaths/min and slightly labored, and blood pressure is 104/70 mm Hg. What looks to be a major portion of the patient's intestines are outside the abdomen.

   a. What steps would you take at the scene?

   (1) _____

   (2) _____

   (3) _____

   b. What steps would you take during transport?

      (1) _____

      (2) _____

      (3) _____

5. A third patient from the car bombing is another young man in considerable respiratory distress. There is a 2-inch wide hole in his right chest through which you can hear air being sucked on inhalation. His skin is warm. His pulse is 108 beats/min and regular, respirations are 30 breaths/min and gasping, and blood pressure is 112/64 mm Hg.

   a. What steps would you take at the scene?

      (1) _____

      (2) _____

      (3) _____

   b. What steps would you take during transport?

      (1) _____

      (2) _____

      (3) _____

6. A 59-year-old man was the driver of a car that plowed into a bridge abutment in the early hours of the morning. The patient is conscious, but very restless. He is sweating profusely. His chest is stable (it's too dark to see whether there are bruises). He can move all his extremities. His pulse is 82 beats/min, respirations are 28 breaths/min, and blood pressure is 100/70 mm Hg.

   a. What steps would you take at the scene?

      (1) _____

      (2) _____

      (3) _____

      (4) _____

      (5) _____

   b. What steps would you take during transport?

      (1) _____

      (2) _____

      (3) _____

      (4) _____

True/False

If you believe the statement to be more true than false, write the letter "T" in the space provided. If you believe the statement to be more false than true, write the letter "F."

_____ **1.** The patient with obstructive shock may have jugular vein distention.

_____ **2.** Cardiogenic shock can lead to warm skin and hypertension.

_____ **3.** Severe bacterial infection can lead to septic shock.

_____ **4.** Simple fainting is also called psychogenic shock.

_____ **5.** The capacitance vessels are the small arterioles.

_____ **6.** When a patient is in "cold shock," he or she may benefit from epinephrine.

_____ **7.** Neurogenic shock usually results from spinal cord injury.

_____ **8.** Sensitization means developing a heightened reaction to a substance.

_____ **9.** Recurrent large areas of subcutaneous edema of sudden onset, usually disappearing within 24 hours and mainly seen in young women, are called angioedema.

_____ **10.** Positive chronotrophic effects will increase the velocity of the heart's conduction.

Short Answer

Complete this section with short written answers using the space provided.

1. List what each of the following could indicate using the acronym M-T-SHIP:

   M: _____

   T: _____

   S: _____

   H: _____

   I: _____

   P: _____

2. Karl Weick's "five-step process" for communicating intuitive decisions and obtaining feedback from team members includes:

   a. _____

   b. _____

   c. _____

   d. _____

   e. _____

Fill-in-the-Table

Fill in the missing parts of the tables.

1.

The "H and T" Questions of Cardiac Arrest	
Reversible Causes of Cardiac Arrest	**Ask your team . . .**
Hypovolemia	Does this patient have any evidence of internal or external bleeding or fluid loss?
_____	How well is the patient oxygenating? Could there have been a respiratory event that led to this cardiac arrest?
Hydrogen ion (acidosis)	Is there any reason for metabolic or respiratory acidosis in this patient?
_____	Does this patient undergo renal dialysis? Might the electrolytes be altered (ie, is the patient on a liquid diet)?
Hypothermia	Does the patient feel cold to touch? If so, obtain the core body temperature.
_____	Is the patient a diabetic? What is the blood glucose level?
Tension pneumothorax	Does the patient have bilateral lung sounds? Is the patient becoming difficult to ventilate? Consider the need for chest decompression.
_____	Is there penetrating trauma to the patient's heart? Consider the need for pericardiocentesis (in the ED).
Toxins	Consider substance abuse (ie, narcotics or opiates). Consider naloxone (Narcan).
_____	Does the patient have a history of blood clots? Is the patient a smoker and/or take birth control? Has the patient had a recent long bone immobilization?
Thrombosis (coronary)	Does the patient have a large AMI developing? Is this patient a candidate for PCI?
_____	Is there a mechanism of injury for life-threatening trauma?

2.

Compensated Versus Decompensated Shock	
Compensated Shock	**Decompensated Shock**
• Agitation, anxiety, restlessness	• Altered mental status (verbal to unresponsive)*
• _____	• _____
• Weak, rapid (thready) pulse	• _____
• Clammy (cool, moist) skin	• Thready or absent peripheral pulses
• _____	• Ashen, mottled, or cyanotic skin
• _____	• _____
• Nausea, vomiting	• Diminished urine output (oliguria)
• Delayed capillary refill in infants and children	• _____
• _____	
• _____	
*Mental status changes are late indicators.	

3.

Types of Shock			
Types of Shock	**Examples of Potential Causes**	**Signs and Symptoms**	**Assessment and Treatment**
_____	Inadequate heart function Disease of muscle tissue Impaired electrical system Disease or injury	Chest pain Irregular pulse Weak pulse Low blood pressure Cyanosis (lips, under nails) Cool, clammy skin Anxiety Rales Pulmonary edema	_____

_____	Mechanical obstruction of the cardiac muscle causing a decrease in cardiac output
	1. Tension pneumothorax
	2. Cardiac tamponade
		Dependent on cause:
		• Dyspnea
		• Rapid, weak pulse
		• Rapid, shallow breaths
		• Decreased lung compliance
		• Unilateral, decreased, or absent breath sounds
		• Decreased blood pressure
		• Jugular vein distention
		• Subcutaneous emphysema
		• Cyanosis
		• Tracheal deviation toward affected side
		• Beck triad (cardiac tamponade):
		  • Jugular vein distention
		  • Narrowing pulse pressure
		  • Muffled heart tones
			_____

_____	Severe bacterial infection	Warm skin Tachycardia Low blood pressure	_____
_____	Cervical or thoracic spinal cord injury, which causes widespread blood vessel dilation	Bradycardia (slow pulse) or normal pulse Low blood pressure Signs of neck injury	_____

(Continued)

| Types of Shock | | | |
Types of Shock	Examples of Potential Causes	Signs and Symptoms	Assessment and Treatment
_____	Extreme life-threatening allergic reaction	Can develop within seconds Mild itching or rash Burning skin Vascular dilation Generalized edema Coma Rapid death	_____ _____ _____ _____
_____	Temporary, generalized vascular dilation Anxiety, bad news, sight of injury or blood, prospect of medical treatment, severe pain, illness, tiredness	Rapid pulse Normal or low blood pressure	_____ _____
_____	Loss of blood or fluid	Rapid, weak pulse Low blood pressure Change in mental status Cyanosis (lips, under nails) Cool, clammy skin Increased respiratory rate	_____ _____ _____
_____	Severe chest injury, airway obstruction	Rapid, weak pulse Low blood pressure Change in mental status Cyanosis (lips, under nails) Cool, clammy skin Increased respiratory rate	_____ _____ _____

Obstetrics

Matching

Match each of the items in the left column to the appropriate term in the right column.

_____ **1.** Expulsion of the fetus, from any cause, before the 20th week of gestation.

_____ **2.** A premature separation of the placenta from the wall of the uterus.

_____ **3.** A watery fluid that provides the fetus with a weightless environment in which to develop.

_____ **4.** An extremely rare, life-threatening condition that occurs when amniotic fluid and fetal cells enter the pregnant woman's pulmonary and circulatory system through the placenta via the umbilical veins, causing an exaggerated allergic response from the woman's body.

_____ **5.** An overgrowth of bacteria in the vagina, characterized by itching, burning, or pain and possibly a "fishy" smelling discharge.

_____ **6.** The term for an oocyte once it has been fertilized and multiplies into cells.

_____ **7.** A vaginal infection that is not technically a sexually transmitted infection, and which can occur in a pregnant or nonpregnant female, but which is more common in pregnancy; also called thrush or a yeast infection.

_____ **8.** A scoring system for assessing the status of a newborn that assigns a number value to each of five areas of assessment.

_____ **9.** A situation in which the head of the fetus is larger than the woman's pelvis; in most cases, cesarean section is required for such a delivery.

_____ **10.** The interior of the cervix.

_____ **11.** The narrowest portion of the uterus that opens into the vagina.

_____ **12.** The sexually transmitted disease with the highest incidence; signs and symptoms include inflammation of the urethra, epididymis, cervix, and fallopian tubes, and discharge from the urethra.

_____ **13.** A blood pressure that is equal to or greater than 140/90 mm Hg, which exists prior to pregnancy, occurs before the 20th week of pregnancy, or continues to persist postpartum.

_____ **14.** The dome-shaped top of the uterus.

_____ **15.** Expulsion of all products of conception from the uterus.

_____ **16.** The remains of a follicle after an oocyte has been released; it secretes progesterone.

A. Human papilloma virus (HPV)

B. Human immunodeficiency virus (HIV)

C. Herpes

D. Habitual abortion

E. Gravidity

F. Oocyte

G. Nuchal cord

H. Myometrium

I. Meconium

J. Lightening

K. Gravid

L. Gonorrhea

M. Gestational period

N. Fundus

O. Follicle-stimulating hormone (FSH)

P. Labor

_____ **17.** The appearance of the newborn's body part (usually the head) at the vaginal opening at the beginning of labor.

_____ **18.** A herpesvirus that can produce the symptoms of prolonged high fever, chills, headache, malaise, extreme fatigue, and an enlarged spleen.

_____ **19.** Seizures that result from severe hypertension in a pregnant woman.

_____ **20.** An egg that attaches outside the uterus, typically in a fallopian tube.

_____ **21.** A disease of the liver that occurs only during pregnancy, in which hormones affect the gallbladder by slowing down or blocking the normal bile flow from the liver; the most common symptom is profuse, painful itching, particularly of the hands and feet.

_____ **22.** Thinning and shortening of the cervix; this is a normal process that occurs as the uterus contracts.

_____ **23.** Intentional expulsion of the fetus.

_____ **24.** The fetus in the earliest stages after fertilization.

_____ **25.** The innermost layers of tissue in the uterus.

_____ **26.** A situation in which a fetus is large, usually defined as weighing more than 4,500 grams or almost 9 pounds, also known as "large for gestational age."

_____ **27.** The developing, unborn infant inside the uterus.

_____ **28.** The stage of labor that begins with the onset of regular labor pains and crampy abdominal pains, during which the uterus contracts and the cervix effaces.

_____ **29.** A hormone produced by the anterior pituitary gland that is important in the menstrual cycle.

_____ **30.** The time that it takes for the fetus to develop in utero, normally 38 weeks.

_____ **31.** A sexually transmitted disease that results in infection with signs and symptoms that include pus-containing discharge from the urethra and painful urination in men, and signs and symptoms of an acute abdomen in women.

_____ **32.** An incision in the perineal skin made to prevent tearing during childbirth.

_____ **33.** The vehicles of transportation of the ova from the ovaries to the uterus; also called the oviducts.

_____ **34.** The fluid-filled, baglike membrane in which the fetus develops.

_____ **35.** The total number of times pregnant, including the current pregnancy.

_____ **36.** A term used to refer to the number of times a woman has been pregnant, regardless of the outcome.

_____ **37.** The middle layer of tissue in the uterus.

_____ **38.** A situation in which the umbilical cord is wrapped around the fetus's neck; cord compression may occur during labor, causing the fetal heart rate to slow and resulting in fetal distress.

_____ **39.** Three or more consecutive pregnancies that end in miscarriage.

Q. Incomplete abortion

R. Imminent abortion

S. Hyperemesis gravidarum

T. Hydramnios

U. First stage of labor

V. Fetus

W. Fetal macrosomia

X. Fallopian tubes

Y. Episiotomy

Z. Endometrium

AA. Cervical canal

BB. Cephalopelvic disproportion

CC. Candidiasis

DD. Breech presentation

EE. Abortion

FF. Abruptio placenta

GG. Amniotic fluid

HH. Amniotic fluid embolism

II. Amniotic sac

JJ. Bloody show

KK. Blastocyst

LL. Bacterial vaginosis

MM. Apgar scoring system

_____ **40.** An infection of the genitals, buttocks, or anal area caused by herpes simplex virus, type 1 or type 2.

_____ **41.** An infection that causes acquired immune deficiency syndrome (AIDS).

_____ **42.** The most common sexually transmitted disease, which can cause genital warts and some types of cancer.

_____ **43.** A spontaneous abortion that cannot be prevented.

_____ **44.** Expulsion of the fetus that results in some products of conception remaining in the uterus.

_____ **45.** The mechanism by which the fetus and the placenta are expelled from the uterus.

_____ **46.** A plug of mucus, sometimes mixed with blood, that is expelled from the dilating cervix and discharged from the vagina.

_____ **47.** A delivery in which the buttocks come out first.

_____ **48.** In pregnancy, a feeling of relief of pressure in the upper abdomen; a premonitory sign of labor.

_____ **49.** A dark, greenish black material in the amniotic fluid that indicates fetal distress; can be aspirated into the fetus's lungs during delivery; the fetus's first bowel movement.

_____ **50.** An egg produced from the female ovary.

_____ **51.** A condition in which there is too much amniotic fluid, also known as polyhydramnios.

_____ **52.** A condition of persistent nausea and vomiting during pregnancy.

NN. Cervix

OO. Corpus luteum

PP. Complete abortion

QQ. Chronic hypertension

RR. Cholestasis

SS. Chlamydia

TT. Crowning

UU. Cytomegalovirus (CMV)

VV. Eclampsia

WW. Ectopic pregnancy

XX. Effacement

YY. Elective abortion

ZZ. Embryo

Multiple Choice

Read each item carefully, and then select the best response.

1. An abortion that occurs naturally and affects 1 in every 5 pregnancies is called a/an:
   A. spontaneous abortion.
   B. septic abortion.
   C. threatened abortion.
   D. incomplete abortion.

2. What is the condition in which the placenta is implanted low in the uterus and, as it grows, it partially obscures the cervical canal?
   A. Abruptio placenta
   B. Molar pregnancy
   C. Pseudocyesis
   D. Placenta previa

3. Which of the following words describes a woman who has had two or more pregnancies?
   A. Multigravida
   B. Primipara
   C. Multipara
   D. Parity

4. When the baby's head enters the birth canal, the _____ stage of labor begins.
   A. fourth
   B. third
   C. second
   D. first

5. The Apgar scoring system is an evaluation tool for the newborn's vital functions and is recommended to be taken at what intervals after birth?
   A. 2 minutes and 10 minutes
   B. 1 minute and 5 minutes
   C. 5 minutes and 10 minutes
   D. 1 minute and 2 minutes

6. _____ of blood loss after delivery is considered postpartum hemorrhage.
   A. 1,000 mL
   B. 150 mL
   C. 750 mL
   D. 500 mL

7. What medication can be used to control postpartum hemorrhage in the prehospital setting?
   A. Oxytocin
   B. Terbutaline
   C. Magnesium sulfate
   D. Diphenhydramine

8. The fallopian tube is composed of three layers of tissues. _____ is NOT one of these layers.
   A. Mucosa
   B. Muscularis
   C. Serosa
   D. Fundus

9. The normal gestational period for an infant to develop in the uterus is how many weeks?
   A. 30
   B. 32
   C. 38
   D. 42

10. A pregnant woman's heart rate gradually increases during pregnancy by an average of how many beats/min by term?
    A. 15 to 20 beats/min
    B. 5 to 10 beats/min
    C. 20 to 25 beats/min
    D. 15 to 30 beats/min

Labeling

Label the following diagram with the correct terms.

1. Structures of the Pregnant Uterus

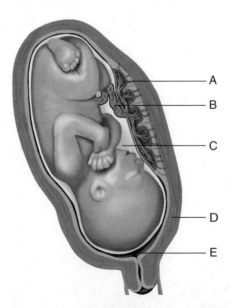

A. _____

B. _____

C. _____

D. _____

E. _____

Fill-in-the-Blank

Read each item carefully, and then complete the statement by filling in the missing word(s).

1. The inner lining of the uterus is called the _____.

2. The _____ _____ connects the placenta to the fetus.

3. A pregnant woman's heart rate gradually _____ during pregnancy.

4. _____ is the most serious of the hypertension disorders that occurs during pregnancy.

5. A/an _____ _____ occurs naturally, affecting about 1 in every 5 pregnancies.

6. _____ _____ is when the placenta is implanted low in the uterus and, as it grows, it partially or fully obscures the cervical canal.

7. _____ is a term used to describe a woman who has had two or more pregnancies.

8. The _____ _____ of labor begins as the baby's head enters the birth canal.

9. In a/an _____ presentation, the fetus lies crosswise in the uterus and may wave at the paramedic with one hand protruding from the vagina.

10. _____ _____ is a drug used in pregnancy as the principal management for eclampsia.

Identify

In the following case study, list the chief complaint, vital signs, and pertinent findings.

You are called to a private residence for a report of a pregnant patient who has vaginal bleeding. The patient is lying in bed, and when you ask what is wrong she tells you, "I am bleeding from my vagina." You see blood on the sheets. You and your partner start a quick assessment. You take the vital signs and your partner obtains a SAMPLE history. The patient is 35 years old and states she started to bleed about half an hour ago. Upon questioning, she tells you there is no pain, the blood was bright red, this is her third pregnancy, and she is in her eighth month. Both the previous pregnancies were full term and delivered by cesarean section. She states that she had strong contractions, but they have decreased. She feels weak and asks if she can have a drink of water. She has no allergies, is taking vitamin supplements per doctor's orders, has no significant past medical history, and had a light breakfast of toast and juice about 2 hours ago. Your partner reports the pulse to be 110 beats/min and thready, respirations are 24 breaths/min, blood pressure is 100/70 mm Hg, and she is pale and diaphoretic. The patient tells you that the blood pressure reading you just measured is lower than the pressure the doctor measured last week at her checkup appointment. You put the patient on 100% supplemental oxygen using a nonrebreathing mask, place a loose trauma pad over the vagina, prepare for immediate transport, start a large-bore IV in the ambulance, contact medical control to discuss the use of magnesium sulfate (some EMS systems may use in this case), and notify the hospital so they can be properly prepared upon your arrival. You arrive at the receiving facility in 15 minutes and are told to go immediately to the delivery room. Later that evening while delivering another patient to the same hospital, you are informed that the mother delivered, and although the baby's birth weight is low, both the mother and the baby are expected to be fine.

1. Chief complaint:

   _____

   _____

2. Vital signs:

   _____

   _____

3. Pertinent findings:

   _____

   _____

Complete the Patient Care Report (PCR)

Reread the incident scenario in the preceding Identify exercise and then complete the following PCR for the patient.

EMS Patient Care Report (PCR)					
Date:	**Incident No.:**	**Nature of Call:**		**Location:**	
Dispatched:	**En Route:**	**At Scene:**	**Transport:**	**At Hospital:**	**In Service:**
Patient Information					
Age:		**Allergies:**			
Sex:		**Medications:**			
Weight (in kg [lb]):		**Past Medical History:**			
		Chief Complaint:			
Vital Signs					
Time:	**BP:**	**Pulse:**	**Respirations:**		**SpO₂:**
Time:	**BP:**	**Pulse:**	**Respirations:**		**SpO₂:**
Time:	**BP:**	**Pulse:**	**Respirations:**		**SpO₂:**
EMS Treatment **(circle all that apply)**					
Oxygen @ _____ L/min via (circle one): NC NRM Bag-Mask Device		**Assisted Ventilation**	**Airway Adjunct**		**CPR**
Defibrillation	**Bleeding Control**	**Bandaging**	**Splinting**		**Other**
Narrative					

Ambulance Calls

The following case scenarios provide an opportunity to explore the concerns associated with patient management and paramedic care. Read each scenario, and then answer each question.

1. A 22-year-old woman calls for an ambulance because of vaginal bleeding. She states that she is "about 3 months pregnant" and that the bleeding started yesterday, when she thinks she passed some tissue. She has used about 10 sanitary napkins since then. On examination, her skin feels cool and wet. Her pulse is 120 beats/min and weak, and her blood pressure is 90/60 mm Hg.

   a. This woman is likely experiencing a/an _____ abortion.
      A. threatened
      B. inevitable
      C. incomplete
      D. missed
      E. septic

   b. List the steps in the prehospital management of this patient.

      (1) _____

      (2) _____

      (3) _____

      (4) _____

      (5) _____

      (6) _____

      (7) _____

2. A 32-year-old woman calls for an ambulance because she is "feeling poorly." She states that she is "about 6 months along" in a pregnancy. She has not had any prenatal care. She had some vaginal bleeding "early on," but it lasted only a few days and then stopped. Now, for several days, the patient has felt vaguely unwell. She has had a brownish vaginal discharge that smells rank, and "things are very quiet in there." On physical examination, the patient does not appear to be in any distress. Her pulse is 74 beats/min and regular, respirations are 18 breaths/min and unlabored, and blood pressure is 120/80 mm Hg. On abdominal examination, you can feel the uterine fundus just above the pelvic brim; it feels quite hard. You are not able to hear fetal heart tones, but the room is noisy, so you are not sure what to make of that finding.

   a. This woman is likely experiencing a/an _____ abortion.
      A. threatened
      B. inevitable
      C. incomplete
      D. missed
      E. septic

   b. Describe the prehospital management required for this patient.

      _____

      _____

3. A 20-year-old primigravida calls for an ambulance because of vaginal bleeding. She states that she is in her fourth month of pregnancy and has been fine up to now, but this morning she noticed some bleeding. She denies abdominal pain or cramping. On physical examination, there are no abnormal findings.

   a. This woman is likely experiencing a/an _____ abortion.
      A. threatened
      B. inevitable
      C. incomplete
      D. missed
      E. septic

b. Describe the prehospital management required for this patient.

_____

_____

4. You are called to a suburban home for a "sick girl." The patient is a 16-year-old girl with a high fever. She insists on giving you her history privately, without her parents in the room. After her parents exit, the girl tells you that she had gone that morning to "some hole in the wall" to have an abortion. A few hours after she got home, she started to feel sick, and she has been having a bad-smelling, bloody vaginal discharge ever since. On examination, she looks very ill. Her pulse is 120 beats/min and weak, respirations are 28 breaths/min and shallow, blood pressure is 80/60 mm Hg, and oral temperature is 40°C (104°F).
   a. This woman is likely experiencing a/an _____ abortion.
      A. threatened
      B. inevitable
      C. incomplete
      D. missed
      E. septic
   b. List the steps in the prehospital management of this patient.
      (1) _____
      (2) _____
      (3) _____
      (4) _____
      (5) _____
      (6) _____

5. You are called to the home of a weeping 26-year-old woman in the 15th week of pregnancy. "It's happening again," she sobs, "I just know it's happening again." She tells you that she has had three miscarriages in the past and that this morning she started having severe abdominal cramps and bleeding, "just like all the other times." She has used six sanitary napkins since the bleeding started about 3 hours ago. On physical examination, she is very distraught. Her pulse is 110 beats/min and regular, respirations are 24 breaths/min and unlabored, blood pressure is 110/70 mm Hg, and she is febrile. On palpating the abdomen, you can feel the uterine contractions.
   a. This woman is likely experiencing a/an _____ abortion.
      A. threatened
      B. inevitable
      C. incomplete
      D. missed
      E. septic
   b. List the steps in the prehospital management of this patient.
      (1) _____
      (2) _____
      (3) _____
      (4) _____
      (5) _____

6. You are called to the home of a 36-year-old grand multipara whose chief complaint is bleeding. She is in her 11th pregnancy and "due any day now." She states that the bleeding, a bright red blood, started a few hours ago without any warning. She has not had any cramps or other symptoms, and "the baby is still kicking like a soccer player." On physical examination, the woman looks a little pale and apprehensive. Her pulse is 124 beats/min and regular,

respirations are 28 breaths/min and unlabored, and blood pressure is 100/68 mm Hg; she is afebrile. On gentle palpation, you find the abdomen soft. The fundus is at the level of the xiphoid, and fetal heart tones are audible. The fetal heart rate is 140 beats/min.

a. List three possible causes of this woman's bleeding.

(1) _____

(2) _____

(3) _____

b. Of those three causes, which do you think is the most likely cause in her case?

_____

c. What signs led you to this diagnosis?

(1) _____

(2) _____

(3) _____

(4) _____

d. List the steps you will take in managing this patient.

(1) _____

(2) _____

(3) _____

(4) _____

(5) _____

(6) _____

(7) _____

7. You are called to see a 28-year-old woman in her 35th week of pregnancy after she had a "fainting spell." The patient's husband greets you at the door and tells you, "We were just sitting there talking—Agnes was lying in bed and I was sitting in the chair—and suddenly I look over and I see that she's out cold. Not sleeping, just out." The patient has meanwhile regained consciousness. She says she feels rather dizzy and has a slight headache, but otherwise feels all right. She denies vaginal bleeding. On physical examination, her pulse is 104 beats/min and regular, her respirations are 24 breaths/min and unlabored, and her blood pressure is 90/60 mm Hg. You have her roll onto her side and recheck her vitals a couple of minutes later; her pulse is now 88 beats/min and her blood pressure is 120/72 mm Hg. Her fundus is nearly at the level of the xiphoid, and fetal heart tones are present at a rate of 160 beats/min.

a. This woman is likely experiencing:

A. an inevitable abortion.

B. preeclampsia.

C. eclampsia.

D. abruptio placenta.

E. supine hypotensive syndrome.

b. List the steps in the prehospital care of this patient.

(1) _____

(2) _____

(3) _____

(4) _____

(5) _____

8. You are called to a downtown department store, where an obviously pregnant woman has fallen and twisted her ankle. You find her surrounded by a knot of agitated people, none of them more agitated than the store manager. As you are checking the woman's pedal pulses, you notice that *both* ankles are swollen, not just the one she injured. You decide you had better get a set of vital signs because you vaguely remember learning that vital signs should be measured in *every* patient, especially every *pregnant* patient. In this woman, you find the pulse is 110 beats/min and regular, respirations are 20 breaths/min and unlabored, and blood pressure is 150/90 mm Hg. As you are taking the radial pulse, you notice that the patient's hands seem puffy. It is too noisy in the store to even bother trying to listen for fetal heart tones, but the woman tells you that the baby is "kicking away."

a. This woman is likely experiencing:

    A. an inevitable abortion.

    B. preeclampsia.

    C. eclampsia.

    D. abruptio placenta.

    E. supine hypotensive syndrome.

b. List the steps in the prehospital care of this patient.

(1) _____

(2) _____

(3) _____

c. En route to the hospital, you find yourself locked in a traffic jam on the freeway. Meanwhile, your patient starts complaining of cramping abdominal pains. "I've never had a baby before," she says, "but I think these are labor pains." While you look helplessly at the line of cars stretching endlessly in front of and behind the ambulance, the woman's eyes suddenly roll back and she has a grand mal seizure. What steps will you take *now*?

(1) _____

(2) _____

(3) _____

(4) _____

(5) _____

9. A 26-year-old woman in her 30th week of pregnancy was the driver of a car that skidded off the road and plowed head-on into a tree. The woman was wearing a shoulder/lap seat belt. Sitting in the passenger seat of the same car was a woman in her 28th week of pregnancy (they were returning together from a natural childbirth class), also wearing a seat belt. En route to the call, you try to review in your mind the injuries you will need to look for in particular because you remember that pregnancy makes a woman more vulnerable to trauma.

a. List five anatomic or physiologic changes of pregnancy that affect a woman's susceptibility or response to trauma.

(1) _____

(2) _____

(3) _____

(4) _____

(5) _____

b. On reaching the scene of the accident, you find the driver of the car conscious, still sitting behind the wheel of the car. She complains of thirst. On physical examination, her skin is cool and moist. Her pulse is 120 beats/min and regular, respirations are 24 breaths/min and shallow, and blood pressure is 110/68 mm Hg. There is a steering wheel bruise on the upper abdomen. The abdomen is not particularly tender, and it is not rigid. The conditions are too noisy to try to hear fetal heart tones. List the steps in managing this patient.

(1) _____

(2) _____

(3) _____

(4) _____

(5) _____

(6) _____

(7) _____

(8) _____

c. The front-seat passenger is also fully conscious. She complains of "whiplash," but otherwise thinks she feels all right. "At least the baby's all right," she says. "I can feel him moving around." On physical examination, her skin is warm and moist. Her pulse is 100 beats/min and regular, respirations are 20 breaths/min and unlabored, and her blood pressure is 124/70 mm Hg. You do not find any evidence of injury. Can you conclude that there has been no injury to the fetus? Explain the reason for your answer.

_____

_____

_____

_____

10. For each of the following cases, indicate one of the following:

T There is time to transport the woman to the hospital for delivery.

D You will have to assist in emergency delivery in the field.

For each case that you decide requires prehospital delivery, indicate what, if any, complications you must anticipate.

_____ **a.** A 20-year-old nullipara (gravida 1, para 0) in her first pregnancy. She says her water broke about 6 hours ago. Now her contractions are about 2 minutes apart, and she feels a need to move her bowels. You are 20 minutes from the hospital. What, if any, complications may occur?

_____

_____

_____ **b.** A 32-year-old multipara (gravida 10, para 8) who has been in labor about 5 hours. Her contractions are 3 minutes apart. She says she thinks the baby's coming. You are 10 minutes from the hospital. What, if any, complications may occur?

_____

_____

_____ **c.** A 25-year-old nullipara (gravida 1, para 0) who has been in labor for 9 hours. Her contractions are 4 to 5 minutes apart. You are 20 minutes from the hospital. What, if any, complications may occur?

_____

_____

_____ **d.** A 30-year-old multipara (gravida 4, para 3) who has been in labor for 6 hours. She had two of her three children by cesarean section. Her contractions are 2 minutes apart, and she is crowning. You are 5 minutes from the hospital. What, if any, complications may occur?

_____

_____

_____ **e.** A 28-year-old nullipara (gravida 1, para 0) whose contractions started 24 hours ago. They do not come at regular intervals, and they have not gotten much more intense since they started. You are 25 minutes from the hospital. What, if any, complications may occur?

_____

_____

_____ **f.** A 24-year-old multipara (gravida 3, para 2) who announces, as you enter her apartment, "Hurry, the twins are coming any minute!" She says she has been in labor "quite a while," and you time her contractions as coming less than 2 minutes apart. You are 20 minutes from the hospital. What, if any, complications may occur?

_____

_____

11. You are assisting in the delivery of a baby in the lingerie section of a downtown department store.
a. The baby's head delivers spontaneously, and you notice that it is covered with a membrane. What should you do?

_____

_____

b. You deal with that problem successfully. The next thing you notice is that the umbilical cord is wound tightly around the baby's neck. What should you do about that?

_____

_____

c. List the steps in carrying out the remainder of the delivery (second and third stages).

(1) _____

(2) _____

(3) _____

(4) _____

(5) _____

(6) _____

(7) _____

(8) _____

(9) _____

12. During another one of your weekends off at the ski lodge, when you are cheerfully snowed in, one of the other guests arrives in the lounge and asks, "Does anyone here know anything about delivering a baby? My wife seems to be in labor." You shrivel up into a corner of your chair, hoping someone else will come forward, but there don't seem to be any obstetricians among the skiers. So, with a sigh, you stand up and follow the distraught husband to his room. There you find a woman in active labor, already crowning. Inspecting the presenting part, you note that it looks awfully smooth, and it has a sort of crack running down the middle.

a. What are you dealing with?

_____

_____

b. Describe how you will manage this case.

(1) _____

_____

(2) _____

_____

(3) _____

_____

(4) _____

_____

(5) _____

_____

(6) _____

_____

(7) _____

_____

13. The day after you get back to work, your very first call is another "possible OB." The patient is a 24-year-old woman in her first pregnancy whose labor started about 10 hours earlier. "This wasn't supposed to happen for another month and a half," she tells you. The contractions are now about 2 minutes apart. When you inspect her to see whether she is crowning, you see a short length of umbilical cord protruding from her vagina. Describe how you will manage this case.

a. _____

b. _____

c. _____

d. _____

e. _____

f. _____

g. _____

14. You are called to the home of a 30-year-old gravida 6, para 5, who has gone into labor. "It's twins," she announces as soon as you come in the door. "I'm carrying twins, and they're coming at any moment. I can feel it." And indeed, when you examine the woman, you find that she is crowning.

a. Describe the special measures necessary in this case.

(1) _____

(2) _____

b. After delivery of the placenta, the mother continues bleeding quite briskly from her vagina. Did this woman have any risk factors for postpartum hemorrhage? If so, what were they?

_____

_____

c. List three other risk factors for postpartum hemorrhage.

(1) _____

(2) _____

(3) _____

d. Describe how you will manage this situation.

(1) _____

(2) _____

(3) _____

(4) _____

(5) _____

(6) _____

True/False

If you believe the statement to be more true than false, write the letter "T" in the space provided. If you believe the statement to be more false than true, write the letter "F."

_____ **1.** If you are transporting a woman in labor, and she begins crowning when you are only a minute or two from the hospital, you should instruct her to cross her legs until you reach the emergency department.

_____ **2.** If the fetal heart rate is less than 120 beats/min, the fetus is in danger.

_____ **3.** A woman should be discouraged from sitting up or squatting for delivery of her baby because those positions are counter to natural physiology and increase the demand on the mother's energy.

_____ **4.** If the baby is coming fast, it is more important to control the delivery than it is to drape the mother with sterile towels.

_____ **5.** If the cut ends of the umbilical cord are oozing blood, you should unclamp them and reapply the clamps more tightly.

_____ **6.** If the placenta has not delivered within 20 minutes of the baby's delivery, you should exert gentle traction on the umbilical cord while you vigorously massage the uterus.

_____ **7.** With the exception of buttocks breech, all other abnormal presentations must be delivered in the hospital.

Short Answer

Complete this section with short written answers using the space provided.

By the second or third week of pregnancy, the placenta starts to develop inside the maternal uterus. The placenta is a specialized organ of pregnancy whose overall task is to nurture the developing fetus. List four specific functions that the placenta carries out for the fetus.

a. _____

b. _____

c. _____

d. _____

Fill-in-the-Table

Fill in the missing parts of the following tables.

1. Fill in the amount of time needed for the three stages of labor for a nullipara and for a multipara.

The Stages of Labor: Nullipara Versus Multipara		
Stages of Labor	**Nullipara**	**Multipara**
First stage	_____	_____
Second stage	_____	_____
Third stage	_____	_____

2. Fill in the missing information in distinguishing false labor from true labor.

False Labor Versus True Labor		
Parameter	**True Labor**	**False Labor**
Contractions	_____	Irregularly spaced
Interval between contractions	Gradually shortens	_____
Intensity of contractions	_____	Stays the same
Effects of analgesics	Do not abolish the pain	_____
Cervical changes	_____	No changes

Neonatal Care

Matching

Match each of the definitions in the left column to the appropriate term in the right column.

_____ **1.** Scale used to assess the status of a newborn 1 and 5 minutes after birth (ranges 0 to 10).

_____ **2.** Intermittent outward movements of the nostrils with each inspiration; indicates an increase in the work needed to breathe.

_____ **3.** Infant within the first month after birth.

_____ **4.** Conditions of severely deficient supply of oxygen to the body leading to end organ damage.

_____ **5.** A narrowing or blockage of the nasal airway by membranous or bony tissue; a congenital condition, meaning it is present at birth.

_____ **6.** A fissure or hole in the roof of the mouth that forms a communicating pathway between the mouth and nasal cavities.

_____ **7.** Low or poor muscle tone (floppy).

_____ **8.** The most common birth defect; associated with hypoxia in the newborn period requiring intervention during the first months of life.

_____ **9.** Lack of movement at the shoulder due to nerve injury resulting from the stretching of the cervical nerve roots (C5 and C6 most commonly) during delivery of the newborn's head during birth. The effect is usually transient, but can be permanent.

_____ **10.** An opening in the septum of the heart that closes after birth.

_____ **11.** Seizure activity that is bilateral, synchronous, and nonmigratory.

_____ **12.** Noises heard when an infant is having difficulty breathing; short inarticulate guttural sounds as effort is expended.

_____ **13.** Underdevelopment of the aorta, aortic valve, left ventricle, and mitral valve; this defect involves the entire left side of the heart.

_____ **14.** Marked hypertrophy and hyperplasia of the two (circular and longitudinal) muscular layers of the pylorus, resulting in the pylorus becoming thick and obstructing the end of the stomach.

_____ **15.** A congenital condition in which part of the bowel does not develop.

_____ **16.** An event where one part of the intestine folds into another part of the intestines, leading to a blockage.

_____ **17.** A paroxysmal alteration in neurologic function (ie, behavioral and/or autonomic functions).

_____ **18.** An injury of childbirth affecting the spinal nerves C7, C8, and T1 of the brachial plexus. It can be contrasted to Erb palsy, which affects C5 and C6.

A. Tetralogy of Fallot

B. Surfactant

C. Retinopathy of prematurity

D. Total anomalous pulmonary venous return (TAPER)

E. Seizure

F. Umbilical vein

G. Tricuspid atresia

H. Acrocyanosis

I. Asphyxia

J. Choanal atresia

K. Congenital heart disease (CHD)

L. Hypotonia

M. Generalized seizure

N. Erb palsy

O. Grunting

P. Hypoplastic left heart syndrome

Q. Cleft palate

R. Atrial septal defect

_____ 19. A dark green fecal material that accumulates in the fetal intestines and is discharged around the time of birth.

_____ 20. A situation in which the ductus arteriosus, which assists in fetal circulation, does not transition as it should after birth to become the ligamentum arteriosum; the result is that the connection between the pulmonary artery and the aorta remains, allowing oxygenated blood to move back into the heart rather than all of it moving out of the aorta and into the systemic circulation.

_____ 21. Delayed transition from fetal to neonatal circulation.

_____ 22. A rare congenital defect in which the four pulmonary veins do not connect to the left atrium; instead, the pulmonary veins connect to the right atrium, resulting in diminished oxygen and an increased load on the right ventricle.

_____ 23. Abnormal location of the placenta in the lower part of the uterus, near or over the cervix.

_____ 24. A term used to describe an infant delivered at less than 37 completed weeks.

_____ 25. Apnea caused by oxygen deprivation; usually corrected with stimulation, such as drying or slapping the newborn's feet. Primary apnea is typically preceded by an initial period of rapid breathing.

_____ 26. Elevated blood pressure in the pulmonary arteries from constriction; causes problems with the blood flow in the lungs, and makes the heart work harder.

_____ 27. A decrease in the amount of oxygen delivered to the extremities. The hands and feet turn blue because of narrowing of small arterioles toward the end of the arms and legs.

_____ 28. An excessive amount of amniotic fluid; may cause preterm labor.

_____ 29. Any pregnancy that lasts more than 42 weeks.

_____ 30. A disease of the eye that affects prematurely born infants; thought to be caused by disorganized growth of retinal blood vessels resulting in scarring and retinal detachment; can lead to blindness in serious cases.

_____ 31. A substance formed in the lungs that helps keep the small air sacs or alveoli from collapsing and sticking together; a low level in a premature infant contributes to respiratory distress syndrome.

_____ 32. A hole in the atrial septal wall that allows oxygenated and deoxygenated blood to mix; patients with this hole have a higher incidence of stroke.

_____ 33. A cardiac anomaly that consists of four defects: a ventricular septal defect, pulmonary stenosis, right ventricular hypertrophy, and an overriding aorta.

_____ 34. The absence of a tricuspid valve, which normally separates the right atrium and the right ventricle.

_____ 35. The blood vessel in the umbilical cord used to administer emergency medications.

S. Apgar score

T. Foramen ovale

U. Infantile hypertrophic pyloric stenosis

V. Klumpke paralysis

W. Neonate

X. Patent ductus arteriosus

Y. Pulmonary hypertension

Z. Primary apnea

AA. Nasal flaring

BB. Meconium

CC. Polyhydramnios

DD. Placenta previa

EE. Intestinal atresia

FF. Intussusception

GG. Persistent pulmonary hypertension

HH. Preterm

II. Post-term

Multiple Choice

Read each item carefully, and then select the best response.

1. As the baby is delivered, a rapid series of events must occur to enable the baby to breathe; this process is called fetal:
   A. transportation.
   B. transposition.
   C. transmission.
   D. transition.

2. An infant delivered at less than 37 weeks of gestation is considered:
   A. preterm.
   B. term.
   C. post-term.
   D. None of the above

3. The Apgar score, named after Dr. Virginia Apgar, who developed this measure in 1953, helps determine the need for and the effectiveness of resuscitation. The Apgar score is determined on the basis of the newborn's condition at _____ minutes after birth.
   A. 2 and 10
   B. 5 and 10
   C. 1 and 5
   D. 1 and 3

4. Fewer than 1% of deliveries involve bradycardia that requires treatment with chest compressions. The most common etiology for bradycardia in a neonate is:
   A. fetal alcohol syndrome.
   B. maternal drug abuse.
   C. hypoxia.
   D. prolapsed cord.

5. Infants do not normally pass stool before birth, but if they do and then inhale the meconium-stained amniotic fluid either in utero or at delivery, their airways may become plugged and hypoxia may ensue. This, in turn, can lead to:
   A. atelectasis.
   B. pneumonitis.
   C. pneumothorax.
   D. All of the above

6. A fluid bolus in an infant consists of _____ mL/kg of normal saline IV given over 5 to 10 minutes.
   A. 10
   B. 15
   C. 5
   D. 20

7. After ensuring the patency of the airway, as necessary, dry, stimulate, and reposition the newborn infant. Flick the soles of the baby's feet and:
   A. begin chest compressions.
   B. slap the baby's buttocks.
   C. aggressively rub the baby's back.
   D. assess the pulse and ventilations.

8. A diagnosis of diaphragmatic hernia is suspected clinically in a newborn with:
   A. apnea.
   B. heart sounds shifted to the left.
   C. scaphoid abdomen.
   D. All of the above

9. Primary apnea is often characterized by:
   A. hypoxia, rapid breathing, apnea, and bradycardia.
   B. hypoxia, apnea, and bradycardia.
   C. apnea and bradycardia.
   D. None of the above

10. The lungs of a premature infant are weak, so use:
   A. the maximum allowable ventilatory pressure to expand lung tissue.
   B. mechanical devices to administer positive-pressure ventilation (PPV).
   C. small puffs from your cheek with a pocket mask to ventilate.
   D. the minimum pressure necessary to move the chest when you are providing PPV.

Labeling

The following is the algorithm used for the resuscitation of a distressed newborn. Fill in the missing information in the boxes of the algorithm below.

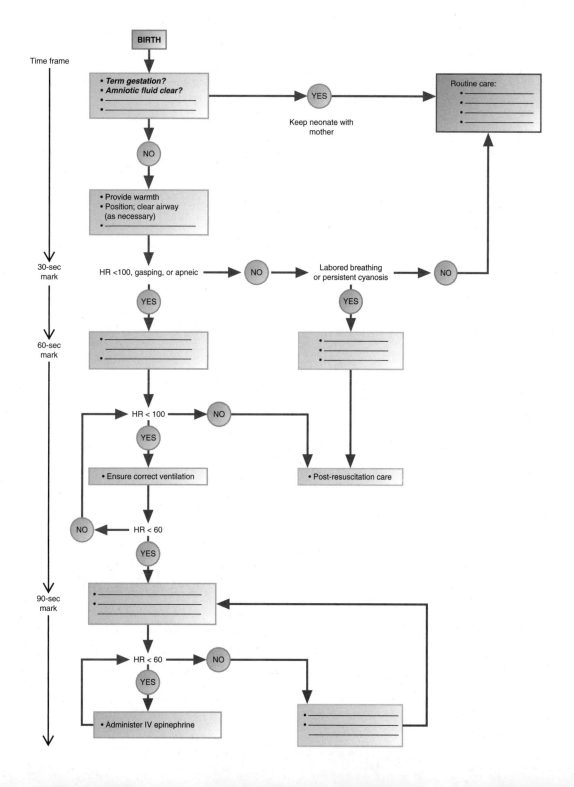

Fill-in-the-Blank

Read each item carefully, and then complete the statement by filling in the missing word(s).

1. During fetal _____, the newborn's lungs need to expand with air within seconds. As the baby's lungs become filled with air, the _____ pressure drops and blood begins to flow to the lungs, picking up _____.

2. An infant delivered at less than _____ completed weeks of gestation is considered preterm; an infant born at _____ to _____ weeks of gestation is described as term; and an infant born at more than _____ weeks of gestation is described as post-term.

3. If the _____ _____ comes out ahead of the baby, the _____ _____ through the umbilical cord may be cut off. In this case, relieving _____ on the cord can be lifesaving.

4. All newborns are _____ immediately after birth. If the newborn remains _____ and quickly becomes pink, ongoing observation and continued _____ with direct skin-to-skin contact with the mother should be maintained while on the way to a local hospital.

5. You should use caution when squeezing the ventilation bag to avoid inadvertently delivering too much volume, potentially resulting in a/an _____. After providing 30 seconds of adequate ventilation by PPV with 100% supplemental oxygen via a bag-mask device, check the infant's pulse. If the rate is less than 60 beats/min, begin chest _____. Effective chest compressions should result in _____ pulses.

6. Oral airways are _____ used for neonates, but they can be lifesaving if airway _____ leads to respiratory failure. Bilateral _____ _____ can be rapidly fatal, but usually responds to placement of an oral airway.

7. Gastric _____ using a/an _____ tube is indicated for prolonged bag-mask ventilation, if abdominal distention is impeding ventilation, or in the presence of a/an _____ hernia.

8. Jitteriness is often confused with a/an _____. Jitteriness is characteristically a disorder of the _____ and is rarely seen at a later age.

9. In many newborns with serious life-threatening _____, the core _____ may actually drop; these infants are at a higher risk for _____ and _____ acidosis.

10. Symptoms of _____ may include cyanosis, _____, irritability, poor sucking or _____, and hypothermia. These symptoms may also be associated with _____, tremors, twitching or _____, and coma.

11. Vomiting _____, occasionally _____ streaked, in the first few hours of life is not _____.

12. _____ should not be administered in the field. The infant may be dehydrated, however, and may need fluid _____. Dry mucous membranes, tachycardia, or a sunken _____ are clues that the patient needs hydration.

13. _____ in a newborn is often a result of _____ ventilation and usually responds to effective PPV. If _____ continues, there could be persistent bradycardia.

14. Because the average _____ _____ cannot provide the specially trained doctors and nurses or the specialized _____ needed for such care, it sometimes becomes necessary to transfer the critically ill infant to a/an _____ _____, where the infant may benefit from highly skilled personnel and sophisticated equipment.

15. The most common cause of acute diarrhea in children is _____ _____.

Identify

In the following case studies, identify the appropriate resuscitation steps.

1. You are dispatched to the scene of a full-term pregnancy. Mom is in active labor and the baby is crowning. You have appropriately decided to move her to your advanced life support unit with the heater turned on and have requested a second unit in the event of complications. To your surprise, you discover the presentation of a prolapsed cord.

   a. How do you treat this emergency?

      (1) _____

      (2) _____

      (3) _____

      (4) _____

(5) _____

(6) _____

(7) _____

2. After assisting in the delivery of a full-term newborn boy, you bulb suction the infant's mouth and nose, and dry and stimulate the baby.

    a. After 30 seconds, the baby is centrally cyanotic of the trunk and mucous membranes. What treatment would you now initiate?

        (1) _____

        (2) _____

    b. After 30 seconds of adequate ventilation by PPV with 100% supplemental oxygen via a bag-mask device, the infant's pulse rate is less than 60 beats/min. What treatment would you now initiate?

        (1) _____

        (2) _____

        (3) _____

Ambulance Calls

The following case scenarios provide an opportunity to explore the concerns associated with patient management and paramedic care. Read each scenario, and then answer each question.

    1. You are called to attend a 38-year-old woman who is in active labor at home. She has not had any prenatal care. She tells you that "this baby is a month late according to my calendar and is sure a long time in coming." Her contractions started about 10 hours ago and are now 2 minutes apart. Her "bag of waters" broke 10 minutes before your arrival, and you notice greenish stains on the bedclothes. The woman says she feels as if she has to move her bowels.

    a. Are there any indications that this may be a complicated delivery or that you may have problems with the baby after delivery? _____

        If so, list the risk factors in this delivery.

        (1) _____

        (2) _____

        (3) _____

        (4) _____

        (5) _____

    b. List four other risk factors, not present in this case, that indicate a high likelihood of complications during delivery or immediately thereafter.

        (1) _____

        (2) _____

        (3) _____

        (4) _____

    c. You immediately set up for delivery—and none too soon! You scarcely have your gloves on before the baby is crowning, and a moment later, the head is delivered. It is covered with a thick, greenish substance. List the steps you would take at this point.

        (1) _____

        (2) _____

d. What further steps should you take when the baby is fully delivered?

(1) _____

(2) _____

(3) _____

(4) _____

(5) _____

2. You are called to a movie theater where a 23-year-old woman who is gravida 4, para 3, went into active labor while watching *Return of the Spider Monster*. You find the patient in a cold, drafty ladies' room, sitting on the floor, panting. "I'm only in my seventh month," she says. "This can't be happening." As she makes that statement, the baby's head delivers spontaneously. You scramble to the floor to control the rest of the delivery. Within seconds, you find yourself holding a very red, wrinkled, little baby.

a. List in sequence the steps you would take at this point.

(1) _____

(2) _____

(3) _____

(4) _____

b. At what point would you clamp and cut the baby's umbilical cord? (Explain the reasoning behind your answer.)

_____

_____

_____

c. What steps can you take to prevent the baby from becoming hypothermic?

(1) _____

(2) _____

(3) _____

(4) _____

(5) _____

d. What other special measures should be taken in caring for this baby, besides ensuring that it stays warm?

(1) _____

(2) _____

(3) _____

3. You are called to a downtown apartment for a "sick woman." You arrive to find a teenage girl sitting on the toilet, having given birth only seconds before. The placenta has not yet delivered. You quickly remove the newborn from the toilet.

a. List the steps you would take at this point.

(1) _____

(2) _____

(3) _____

(4) _____

(5) _____

b. What would be the indications for starting artificial ventilation on this baby?

(1) _____

(2) _____

(3) _____

c. As it turns out, the baby has one of those indications, so you start artificial ventilation with a bag-mask device and 100% supplemental oxygen. After a minute, you reassess the baby and find that its heart rate is 84 beats/min. What should you do now?

_____

_____

_____

d. After another minute or so, you reassess again. The baby's heart rate is now 56 beats/min. What should you do now?

_____

_____

_____

_____

e. Under what circumstances should you administer epinephrine to this baby?

(1) _____

(2) _____

f. If ordered to give epinephrine, what dosage will you give? (The baby weighs 3 kg.)

_____

True/False

If you believe the statement to be more true than false, write the letter "T" in the space provided. If you believe the statement to be more false than true, write the letter "F."

_____ **1.** Prolonged oropharyngeal suctioning may stimulate the vagus nerve in a newborn and cause severe bradycardia.

_____ **2.** Even slight meconium staining of the amniotic fluid indicates a need to intubate the newborn immediately after delivery.

_____ **3.** If you are concerned that the fetal heart rate is too low at any point during labor, you should roll the mother onto her side and give her supplemental oxygen to breathe.

_____ **4.** The typical umbilical cord has two arteries and one vein.

_____ **5.** Infants may die of cold exposure at temperatures adults find comfortable.

_____ **6.** Most newborns who require resuscitation will need cardiopulmonary resuscitation (CPR).

_____ **7.** The umbilical vein is a large, thin-walled vessel usually found at the 4 o'clock position, as compared to the two thick-walled umbilical arteries usually found at 12 and 8 o'clock.

_____ **8.** Birth injuries account for 20% to 30% of all infant deaths.

_____ **9.** A normal number of stools per day for an infant is five to six, especially if the infant is breastfeeding, when infants often produce stool after every feeding.

_____ **10.** Meconium-stained amniotic fluid, which is present in 10% to 15% of deliveries, carries a high risk of morbidity.

Short Answer

Complete this section with short written answers using the space provided.

1. Neonatal IV access under the best circumstances can be difficult and stressful. An important alternative is catheterization of the umbilical vein. Detail the steps necessary to perform this task.

   a. _____

   b. _____

   c. _____

   d. _____

   e. _____

2. One of the most important skills that a paramedic must acquire and maintain is the ability to intubate neonates. Describe the steps necessary to properly intubate a neonate.

   a. _____

   b. _____

   c. _____

Fill-in-the-Table

Complete the following table by filling in the causes of neonatal seizures.

Causes of Neonatal Seizures
• Hypoxic ischemic encephalopathy
• _____
• _____
• _____
• _____
• _____
• Development defects
• Hypocalcemia
• _____
• _____
• _____

Problem Solving

Practice your calculation skills by solving the following math problems using the Apgar score.

You have just assisted in the delivery of a full-term newborn.

1. At 1 minute, the baby is centrally blue and pale, and the pulse rate is 100 beats/min; the baby grimaces, has some extremity flexion, and has a slow and irregular respiratory effort. The Apgar score is _____.

2. At 5 minutes, the baby is pink with blue extremities, has a pulse rate of 120 beats/min, is actively crying with a strong effort, and has active motion. The Apgar score is _____.

Skill Drills

Test your knowledge of skill drills by placing the following photos in the correct order. Number the first step with a "1," the second step with a "2," and so forth.

1. Intubating a Newborn

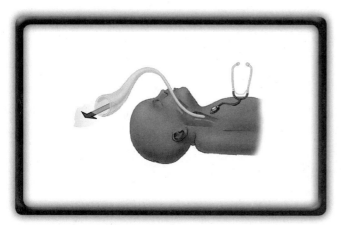

_____ Confirm placement. Observe chest rise, auscultate laterally and high on the chest, note mist in the endotracheal (ET) tube, note equal breath sounds on both sides, and observe for clinical improvement. Monitor ET_{CO_2} via waveform capnography and consider using pulse oximetry.

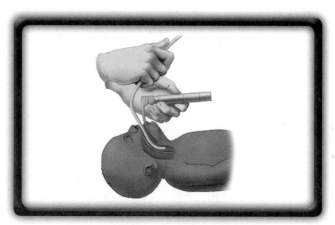

_____ Place the laryngoscope blade in the oropharynx. Visualize the vocal cords. Place the ET tube between the vocal cords until the black line on the ET tube is at the level of the cords.

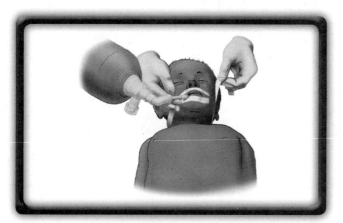

_____ Tape the ET tube in place. Monitor the newborn closely for complications.

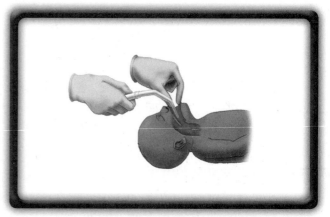

_____ Suction the oropharynx if there are copious secretions that prevent adequate ventilation. Avoid deep suctioning and provider bag-mask ventilation if bradycardia results.

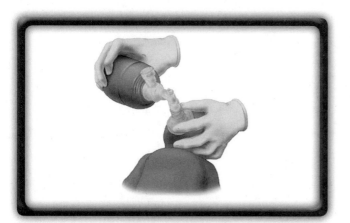

_____ Preoxygenate the newborn by bag-mask ventilation to an oxygen saturation greater than 95%.

Pediatric Emergencies

Matching

Part I

Match the following statements with the age group(s) most applicable to each. The statements may apply to more than one age group.

_____ **1.** Don't let your guard down regarding scene safety.

_____ **2.** They can be distracted by jangling keys and cooing noises.

_____ **3.** Give them appropriate choices and control whenever possible, and provide ongoing reassurance and encouragement.

_____ **4.** Assessment begins with observation of their interactions with the caregiver, vocalizations, and mobility, measured through the Pediatric Assessment Triangle.

_____ **5.** They should be examined on mother's lap if stable.

_____ **6.** They can provide at least some of the history.

_____ **7.** During the first months of life, they do not do very much other than eat, sleep, and cry.

_____ **8.** Tailor the physical exam to their age and developmental stage.

_____ **9.** Friends are key support figures, and this is a time of experimentation and risk-taking behaviors.

_____ **10.** Child abuse or maltreatment comes in many forms: physical abuse, sexual abuse, emotional abuse, and child neglect.

_____ **11.** They become much more analytic and capable of abstract thought. At this age, they can understand cause and effect.

_____ **12.** Use play and distraction techniques whenever possible.

_____ **13.** Make sure your hands and stethoscope are warm.

_____ **14.** Once secondary sexual characteristics have developed, they should be treated as an adult.

_____ **15.** They will be able to tell you what hurts and may have a story to share about the illness or injury.

A. Neonates and infants

B. Toddlers

C. Preschoolers

D. School-age children

E. Adolescents

Part II

Match the definitions in the left column with the most appropriate term in the right column.

_____ **1.** An unexpected, sudden episode of color change, tone change, or apnea that requires mouth-to-mouth resuscitation or vigorous stimulation.

_____ **2.** Inflammation of the epiglottis.

_____ **3.** A tube that is surgically placed directly into the patient's stomach through the skin in order to provide nutrition or medications.

_____ **4.** An invasive exudative bacterial infection of the soft tissues of the trachea.

A. Meckel diverticulum

B. Malrotation with volvulus

C. Intussusception

D. Inborn errors of metabolism

_____ **5.** A condition that occurs when there is a twisting of the bowel around its mesenteric attachments to the abdominal wall.

_____ **6.** A method of delivering oxygen by holding a face mask or similar device near an infant's or a child's face; used when a nonrebreathing mask is not tolerated.

_____ **7.** A catheter inserted into the vena cava to permit intermittent or continuous monitoring of central venous pressure and to facilitate obtaining blood samples for chemical analysis.

_____ **8.** Any improper or excessive action that injures or otherwise harms a child or infant; it includes physical abuse, sexual abuse, neglect, and emotional abuse.

_____ **9.** Seizures characterized by alteration of consciousness with or without complex focal motor activity.

_____ **10.** Inadequate production of cortisol and aldosterone by the adrenal gland.

_____ **11.** Abnormalities of the heart during development, many of which lead to cyanosis.

_____ **12.** A common disease of childhood due to upper airway obstruction and characterized by stridor, hoarseness, and a barking cough.

_____ **13.** A genetic disease that primarily affects the respiratory and digestive systems.

_____ **14.** A pathologic state in which there is an imperfect match between the areas of the lung being ventilated and the areas being perfused.

_____ **15.** A condition in which the heart becomes weakened and enlarged, making it less efficient and causing a negative impact to the pulmonary, hepatic, and other systems.

_____ **16.** The seizures characterized by manifestations that indicate involvement of both cerebral hemispheres.

_____ **17.** A short, low-pitched sound at the end of exhalation, present in children with moderate to severe hypoxia; reflects poor gas exchange because of fluid in the lower airways and air sacs.

_____ **18.** A bleeding disorder that is primarily hereditary, in which clotting does not occur or occurs insufficiently.

_____ **19.** The increased accumulation of cerebrospinal fluid within the ventricles of the brain.

_____ **20.** A condition in which the heart muscle is unusually thick, which means that the heart has to pump harder to get blood to leave.

_____ **21.** An agency that is the community legal organization responsible for protection, rehabilitation, and prevention of child maltreatment and neglect; it has the legal authority to temporarily remove children from homes if there is a reason to believe they are at risk for injury or neglect and to secure foster placement.

_____ **22.** An unusual form of seizure that occurs in association with a rapid increase in body temperature.

_____ **23.** Skin pulling between and around the ribs and clavicles during inhalation; a sign of respiratory distress.

_____ **24.** A brief, self-limiting, generalized seizure in a previously healthy child between ages 6 months and 6 years that is associated with the onset of or sudden increase in fever.

E. Hypopituitarism

F. Hypertrophic cardiomyopathy

G. Hydrocephalus

H. Hemophilia

I. Generalized seizures

J. Grunting

K. Gastrostomy tube

L. Dilated cardiomyopathy

M. Epiglottitis

N. Absence seizures

O. Acrocyanosis

P. Croup

Q. Cystic fibrosis

R. Apparent life-threatening event

S. Central venous catheter

T. Bronchopulmonary dysplasia

U. Bronchiolitis

V. Blow-by technique

W. Bacterial tracheitis

X. Congenital heart disease

_____ **25.** A condition in which the pituitary gland does not produce normal amounts of some or all of its hormones. It can be congenital; can be secondary to tumors, infection, or strokes; or can develop after trauma or radiation therapy.

_____ **26.** A group of congenital conditions that cause either accumulation of toxins or disorders of energy metabolism in the neonate. These conditions are characterized by an infant's failure to thrive and by vague signs such as poor feeding.

_____ **27.** A condition seen in children younger than 2 years, characterized by dyspnea and wheezing.

_____ **28.** A spectrum of lung conditions found in premature neonates who require long periods of high-concentration oxygen and ventilator support, ranging from mild reactive airways to debilitating chronic lung disease.

_____ **29.** Telescoping of the intestines into themselves.

_____ **30.** One of the most common congenital malformations of the small intestines, which presents with painless rectal bleeding.

_____ **31.** Inflammation of the myocardium.

_____ **32.** A stiff or painful neck; commonly associated with meningitis.

_____ **33.** Areas where cartilage is transformed through calcification into a new area of bone.

_____ **34.** The inadequate production or absence of the pituitary hormones, including adrenocorticotrophic hormone, cortisol, thyroxine, lueteinizing hormone, follicle-stimulating hormone, estrogen, testosterone, growth-hormone, and antidiuretic hormone.

_____ **35.** The type of seizures characterized by a brief lapse of attention in which the patient may stare and not respond; formerly known as petit mal seizures.

_____ **36.** Cyanosis of the extremities.

_____ **37.** An acute infectious disease characterized by catarrhal stage, followed by a paroxysmal cough that ends in a whooping inspiration; also called whooping cough.

_____ **38.** Characterized by small purplish, nonblanching spots on the skin.

_____ **39.** Inflammation of the meningeal coverings of the brain and spinal cord; usually caused by a virus or bacterium; the viral type is less severe than the bacterial; the bacterial type can result in brain damage, hearing loss, learning disability, or death.

_____ **40.** Pertaining to bruising of the skin.

_____ **41.** Hypertrophy of the pyloric sphincter of the stomach; ultimately leads to intestinal obstruction, often in infants.

_____ **42.** A virus that affects the upper and lower respiratory tracts, but disease, namely pneumonia and bronchiolitis, is more prevalent in the lower respiratory tract.

_____ **43.** The abrupt and unexplained death of an apparently healthy child younger than 1 year.

_____ **44.** A condition in which the skin slowly retracts after being pinched and pulled away slightly from the body; a sign of dehydration.

_____ **45.** A reduction in the number of platelets in the blood.

Y. Congenital adrenal hyperplasia

Z. Complex partial seizures

AA. Complex febrile seizures

BB. Child protective services (CPS)

CC. Child abuse

DD. Meningitis

EE. Nuchal rigidity

FF. Panhypopituitarism

GG. Ossification centers

HH. Myocarditis

II. Simple febrile seizures

JJ. Sudden infant death syndrome (SIDS)

KK. Partial seizures

LL. Retractions

MM. Respiratory syncytial virus

NN. Pyloric stenosis

OO. Purpuric

PP. Petechial

QQ. Pertussis

RR. Pediatric Assessment Triangle (PAT)

SS. Thrombocytopenia

_____ **46.** Seizures that feature rhythmic back-and-forth motion of an extremity and body stiffness.

_____ **47.** An abnormal position to keep the airway open; involves leaning forward onto two arms stretched forward.

_____ **48.** Narrowing of the diameter of the blood vessels.

_____ **49.** A surgically inserted tube draining cerebrospinal fluid from the cerebral ventricles into a body cavity, often the peritoneal cavity or the right atrium.

_____ **50.** Seizures that involve only one part of the brain.

_____ **51.** An assessment tool that allows rapid formation of a general impression of the type and level of illness or injury in an infant or child without touching him or her; consists of assessing appearance, work of breathing, and circulation to the skin.

_____ **52.** The most common heritable disorder of coagulation. Its presentation can mimic hemophilia A.

TT. Tenting

UU. Tonic-clonic seizures

VV. Tripoding

WW. Vasoconstriction

XX. Von Willebrand disease

YY. Ventricular shunt

ZZ. Ventilation-perfusion mismatch

Multiple Choice

Read each item carefully, and then select the best response.

1. Although child abuse can generate a big emotional response from the emergency medical services (EMS) crew, remember that your primary focus should be:
  A. documenting the suspected abuse for further prosecution.
  B. separating the patient from the suspected abuser.
  C. the trauma assessment, management, and ensuring the safety of the child.
  D. properly securing the crime scene for investigators.

2. A child's developmental stage affects his or her response to injury. As a result:
  A. being strapped to a backboard may be considered fun.
  B. a paramedic could turn an activity as serious as immobilizing a child's spine on a backboard into a "game."
  C. being immobilized on a backboard may be terrifying and anxiety provoking.
  D. children should never be strapped or immobilized on a backboard.

3. All of the following injury patterns may be more common in pediatric patients, EXCEPT:
  A. blunt force trauma.
  B. falls.
  C. skull fractures.
  D. joint dislocations.

4. PAT is an acronym:
  A. developed from a common children's book to help soothe a sick or injured child.
  B. developed to remember the proper methods of conducting a hands-on assessment of a child.
  C. that stands for *palpating a tender* abdomen.
  D. that stands for the *Pediatric Assessment Triangle*.

5. One of the best ways to assess a pediatric patient's oxygenation status is to:
  A. evaluate the child's respiratory rate.
  B. evaluate the work of breathing.
  C. auscultate the lung.
  D. obtain the pulse.

6. Abnormal positioning and retractions are physical signs of increased work of breathing that can easily be assessed without touching the patient. All of the following are signs of increased work of breathing, EXCEPT:
  A. the sniffing position.
  B. tripoding
  C. retractions.
  D. All of the above are signs of increased work of breathing.

7. A child with an ominous mechanism of injury includes a/an:
   A. unstable or compromised airway from a motor vehicle crash.
   B. isolated extremity fracture from a fall.
   C. conscious, alert child who crashed his or her bicycle while wearing a helmet that cracked.
   D. skateboarder with an obvious fractured wrist.

8. Paramedics may encounter children with special health care needs. These may include:
   A. physical, developmental, and learning disabilities.
   B. tracheostomy tubes and artificial ventilators.
   C. gastrostomy tubes (G-tubes).
   D. All of the above

9. The federally funded program that was created more than 20 years ago in an effort to reduce child disability and death caused by severe illness and injury is known as:
   A. the Department of Transportation (DOT) curriculum.
   B. NHYSA.
   C. EMSC.
   D. TSA.

10. Inserting an oral airway in a child is similar to inserting an airway in an adult, EXCEPT:
    A. you use a different method for determining the proper size.
    B. it should not be used in the presence of ingested caustics.
    C. it is inserted in an inverted manner, and then flipped over into the correct position.
    D. you must take care to avoid injuring the hard palate.

11. Which type of child abuse has the greatest incidence?
    A. Physical
    B. Sexual
    C. Neglect
    D. Psychological

12. Which of the following is NOT a risk factor for child abuse?
    A. Child with disability
    B. Disorganized family structure
    C. Parent was abused
    D. Financial stability

13. You are called to the scene of a 4-year-old child injured inside a residence. You enter the house and find the child and a parent. You assess the child and become suspicious about the injury. Your partner interviews the parent. Which of the following is a red flag for child abuse by a caregiver?
    A. The caregiver overreacts to the child's condition.
    B. The caregiver seems forthcoming about what happened.
    C. The caregiver is enraged about care being provided by EMS.
    D. The caregiver seems concerned.

14. You have completed a call where there is a high suspicion of child abuse. When you write the patient care report, what type of information is helpful to include for child protective services when they review the report?
    A. Subjective
    B. Speculative
    C. Conjecture
    D. Objective

15. You have been called to a residence where there is a 5-year-old boy who reportedly fell while running and hit his forehead. He has a bruise and an abrasion. While you do an assessment to determine if there are any additional injuries, you notice the boy has numerous bruises of different colors. Which location of bruises on the child would make you MOST suspicious of child abuse?
    A. Knees
    B. Arms
    C. Lower legs
    D. Back

Labeling

On the following diagram, indicate the technique for measuring the distance to insert an NG or OG tube.

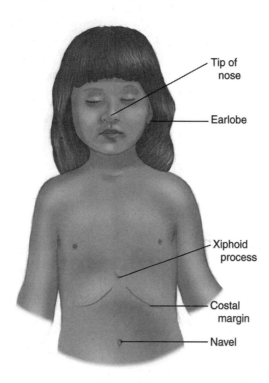

- Tip of nose
- Earlobe
- Xiphoid process
- Costal margin
- Navel

Fill-in-the-Blank

Read each item carefully, and then complete the statement by filling in the missing word(s).

1. A nasopharyngeal (nasal) airway is usually well _____ and is not as likely as the _____ airway to cause vomiting.

2. The _____ - _____ _____ can be used for a child with mild respiratory distress who will not tolerate a facial mask.

3. Bag-mask ventilation is _____ the first step in assisted _____, and it represents definitive _____ _____ for many patients.

4. Potential complications of pediatric intubation include damage to _____ and oral structures, _____ of gastric contents, and incorrect _____.

5. Because stimulation of the _____ nervous system and _____ can occur during intubation, the paramedic should apply a/an _____ monitor and a/an _____ _____.

6. The types of shock you may encounter are the same in adults and children: _____, _____, and _____.

7. A pediatric patient with _____ shock will often appear listless or lethargic and may have compensatory _____. The child may appear _____, _____, or _____.

8. Further assessment of a pediatric patient in shock may identify signs of dehydration such as: _____ _____, dry _____ _____, poor skin _____, or _____ capillary refill with cool extremities.

9. Complications associated with intraosseous infusion may include _____ _____, growth plate _____, and bone inflammation caused by _____.

10. Cardiogenic shock is _____ in the pediatric population but may be present in children with underlying _____ heart disease or _____ disturbances.

Identify

In the following case studies, list the chief complaint, vital signs, and pertinent negatives.

1. It's about 3:30 AM and you are dispatched priority one for a 2-year-old with difficulty breathing. As you approach the residence, you notice a family member frantically trying to wave you down. You think to yourself that this doesn't look good. You grab your pediatric gear and cardiac monitor and then quickly enter the house. Once inside, you are told that the girl woke the whole household with this terrible barky cough. She is sitting on her mother's lap. The mother states that the child has been irritable for several days with symptoms consistent with an upper respiratory infection: coughing, runny nose, and sneezing. The child has audible stridor, a "seal-like" barking cough, and is conscious and alert. She has an oxygen saturation of 95% on ambient room air. She also has a normal capillary refill. You attempt to take her blood pressure and she begins to get agitated and cling to her mother.

   a. Chief complaint:

   _____

   _____

   b. Vital signs:

   _____

   _____

   c. Pertinent negatives:

   _____

   _____

2. Today is your turn on medivac duty. Medcom dispatches you to intercept a ground ambulance about 25 minutes to the west. As you lift off, you discover that this patient is only 1 week old and was the survivor of a motor vehicle crash involving a fatality. You and your crew arrive on the scene several minutes before the ambulance arrives. The state police are on scene securing the landing zone. They advise you that the patient's mother was holding the baby and both were unrestrained and ejected on impact. The mother suffered fatal injuries. You are thinking the worst and begin to set up your pediatric resuscitation equipment. When the ambulance arrives, you are quickly handed the neonatal trauma patient. The baby has oxygen in place, appears to be wrapped well, and is thoroughly secured with a vacuum splint conforming to his tiny body. The baby appears to be sleeping peacefully and has only a small forehead abrasion. You begin the primary assessment as you begin your flight to the trauma center. The assessment indicates an infant with no visible distress. The baby has an intact airway and is breathing at 30 breaths/min, he has an apical pulse rate at 150 beats/min, his skin color appears normal, and the skin is warm and dry. Lung sounds are clear and equal. Oxygen saturation is 96%. Remarkably, there doesn't appear to be any noticeable external bleeding. In fact, the assessment is totally unremarkable. After a "not so routine" mechanism of injury, the infant is safely delivered to the regional trauma center.

   a. Chief complaint:

   _____

   _____

b. Vital signs:

_____

_____

c. Pertinent negatives:

_____

_____

3. While working in the ALS "fly car," you are dispatched priority one on a mutual assist with a local BLS ambulance. They request that you meet them while they begin the response to the local pediatric emergency department. They state that they are treating a 2½-year-old girl in "status." You arrange a safe place to meet the ambulance and secure your vehicle. As you await their arrival, you prepare your pediatric ALS equipment and begin reviewing protocols. Once on the ambulance, you notice the small patient secured to the cot. Mom is in the front passenger's seat. The child has recently been sick with an upper respiratory infection and low-grade fever. Nothing like this has ever happened before. The child suddenly appeared to go into convulsions after being given oral pediatric acetaminophen for an elevation in her fever. The BLS crew states that the patient was actively seizing on their arrival. They initiated high-flow supplemental oxygen with a pediatric nonrebreathing face mask, requested ALS, and initiated transport. On your arrival, the patient is postictal, with the following vital signs: ashen skin that is warm and dry, and a rectal temperature of 100.3°F. The patient responds to pain. Her oxygen saturation is 98%. Pupils are sluggish but equal. The patient has equal bilateral breath sounds. The remainder of the exam is unremarkable. The patient's mother denies any other medications, history, or allergies to medications. She further denies any recent injury or trauma to the child.

a. Chief complaint:

_____

_____

b. Vital signs:

_____

_____

c. Pertinent negatives:

_____

_____

Complete the Patient Care Report (PCR)

Reread the first incident scenario in the preceding Identify exercises and then complete the following PCR for the patient.

EMS Patient Care Report (PCR)					
Date:	Incident No.:	Nature of Call:		Location:	
Dispatched:	En Route:	At Scene:	Transport:	At Hospital:	In Service:
Patient Information					
Age: Sex: Weight (in kg [lb]):			Allergies: Medications: Past Medical History: Chief Complaint:		
Vital Signs					
Time:	BP:	Pulse:	Respirations:		SpO$_2$:
Time:	BP:	Pulse:	Respirations:		SpO$_2$:
Time:	BP:	Pulse:	Respirations:		SpO$_2$:
EMS Treatment (circle all that apply)					
Oxygen @ _____ L/min via (circle one): NC NRM Bag-Mask Device		Assisted Ventilation	Airway Adjunct		CPR
Defibrillation	Bleeding Control	Bandaging	Splinting		Other
Narrative					

Ambulance Calls

The following case scenarios provide an opportunity to explore the concerns associated with patient management and paramedic care. Read each scenario, and then answer each question.

1. You are called to the scene of a collision in which a 6-year-old child was struck by a car as he darted into the street in front of his home. The child is lying in the street surrounded by a small group of people, including his very distraught parents.

   a. Given the mechanism of injury, list at least three injuries you must look for in particular in this child.

      (1) _____

      (2) _____

      (3) _____

   b. As you are kneeling beside the injured child, carefully going through the steps of the primary assessment, the child's father (who looks like a pro wrestler) charges over and starts shouting at you: "What the h—do you think you're doing with my kid? Stop messing around and take him to a *hospital*. Can't you see he's hurt bad? He's going to die here while you dingbats muck about." [The father's actual comments are less polite but cannot be quoted verbatim in a workbook.]

     (1) What are your feelings at this moment?

     _____

     _____

     (2) How will you deal with this situation?

       (a) _____

       (b) _____

       (c) _____

       (d) _____

   c. On checking the child's vital signs, you find the following: pulse is 120 beats/min and regular; respirations are 24 breaths/min and unlabored; blood pressure is 90/60 mm Hg. Which of the following conclusions can be drawn from those vital signs?

     (1) The child is going into shock.

     (2) The child has increasing intracranial pressure.

     (3) The vital signs are normal for a child of that age.

     (4) There is probably significant intrathoracic injury.

     (5) There is probably significant intra-abdominal bleeding.

2. You are called around 1:00 AM for a child who "can't breathe." A haggard father greets you at the door and tells you that his 2-year-old Tammy has had "a little cold" for a couple of days but otherwise seemed fine. ("It didn't slow her down a bit.") Tonight, however, she began coughing, and the cough kept getting worse. Indeed, even as you are walking toward the child's room, you can hear a loud barking noise. On reaching Tammy's room, you see a very agitated 2-year-old struggling in her mother's lap. Her nostrils are flaring with each inhalation, and there are retractions of her neck muscles. Her lips are bluish. She flails and has a fit of dry coughing as you start to come near. Eventually, you manage to measure a pulse of 160 beats/min and a respiratory rate of 52 breaths/min. When you try to auscultate the child's chest, however, she grabs your stethoscope and yanks it out of your ears.

   a. The vital signs are _____ (normal or abnormal?) for a child of this age.

   b. The most likely diagnosis is _____.

   c. What steps will you take in managing this child?

      (1) _____

      (2) _____

      (3) _____

      (4) _____

      (5) _____

3. You are called for a 4-month-old infant in respiratory distress. His mother says that he's been "off his feed" for a couple of days and has been sneezing a lot. On examination, you notice that the baby seems to be breathing like a rabbit. The pulse is 180 beats/min, respirations are 60 breaths/min, and blood pressure is 90/60 mm Hg. There is diffuse wheezing throughout the chest.

   a. The vital signs are _____ (normal or abnormal?) for a child of this age.

   b. The most likely diagnosis is _____.

   c. What steps will you take in managing this child?

      (1) _____

      (2) _____

      (3) _____

      (4) _____

      (5) _____

      (6) _____

4. You are called for a 2½-year-old having difficulty breathing. The mother says that she left little Bobby playing quietly in his room, and when she returned half an hour later, she found him in severe respiratory distress. She thinks he's had a slight respiratory infection, nothing serious. "You know, it's just one runny nose after another all winter with them. Each one gives it to the others, and I've got five little ones—so I can't always keep track of who has a runny nose."

You find Bobby in severe respiratory distress. He makes high-pitched squeaks when he tries to inhale, and his eyes look like they are popping out of his head. His lips are blue. You place the back of your hand on his forehead and note that the skin does not feel abnormally warm.

   a. The most likely diagnosis is _____.

   b. What steps will you take in managing this child?

      (1) _____
         _____

      (2) _____
         _____

      (3) _____
         _____

      (4) _____
         _____

      (5) _____
         _____

      (6) _____
         _____

      (7) _____
         _____

c. As you are in the middle of treating this child's respiratory problem, he becomes pulseless and apneic. What is the depth and rate of chest compressions that you must perform?

_____

_____

d. Where will you check for a pulse?

_____

_____

e. You find that the pulse is absent. What is the correct compression point for external chest compressions?

_____

_____

f. The monitor shows ventricular fibrillation. Assuming that the child weighs 12 kg, what is the defibrillation dosage? _____ joules

g. Which drugs may be given by intraosseous (IO) infusion if you can't get an IV line established right away?

_____

_____

5. You are called to see a 4-year-old who is "very sick." His mother says that he was fine until a few hours ago when he began complaining of a sore throat. Since then, he would not eat or drink anything, and he is very feverish. You find the child sitting very still, bolt upright in bed, with his chin thrust forward. He does not reply to your questions, but only nods or shakes his head slightly. Saliva is dribbling out of the corners of his mouth. His skin feels very hot. His pulse is 140 beats/min, respirations are 40 breaths/min and quiet, blood pressure is 90/60 mm Hg. The chest is clear.

    a. The vital signs are _____ (normal or abnormal?) for a child of this age.

    b. The most likely diagnosis is _____.

    c. What steps will you take in managing this child?

        (1) _____

        (2) _____

        (3) _____

        (4) _____

        (5) _____

    d. What is the special danger threatening this child?

_____

_____

6. You are called to a field about 6 miles outside of town where a 6-year-old child in the first-grade nature study class is having difficulty breathing. The teacher says that she noticed him lagging behind the others several times during the morning, and finally she found him sitting by himself under a tree, struggling to breathe. You find the child still sitting under the tree, but apparently dozing. It is difficult to wake him, and when he does open his eyes, he just stares at you blankly. When you ask him whether he has taken any medicine today, he just shakes his head and seems to doze again.

On examination, the child's pulse is 160 beats/min and somewhat weak, respirations are 52 breaths/min and shallow, and blood pressure is 90/60 mm Hg on exhalation and 50 systolic during inhalation. The lips look bluish. There is retraction of the neck muscles. The chest does not seem to move with respiration, and it sounds like an empty barrel when you tap on it. You can hardly hear any breath sounds at all. On the child's wrist is a medical identification bracelet inscribed "asthmatic."

a. List five signs that suggest this child is having a very serious asthmatic attack.

(1) _____

(2) _____

(3) _____

(4) _____

(5) _____

b. List the steps you would take in managing this case.

(1) _____

(2) _____

(3) _____

(4) _____

(5) _____

(6) _____

7. The very same evening, you are called to see a child who is "short of breath." The child is a known asthmatic.

a. List five questions you would ask the child and his parents in taking the history.

(1) _____

(2) _____

(3) _____

(4) _____

(5) _____

b. Your protocol calls for administering albuterol for an acute asthmatic attack.

(1) What are the relevant *contraindications* to albuterol?

_____

_____

(2) What are the possible adverse *side effects* of albuterol?

_____

_____

(3) What is the correct *dosage*, and how is the drug administered?

_____

_____

8. You are called to a downtown apartment for a "very sick baby." A frightened-looking young mother greets you at the door and hurries you into the bedroom, where a baby is lying very still in its crib. You observe at once that the baby's color is grayish and that it is not breathing. When you touch the baby to open the airway, you can feel that the skin is cold. Describe what you will do from this point on.

_____

_____

_____

_____

9. You are called for a 2-year-old child who is "having a fit." En route to the call, you review in your mind the possible causes of seizures in children.

   A. List five causes of seizures in children.

     (1) _____

     (2) _____

     (3) _____

     (4) _____

     (5) _____

   b. List five questions you should ask in taking the child's history.

     (1) _____

     (2) _____

     (3) _____

     (4) _____

     (5) _____

   c. List five things you would look for in particular in examining the child.

     (1) _____

     (2) _____

     (3) _____

     (4) _____

     (5) _____

   d. You learn that the child has never had a seizure before. On examining him, you find that he is no longer seizing but is still somewhat drowsy. His skin is very hot, so you take an axillary temperature and get a reading of 39°C (102.2°F). The pupils are equal and reactive. The neck is supple. The chest is clear. Describe how you would manage this case.

     (1) _____

     (2) _____

10. You are summoned to a local high school where a 14-year-old girl is having a seizure. The school nurse tells you that the child has never had a seizure in school before. This seizure came on while the girl was in the auditorium watching a movie. The seizure lasted about 5 minutes. One of the teachers then carried the girl to the nurse's office. The nurse was in the middle of trying to contact the girl's mother when the child had another grand mal seizure. Now, as you are speaking with the nurse, you witness a third grand mal seizure that lasts about 6 minutes.

   a. List the steps in treating this patient.

     (1) _____

     (2) _____

     (3) _____

     (4) _____

     (5) _____

     (6) _____

     (7) _____

b. What drug is used in the emergency treatment of repeated seizures, and what are its contraindications?

_____

_____

c. What are the possible adverse side effects?

_____

_____

11. You are called to attend to a 10-month-old baby who sustained burns to the foot when he "stepped on a cigarette." Something about the story sounds "fishy" to you, and you find yourself on the alert for evidence that the child has been abused.

a. What's "fishy" about the story?

_____

_____

b. List 10 possible clues that might substantiate your suspicion that a child has been abused.

(1) _____

(2) _____

(3) _____

(4) _____

(5) _____

(6) _____

(7) _____

(8) _____

(9) _____

(10) _____

c. By the time you finish examining the child, you are privately convinced that the baby was deliberately burned and that, furthermore, he has been burned and beaten in the past. How should you manage this case?

(1) _____

(2) _____

(3) _____

(4) _____

(5) _____

d. Suppose the child's parent refuses to allow the child to be transported to the hospital? What should you do then?

(1) _____

(2) _____

(3) _____

12. You are called to treat an 18-month-old baby who fell off a second-floor balcony to the ground 5 meters (about 15 feet) below. On examination, you find the baby conscious but drowsy. Vital signs are a pulse of 80 beats/min and regular, respirations are 16 breaths/min, and blood pressure is 100/70 mm Hg. There is a bruise on the left forehead.

The pupils are equal and reactive to light. The point of maximal impulse (PMI) is in the midclavicular line. Breath sounds are equal bilaterally. The abdomen does not appear distended. The baby is moving all extremities. List the steps in the prehospital management of this case.

a. _____

b. _____

c. _____

d. _____

e. _____

f. _____

13. You are called to the scene of a motor vehicle collision on the interstate highway in which a car jumped the median divider and plowed head-on into an oncoming vehicle. Among the injured are two children, both backseat passengers in the vehicle that was hit. Both children have been removed from the wrecked car by well-meaning bystanders.

a. The first child is about 4 years old and is lying listlessly on the ground. His skin feels cool. His pulse is 160 beats/min and difficult to palpate, his respirations are 48 breaths/min, and his blood pressure is 90/60 mm Hg on both inhalation and exhalation. You find no signs of head injury. The pupils are equal and reactive. The neck veins are not distended. The PMI is in the midclavicular line. There are no bruises on the chest. Breath sounds are impossible to hear due to all the noise. There is a seat belt mark across the anterior abdomen, which looks somewhat distended. Capillary refill takes 3 seconds. The right arm appears broken. List the steps in the prehospital management of this case.

(1) _____

(2) _____

(3) _____

(4) _____

(5) _____

(6) _____

(7) _____

b. The second child looks to be about 2 years old and is gasping for breath. The upper airway seems clear, but not much air is moving in and out of the chest. The lips are bluish. The trachea seems to be slanting to the left. It is impossible to auscultate breath sounds due to all the noise at the scene. The PMI is in the anterior axillary line. The abdomen looks slightly distended but not bruised. List the steps in the prehospital management of this case.

(1) _____

(2) _____

(3) _____

(4) _____

(5) _____

(6) _____

(7) _____

(8) _____

14. You are called to the scene of a smoky house fire just as one of the fire fighters is emerging from the building carrying a baby. "He was in the thick of it," the fire fighter tells you. "Out cold when I found him." The baby still seems very drowsy.

   a. Should this infant be intubated? Why or why not?

   _____

   _____

   b. List five indications for the immediate intubation of an infant or small child who has been in a fire.

   (1) _____

   (2) _____

   (3) _____

   (4) _____

   (5) _____

15. You are all settled in to watch a football game on your day off when a neighbor comes running in, carrying her lethargic 2-year-old. "Johnny's choking on peanuts!" she wails.

   "Did what?" you ask, not really wanting to know the answer.

   "He's choking. Help, do something, he's turning blue!"

   a. What is the recommended method to relieve a severe airway obstruction in a conscious child?

   _____

   _____

   b. List the steps you would take to achieve this.

   (1) _____

   _____

   (2) _____

   _____

   (3) _____

   _____

   (4) _____

   _____

   (5) _____

   _____

   (6) _____

   _____

True/False

If you believe the statement to be more true than false, write the letter "T" in the space provided. If you believe the statement to be more false than true, write the letter "F."

_____ **1.** A child who is seriously ill or injured will always be agitated and showing clear signs of distress.

_____ **2.** A sunken anterior fontanelle in an infant suggests meningitis or a head injury.

_____ **3.** Neonates and infants can easily communicate their needs when they are in pain.

_____ **4.** Grunting is a sign of respiratory distress in infants.

_____ **5.** An infant falling from a height is most likely to sustain injury to the head.

_____ **6.** The method of choice for opening the airway of a small child who has been struck by a car is the head tilt–chin lift method.

_____ **7.** To insert an oropharyngeal airway in a small child, introduce the airway tip-upward, and then rotate it 180° and slide it into place.

_____ **8.** Hypotension is an early response to blood loss in infants and small children.

_____ **9.** The first step in assembling the equipment for pediatric intubation is to check the cuff on the endotracheal tube you have selected.

_____ **10.** A straight blade is preferred for pediatric intubation.

_____ **11.** In intubating infants, the laryngoscope blade is slipped beneath the epiglottis, to lift it up, rather than into the vallecula.

_____ **12.** The narrowest point in an infant's airway is the opening between the vocal cords.

_____ **13.** Initial burn management begins with removal of burning clothing and support of the ABCs.

_____ **14.** Pediatric trauma victims must have a rigid cervical collar in place prior to transport.

_____ **15.** Sinus tachycardia, a pulse rate higher than normal for age, is common in children.

Short Answer

Complete this section with short written answers using the space provided.

1. List six signs suggestive of hypovolemic shock in infants and small children.

   a. _____

   b. _____

   c. _____

   d. _____

   e. _____

   f. _____

2. Upon completing the primary assessment of any seriously injured person, of any age, the paramedic must make a decision whether to transport at once or to proceed to the secondary assessment. List 10 indications for immediate transport ("load-and-go") of injured infants and children.

   a. _____

   b. _____

   c. _____

   d. _____

   e. _____

   f. _____

   g. _____

   h. _____

   i. _____

   j. _____

Fill-in-the-Table

Fill in the missing parts of the following tables.

1. In examining an injured infant or child, you must know exactly what you are looking for so that each second spent on the physical exam is well invested. In the following table, indicate what in particular you would be looking for as you examine each part of the body areas mentioned.

Pediatric Physical Examination	
Body Area	**What I Am Looking for in Particular**
Head	• _____ • _____ • _____
Neck	• _____ • _____
Chest	• _____ • _____ • _____
Abdomen	• _____ • _____
Extremities	• _____ • _____ • _____

2. In the following table, provide the normal respiratory rate for each pediatric age group.

Pediatric Respiratory Rates	
Age	**Respiratory Rate (breaths/min)**
Infant	
Toddler	
Preschool-aged child	
School-aged child	
Adolescent	

3. In the following table, provide the normal pulse rate for each pediatric age group.

Pediatric Pulse Rates	
Age	**Pulse Rate (beats/min)**
Infant	
Toddler	
Preschool-aged child	
School-aged child	
Adolescent	

4. In the following table, provide the normal blood pressure for each pediatric age group.

Normal Blood Pressure for Age	
Age	Minimal Systolic Blood Pressure (mm Hg)
Infant	
Toddler	
Preschool-aged child	
School-aged child	
Adolescent	

5. In the following table, describe what the letters in the CHILD ABUSE mnemonic represent.

CHILD ABUSE Mnemonic	
Mnemonic	What the Letter Represents
C	_____
H	History consistent with injuries
I	_____
L	Lack of supervision
D	_____
A	Affect
B	_____
U	Unusual injury patterns
S	_____
E	Environmental clues

Problem Solving

Practice your calculation skills by solving the following math problems.

1. For children 1 to 10 years old, one would calculate the lower limit of acceptable blood pressure for age using the following formula:

$$\text{Minimal systolic blood pressure} = 80 + (2 \times \text{age in years})$$

a. You are evaluating a pediatric trauma patient. His age is 6 years. What would you estimate a normal systolic blood pressure to be?

b. This patient is a 10-year-old asthmatic. What would you estimate a normal systolic blood pressure to be?

c. On arrival, you have an unconscious pediatric patient. You estimate his age to be 5 or 6 years. What would normal blood pressure be for a patient this age?

2. One would calculate the endotracheal tube size for a child older than 1 year as follows:

$$(Age + 16) \div 4 = \text{Size of ET tube (in mm)}$$

   a. Calculate the appropriate ET tube size of a 6-year-old child.

   b. Calculate the appropriate ET tube size of a 9-year-old child.

3. You have been called to the scene for a 4-year-old child who is unconscious and unresponsive after being shocked by an electrical outlet. He is also pulseless and apneic.
   a. He weighs 40 pounds. Appropriate two-person BLS is in progress on your arrival. You attach the patient to your defibrillator/monitor and notice ventricular fibrillation. What energy setting would you use to administer defibrillations?

   _____

   _____

   b. How much energy should be used on subsequent defibrillations?

   _____

   _____

4. You have now been called to the scene for a 6-year-old girl who has severe anaphylaxis after ingesting peanuts at the ball game. The child is anxious, and she has an increased work of breathing, and poor circulation. She weighs 60 lb.
   a. As the paramedic in charge, you decide that among all your other treatment priorities, this patient requires epinephrine. How will you administer this drug and at what dose?

   _____

   _____

   b. This patient further requires the administration of diphenhydramine (Benadryl). How will you administer this drug and at what dose?

   _____

   _____

   c. Fortunately, your patient is beginning to improve, but she's still wheezing. What drug would you consider and at what dose?

   _____

   _____

Skill Drills

Test your knowledge of skill drills by filling in the correct words in the photo captions.

1. One-Person Bag-Mask Ventilation for a Child

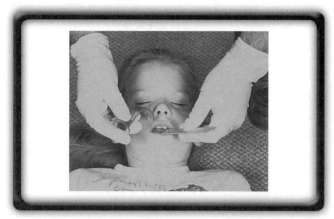

Step 1: Open the _____, and _____ the appropriate airway adjunct.

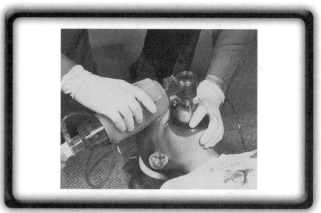

Step 2: Hold the _____ on the patient's face with a one-handed _____ _____-_____ _____ technique (E-C clamp). Ensure a good _____ - _____ - _____ seal while maintaining the airway.

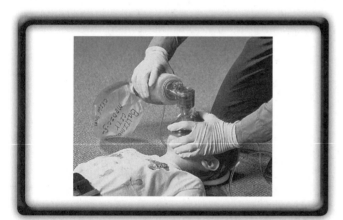

Step 3: Squeeze the bag using the correct _____ rate of _____ to _____ breaths/min for children. Allow adequate time for exhalation.

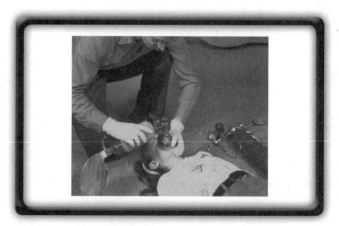

Step 4: Assess effectiveness of ventilation by assessing _____ rise and fall of the _____.

Geriatric Emergencies

Matching

Match each of definitions in the left column to the appropriate term in the right column.

_____ **1.** Organizations that investigate cases involving abuse and neglect and provide case management services in some cases.

_____ **2.** The assessment and treatment of disease in someone 65 years or older.

_____ **3.** A chronic deterioration of mental functions.

_____ **4.** A progressive organic condition in which neurons die, causing dementia.

_____ **5.** A condition in which the aortic valve thickens due to fibrosis and calcification, obstructing blood flow from the left ventricle.

_____ **6.** A condition in which the aortic valve does not open fully, decreasing blood flow from the heart.

_____ **7.** A decrease in bone mass and density.

_____ **8.** A pathologic condition in which the arterial walls become thickened and inelastic.

_____ **9.** A disorder in which cholesterol and calcium build up inside the walls of the blood vessels, forming plaque, which eventually leads to partial or complete blockage of blood flow.

_____ **10.** An acute confusional state characterized by global impairment of thinking, perception, judgment, and memory.

_____ **11.** Sadness from loss, grieving.

_____ **12.** A clouding of the lens of the eye, or its surrounding transparent membrane; normally a result of age.

_____ **13.** An acute inflammation in the skin caused by a bacterial infection.

_____ **14.** A disease of the eye caused by an increase in intraocular pressure; when severe enough, this may damage the optic nerve and potentially cause permanent loss of vision.

_____ **15.** Shingles; a contagious condition caused by the reactivation of the varicella virus or nerve roots.

_____ **16.** A tendency to constancy or stability in the body's internal milieu.

_____ **17.** An organization that provides end-of-life care to patients with terminal illnesses and their families.

_____ **18.** An inner ear disorder in which endolymphatic rupture creates increased pressure in the cochlear duct, which then leads to damage to the organ of Corti and the semicircular canal; symptoms include severe vertigo, tinnitus, and sensori-neuronal hearing loss.

_____ **19.** A formula used to determine the number of older people in a society as compared with the number of potential workers who are theoretically capable of providing resources to sustain the whole population. It is the number of older people (65 years and older) for every 100 adults (potential caregivers) between the ages of 18 and 64 years.

A. Spondylosis

B. Adult protective services

C. Delirium

D. Cellulitis

E. Dementia

F. Presbycusis

G. Herpes zoster

H. Homeostasis

I. Meniere disease

J. Geriatrics

K. Osteoporosis

L. Alzheimer disease

M. Rheumatoid arthritis

N. Sepsis

O. Parkinson disease

P. Arteriosclerosis

Q. Aortic sclerosis

R. Bereavement

S. Aortic stenosis

_____ **20.** The degeneration of a joint surface caused by wear and tear that leads to pain and stiffness.

_____ **21.** A neurologic condition in which the portion of the brain responsible for production of dopamine has been damaged or overused, resulting in tremors.

_____ **22.** The use of multiple medications.

_____ **23.** Progressive hearing loss, particularly in the high frequencies, along with lessened ability to discriminate between a particular sound and background noise.

_____ **24.** Ulcers that occur when pressure is applied to body tissue, resulting in a lack of perfusion and ultimately necrosis.

_____ **25.** The ability to perceive the position and movement of one's body or limbs.

_____ **26.** An inflammatory disorder that affects the entire body and leads to degeneration and deformation of joints.

_____ **27.** A disease state that results from the presence of microorganisms or their toxic products in the bloodstream.

_____ **28.** Degenerative condition resulting in decreased mobility of vertebral joints and compression of neural elements.

T. Hospice

U. Cataracts

V. Glaucoma

W. Osteoarthritis

X. Old-age dependency ratio

Y. Polypharmacy

Z. Proprioception

AA. Atherosclerosis

BB. Pressure ulcers

Multiple Choice

Read each item carefully, and then select the best response.

1. Geriatrics is the assessment and treatment of disease in someone _____ years or older.
  A. 55
  B. 65
  C. 75
  D. None of the above

2. A 35-year-old is aging just as fast as an 85-year-old, but the older person exhibits the cumulative results of a _____ process.
  A. longer
  B. shorter
  C. degenerative
  D. cumulative

3. Over time, cardiac output declines, mostly as a result of a/an _____ stroke volume.
  A. increasing
  B. strengthening
  C. decreasing
  D. weakening

4. Musculoskeletal changes, such as _____, may also affect pulmonary function by limiting lung volume and maximal inspiratory pressure.
  A. kyphosis
  B. osteoporosis
  C. decreased bone mass
  D. arthritis

5. Incontinence is not a normal part of aging and can lead to:
  A. skin irritation.
  B. skin breakdown.
  C. urinary tract infections.
  D. All of the above

6. _____ enables us to maintain postural stability by using a variety of receptors in the joints and information provided by the eyes. As these mechanisms fail with age, people become less steady on their feet, and the tendency to fall increases markedly.
   A. Balance
   B. Posture
   C. Proprioception
   D. Homeostasis

7. Elderly patients are much more vulnerable to the following temperature stresses, EXCEPT:
   A. heat exhaustion.
   B. hypothermia.
   C. the absence of a febrile response to illness.
   D. hormonal temperature effects.

8. Chronic obstructive pulmonary disease (COPD) includes all of the following, EXCEPT:
   A. chronic asthma.
   B. chronic bronchitis.
   C. emphysema.
   D. diuretic intolerant edema.

9. The extent of bone loss that a person undergoes is influenced by numerous factors, including:
   A. genetics, smoking, and level of activity.
   B. age, sex, and genetics.
   C. age, skin condition, and diet.
   D. smoking, age, and skin condition.

10. Some patients fear that mentioning a symptom will lead to a diagnosis or treatment that will jeopardize their independence. "If I mention those pains in my stomach," the older person may reason:
   A. "they'll put me in that nursing home to die."
   B. "my kids will think I'm going to die, and they'll start fighting over the money."
   C. "they'll put me in the hospital, and I can't afford another hospitalization and more prescriptions."
   D. "they'll put me in the hospital, and I may never come out of that place again."

Labeling

Label the components of the GI system and place as asterisk (*) next to the primary location(s) for GI bleeding.

1. Lower Gastrointestinal (GI) System

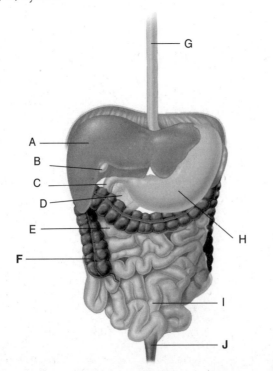

A. _____

B. _____

C. _____

D. _____

E. _____

F. _____

G. _____

H. _____

I. _____

J. _____

2. Upper GI System

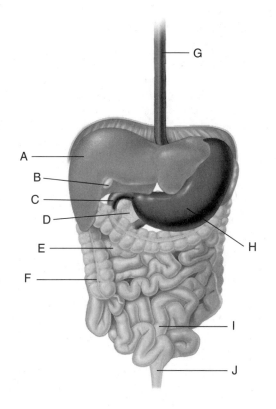

A. _____

B. _____

C. _____

D. _____

E. _____

F. _____

G. _____

H. _____

I. _____

J. _____

Fill-in-the-Blank

Read each item carefully, and then complete the statement by filling in the missing word(s).

1. _____ people constitute an ever-increasing proportion of patients in the health care system, particularly the _____ care sector.

2. There is a widespread tendency to attribute genuine disease symptoms to "_____ _____ _____" and to neglect their treatment.

3. The heart _____ with age, probably in response to the chronically increased afterload imposed by stiffened blood vessels.

4. A person's _____ capacity also undergoes significant _____ with age, largely because of decreases in the elasticity of the lungs and in the size and strength of the respiratory muscles.

5. As a person ages, the kidneys shrink in size. This decline in weight results from a loss of functioning _____ _____, which translates into a smaller effective _____ surface.

6. The decrease in _____ may lead to malnutrition. Other changes in the mouth include a reduction in the volume of _____, with a resulting _____ of the mouth.

7. Narrowing of the _____ disks and _____ of the vertebrae contribute to a decrease in _____ as a person ages, along with changes in posture.

8. A hearing-related impairment noted in the elderly population is _____ _____. Onset of symptoms usually occurs in early middle age, with symptoms presenting in _____ that last several _____ at a time.

9. _____ and loss of _____ of the skin are the most visible signs of aging. Wrinkling occurs because the skin becomes thinner, _____, less elastic, and more _____.

10. Heart attack is the major cause of _____ and _____ in people older than 65 years, and its potential for mortality increases significantly after a person reaches _____ years.

Identify

In the following case studies, list the chief complaint, vital signs, and pertinent negatives.

1. On arrival to the Adult Day Care Center, you discover an 84-year-old woman who has "fallen." She normally walks with the assistance of a cane or walker. She is lying on a deeply carpeted floor and is conscious, alert, and complaining of right-sided midthigh pain. The fall was reportedly not witnessed. Her aide was assisting another client when the fall occurred. Your patient does not have a good recollection of what happened. She denies chest pain, shortness of breath, dizziness, nausea, or vomiting. She also denies tripping and falling. The area appears clear of obstacles, rugs, or other obvious trip hazards. Your physical exam is as previously indicated. You notice some inward rotation and shortening of the extremity. Her pulse is 84 beats/min and very irregular. Her oxygen saturation is 88% on room air. Her blood pressure is 106/86 mm Hg. The patient's skin turgor is poor, with a delayed capillary refill of > 2 seconds. Pupils are Equal And Round, Regular in size, and reactive to Light (PEARRL). An electrocardiogram (ECG) shows a sinus rhythm with frequent premature ventricular contractions (PVCs) and short runs of ventricular tachycardia.

   a. Chief complaint:

   _____

   _____

   b. Vital signs:

   _____

   _____

   c. Pertinent negatives:

   _____

   _____

2. It's early afternoon on a clear and warm spring day. You are dispatched to the parking lot of a local supermarket for a reported motor vehicle crash. On arrival, you discover an elderly man who is 92 years old. He is the driver of a vehicle that struck several parked cars. Bystanders state that the patient appears to be either sleeping or unconscious. You find the patient to be conscious but not alert to person, place, time, or purpose. The police identify his home phone number and call it. A pleasant-sounding elderly woman answers and states that her husband left home over an hour ago to pick up some groceries. She states that he has a problem with "sugar" and wonders if he has his hearing aids in place. As you begin examining the patient and taking his history, it becomes obvious that he is not wearing hearing aids. There is minimally detectable damage to the vehicle as well as the vehicles that were struck. The patient was found not to be wearing his seat belt. He does have a medical identification bracelet on and it indicates extensive cardiac and diabetic history. Vital signs indicate a blood glucose level of 66 mg/dL. His pulse rate is 92 beats/min and regular, and blood pressure is 160/72 mm Hg. His skin is warm and moist, his capillary refill is normal, and he has oxygen saturation of 96% on room air. The patient is able to maintain his own airway and gag reflex. He was initially assisted with oral glucose by the EMRs at the scene. He is becoming increasingly alert and oriented and denies any injury.

   a. Chief complaint:

   _____

   _____

   b. Vital signs:

   _____

   _____

   c. Pertinent negatives:

   _____

   _____

Complete the Patient Care Report (PCR)

Reread the first incident scenario in the preceding Identify exercises and then complete the following PCR for the patient.

EMS Patient Care Report (PCR)					
Date:	Incident No.:	Nature of Call:		Location:	
Dispatched:	En Route:	At Scene:	Transport:	At Hospital:	In Service:
Patient Information					
Age:			Allergies:		
Sex:			Medications:		
Weight (in kg [lb]):			Past Medical History:		
			Chief Complaint:		
Vital Signs					
Time:	BP:	Pulse:		Respirations:	SpO$_2$:
Time:	BP:	Pulse:		Respirations:	SpO$_2$:
Time:	BP:	Pulse:		Respirations:	SpO$_2$:
EMS Treatment (circle all that apply)					
Oxygen @ _____ L/min via (circle one): NC NRM Bag-Mask Device		Assisted Ventilation	Airway Adjunct		CPR
Defibrillation	Bleeding Control	Bandaging	Splinting		Other
Narrative					

Ambulance Calls

The following case scenarios provide an opportunity to explore the concerns associated with patient management and paramedic care. Read each scenario, and then answer each question.

1. One way to try to ensure that you don't miss anything important in the patient's history is to ask some general screening questions, irrespective of the patient's chief complaint. Suppose an 80-year-old woman has called for an ambulance because she feels "tired and weak." List 10 general screening questions you would ask to assess the status of her major organ systems.

   a. _____

   b. _____

   c. _____

   d. _____

   e. _____

   f. _____

   g. _____

   h. _____

   i. _____

   j. _____

2. You are called to the apartment of a 78-year-old woman who fell down.
   a. List five questions you would ask in taking the history of the present illness.

      (1) _____

      (2) _____

      (3) _____

      (4) _____

      (5) _____

   b. List the information you should obtain about the patient's past (other) medical history.

      (1) _____

      (2) _____

      (3) _____

      (4) _____

   c. List six things you would look for in particular in performing the physical examination.

      (1) _____

      (2) _____

      (3) _____

      (4) _____

      (5) _____

      (6) _____

d. While conducting the physical examination, you will of course be alert for signs or symptoms of those injuries to which older people are particularly vulnerable. List three injuries to which elderly patients are more susceptible.

(1) _____

(2) _____

(3) _____

3. You are called to a shopping center where an elderly man tripped on a potted plant and fell, sustaining a minor laceration to his arm. As you are applying a dressing to the laceration, you notice that he seems very listless and depressed. List five factors related to geriatric suicide.

a. _____

b. _____

c. _____

d. _____

e. _____

True/False

The public (and also, regrettably, health care professionals) holds many widespread misconceptions about the elderly and the process of aging that result in inaccurate stereotypes of elderly persons. If you believe the statement to be more true than false, write the letter "T" in the space provided. If you believe the statement to be more false than true, write the letter "F."

_____ **1.** The rate of aging is the same in a 35-year-old as it is in an 85-year-old.

_____ **2.** Mental deterioration and some degree of dementia are an inevitable part of the aging process.

_____ **3.** Elderly people are more likely than younger individuals to seek emergency care for minor, nonserious complaints.

_____ **4.** The pain mechanism is often depressed among the elderly.

_____ **5.** The possibility of hearing loss increases with age.

_____ **6.** Sweat gland activity increases, hindering the ability to sweat and to regulate heat.

_____ **7.** A specific illness or injury in elderly people is more likely to result in generalized deterioration.

_____ **8.** Cellulitis is an acute inflammation in the skin caused by a viral infection. This condition usually affects the lower extremities.

_____ **9.** Elderly patients must always be placed in a traction splint for a femoral fracture.

_____ **10.** One clue to elder abuse is unexplained injuries that do not fit the stated cause.

Short Answer

Complete this section with short written answers using the space provided.

1. Patients older than 65 years of age account for one third of all ambulance calls today. As the population continues to age, that percentage can be expected to increase. It is therefore important for paramedics to understand the special problems and challenges posed by caring for the elderly. List five characteristics of the elderly that make it particularly challenging to diagnose their problems correctly and provide them with appropriate care.

a. _____

b. _____

c. _____

d. _____

e. _____

2. The process of aging in our society is nearly always accompanied by social and psychological stresses that may have an enormous impact on health. List two potentially stressful changes that tend to occur in a person's life as he or she approaches the "golden age."

a. _____

b. _____

3. The normal aging process produces changes in nearly every organ system of the body. It is important to know what constitutes a *normal* age-related change so that such a change will not be mistaken for a sign of disease (and, conversely, so that signs of disease will not be disregarded as "just part of getting old"). For each of the following organ systems, list two changes in structure or function that occur as a normal consequence of aging.

a. Cardiovascular

(1) _____

(2) _____

b. Respiratory

(1) _____

(2) _____

c. Renal

(1) _____

(2) _____

d. Digestive

(1) _____

(2) _____

e. Musculoskeletal

(1) _____

(2) _____

f. Nervous

(1) _____

(2) _____

g. Homeostatic

(1) _____

(2) _____

4. In younger patients, the chief complaint often has considerable value in localizing the patient's underlying problem. A middle-aged man suffering an acute myocardial infarction, for example, will usually complain of pain or discomfort in his chest, while a young person with pneumonia usually will have a cough and a fever. Among the elderly, on the other hand, the response to serious illness tends to be less specific. List four responses to illness common among seriously ill elderly patients.

a. _____

b. _____

c. _____

d. _____

5. Obtaining an accurate history from an elderly patient requires considerable skill because there are a number of obstacles to history taking among the elderly that do not exist when you talk with younger patients. List four obstacles to obtaining a medical history from an elderly person, and indicate what steps you can take to overcome each of them.

   a. Obstacle:

   _____

   _____

   What I can do to try to overcome the obstacle:

   _____

   _____

   b. Obstacle:

   _____

   _____

   What I can do to try to overcome the obstacle:

   _____

   _____

   c. Obstacle:

   _____

   _____

   What I can do to try to overcome the obstacle:

   _____

   _____

   d. Obstacle:

   _____

   _____

   What I can do to try to overcome the obstacle:

   _____

   _____

6. In a middle-aged patient, the clinical presentation of such conditions as acute myocardial infarction or congestive heart failure is usually straightforward. In an elderly person with the same problem, the clinical presentation may be much less clear-cut. List at least two signs or symptoms that are commonly part of the clinical presentation of acute myocardial infarction and of congestive heart failure in the elderly.

Condition	Possible Signs and Symptoms in the Elderly
Acute myocardial infarction	
Congestive heart failure	

7. One of the most common presenting symptoms among the elderly is an acute confusional state (delirium). Complete the list of conditions likely to present as delirium in the elderly, which are represented by the letters in the acronym DELIRIUMS below:

D: _____

E: _____

L: _____

I: _____

R: _____

I: _____

U: _____

M: _____

S: _____

Fill-in-the-Table

Fill in the missing parts of the following tables.

1.

Causes of Falls in the Elderly	
Cause	Clues to Suggest This Cause
_____	Obvious environmental hazard at the scene, such as poor lighting, scatter rugs, uneven sidewalk, ice or other slippery surface
_____	Sudden fall; patient found on the ground somewhat confused, often temporarily paralyzed and unable to get up; no premonitory symptoms
_____	Fall when getting up from a recumbent or sitting position (Check medications the patient is taking, and ask about occult blood loss, such as presence of black stools. Measure blood pressure in recumbent and sitting positions.)
_____	Marked bradycardia or tachydysrhythmias
_____	Other characteristic signs of stroke, such as hemiparesis, hemiplegia, or aphasia
_____	Patient felt something snap before falling

2.

Drugs Most Commonly Causing Toxic Reactions in Elderly People	
Medication	**Symptoms**
Anti-inflammatory agents (NSAIDs, steroids)	Drowsiness, dizziness, confusion, anxiety, bradypnea, tachypnea, GI bleeding
_____	GI signs, altered mental status, seizures, coma
Anticholinergics and antihistamines	Urination difficulty, constipation, drowsiness, restlessness, irritability, hypertension
_____	Ecchymosis, epistaxis, hematuria, abdominal pain, vomiting, fecal blood
Antidysrhythmics (amiodarone, lidocaine)	Restlessness, hypotension, bradycardia, tachycardia, palpitations, angina
_____	Confusion, delirium, disorientation, memory impairment
Antihypertensives (diuretics, alpha blockers, beta blockers; angiotensin-converting enzyme inhibitors)	Hypotension, palpitations, angina, fluid retention, headache
_____	Drowsiness, tachycardia, dizziness, restlessness
Digoxin	Headache, fatigue, malaise, drowsiness, depression
_____	Hypoglycemia presenting as confusion
Narcotics	Delirium, respiratory depression, apnea, involuntary muscle movements
_____	Incoordination, dizziness, disturbances in cognitive function

Patients With Special Challenges

Matching

Match each of the terms in the right column to the appropriate definition in the left column.

_____ **1.** Any form of maltreatment that results in harm or loss. Maltreatment may be physical, sexual, psychological, or financial/material.

_____ **2.** Increased intraocular pressure that leads to ocular pain and decreased visual acuity; sudden onset is a medical emergency.

_____ **3.** The medical specialty dedicated to prevention and treatment of obesity.

_____ **4.** Excessive growth and division of abnormal cells within the body that can occur in many body systems, tissues, and organs, and that can progress rapidly and cause death in a relatively short period of time.

_____ **5.** Refusal or failure on the part of the caregiver to provide life necessities, such as food, water, clothing, shelter, personal hygiene, medicine, comfort, and personal safety.

_____ **6.** An eye condition caused by a clouding of the lens, leading to decreased vision.

_____ **7.** A disorder in which patients have difficulty interpreting speech and differentiating it from other sounds that are present.

_____ **8.** The surgical establishment of an opening between the colon and the surface of the body for the purpose of providing drainage of the bowel.

_____ **9.** A sickness that a patient cannot be cured of; death is imminent.

_____ **10.** A device that converts energy or pressure into electrical signals.

_____ **11.** A traumatic insult to the brain capable of producing physical, intellectual, emotional, social, and vocational changes.

_____ **12.** Medical treatment aimed at symptom relief and providing comfort for the patient.

_____ **13.** A type of hearing impairment due to problems with the middle ear bones' ability to conduct sounds from the outer ear to the inner ear.

_____ **14.** A psychological condition in which stress or mental conflict is converted into physical complaints.

_____ **15.** The cultural practice of placing warm cups on the skin to pull out illness from the body. The red, flat, rounded skin lesions are often more intensely red at the borders.

_____ **16.** A slow-growing, benign tumor of the vestibular cochlear nerve that can lead to loss of hearing in the affected ear.

_____ **17.** A genetic disorder of the endocrine system that makes it difficult for chloride to move through cells; primarily targets the respiratory and digestive systems.

_____ **18.** A complete or partial hearing loss.

A. Cerebrospinal fluid shunt

B. Central auditory processing disorder

C. Cancer

D. Autism

E. Asynchrony

F. Acute angle-closure glaucoma

G. Abuse

H. Fistula

I. Dysarthria

J. Dialysis

K. Developmental delay

L. Cystic fibrosis

M. Cupping

N. Conductive hearing loss

O. Colostomy

P. Glaucoma

Q. Heparinized solution

R. Hydrocephalus

_____ **19.** A broad term that describes an infant or child's failure to reach a particular developmental milestone by the expected time.

_____ **20.** Insufficient development of a portion of the brain, resulting in some level of dysfunction or impairment.

_____ **21.** Medical treatment aimed at curing an illness.

_____ **22.** A medical process by which a patient's blood is cleansed of excess toxins by passing through a special machine.

_____ **23.** A condition characterized by normal function of the structures of the ear without a corresponding stimulation of auditory centers of the brain; also called auditory dyssynchrony.

_____ **24.** A developmental disorder characterized by impairments of social interaction; may include severe behavioral problems, repetitive motor activities, and impairment in verbal and nonverbal skills.

_____ **25.** A speech disorder caused by neuromuscular disturbance that causes speech to become slow and slurred.

_____ **26.** A form of abuse that may be verbal (such as ridicule, threats, blaming, or humiliation), or nonverbal (caregiver ignores the victim or isolates the victim from others); causes a substantial change in the victim's behavior, emotional response, or cognitive function, or may manifest as a variety of mental illnesses.

_____ **27.** A surgical connection between an artery and a vein.

_____ **28.** An eye condition caused by increased intraocular pressure.

_____ **29.** A form of dialysis in which blood is removed from the patient through a catheter or fistula, and then returns to the body through another needle, removing various toxins, electrolytes, and fluids in the process.

_____ **30.** A developmental condition in which damage is done to the brain. It presents during infancy as a delay in walking or crawling and can take on a spastic form in which muscles are in a nearly constant state of contraction.

_____ **31.** A tube placed in the body to relieve pressure by drawing excess cerebrospinal fluid away from the brain or spinal cord.

_____ **32.** A saline solution mixed with heparin, an anticoagulant used to prevent blood clots from forming.

_____ **33.** A program and philosophy that attempt to help the patient maximize the quality of remaining life by providing social and emotional support, treating discomfort with pharmacologic and nonpharmacologic approaches, and helping patients and families cope with the prospect of impending death.

_____ **34.** A medical condition in which there is an abnormal buildup of cerebrospinal fluid in the skull; this can be acquired (occurring after birth) or congenital (developing before birth).

_____ **35.** Disruption or loss of normal gastrointestinal motility.

_____ **36.** A balloon that is inserted into the aorta and connected to a pump via a catheter; this therapy helps to increase the blood flow to the coronary arteries during diastole (inflation) and decrease afterload of blood from the left ventricle (deflation).

_____ **37.** A type of disability in which difficulties with reading, spelling, or writing cause a person to fall behind expectations for a given age.

_____ **38.** A neurologic impairment in which the brain is intermittently unable to carry out the command for speech or other tasks.

S. Intra-aortic balloon pump

T. Multiple sclerosis

U. Mental retardation

V. Mandatory reporter

W. Urostomy

X. Transducer

Y. Systemic lupus erythematosus

Z. Spina bifida

AA. Spastic paralysis

BB. Rheumatoid arthritis

CC. Quadriplegia

DD. Muscular dystrophy

EE. Myasthenia gravis

FF. Neglect

GG. Osteoarthritis

HH. Peritoneal dialysis

II. Poliomyelitis

JJ. Mongolian spots

KK. Meniere disease

LL. Language-based learning disability

_____ **39.** Disturbance or lack of synchronization.

_____ **40.** A category of professional required by some states to report suspicions of child maltreatment. Prehospital professionals may be included.

_____ **41.** Lesions that resemble bruises, typically on the buttocks or back, that are present at birth on many infants of Asian or African origin.

_____ **42.** An autoimmune condition in which the body attacks the myelin that insulates the brain and spinal cord, causing scarring.

_____ **43.** A broad term that describes a category of incurable genetic diseases that cause a slow, progressive degeneration of the muscle fibers.

_____ **44.** A condition in which the body generates antibodies against its own acetylcholine receptors, causing muscle weakness, often in the face.

_____ **45.** A complication of myasthenia gravis in which weakened respiratory muscles lead to respiratory failure.

_____ **46.** A genetic chromosomal defect that can occur during fetal development and that results in mental retardation and certain physical characteristics, such as a round head with a flat occiput and slanted, wide-set eyes.

_____ **47.** A term used when a person has a body mass index of greater than 30 kg per meters squared (kg/m²).

_____ **48.** The degeneration of a joint surface caused by wear and tear that leads to pain and stiffness.

_____ **49.** Medical care aimed at relief of pain and suffering in terminally ill patients.

_____ **50.** A type of dialysis in which a special solution is instilled through a catheter into the patient's abdomen, and that draws toxins, electrolytes, and other fluids from the body through the peritoneal membrane.

_____ **51.** A category of disorders that impact a person's ability to produce sounds that combine into spoken words.

_____ **52.** A viral infection that attacks and destroys motor axons. The disease can cause weakness, paralysis, and respiratory arrest. Because an effective vaccine has been developed, the incident of the disease is now rare.

_____ **53.** Paralysis of upper and lower extremities.

_____ **54.** Any eye disorder in which the retina becomes diseased, leading to partial or total vision loss.

_____ **55.** An inflammatory disorder that affects the entire body and leads to degeneration and deformation of joints.

_____ **56.** A condition characterized by delayed language developmental milestones, resulting in the person repeatedly using irrelevant phrases out of context, confusing word pairs, and having trouble following conversations.

_____ **57.** A permanent lack of hearing caused by a lesion or damage of the inner ear.

_____ **58.** A chronic form of paralysis in which the affected muscles experience continued spasm.

_____ **59.** A form of cerebral palsy in which all four limbs are affected.

MM. Ileus

NN. Hospice

OO. Hemodialysis

PP. Emotional abuse

QQ. Down syndrome

RR. Developmental disability

SS. Deafness

TT. Curative care

UU. Comfort care

VV. Conversion disorder

WW. Cerebral palsy

XX. Cataract

YY. Bariatrics

ZZ. Auditory neuropathy

AAA. Apraxia

BBB. Acoustic neuroma

CCC. Traumatic brain injury

DDD. Terminal illness

EEE. Surrogate decision maker

FFF. Spastic tetraplegia

GGG. Stoma

_____ **60.** A developmental anomaly in which a portion of the spinal cord or meninges protrudes outside the spinal column or even outside the body, usually in the area of the lumbar spine (the lower third of the spine); also called myelomeningocele.

_____ **61.** An inner ear disorder that causes vertigo, tinnitus, and hearing impairment.

_____ **62.** A primarily cognitive disorder that appears during childhood and is accompanied by lack of adaptive behaviors, such as the ability to live and function independently or interact successfully with others; the person generally has an intelligence quotient below 70; also known as intellectual disability.

_____ **63.** A surgical opening, such as into the abdominal wall or trachea.

_____ **64.** A person legally authorized to make health care decisions on behalf of a patient who is incapable of making or communicating the decision on his or her own.

_____ **65.** A multisystem autoimmune disease.

_____ **66.** A surgically constructed opening for the urinary system.

HHH. Semantic pragmatic disorder

III. Sensorineural hearing loss

JJJ. Retinopathy

KKK. Myasthenic crisis

LLL. Obese

MMM. Palliative care

NNN. Phonologic process disorders

Multiple Choice

Read each item carefully, and then select the best response.

1. Which of the following would be considered speech impairments?
   A. Articulation disorders
   B. Language disorders
   C. Fluency disorders
   D. All of the above

2. When establishing communication with a patient with speech impairment, the paramedic should do which of the following?
   A. Ask the patient how he or she would be comfortable communicating.
   B. Use an interpreter.
   C. Be patient because communicating is going to take time.
   D. All of the above

3. It is estimated that _____ million children and up to _____ million elderly adults are victimized by abuse each year.
   A. 3; 2
   B. 4; 1
   C. 5; 2
   D. 6; 2

4. The different types of paralysis include all of the following, EXCEPT:
   A. spastic paralysis.
   B. quadriplegia.
   C. myasthenia gravis.
   D. paraplegia.

5. All of the following are helpful tips when moving a morbidly obese patient, EXCEPT:
   A. treat the patient with dignity and respect.
   B. avoid trying to lift the patient by only one limb, which would risk injury to the person's overtaxed joints.
   C. follow up on the patient's carefully monitored diet.
   D. coordinate and communicate all moves to all team members *prior* to starting.

6. Patients with Down syndrome are at greater risk for which of the following medical conditions?
   A. Hearing and vision problems
   B. Medical complications that affect the cardiovascular, sensory, endocrine, orthopedic, dental, and gastrointestinal systems
   C. Enlarged tongue and dental anomalies that can lead to speech abnormalities
   D. All of the above

7. As health care providers, you and your team will often be called on to assist a patient who has a terminal illness. Each of the following are examples of terminal illnesses, EXCEPT:
   A. liver failure.
   B. Lou Gehrig disease.
   C. pulmonary disease.
   D. type II diabetes.

8. Cancer frequently targets organs and body systems such as the liver and:
   A. the brain.
   B. the colon.
   C. the skin.
   D. All of the above

9. Which of the following devices serves as a long-term replacement for an endotracheal tube in a patient who has a chronic condition?
   A. A ventricular assist device
   B. A tracheostomy tube
   C. An obturator
   D. A stoma

10. You are treating a 62-year-old man who is complaining of chest pain for the past 35 minutes. You have decided to administer aspirin, nitroglycerin, and morphine, as well as oxygen, and to start a medication IV line. The patient has been receiving treatments through a long-term vascular access device in his chest. If there are still distal IV sites available, why should the paramedic avoid using the long-term device in the chest?
    A. The device may be inserted directly into an artery, rather than a vein.
    B. It may require a special needle to access the port.
    C. The device may be maintained with a high dose of anticoagulant.
    D. All of the above

Labeling

Label the following diagrams with the correct terms.

1. American Sign Language (ASL) Signs

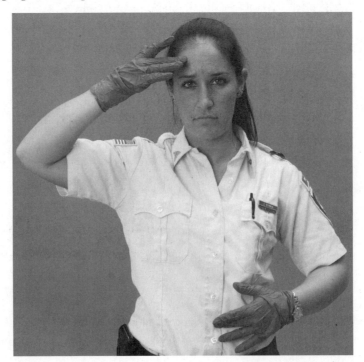

A. _____

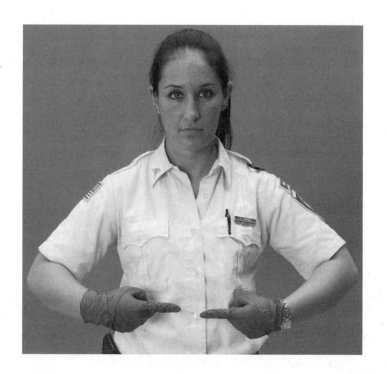

B. _____

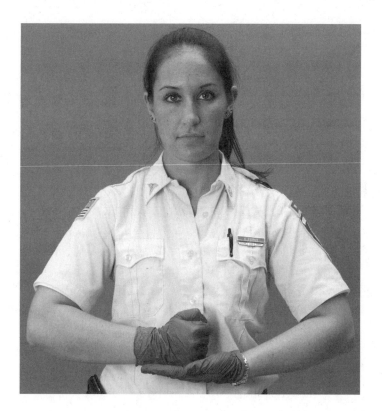

C. _____

2. Vessels and Structures in the Extremity of a Dialysis Patient

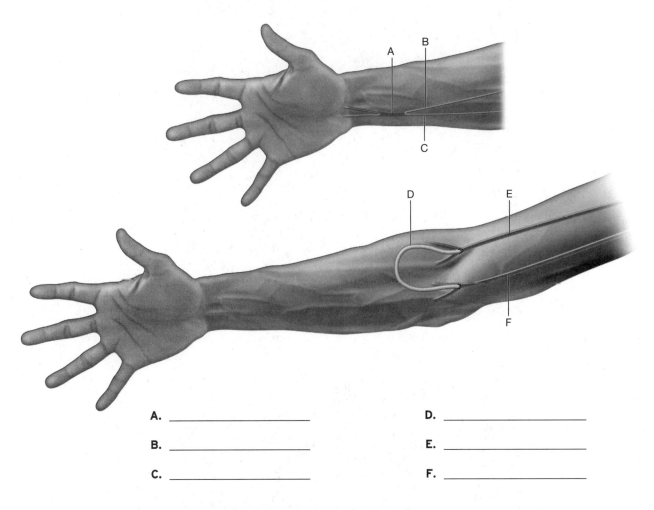

A. _____

B. _____

C. _____

D. _____

E. _____

F. _____

Fill-in-the-Blank

Read each item carefully, and then complete the statement by filling in the missing word(s).

1. Hearing challenges are generally classified into two types: _____ and _____ deafness.

2. Hearing _____ may be _____ or acquired.

3. Speech impairment may be divided into disorders impacting _____, voice _____, fluency, and _____.

4. Autistic patients may present with a/an _____-_____ disorder of speech.

5. _____ is the most common type of arthritis. It is caused by _____ loss or abnormal bone growth, usually in response to _____ or excess "wear and tear" on a joint over time.

6. The medical specialty of _____ has emerged in response to the widespread and profound incidence of adult and childhood _____.

7. Myelomeningocele, also known as _____ _____, is a birth defect caused by improper development of the _____ _____ tube consisting of the brain and spinal cord.

8. Infants and young children may be diagnosed with _____ _____ (_____), a genetic disorder that is characterized by increased production of mucus in the lungs and digestive tract. This disorder is caused by a _____ _____ gene, inherited from each parent.

9. Cerebral palsy generally produces _____ _____ muscle function or _____ .

10. Spina bifida is the most common permanently disabling _____ _____. In this disorder, during the first month of _____, the fetus's spinal _____ does not close properly or completely and vertebrae do not _____.

Identify

In the following case studies, list the chief complaint, the history of the present illness, and other medical history.

1. You have been called to the scene by distraught family members. The patient is becoming increasingly disoriented and appears unresponsive. The patient is exhibiting an irregular breathing pattern with periods of apnea. His blood pressure is about 70/palp, and his pulse is very fast and erratic. Some family members have what appears to be a valid prehospital do not resuscitate (DNR) order.

   a. Chief complaint:

   _____

   _____

   b. History of the present illness:

   _____

   _____

   c. Other medical history:

   _____

   _____

2. You are responding to a call to an adult group home for adults with disabilities. The nature of the call is for a patient with seizures. On arrival, you are met by staff members who have the patient's complete chart. The patient has a history of Down syndrome and a seizure disorder. The patient is on multiple medications and has been given rectal diazepam (Diastat).

   a. Chief complaint:

   _____

   _____

   b. History of the present illness:

   _____

   _____

   c. Other medical history:

   _____

   _____

3. Your patient has a chief complaint of fever. The patient's home health aide states that the patient's urine has been cloudy and he's suddenly developed a fever of 101.3°F. He is conscious and alert, and his vitals are a blood pressure of 110/70 mm Hg and a heart rate of 108 beats/min. He is always confined to a wheelchair. He communicates with a writing board. He is a quadriplegic and has a Foley catheter, tracheotomy, colostomy, and feeding tube. He is taking an antibiotic and a steroid medicine.

   a. Chief complaint:

   _____

   _____

   b. History of the present illness:

   _____

   _____

   c. Other medical history:

   _____

   _____

Complete the Patient Care Report (PCR)

Reread incident scenario 3 in the preceding Identify exercises, and then complete the following PCR for the patient.

EMS Patient Care Report (PCR)					
Date:	**Incident No.:**	**Nature of Call:**		**Location:**	
Dispatched:	**En Route:**	**At Scene:**	**Transport:**	**At Hospital:**	**In Service:**

Patient Information			
Age:		**Allergies:**	
Sex:		**Medications:**	
Weight (in kg [lb]):		**Past Medical History:**	
		Chief Complaint:	

Vital Signs				
Time:	**BP:**	**Pulse:**	**Respirations:**	**SpO$_2$:**
Time:	**BP:**	**Pulse:**	**Respirations:**	**SpO$_2$:**
Time:	**BP:**	**Pulse:**	**Respirations:**	**SpO$_2$:**

EMS Treatment (circle all that apply)				
Oxygen @ _____ L/min via (circle one): NC NRM Bag-Mask Device		**Assisted Ventilation**	**Airway Adjunct**	**CPR**
Defibrillation	**Bleeding Control**	**Bandaging**	**Splinting**	**Other**

Narrative

Ambulance Calls

The following case scenarios provide an opportunity to explore the concerns associated with patient management and paramedic care. Read each scenario, and then answer each question.

1. You receive an "alpha" response for a patient with chronic pain. On arrival, you note the wheelchair ramp in front of the apartment. Once inside you recognize your patient. You have provided care for her in the past. She is 36 years old and is complaining of severe lower back pain and requesting transportation to the medical center. She is somewhat difficult to interact with and is not very polite. Despite that, you continue to be professional and initiate care. She has a history of spina bifida and is seated in her motorized wheelchair. She is covered in a blanket.

   a. What can you do to help alleviate her discomfort during transfer from her wheelchair to the cot?

   _____

   _____

   b. Based on your knowledge of spina bifida, what other medical issues may be present?

   _____

   _____

2. Tonight you are working a special event at the civic center. It's the concert of a popular country singer. The place is packed. Other than a couple of requests for ice packs and ear plugs, the event has been uneventful. Suddenly, security requests EMS to section 103 for a person having a seizure. Your patient is a 12-year-old girl with her mom. The patient has Down syndrome and a seizure disorder. The seizure is over by the time you arrive, but the patient appears postictal and has a large amount of saliva and snoring-type respirations.

   a. How would you go about treating the patient?

   _____

   _____

   b. What are the characteristic physical features of someone with Down syndrome?

   _____

   _____

True/False

If you believe the statement to be more true than false, write the letter "T" in the space provided. If you believe the statement to be more false than true, write the letter "F."

_____ **1.** Whatever the source of the challenge, patients with special needs will require you to adapt your assessment and management to accommodate their needs.

_____ **2.** A method of instilling a special solution through a catheter into the renal patient's abdomen is referred to as hemodialysis.

_____ **3.** Cortical visual impairment involves total visual impairment.

_____ **4.** A phonologic process disorder impacts a person's ability to produce sounds that combine into spoken words.

_____ **5.** Patients with nearsightedness have an impairment known as myopia.

_____ **6.** It is not necessary to modify patient assessment techniques for the patient with a cognitive impairment.

_____ **7.** Patients with mental impairments view all strangers, especially paramedics in uniform, in a friendly and calm manner.

_____ **8.** Cystic fibrosis is a chronic dysfunction of the endocrine system that targets multiple body systems but primarily the respiratory and digestive systems.

_____ **9.** Muscular dystrophy is an acquired muscular disease that causes degeneration of the muscle fibers. In many cases, the destroyed fibers are replaced by fat or connective tissue.

_____ **10.** Patients with myasthenia gravis have facial and throat muscles that could become so weak that the patient suffers an acute onset of respiratory failure. In such a case, you need to intervene immediately with airway management, ventilatory support, and possibly intubation.

Short Answer

Complete this section with short written answers using the space provided.

1. Oftentimes, paramedics treat patients who are hesitant about allowing transport. One of the primary reasons encountered is the financial concern voiced by patients. This is a legitimate patient concern and one that often must be addressed in the prehospital environment.

   a. Describe how you could go about getting a patient with financial concerns to go to the emergency department.

   _____

   _____

   b. Are there any free clinics in your response area to which you could refer patients?

   _____

   _____

   c. Are you legally and medically allowed to transport to these clinics?

   _____

   _____

   d. Are hospitals required to evaluate the patients you bring them?

   _____

   _____

2. Many of the patients a paramedic encounters have hearing impairments. Sometimes this impairment is readily noticeable.

   a. What clues would indicate to you that your patient has a hearing impairment?

   (1) _____

   (2) _____

   (3) _____

   b. How would you go about communicating with someone with a hearing impairment?

   (1) _____

   (2) _____

   (3) _____

   (4) _____

   (5) _____

   (6) _____

   (7) _____

   (8) _____

3. Transporting obese patients can be particularly challenging for paramedic crews. Describe strategies that would be helpful to the patient and the EMS providers.

   a. _____

   b. _____

   c. _____

   d. _____

   e. _____

f. _____

g. _____

4. You respond to a car crash. On arrival, you discover a frightened but apparently uninjured rear-seat passenger. Everyone else appears to be out of the car walking around. You discover that the passenger has a visual impairment.

  a. What are some of the causes of visual impairments?

    (1) _____

    (2) _____

    (3) _____

    (4) _____

    (5) _____

  b. What can paramedics do to alleviate some of the fears felt by patients with visual impairments?

    (1) _____

    (2) _____

    (3) _____

    (4) _____

Fill-in-the-Table

Fill in the missing parts of the tables.

1. A special need is identified in the left column. Use the right column to describe a particular patient care need based on the special need identified.

Care Needs for Special Needs Patients	
Special Need	**Associated Patient Care Need**
Speech impairments	_____
Visual impairments	_____
Paralysis	_____
Obesity	_____
Developmental disabilities	_____
Pathologic challenges	_____

2. Complete the list of obesity causes.

Causes of Obesity	
Primary Causes	• Poor dietary choices • _____ • _____
Secondary Causes	• Hormonal changes • _____ • Low basal metabolic rate • _____ • _____ • Declining smoking • _____

CHAPTER

46

Transport Operations

Matching

Part I

Match each of the numbered items to the appropriate type of ambulance transport.

Your air ambulance transports to a regional trauma center. Your ground ambulance transports to a community hospital. Choose the correct transportation for your patient.

A. Air ambulance
G. Ground ambulance

_____ **1.** 50-year-old in cardiac arrest

_____ **2.** 8-year-old having an asthma attack

_____ **3.** 22-year-old thrown from a rollover crash

_____ **4.** 44-year-old with amputation of the left hand

_____ **5.** 26-year-old mountain climber who fell approximately 50 feet

_____ **6.** 24-year-old with a breech presentation delivery

_____ **7.** 56-year-old with an active upper gastrointestinal bleed

_____ **8.** 18-year-old with a broken femur from an all-terrain vehicle crash

_____ **9.** 2-year-old near drowning (submersion) victim who fell through ice at the local pond

_____ **10.** 34-year-old with a broken ankle from a football game

Part II

Match each of the definitions in the left column to the appropriate term in the right column.

_____ **1.** A sensation that, when an operator depresses the brake pedal, the steering wheel is being pulled to the left or the right.

_____ **2.** A person who assists a driver in backing up an ambulance to compensate for blind spots at the back of the vehicle.

_____ **3.** A sensation of looseness or sloppiness in a vehicle's steering.

_____ **4.** Keeping a safe distance between your vehicle and other vehicles on any side of you.

_____ **5.** Federal standards that regulate the design and manufacturing guidelines of emergency ambulances.

_____ **6.** A finding that when the operator lets go of the steering wheel, a vehicle consistently wanders to the left or right.

_____ **7.** The process of removing dirt, dust, blood, or other visible contaminants from a surface.

_____ **8.** Driving with awareness and responsibility for other drivers on the roadway when you are operating an ambulance in the emergency mode, and making sure that other drivers are aware of your approach.

_____ **9.** Extra heavy-duty vehicle.

_____ **10.** Standard van, forward-control integral cab-body ambulance.

_____ **11.** Specialty van, forward-control integral cab-body ambulance.

_____ **12.** The killing of pathogenic agents by using potent means of disinfection.

A. Wheel wobble

B. Strategic deployment

C. Steering play

D. Spotter

E. Steering pull

F. Type II ambulance

G. Sterilization

H. Type I ambulance

I. Type III ambulance

J. Wheel bounce

K. Posting

L. Medevac

_____ **13.** Medical evacuation of a patient by helicopter.

_____ **14.** Fixed-wing aircraft and helicopters that have been modified for medical care; used to evacuate and transport patients with life-threatening injuries to treatment facilities.

_____ **15.** A chirping or squealing sound, synchronous with engine speed.

_____ **16.** To remove or neutralize radiation, chemical, or other hazardous material from clothing, equipment, vehicles, and personnel.

_____ **17.** The killing of pathogenic agents by direct application of chemicals.

_____ **18.** Areas of the road that are blocked from your sight by your own vehicle or mirrors.

_____ **19.** A sensation that an ambulance has lost its power brakes.

_____ **20.** A time of day or a day of the week when the call volume is at its highest.

_____ **21.** The placement of an ambulance at a specific geographic location in order to cover larger areas of territory and reduce response times.

_____ **22.** A drift that is persistent enough that an operator can feel a tug on the steering wheel.

_____ **23.** A process, such as heating, that removes microbial contamination.

_____ **24.** The staging of ambulances to strategic locations within a service area to allow for coverage of emergency calls.

_____ **25.** Conventional, truck-cab chassis with a modular ambulance body that can be transferred to a new chassis as needed.

_____ **26.** A vibration, synchronous with road speed, that can be felt in the steering wheel.

_____ **27.** A condition in which the tires of a vehicle may be lifted off the road surface as water "piles up" under them, making the vehicle feel as though it is floating.

_____ **28.** Designated location for the landing of air ambulances.

_____ **29.** A common finding at low speeds when a vehicle has a bent wheel.

M. Hydroplaning

N. Heavy-duty ambulance

O. Drift

P. Disinfection

Q. Cushion of safety

R. Air ambulance

S. Belt noise

T. Cleaning

U. Brake pull

V. Brake fade

W. Blind spots

X. Decontaminate

Y. DOT KKK 1822

Z. Due regard

AA. High-level disinfection

BB. Peak loads

CC. Landing zone

Multiple Choice

Read each item carefully, and then select the best response.

1. The design and manufacturing specifications outlined in KKK 1822 federal guidelines are developed by the:
   A. American Heart Association.
   B. General Services Administration.
   C. Bureau of Transport.
   D. National Fire Protection Association.

2. Which of the following should be done at the beginning of each shift?
   A. Change the oil in the ambulance.
   B. Complete an ambulance equipment/supply checklist.
   C. Wash the ambulance.
   D. Replace the supplies that were used the day before.

3. When leaving the scene, what should you tell family members who are following you to the hospital?
   A. Drive as fast as you can with your flashers on.
   B. Follow the ambulance with your flashers on.
   C. Drive normally and do not follow the ambulance.
   D. Don't come until the doctor has called you.

4. What can happen to the grass on the side of the road if you park the ambulance on it?
   A. Nothing.
   B. It can catch fire.
   C. It can die from the fumes of the ambulance.
   D. It can clog up the underside of the ambulance and cause the ambulance to stop running.

5. What should you use when backing up an ambulance?
   A. The mirrors
   B. The guidance system that beeps when you are about to run into something
   C. The mirrors and a spotter
   D. Never back up an ambulance; always park so you can leave without backing up.

6. Each of the following are considered advantages of using an air ambulance, EXCEPT:
   A. they can provide access to remote areas.
   B. they are used when rapid transport is needed.
   C. they can carry many caregivers.
   D. specialized skills or equipment are needed.

7. How big should the standard landing zone be for a typical helicopter?
   A. 50 × 50 feet
   B. 75 × 75 feet
   C. 100 × 100 feet
   D. 100 × 100 yards

8. What type of light should you use to mark a landing zone?
   A. A strobe light in each corner of the zone
   B. A strobe light in the center of the zone
   C. A spotlight shining straight up in the center of the zone
   D. Blue flares in the center of the zone

9. When should you approach the helicopter after it has landed?
   A. Only after the blades have come to a complete stop
   B. As soon as it touches down
   C. When the pilot or crew on the helicopter signal for you to approach
   D. Never approach; let the crew come to you.

10. Which of the following is NOT a key factor in staffing your ambulances?
   A. Unit cost of each run
   B. Taxpayer subsidies
   C. Response times
   D. The types of calls you will respond to

Labeling

Label the following diagrams with the correct terms.

1. Locations of the Landing Zone
   A. Where to post guard
   B. Pilot's blind area
   C. Pilot's area of vision

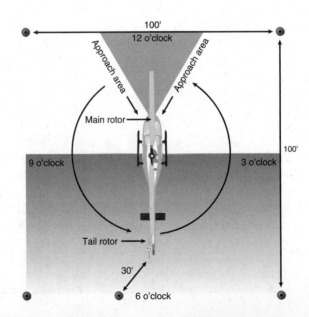

2. Helicopter Hand Signals

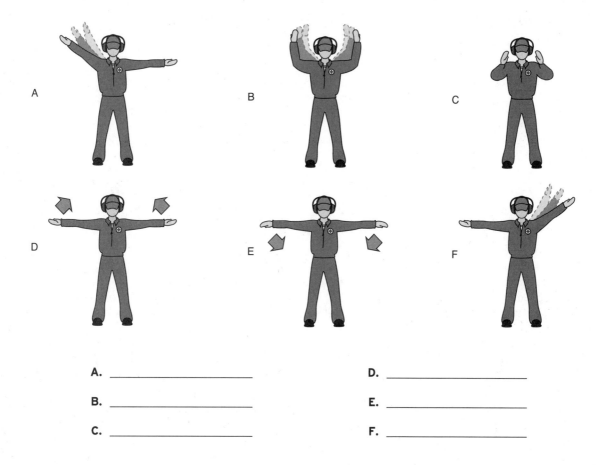

A. _____   D. _____

B. _____   E. _____

C. _____   F. _____

Fill-in-the-Blank

Assume you have been called to the scene of a road crash. Among the equipment listed here, mark an X beside that which you would grab to take along on your first dash from the ambulance to the patient. If any equipment you need has been left off the list, add it at the end and explain why you need it.

One sure way to *waste* time at the scene of a collision (or at any call) is to make a dozen trips back and forth to the ambulance to fetch equipment and supplies that you left behind. Well-organized paramedics take with them everything needed for the primary assessment and first stages of management.

_____ Long-leg air splint   _____ Stethoscope

_____ Drug box   _____ Flashlight

_____ Portable suction unit   _____ Triangular bandages

_____ Oxygen cylinder   _____ Chemical cold packs

_____ OB kit   _____ Cervical collar

_____ Pocket mask   _____ Traction splint

_____ Oropharyngeal airways   _____ Nonrebreathing mask

_____ Intravenous fluid bags   _____ Long backboard/straps

_____ Dressing materials   _____ Oral thermometer

_____ Large-bore IV cannulas   _____ Fire extinguisher

_____ Head immobilizer   _____ Bed pan

_____ Self-adhering roller bandage   _____ Heavy-duty scissors

_____ Selection of board splints   _____ Emesis basin

_____ Wheeled cot stretcher   _____ Handheld radio

_____ ECG monitor   _____ Adhesive bandages

_____ Contact lens remover

Other equipment that might be needed:

_____

_____

Identify

In the following case study, list the chief complaint, vital signs, and pertinent negatives.

Walt and Dave respond to a two-vehicle crash. Their patient is a 41-year-old woman who tried to avoid a car that crossed the centerline on the highway. The SUV she was driving rolled twice and landed on its wheels. The back portion was struck by the oncoming car. Walt is able to gain access through a back door and performs manual stabilization. Dave begins an assessment on the patient. She is conscious and alert and remembers the entire collision. She is complaining of pain in her left shoulder area. The rapid trauma assessment shows a deformity of the left collarbone and bruising beginning around the seat belt marks. Because of the collarbone, a cervical collar won't fit, and so Dave and Walt immobilize the woman on a backboard, pad the neck and head with towels, and then tape them down. Walt first applies supplemental oxygen and then begins baseline vital signs on the woman. He finds that her breathing is 22 breaths/min and shallow with decreased lung sounds on the left. Her pulse is 114 beats/min, and blood pressure is 132/84 mm Hg. The heart monitor shows sinus tachycardia with a few premature ventricular contractions (PVCs) every few minutes. The patient can feel her arms and legs and is rating her pain in the shoulder at a 9/10. Her Pupils are Equal And Round, Regular in size, and react to Light (PEARRL). Skin is warm, but to help with shock, Dave turns the heat on in the unit and places a blanket over her. Walt starts an IV, and they monitor her heart and breathing on the way to the trauma center. Walt does a secondary assessment and a physical exam that turns up a few small scrapes and bruises to her legs. He gets a SAMPLE history just as they pull into the regional trauma center.

a. Chief complaint:

_____

_____

b. Vital signs:

_____

_____

c. Pertinent negatives:

_____

_____

Complete the Patient Care Report (PCR)

Reread the case study in the preceding Identify exercise, and then complete the following PCR for the patient.

EMS Patient Care Report (PCR)					
Date:	**Incident No.:**	**Nature of Call:**		**Location:**	
Dispatched:	**En Route:**	**At Scene:**	**Transport:**	**At Hospital:**	**In Service:**
Patient Information					
Age:		**Allergies:**			
Sex:		**Medications:**			
Weight (in kg [lb]):		**Past Medical History:**			
		Chief Complaint:			
Vital Signs					
Time:	**BP:**	**Pulse:**	**Respirations:**	**SpO$_2$:**	
Time:	**BP:**	**Pulse:**	**Respirations:**	**SpO$_2$:**	
Time:	**BP:**	**Pulse:**	**Respirations:**	**SpO$_2$:**	
EMS Treatment (circle all that apply)					
Oxygen @ _____ L/min via (circle one): NC NRM Bag-Mask Device		**Assisted Ventilation**	**Airway Adjunct**	**CPR**	
Defibrillation	**Bleeding Control**	**Bandaging**	**Splinting**	**Other**	
Narrative					

Ambulance Calls

The following case scenarios provide an opportunity to explore the concerns associated with patient management and paramedic care. Read each scenario, and then answer each question.

1. Unit 2 has been dispatched to a new subdivision for a man who fell off a second-story roof. When Cory and Bill arrive, they find a 22-year-old man unconscious and lying on a large pile of dirt. Cory and Bill don't really like each other much and neither one is willing to concede to the other. They both sprint to the patient to try to be the "lead" medic on the scene. Neither one of them has bothered to take any equipment. The patient is lying on his back. Cory finally performs C-spine stabilization while Bill starts a secondary assessment including a rapid trauma assessment, but that is kind of hard because he has no equipment. Bill sends a worker from the scene to get his orange airway bag out of the squad. After the airway bag arrives, oxygen is applied and Bill does his assessment. The patient doesn't seem to have any broken bones, but is still out cold. One of the workers is trying to tell Cory what happened, but Cory won't listen. He lets the worker know that they are "here" now, and they will handle any medical problems. After about 15 minutes of being on scene, Bill finally has to go get a rigid C-collar, backboard, and cot because the construction workers can't seem to find them even with Bill yelling at them. After they get the patient in the unit, they take vital signs, and they both try to grab the airway bag so that they can intubate. After a few seconds of arguing, they decide to do rock, paper, scissors to pick who gets to intubate. Cory wins and succeeds in intubating, and Bill decides to start a couple of IVs. Bill gives Cory a high-five after he sticks a 14-gauge in the left AC. After they get ready to roll, there is a discussion and another rock, paper, scissors contest to decide who is going to drive. Thirty-four minutes after reaching the scene, they are on the road to the closest hospital. Because their patient is starting to posture, they decide to turn around and head for the trauma center, another 15 minutes away.

   a. What should Cory and Bill have done prior to arriving on the scene?

   _____

   _____

   b. List six questions Cory and Bill should have asked the workers at the scene.

   (1) _____

   (2) _____

   (3) _____

   (4) _____

   (5) _____

   (6) _____

   c. Discuss Cory and Bill's transport decision and what you would have done differently.

   _____

   _____

   _____

   _____

2. Jeff and Larry both show up just a few minutes late for their shift. Both of them were up late the night before watching the Monday night football game on TV. They both agree that because they are late and they each have headaches they will skip the morning check of the squad and go straight for the coffee and aspirin. Right away, they get a call for a woman who has fallen in front of the local grocery store. As they climb into the unit and take off, Jeff can hardly keep the squad on the road. It is doing a shimmy and shake down the road. When they arrive at the grocery store, the patient seems to be okay and doesn't want to go anywhere but home. She denies any pain and

is alert. She states she just stepped off of the curb wrong and lost her balance. The store manager is the one who insisted on calling for an ambulance. Jeff turns off the squad when they decide this is a no-transport and grabs the paperwork for the patient to sign off on. After getting that all cleared up, they jump back into the squad to leave, but it won't start. They miss two calls while waiting for a tow truck. After they get the squad back to the service station, they are really embarrassed to find they were out of gas, and the shimmy they felt earlier was because of low pressure in a back tire. They finally make it back to the station around noon to a very angry supervisor and a stressed-out crew number 2 who had to cover calls for Jeff and Larry.

a.   Why should you check your squad at the beginning of every shift?

_____

_____

b.   What visual factors would you check before jumping in and running a call?

_____

_____

True/False

If you believe the statement to be more true than false, write the letter "T" in the space provided. If you believe the statement to be more false than true, write the letter "F."

_____   **1.**   The standards for ambulances are determined by the Food and Drug Administration (FDA).

_____   **2.**   Original guidelines called for ambulances to be painted orange and white.

_____   **3.**   The DOT KKK 1822 standards developed the three main types of ambulances.

_____   **4.**   The defibrillator and pulse oximeter do not need to be tested.

_____   **5.**   Brake fade is tested before driving the ambulance.

_____   **6.**   The Commission on Accreditation of Ambulance Services (CAAS) recommends that urban response time should be less than 8 minutes.

_____   **7.**   One of the system status management (SSM) goals is to have a paramedic in every unit.

_____   **8.**   A paramedic should always act as an advocate for the patient.

_____   **9.**   Due regard states that if you have your lights and sirens on, you have the right of way and can break the traffic laws.

_____   **10.**   Patient cost is a disadvantage of using an air ambulance.

Short Answer

Complete this section with short written answers using the space provided.

Only 1 out of 10 trauma patients is critically injured. But for that 1 patient out of 10, every minute that elapses between the time of injury and arrival at the operating suite reduces the patient's chances of survival. For that reason, all those who deal with the case in its pre–operating room phase must act as efficiently as possible. List three ways that you can save seconds, or minutes, of the "golden hour (golden period)" without compromising the care of the patient.

1.   _____

2.   _____

3.   _____

Fill-in-the-Table

Fill in the missing parts of the table.

Advantages and Disadvantages of Using an Air Ambulance	
Advantages	**Disadvantages**
• Specialized skills or equipment are needed	• _____
• _____	• Altitude limitations
• _____	• _____
• Helicopter hospital helipads are available	• Aircraft cabin size
• _____	• Terrain
	• _____
	• Patient's condition
	• Restrictions on the number of caregivers
	• _____

Incident Management and Multiple-Casualty Incidents

Matching

Match each of the terms in the right column to the appropriate description in the left column.

_____ **1.** The process of directing responders to return to their facilities when work at a disaster or multiple-casualty incident has finished, at least for the particular responders.

_____ **2.** In incident command, the person appointed to determine the type of equipment and resources needed for a situation involving extrication or special rescue; also called the rescue supervisor.

_____ **3.** The end of the incident command structure when an incident draws to a close.

_____ **4.** In incident command, when an incident commander turns over command to someone with more experience in a critical area.

_____ **5.** An ongoing or uncontained incident in which rescuers will have to search for patients and then triage or treat them. The situation may produce more patients. Examples include school shootings, tornadoes, a hazardous materials release, and rising floodwaters.

_____ **6.** In incident command, the position that carries out the orders of the commander to help resolve the incident.

_____ **7.** In incident command, the position in an incident responsible for accounting of all expenditures.

_____ **8.** An oral or written plan stating general objectives reflecting the overall strategy for managing an incident.

_____ **9.** The overall leader of the incident command system to whom commanders or leaders of the incident command systems divisions report.

_____ **10.** A system implemented to manage disasters and multiple-casualty incidents in which section chiefs—including finance, logistics, operations, and planning—report to the incident commander.

_____ **11.** In incident command, the position that helps procure and stockpile equipment and supplies during an incident.

_____ **12.** A branch of operations in a unified command system, whose three designated sector positions are triage, treatment, and transport.

_____ **13.** In incident command, the person who works with area medical examiners, coroners, and law enforcement agencies to coordinate the disposition of dead victims.

_____ **14.** An emergency situation that can place great demand on the equipment or personnel of the EMS system or that has the potential to overwhelm your available resources.

_____ **15.** An agreement between neighboring EMS systems to respond to multiple-casualty incidents or disasters in each other's region when local resources are insufficient to handle the response.

A. Triage

B. Logistics

C. Morgue supervisor

D. Staging supervisor

E. Public information officer (PIO)

F. Treatment supervisor

G. Finance

H. Liaison officer

I. Rehabilitation supervisor

J. Extrication supervisor

K. Closed incident

L. JumpSTART triage

M. Demobilization

N. Command

O. Critical incident stress management (CISM)

_____ **16.** A Department of Homeland Security system designed to enable federal, state, and local governments and private-sector and nongovernmental organizations to effectively and efficiently prepare for, prevent, respond to, and recover from domestic incidents, regardless of cause, size, or complexity, including acts of catastrophic terrorism.

_____ **17.** A contained incident in which patients are found in one focal location and the situation is not expected to produce more patients than initially present.

_____ **18.** An area designated by the incident commander, or a designee, in which public information officers from multiple agencies disseminate information about the incident.

_____ **19.** A sorting system for pediatric patients younger than 8 years or weighing less than 100 pounds. There is a minor adaptation for infants because they cannot ambulate on their own.

_____ **20.** In incident command, the person who relays information, concerns, and requests among responding agencies.

_____ **21.** In incident command, the position that oversees the incident, establishes the objectives and priorities, and from there develops a response plan.

_____ **22.** A process that confronts responses to critical incidents and defuses them.

_____ **23.** In incident command, the position that ultimately produces a plan to resolve any incident.

_____ **24.** A type of patient sorting used to rapidly categorize patients; the focus is on speed in locating all patients and determining an initial priority as their condition warrants.

_____ **25.** In incident command, the person who keeps the public informed and relates any information to the press.

_____ **26.** In incident command, the person who establishes an area that provides protection for responders from the elements and the situation.

_____ **27.** In incident command, the person appointed to determine the type of equipment and resources needed for a situation involving extrication or special rescue; also called the extrication supervisor.

_____ **28.** In incident command, the person who gives the "go ahead" to a plan or who may stop an operation when rescuer safety is an issue.

_____ **29.** A type of patient sorting used in the treatment sector that involves retriage of patients.

_____ **30.** A command system in which one person is in charge, generally used with small incidents that involve only one responding agency or one jurisdiction.

_____ **31.** In incident command, the subordinate positions under the commander's direction to which the workload is distributed; the supervisor/worker ratio.

_____ **32.** When individual units or different organizations make independent and often inefficient decisions about the next appropriate action.

_____ **33.** The capabilities of a receiving hospital to handle a large number of unexpected emergency patients, such as those seen in a multiple-casualty incident.

P. Unified command system

Q. Medical incident command

R. Multiple-casualty incident (MCI)

S. Primary triage

T. Mutual aid response

U. Triage supervisor

V. Rescue supervisor

W. Safety officer

X. National Incident Management System (NIMS)

Y. Open incident

Z. Transportation supervisor

AA. Operations

BB. Transfer of command

CC. Secondary triage

DD. Termination of command

EE. START triage

FF. Freelancing

GG. Hospital surge capacity

_____ **34.** In incident command, the person who locates an area to stage equipment and personnel, and tracks unit arrival and deployment from the staging area.

_____ **35.** A patient sorting process that stands for simple triage and rapid treatment and uses a limited assessment of the patient's ability to walk, respiratory status, hemodynamic status, and neurologic status.

_____ **36.** In incident command, the person who coordinates transportation and distribution of patients to appropriate receiving hospitals.

_____ **37.** In incident command, the person responsible for locating, setting up, and supervising the treatment area.

_____ **38.** To sort patients based on the severity of their conditions and prioritize them for care accordingly.

_____ **39.** The person in charge of prioritizing patients, whose primary duty is to ensure that every patient receives initial triage.

_____ **40.** A command system used in larger incidents in which there is a multiagency response or multiple jurisdictions are involved.

HH. Joint information center

II. Incident action plan

JJ. Incident command system (ICS)

KK. Incident commander (IC)

LL. Planning

MM. Span of control

NN. Single command system

Multiple Choice

Read each item carefully, and then select the best response.

1. The ICS is designed to control duplication of effort and:
   A. triaging.
   B. application of triage tags.
   C. freelancing.
   D. communication coding.

2. A large hazardous materials incident would require what kind of command system?
   A. Single command system
   B. Unified command system
   C. Rescue command system
   D. Medical command system

3. When sizing up a multiple-casualty incident (MCI) scene, which of the following questions does NOT fit in scene size-up?
   A. What do I have?
   B. What resources do I need?
   C. Who is coming to help?
   D. What do I need to do?

4. What is the triage supervisor ultimately responsible for?
   A. Triage of every patient
   B. Movement of patients to a treatment sector
   C. Counting and prioritizing all patients
   D. Transportation to the hospitals

5. Where should the rehabilitation area be located?
   A. As close as possible to the treatment area
   B. Next to the media area
   C. Outside
   D. Away from the scene and the media

6. What does the _D_ stand for in the **IDME** mnemonic that applies to triage?
   A. Delayed
   B. Dead
   C. Don't move
   D. Decompensated shock

7. Which of the following is NOT a special consideration during triage?
   A. A hysterical and disruptive patient
   B. An injured rescue worker
   C. Death of a friend
   D. Hazardous material exposure

8. What color triage tag would you give a patient at an MCI who is breathing 4 breaths/min after you have opened the person's airway?
   A. Green
   B. Yellow
   C. Red
   D. Black

9. When arriving on a scene to begin triage, what is a good thing to yell to the patients?
   A. If you can walk, move across the street to the oak tree.
   B. Stay where you are, and we will move all of you.
   C. Everyone just lie still and raise your hand if you think you are okay.
   D. Run for your lives! Clear the area as fast as you can.

10. What is your number one priority at the scene of an MCI?
    A. Triage of patients
    B. Scene safety
    C. Treatment of patients
    D. Setting up the proper sectors

Labeling

Label the following diagrams with the correct terms.

1. Diagram of an MCI

   Label the following areas:
   A. Treatment area
   B. Triage area
   C. Extrication area
   D. Incident area

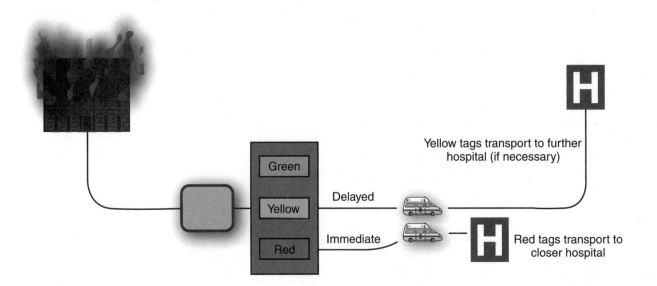

2. The JumpSTART Pediatric MCI Triage Algorithm

Indicate if the following are:

A. Black/Nonsalvageable

B. Red/Immediate

C. Yellow/Delayed

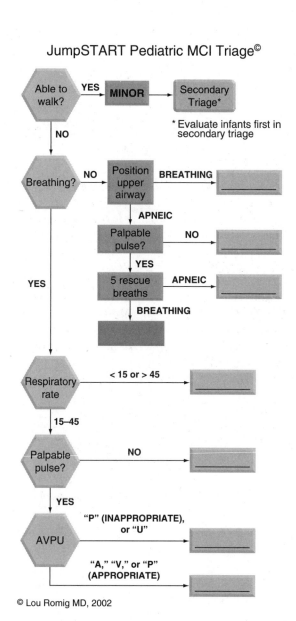

JumpSTART Pediatric MCI Triage©

© Lou Romig MD, 2002

Fill-in-the-Blank

Read each item carefully, and then complete the statement by filling in the missing word(s).

1. A/an _____-_____ _____ refers to any call that involves three or more patients, any situation that places such a great demand on available equipment or personnel that the system would require a/an _____ _____ _____, or any incident that has the potential to create one of the previously mentioned situations.

2. A/an _____ incident is a situation that is expected to produce no more patients than are initially present.

3. The _____ section chief is responsible for documenting all expenditures at the incident that will need to be reimbursed.

4. The three officers that will help incident command (IC) the most are the _____, _____, and _____ officers.

5. _____ is a component of the National Incident Management System (NIMS) that establishes measures for all responders to incorporate into their systems in preparation to respond to all incidents at any time.

6. The _____ supervisor coordinates and distributes patients to the appropriate hospitals.

7. Initial triage done in the field is known as _____, and then the _____ triage is done as the patients are brought to the treatment sector.

8. The *R* in the START triage system stands for _____.

9. _____ START was developed for pediatric patients involved in an MCI.

10. The _____ supervisor is in charge of parking vehicles and collecting supplies to be used at the scene.

Identify

In the following case study, list the chief complaint, vital signs, and pertinent negatives.

You have responded to a blast at a local fertilizer plant. Your patient is a 32-year-old man who is found outside the blast area. He is lying on his side because he has a piece of wood impaled in his left buttock. He is conscious and alert. The wood is sticking out about 6 inches and there is not much blood. He is unable to move because of the wood. Your partner starts the primary assessment and secondary assessment as you apply oxygen. The rapid trauma assessment shows small nicks and cuts on the man's back and legs, but they are all secondary injuries that are not life threatening. He says he was knocked to the ground when the explosion occurred. You are taking no chances and place him in a rigid cervical collar even though you won't be able to lay him flat. He is breathing 20 breaths/min, with an oxygen saturation of 97% and clear lung sounds. Pulse is 98 beats/min and regular, and blood pressure is 136/88 mm Hg. The patient rates his pain at a 7/10. His skin is warm and dry. You stabilize the wood in place and place the patient on a backboard and then use pillows to help stabilize him from rolling off his right side. You get him in the unit, place him on the heart monitor (which shows normal sinus rhythm), and then start an IV on him. You give him 5 mg of morphine for the pain because it is really starting to hurt since you moved him. You opt for the regional trauma center even though it is 7 minutes farther away than the community hospital.

1. Chief complaint:

   _____

   _____

2. Vital signs:

   _____

   _____

3. Pertinent negatives:

   _____

   _____

Ambulance Calls

The following case scenarios provide an opportunity to explore the concerns associated with patient management and paramedic care. Read each scenario, and then answer each question.

1. It is a hot, stuffy day in June in your community of 1,600 people. You are on a volunteer rescue squad in your home community and work for a critical care ground transport company in the city 25 miles away. It is your day off and you are enjoying the weather, but there have been tornado watches issued for your area. Later in the afternoon, the weather begins to get a little more serious, and you switch on your radio to get the latest updates. At 4:30 PM sirens go off indicating a tornado in the area, so you head down to the basement with your kids and the dog. Your wife is

at work at the nursing home. Before you know it, it sounds as if a freight train has hit your home. After everything is quiet, you fight your way out of the basement only to see total devastation of what used to be your community. You check with your neighbors to see if they are okay and decide to leave your kids with them. Because your truck is nowhere to be found, you grab a bike lying in the street and head down to the fire department.

Okay, take a little break here and answer a few questions. Consider working in teams and compare notes after you have answered your questions.

a. List 10 things you would like to have in your emergency kit to take with you.

(1) _____

(2) _____

(3) _____

(4) _____

(5) _____

(6) _____

(7) _____

(8) _____

(9) _____

(10) _____

b. There is a lot of damage in the area, and people are gathering in the streets. What are you going to tell them to do as you ride by on your bicycle?

_____

_____

c. What type of hazards can you expect during the 2-mile ride to the fire station?

_____

_____

2. You finally arrive at the fire department as the rest of your crew gathers; there are 24 emergency responders present. It has been estimated that at least 100 homes were destroyed plus the nursing home, which houses 75 patients. This really worries you because you know your wife was there when the storm hit. The firehouse and the high school two blocks away have not been touched by the twister. You have three ambulances and six fire trucks. Emergency management has two pickups, and the sheriff's office has three cars available. Word has gone out to the surrounding communities asking for all the help you can get.

a. Who should take command of this situation, and where should you set up the command post?

_____

_____

b. What type of buildings can be used for an emergency center for the walking wounded and displaced victims of the storm?

_____

_____

3. This is going to be a long night. Power is out all over town. You quickly begin to break into teams to begin searching for patients. There are many injuries at the nursing home as a result of the large number of people who were unable to get underground. You are sent there to work in the treatment center, and you see around 60 people with injuries over the next 6 hours. Your wife has made it through okay with only minor cuts. She is classified as walking wounded and actually pitches in to help with the patients that are worse. It takes 24 hours for all the homes to be searched, and your town suffers three deaths caused by this tornado. Three days later, most of the power has been restored to the houses that are still standing, and things start to calm down around town. There will be cleanup going on for the next few months, and it will take a couple of years to put everything back together. You are thankful that all the agencies in your town, even though they are small, work well together and have prepared for this type of emergency.

a. List some outside agencies in your area that will be able to help you in the first 3 hours of this disaster.

_____

_____

_____

True/False

If you believe the statement to be more true than false, write the letter "T" in the space provided. If you believe the statement to be more false than true, write the letter "F."

_____ **1.** There will never be physicians on the scene of an MCI.

_____ **2.** The planning section solves problems as they arise at an MCI.

_____ **3.** Critical infrastructures include electricity, water, fuel, and communications systems.

_____ **4.** An open incident is where you have not found all the victims.

_____ **5.** Command functions include triage and treatment functions.

_____ **6.** The safety officer has the power to stop all rescue functions.

_____ **7.** One function of the planning section is the development of an incident action plan.

_____ **8.** Face-to-face communications are the best because of infrastructure problems at the scene of an MCI.

_____ **9.** Yellow tag patients are deemed immediate priority patients because they have the best chance of survival.

_____ **10.** The second step in the START process is triage of the nonwalking patients.

Short Answer

Complete this section with short written answers using the space provided.

1. Discuss the first step of the START triage system.

_____

_____

2. Discuss the second step of the START triage system.

_____

_____

3. Why is the JumpSTART triage system needed for a pediatric patient?

_____

_____

4. Why should you participate in the critical incident stress management in the rehabilitation sector?

_____

_____

Fill-in-the-Table

Fill in the missing parts of the table.

MCI Equipment and Supplies*	
Airway control	PPE (gloves, face shield, HEPA or N-95 mask)
	_____
	Rigid-tip Yankauer and flexible suction catheters
	LMA, Combitube, King-LT, ET tubes*
	_____
	Tube restraint, tape, syringes, stylet*
	End-tidal CO_2 device
Breathing	_____
	Bag-mask device(s) (adult and child), spare masks
	Oxygen delivery devices (nonrebreathing mask, cannula, extension tubing)
	_____
	Large-bore IV catheter for thoracic decompression*
Circulation	_____
	Sphygmomanometer, stethoscope
	Burn dressings, burn sheets, sterile water for irrigation
	_____
	1,000-mL bags of normal saline, IV start kits, catheters*
Disability	_____
	Head beds, wide tape, backboard straps
	_____
Exposure	Space blanket to cover patients
	Scissors
Logistic/Command	Sector vests (triage, treatment, transport, staging, command, rescue)
	Pads of paper, pencils, pens, markers
	_____
	Assessment cards
Note: The items denoted by * could be packaged in an ALS pod.	

48 Vehicle Extrication and Special Rescue

Matching

Match each of the definitions in the left column to the appropriate term in the right column.

_____ **1.** A method of accounting for all personnel at an emergency incident and ensuring that only personnel with specific assignments are permitted to work within the various zones.

_____ **2.** Technique of controlling the rope as it is fed out to climbers.

_____ **3.** Specialized cribbing assemblies made out of wood or plastic in a step configuration.

_____ **4.** A high-risk situation where law enforcement agencies may deploy use of specialized law enforcement tactical units or the special weapons and tactics (SWAT) team.

_____ **5.** A complex rescue incident involving vehicles or machinery, water or ice, rope techniques, a trench or excavation collapse, confined spaces, a structural collapse, wilderness search and rescue, or hazardous materials, and which requires specially trained personnel and special equipment.

_____ **6.** Vehicle design where the body of the vehicle is placed onto a frame skeleton and the frame acts as the foundation for the vehicle. The design consists of two large beams tied together by cross member beams.

_____ **7.** Phenomenon associated with cold water immersion in which reflexes in the body and a lowered metabolic rate help preserve basic body functions.

_____ **8.** A space with limited or restricted access that is not meant for continuous occupancy, such as a manhole, well, or tank.

_____ **9.** A rope rescue operation where the angle of the slope is greater than 45 degrees; rescuers depend on life safety rope rather than a fixed support such as the ground.

_____ **10.** The area immediately surrounding an incident site that is directly dangerous to life and health. All personnel working in this area must wear complete and appropriate protective clothing and equipment. Entry requires approval by the incident commander or a designated sector officer. Complete backup, rescue, and decontamination teams must be in place at the perimeter before operations begin.

_____ **11.** The training level that provides a high level of competency in the various disciplines of technical or hazardous materials rescue for rescuers who will be directly involved in the rescue operation itself.

_____ **12.** A type of glass that is heat-treated so that it will break into small pieces.

A. Wedges

B. Tactical situation

C. Unibody construction

D. Spoil pile

E. Technician

F. Simple access

G. Technical rescue incident (TRI)

H. Self-rescue position

I. Cold protective response

J. Secondary collapse

K. Accountability system

L. Awareness

_____ **13.** An atmospheric concentration of any toxic, corrosive, or asphyxiant substance that poses an immediate threat to life or that could cause irreversible or delayed adverse health effects. The three general types are toxic, flammable, and oxygen-deficient.

M. Body-over-frame construction

_____ **14.** Type of window glazing that incorporates a sheeting material that stops the glass from breaking into shards.

N. Alternative powered vehicles

_____ **15.** A rope rescue operation on a mildly sloping surface (less than 45 degrees) or flat land where rescuers are dependent on the ground for their primary support, and the rope system is a secondary means of support.

O. Belay

_____ **16.** A vehicle that uses fuels other than petroleum or a combination of petroleum and another fuel for power.

P. Search and rescue

_____ **17.** The first level of rescue training provided to all responders, with an emphasis on recognizing the hazards, securing the scene, and calling for appropriate assistance. There is no actual use of rescue skills.

Q. Cold zone

_____ **18.** The technical rescue training level geared toward working in the warm zone of an incident. Training at this level allows responders to directly assist those conducting the rescue operation and to use certain rescue skills and procedures.

R. Confined space

_____ **19.** A method used to ascend rocky faces and ridges; it can be considered a cross between hill climbing and rock climbing.

S. High-angle operations

_____ **20.** The process of locating and removing a patient from the wilderness.

T. Hot zone

_____ **21.** Short lengths of wood that are used to stabilize vehicles.

U. Warm zone

_____ **22.** A condition in which a patient is trapped by debris, soil, or other material and is unable to extricate himself or herself.

V. Tempered glass

_____ **23.** Any tool or equipment operating from human power.

W. Technical rescue team

_____ **24.** A collapse that occurs following the primary collapse. This can occur in trench, excavation, and structural collapse.

X. Shims

_____ **25.** Position used in fast-moving water rescue situations. The rescuer rolls into a face-up arched position with the lower back higher than the feet to avoid objects below the surface. The feet should be together and facing in the direction of travel (feet first), with arms at the sides.

Y. Shoring

_____ **26.** Access that is easily achieved with the use of simple hand tools or force.

Z. Special weapons and tactics (SWAT) team

_____ **27.** Also commonly known as a life vest, this allows the body to float in water.

AA. Step chocks

_____ **28.** To descend on a fixed rope.

BB. Scrambling

_____ **29.** A specialized law enforcement tactical unit.

CC. Rappelling

_____ **30.** The pile of dirt that has been removed from an excavation. The pile may be unstable and prone to collapse.

DD. Complex access

_____ **31.** A group of rescuers specially trained in the various disciplines of technical rescue.

EE. Cribbing

_____ **32.** A vehicle design with no formal frame structure; the body and frame are one piece, which is considered to be the structural integrity of the vehicle.

FF. Entrapment

_____ **33.** Objects that are smaller than wedges used to snug loose cribbing under a load or to fill void spaces.

GG. Hand tool

_____ **34.** A method of supporting a trench wall or building components such as walls, floors, or ceilings using either hydraulic, pneumatic, or wood shoring systems.

HH. Laminated glass

_____ **35.** The area located between the hot zone and the cold zone at an incident. Decontamination stations are located here.

II. Immediately dangerous to life and health (IDLH)

_____ **36.** A safe area for those agencies involved in the operations; the incident commander, command post, EMS providers, and other support functions necessary to control the incident should be located here.

JJ. Operations

_____ **37.** Complicated entry that requires special tools and training and includes breaking windows or using other force.

KK. Low-angle operations

_____ **38.** Used to snug loose cribbing.

LL. Personal flotation device (PFD)

Multiple Choice

Read each item carefully, and then select the best response.

1. Which of the following is NOT considered a technical rescue incident?
   A. Trench collapse
   B. A fender-bender collision
   C. Water rescue
   D. Wilderness search and rescue

2. What is the first priority in a rescue situation?
   A. Mobilizing the correct teams
   B. Following the golden rule of public service
   C. Protecting the patient during the rescue
   D. Ensuring rescuer safety

3. The "A" in the mnemonic FAILURE stands for:
   A. additional medical problems not considered.
   B. additional patients not accounted for.
   C. acclimation to the weather.
   D. additional equipment needed.

4. You find the entry and rescue teams in the _____ zone(s).
   A. cold
   B. warm
   C. hot
   D. warm and hot

5. Which of the following is NOT necessary to know when gathering information about a scene before you arrive?
   A. The road conditions en route to the incident
   B. The nature of the incident
   C. The location of the incident
   D. The specific hazard information

6. Who is in charge of having all of the utilities shut down at a scene?
   A. Dispatcher
   B. Incident command
   C. Police chief
   D. Fire chief

7. Which of the following is NOT a technique for calming a patient during a lengthy rescue?
   A. Allowing time for the patient to respond to you
   B. Lying to the patient to keep him or her calm
   C. Being aware of your body language
   D. Making and keeping eye contact with the patient

8. On a vehicle, the "A" post is:
   A. the post between the front seat and back seat.
   B. the post between the middle seat and back seat.
   C. the post that holds in the windshield.
   D. the post that holds in the back window.

9. When you need to stabilize a vehicle, you use a stout piece of lumber that is 4 inches by 4 inches. This is called:
   A. a step block.
   B. wedging.
   C. a "C block."
   D. cribbing.

10. If you are unable to gain easy access by opening a door to the wrecked vehicle, what is the next best procedure?
   A. Break the windshield
   B. Displace the door
   C. Peel back the roof
   D. Break a side window

Labeling

Label the following diagrams with the correct terms.

1. Label the A, B, and C posts on the vehicle below.

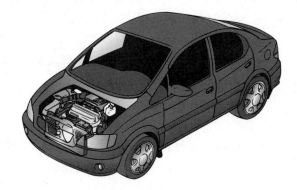

2. Label the following photos with the appropriate type of wood cribbing design.

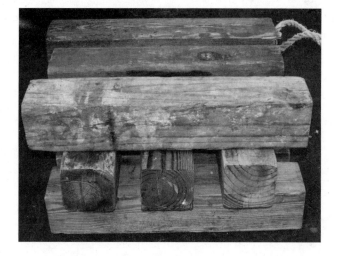

A. _____

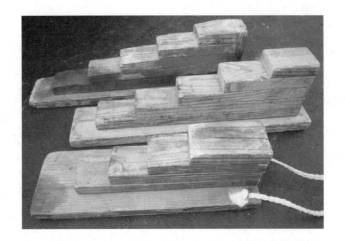

B. _____

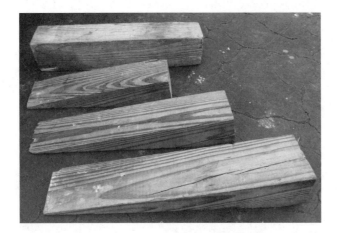

C. _____

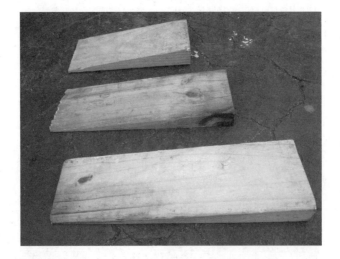

D. _____

Fill-in-the-Blank

Read each item carefully, and then complete the statement by filling in the missing word(s).

1. Before removing a windshield, you should _____ your patient from flying glass.

2. If the air bag on the driver's side has not deployed during the car crash, it poses a/an _____ for the driver and the rescuers.

3. When displacing a roof, you should cut the _____ post(s) and fold back the roof.

4. A/an _____ _____ is a location that is surrounded by a structure that is not designed for continuous occupancy.

5. _____ _____ is a gas that is released when bacteria break down organic material without oxygen. It is flammable, toxic, and colorless.

6. When dealing with an entrapment or trench collapse, the patient is dug out only after _____ has been put in place.

7. If you find yourself being swept away in fast water during a rescue, you should position yourself in the _____-_____ _____.

8. The first thing to do when attempting to help a person during a water rescue is to _____ _____ to the person.

9. When responding to a drowning (submersion), you have only a short time before the rescue becomes a/an _____.

10. You respond to a rescue situation where the patient is down a slope that is less than 45°. This is known as a/an _____-_____ operation.

Identify

In the following case study, list the chief complaint, vital signs, and pertinent negatives.

You are called to a vehicle that has rolled down a 75-foot embankment. The special rappelling team responded and has secured your patient on a backboard and then placed him in a Stokes basket. They pull the basket up the embankment for you to start working on the patient. He was wearing his seat belt when he lost control of the car and rolled. The patient, Jim, is conscious, but unable to answer any questions except for providing his first name. Your partner applies high-flow supplemental oxygen, and you begin a trauma assessment while your partner takes the baseline vitals. Jim has multiple cuts on his face and head, with some blood coming from his left ear. You find instability in the pelvic region and a deformed left arm and collarbone. Jim's blood pressure is 102/68 mm Hg, and pulse is thready in the wrist at a rate of 116 beats/min. His oxygen saturation is 96%, and his breathing is shallow at 24 breaths/min. Lung sounds are slightly diminished on the left side. Jim is cool to the touch and appears very pale. His Pupils are Equal And Round, and Regular in size, but do not react very quickly to light. You know that Jim needs to be at a regional trauma center, and you call for air medical transport. After hooking up the heart monitor, you find that Jim is in sinus tachycardia. Your partner does a halo test on the blood coming from his ear, and it is negative. Jim begins to come around a little more but doesn't remember any of the crash. Your partner starts two large-bore intravenous lines (IVs) with normal saline, while you do a secondary assessment. You find some rigidity in the lower abdomen. After you give a quick report to the helicopter personnel, Jim is flown to the closest regional trauma center.

1. Chief complaint:

   _____

   _____

2. Vital signs:

   _____

   _____

3. Pertinent negatives:

   _____

   _____

Complete the Patient Care Report (PCR)

Reread the case study in the preceding Identify exercise and then complete the following PCR for the patient.

EMS Patient Care Report (PCR)					
Date:	Incident No.:	Nature of Call:			Location:
Dispatched:	En Route:	At Scene:	Transport:	At Hospital:	In Service:

Patient Information	
Age:	Allergies:
Sex:	Medications:
Weight (in kg [lb]):	Past Medical History:
	Chief Complaint:

Vital Signs				
Time:	BP:	Pulse:	Respirations:	SpO$_2$:
Time:	BP:	Pulse:	Respirations:	SpO$_2$:
Time:	BP:	Pulse:	Respirations:	SpO$_2$:

EMS Treatment (circle all that apply)				
Oxygen @ _____ L/min via (circle one): NC NRM Bag-Mask Device		Assisted Ventilation	Airway Adjunct	CPR
Defibrillation	Bleeding Control	Bandaging	Splinting	Other

Narrative

Ambulance Calls

The following case scenario provides an opportunity to explore the concerns associated with patient management and paramedic care. Read the scenario, and then answer each question.

1. You and your crew (two other paramedics) are called to the scene of a highway crash just outside of town. Arriving at the scene, you see a late-model sedan "accordioned" against a utility pole. The windshield is shattered. The driver is unconscious, bleeding, and tightly pinned between the steering wheel and the seat. There are no passengers.

   a. List in order the steps you would take. Include details of how you would reach the patient.

   (1) _____

   _____

   (2) _____

   _____

   (3) _____

   _____

   (4) _____

   _____

   (5) _____

   _____

   (6) _____

   _____

   (7) _____

   _____

   (8) _____

   _____

   b. List the actions you would take after the patient has been transferred to the care of emergency department personnel.

   (1) _____

   (2) _____

True/False

If you believe the statement to be more true than false, write the letter "T" in the space provided. If you believe the statement to be more false than true, write the letter "F."

_____ 1. In an extrication, the primary function of a paramedic is to direct the disentanglement of the patient from the wreckage.

_____ 2. The most efficient access to a patient in a badly damaged vehicle is usually through a window on the passenger side of the vehicle.

_____ 3. Care of the car crash victim should start even before the patient is removed from the vehicle.

_____ 4. The paramedic should treat all downed wires as if they are charged until the power company turns them off.

_____ 5. To protect the scene and the rescuers, place a large emergency vehicle at an angle to provide a barrier against oncoming traffic.

_____ **6.** A disabled vehicle that is upright on four wheels still needs to be stabilized before anyone enters it to reach the injured inside.

_____ **7.** The windshield is another easy way to gain access.

_____ **8.** The most common tool used to remove tempered glass is a flat-head axe.

_____ **9.** Removal of the patient is referred to as disentanglement.

_____ **10.** The air bag energy capacitor can store power for up to 30 minutes.

Short Answer

Complete this section with short written answers using the space provided.

   1. Discuss the three phases of training that you might receive in technical rescue.

     a. Awareness:

_____

_____

     b. Operations:

_____

_____

     c. Technician:

_____

_____

   2. Discuss the five guidelines that are useful when working with a rescue team.

     a.

_____

_____

     b.

_____

     c.

_____

     d.

_____

_____

     e.

_____

_____

3. What gear is considered minimal for a water rescuer?

_____

_____

4. When breaking glass in an automobile, discuss the differences of the glass in the windows versus the windshield.

_____

_____

Fill-in-the-Table

Fill in the missing parts of the table.

1. Write in the correct statement for the letters for the mnemonic "FAILURE."

Failure Mnemonic	
F	_____
A	_____
I	_____
L	_____
U	_____
R	_____
E	_____

Skill Drills

Test your knowledge of skill drills by placing the following photos in the correct order. Number the first step with a "1," the second step with a "2," and so on.

Stabilizing a Suspected Spinal Injury in the Water

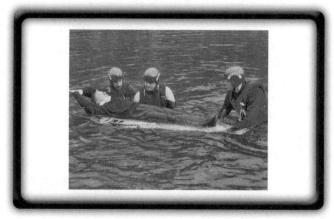

_____ Float a buoyant backboard under the patient as you continue ventilation.

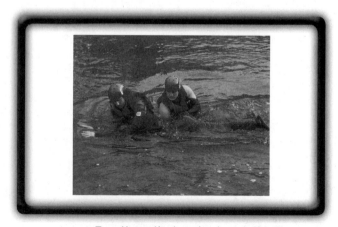

_____ Turn the patient supine by rotating the entire upper half of the patient's body as a single unit.

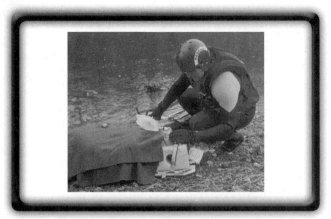

_____ Remove the patient's wet clothes and cover the patient with a blanket. Apply oxygen if breathing adequately; apply positive-pressure ventilation if apneic or breathing inadequately. Begin CPR if breathing and pulse are absent.

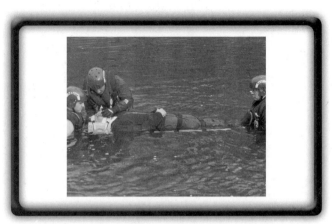

_____ Secure the trunk and head of the patient to the backboard to eliminate motion of the cervical spine.

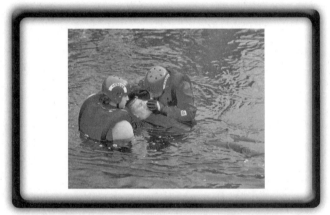

_____ As soon as the patient is turned, begin artificial ventilation using the mouth-to-mouth method or a pocket mask.

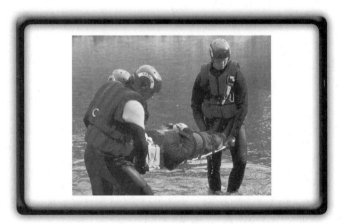

_____ Remove the patient from the water, on the backboard.

Hazardous Materials

Matching

Match each of the items in the right column to the appropriate definition in the left column.

_____ **1.** A type of decontamination that is done with large pads that the hazardous materials team uses to soak up liquid and remove it from the patient.

_____ **2.** Any gas that displaces oxygen from the atmosphere; can be deadly if exposure occurs in a confined space.

_____ **3.** An organization, office, or person responsible for enforcing the requirements of a code or standard, or for approving equipment, materials, an installation, or a procedure.

_____ **4.** A document carried by drivers of commercial vehicles that should provide specific information about what is carried on the vehicle.

_____ **5.** A tool to help predict downward concentrations of hazardous materials based on the input of environmental factors into a computer model.

_____ **6.** A chemical asphyxiant that results in a cellular respiratory failure; this gas ties up hemoglobin to the extent that oxygen in the blood becomes inaccessible to the cells.

_____ **7.** A glass, plastic, or steel nonbulk storage container, ranging in volume from 5 to 15 gallons.

_____ **8.** Bulk packaging that is permanently attached to or forms a part of a motor vehicle, or is not permanently attached to any motor vehicle, and that, because of its size, construction, or attachment to a motor vehicle, is loaded or unloaded without being removed from the motor vehicle.

_____ **9.** Substances that interfere with the use of oxygen at the cellular level.

_____ **10.** A resource available to emergency responders via telephone on a 24-hour basis.

_____ **11.** Any vessel or receptacle that holds material, including storage vessels, pipelines, and packaging.

_____ **12.** A class of chemicals with either high or low pH levels. Exposure can cause severe soft-tissue damage.

_____ **13.** A chemical asphyxiant used in many industrial processes; exposure can occur from by-products of combustion at structural fires.

_____ **14.** Portable, nonbulk, compressed gas containers used to hold liquids and gases. Uninsulated compressed gas cylinders are used to store substances such as nitrogen, argon, helium, and oxygen. They have a range of sizes and internal pressures.

_____ **15.** A controlled area within the warm zone where decontamination takes place.

_____ **16.** A type of decontamination method that uses copious amounts of water to flush the contaminant from the skin or eyes.

A. Solvents

B. Systemic effect

C. Threshold limit value (TLV)

D. Threshold limit value/ short-term exposure limit (TLV-STEL)

E. Toxic products of combustion

F. Upper flammable limit (UFL)

G. Vapor pressure

H. Water soluble

I. Lethal dose (LD)

J. Level B ensemble

K. Level D ensemble

L. Lower flammable limit (LFL)

M. Nonbulk storage vessels

N. Medical monitoring

O. MC-331 pressure cargo tanker

P. SLUDGEM

_____ **17.** A type of decontamination in which as much clothing and equipment as possible are disposed of to reduce the magnitude of the problem.

_____ **18.** The principle that the longer a hazardous material is in contact with the body or the greater the concentration, the greater the effect will most likely be.

_____ **19.** Barrel-like nonbulk storage vessels used to store a wide variety of substances, including food-grade materials, corrosives, flammable liquids, and grease. They may be constructed of low-carbon steel, polyethylene, cardboard, stainless steel, nickel, or other materials.

_____ **20.** Tanks designed to carry dry bulk goods such as powders, pellets, fertilizers, or grain. Such tanks are generally V-shaped with rounded sides that funnel toward the bottom.

_____ **21.** The process of removing the bulk of contaminants off a victim without regard for containment. It is used in potentially life-threatening situations, without the formal establishment of a decontamination corridor.

_____ **22.** The removal or relocation of people who may be affected by an approaching release of hazardous material.

_____ **23.** An expression of a fuel/air mixture, defined by upper and lower limits, that reflects an amount of flammable vapor mixed with a given volume of air.

_____ **24.** The minimum temperature at which a liquid or a solid releases sufficient vapor to form an ignitable mixture with air.

_____ **25.** Any substance that is toxic, poisonous, radioactive, flammable, or explosive and causes injury or death with exposure.

_____ **26.** The federal OSHA regulation that governs hazardous materials waste site and response training. Specifics can be found in Title 29, standard number 1910.120. Subsection (q) is specific to emergency response.

_____ **27.** The minimum temperature at which a fuel, when heated, will ignite in air and continue to burn.

_____ **28.** A phrase that means the atmospheric concentration of any toxic, corrosive, or asphyxiant substance will pose an immediate threat to life, irreversible or delayed adverse effects, or serious interference for a team member attempting to escape from the dangerous atmosphere; a respirator is mandatory.

_____ **29.** A bulk container that serves as both a shipping and a storage vessel. Such tanks hold between 5,000 and 6,000 gallons of product and can be pressurized or nonpressurized. It may be shipped by all modes of transportation.

_____ **30.** Signage at least 3.9 inches on each side that is often required on all four sides of individual packages and boxes that are being transported.

_____ **31.** The concentration of a material in air that, on the basis of laboratory tests (inhalation route), is expected to kill a specified number of the group of test animals when administered over a specified period of time.

_____ **32.** A single dose that causes the death of a specified number of the group of test animals exposed by any route other than inhalation.

_____ **33.** The highest level of protection suit worn by hazardous materials personnel. May also be referred to as fully encapsulating because the suit covers everything, including the breathing apparatus.

Q. Secondary contamination

R. Primary contamination

S. Permissible exposure limit (PEL)

T. Material safety data sheets (MSDS)

U. MC-307/DOT 407 chemical hauler

V. Carboy

W. Absorption

X. Authority having jurisdiction (AHJ)

Y. CAMEO

Z. Carbon monoxide

AA. Bill of lading

BB. Asphyxiant

CC. Cargo tank

DD. CHEMTREC

EE. Corrosives

FF. Cylinders

GG. Dry bulk cargo tanks

_____ **34.** Personal protective equipment that is one step less protective than level A, but provides for a high level of respiratory protection.

_____ **35.** A level of personal protective equipment that provides splash protection.

_____ **36.** The level of protection that fire fighter turnout gear provides.

_____ **37.** An effect of a hazardous material on the body that is limited to the area of contact.

_____ **38.** The minimum amount of gaseous fuel that must be present in the air for the air/fuel mixture to be flammable or explosive.

_____ **39.** The physical process of reducing or removing surface contaminants from large numbers of victims in potentially life-threatening situations in the fastest time possible.

_____ **40.** Information documents that are supposed to be kept on site at workplaces for every potentially hazardous chemical at the workplace.

_____ **41.** A vehicle that typically carries between 6,000 gallons and 10,000 gallons of a product such as gasoline or other flammable and combustible materials. The tank is nonpressurized.

_____ **42.** A tanker with a rounded or horseshoe-shaped tank capable of holding 6,000 to 7,000 gallons of flammable liquid, mild corrosives, and poisons. The tank has a high internal working pressure.

_____ **43.** A tanker that often carries aggressive (highly reactive) acids such as concentrated sulfuric and nitric acid. It is characterized by several heavy-duty reinforcing rings around the tank and holds approximately 6,000 gallons of product.

_____ **44.** A tanker that carries materials such as ammonia, propane, Freon, and butane. This type of tank is commonly constructed of steel and has rounded ends and a single open compartment inside. The liquid volume inside the tank varies, ranging from the 1,000-gallon delivery truck to the full-size 11,000-gallon cargo tank.

_____ **45.** A low-pressure tanker designed to maintain the low temperature required by the cryogens it carries. A boxlike structure containing the tank control valves is typically attached to the rear of the tanker.

_____ **46.** The process of assessing the health status of hazardous materials team members before and after entry to a hazardous incident site.

_____ **47.** A type of decontamination that uses one chemical to change the hazardous material into two less harmful substances; rarely used by hazardous materials teams.

_____ **48.** Any container other than bulk storage containers such as drums, bags, compressed gas cylinders, and cryogenic containers. These vessels hold commonly used commercial and industrial chemicals such as solvents, cleaners, and compounds.

_____ **49.** The maximum concentration of a chemical that a person may be exposed to under OSHA regulations.

_____ **50.** Signage at least 10.8 inches on each side that is often required to be on all four sides of transport vehicles identifying the hazardous contents of the vehicle.

_____ **51.** An exposure that occurs with direct contact with the hazardous material.

HH. Dose effect

II. Dilution

JJ. Lethal concentration

KK. Intermodal tanks

LL. Ignition temperature

MM. Hazardous material

NN. Water reactive

OO. Flammable range

PP. Emergency decontamination

QQ. MC-312/DOT 412 corrosive trailer

RR. MC-306/DOT 406 flammable liquid tanker

SS. Mass decontamination

TT. Local effect

UU. Level C ensemble

VV. Level A ensemble

WW. MC-338 cryogenic tanker

XX. Neutralization

YY. Placards

_____ **52.** An engineered method to control spilled or released product if the main containment vessel fails.

_____ **53.** Exposure to a hazardous material by contact with a contaminated person or object.

_____ **54.** A method of safeguarding people located near or in a hazardous area by keeping them in a safe atmosphere, usually inside structures.

_____ **55.** A mnemonic that stands for salivation, lacrimation, urination, defecation, gastrointestinal activity, emesis, miosis, which are the signs and symptoms that can be produced by exposure to organophosphate and carbamate pesticides or other nerve-stimulating agents.

_____ **56.** Substances that are capable of dissolving other substances.

_____ **57.** The measure that indicates whether a hazardous material will sink or float in water.

_____ **58.** A physiologic effect on the entire body or one of the body's systems.

_____ **59.** A multistep process of carefully scrubbing and washing contaminants off a person or object, collecting runoff water, and collecting and properly handling all items.

_____ **60.** The concentration of substance that is supposed to be safe for exposure no more than 8 hours per day and 40 hours per week.

_____ **61.** The maximum concentration of hazardous materials to which a worker should not be exposed, even for an instant.

_____ **62.** The concentration of a substance that a worker can be exposed to for up to 15 minutes but no more than four times per day with at least 1 hour between each exposure.

_____ **63.** The concentration at which direct or airborne contact with a material could result in possible and significant exposure from absorption through the skin, mucous membranes, and eyes.

_____ **64.** Hazardous chemical compounds that are released when a material decomposes under heat.

_____ **65.** A high-volume transportation device made up of several individual compressed gas cylinders banded together and affixed to a trailer. It carries compressed gases such as hydrogen, oxygen, helium, and methane, and it may carry several different gases in individual tubes.

_____ **66.** The maximum amount of gaseous fuel that can be present in the air if the air/fuel mixture is to be flammable or explosive.

_____ **67.** The weight of an airborne concentration (vapor or gas) as compared with an equal volume of dry air.

_____ **68.** For the purpose of this chapter, the pressure associated with liquids held inside any type of closed container.

_____ **69.** A property that indicates that a material will undergo a chemical reaction (for example, explosion) when mixed with water.

_____ **70.** A property that indicates that a material can be dissolved in water.

_____ **71.** A cargo document kept by the conductor of a train; also referred to as a consist.

ZZ. Secondary containment

AAA. Shelter-in-place

BBB. Specific gravity

CCC. Technical decontamination

DDD. Threshold limit value/skin

EEE. Waybill

FFF. Tube trailer

GGG. Vapor density

HHH. Labels

III. Immediately dangerous to life and health (IDLH)

JJJ. HAZWOPER

KKK. Flash point

LLL. Evacuation

MMM. Chemical asphyxiants

NNN. Container

OOO. Cyanide

PPP. Decontamination corridor

QQQ. Disposal

RRR. Drums

SSS. Threshold limit value/ceiling (TLV/C)

Multiple Choice

Read each item carefully, and then select the best response.

1. You can learn a great deal from a pesticide label. Of the following, which would NOT be found on a label?
   A. The EPA registration number
   B. The UN Classification number
   C. The active ingredients
   D. The total amount of product in the container

2. As a hazardous liquid is heated or burns, it often is converted to a/an:
   A. gas.
   B. inert, safe by-product.
   C. diluted nontoxic product.
   D. deadly solid.

3. The threshold limit value (TLV) is the maximum concentration of a toxin to which someone can be exposed in:
   A. 1 hour.
   B. 24 hours.
   C. 1 year.
   D. a 40-hour work week.

4. Emergency decontamination should be performed:
   A. at each and every hazardous materials incident.
   B. only if a qualified decontamination team is responding.
   C. only after appropriate PPE has been donned.
   D. after a series of containment pools have been set up.

5. To prepare an ambulance for the transportation of contaminated patients, paramedics should do all of the following, EXCEPT:
   A. remove all unnecessary equipment, including the cot mattress.
   B. use as much disposable equipment as necessary.
   C. wrap the patient in a plastic barrier.
   D. line the interior of the ambulance with plastic sheets.

6. A paramedic should have a working knowledge of hazardous materials spills and properly providing care for injured patients. This knowledge should include training to which of the following levels?
   A. Technician
   B. Awareness
   C. Operations
   D. EMS operations

7. Material safety data sheets (MSDS) provide a considerable amount of useful information to emergency responders. Of the following, which is NOT provided on the MSDS?
   A. The name of hazardous material
   B. The appropriate first aid measures
   C. The appropriate mode of transportation
   D. The contact information

8. Hazardous materials teams have many high-tech tools at their disposal. These tools include all of the following, EXCEPT:
   A. Computer-Aided Management of Emergency Operations (CAMEO).
   B. air-monitoring equipment.
   C. colorimetric devices.
   D. self-contained breathing apparatus (SCBA).

9. Which of the following steps must be performed by paramedics who discover that a routine-sounding call is a hazardous materials incident?
   A. Isolate the incident as much as possible using the guidelines in the *Emergency Response Guidebook* (ERG).
   B. Remain in the hot zone to evacuate injured patients.
   C. Approach and position your unit downwind from the incident.
   D. Don Level A protection and begin setting up the decontamination corridor.

10. Paramedics need to balance the risk/benefit of invasive procedures for hazardous materials patients because:
   A. IVs may help contamination pass the skin barrier.
   B. PASG/MAST would become contaminated and have to be incinerated.
   C. endotracheal tubes may cause upper airway obstruction as the plastic vaporizes.
   D. There is no known risk; paramedics need to perform patient care as normal.

Fill-in-the-Blank

Read each item carefully, and then complete the statement by filling in the missing word(s).

1. With _____ _____, you will not use rescue skills.

2. When you first arrive at a call and recognize a hazardous materials incident, your most important job will be to _____ _____ _____.

3. All EMS personnel should receive appropriate hazardous materials response training, based on the needs and requirements of the _____ _____ _____ and the local EMS agency.

4. Responding paramedics must gather as much _____ as possible when calling for the hazardous materials team.

5. If you are responding to an incident that involves a/an _____ setting in which _____ may be in use or accidentally released, you should have a high index of suspicion of hazardous materials.

6. Other good sources of information for identifying hazardous materials include the _____ _____ _____, which should be carried by the truck driver in the cab, and the _____ or "consist" that is carried by the conductor of a train.

7. There are two basic types of contamination: _____ and _____.

8. _____ _____ is the direct exposure of a patient to a hazardous material.

9. _____ _____ takes place when a hazardous material is transferred to a person from another person or from contaminated objects.

10. A/an _____ _____ may be described as a reddening of the skin or formation of blisters. Some chemicals may have a/an _____ effect on your patient.

Identify

1. Respond to the following questions by basing your answers on the following *Emergency Response Guidebook* (*ERG*) information.

GUIDE 123 | GASES - TOXIC AND/OR CORROSIVE | **ERG2004**

POTENTIAL HAZARDS

HEALTH
- **TOXIC; may be fatal if inhaled or absorbed through skin.**
- Vapors may be irritating.
- Contact with gas or liquefied gas may cause burns, severe injury and/or frostbite.
- Fire will produce irritating, corrosive and/or toxic gases.
- Runoff from fire control may cause pollution.

FIRE OR EXPLOSION
- Some may burn, but none ignite readily.
- Vapors from liquefied gas are initially heavier than air and spread along ground.
- Cylinders exposed to fire may vent and release toxic and/or corrosive gas through pressure relief devices.
- Containers may explode when heated.
- Ruptured cylinders may rocket.

PUBLIC SAFETY
- **CALL Emergency Response Telephone Number on Shipping Paper first. If Shipping Paper not available or no answer, refer to appropriate telephone number listed on the inside back cover.**
- As an immediate precautionary measure, isolate spill or leak area for at least 100 meters (330 feet) in all directions.
- Keep unauthorized personnel away.
- Stay upwind.
- Many gases are heavier than air and will spread along ground and collect in low or confined areas (sewers, basements, tanks).
- Keep out of low areas.
- Ventilate closed spaces before entering.

PROTECTIVE CLOTHING
- Wear positive pressure self-contained breathing apparatus (SCBA).
- Wear chemical protective clothing that is specifically recommended by the manufacturer. It may provide little or no thermal protection.
- Structural firefighters' protective clothing provides limited protection in fire situations ONLY; it is not effective in spill situations where direct contact with the substance is possible.

EVACUATION
Spill
- See the Table of Initial Isolation and Protective Action Distances for highlighted substances. For non-highlighted substances, increase, in the downwind direction, as necessary, the isolation distance shown under "PUBLIC SAFETY".

Fire
- If tank, rail car or tank truck is involved in a fire, ISOLATE for 800 meters (1/2 mile) in all directions; also, consider initial evacuation for 800 meters (1/2 mile) in all directions.

Page 194

a. How dangerous of a substance is this?

_____

_____

b. What type of PPE should you be wearing if you are working in the "inner circle"?

_____

_____

c. Based on the preceding information, what should you do regarding your location and staging area?

_____

_____

2. Identify the four levels of personal protective equipment (PPE) for hazardous materials scenes (Levels A–D), and then indicate their uses.

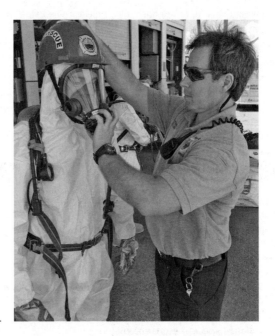

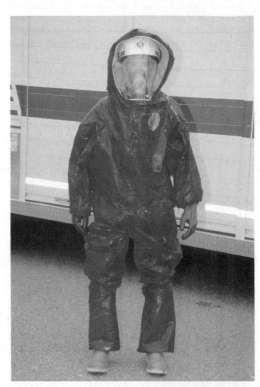

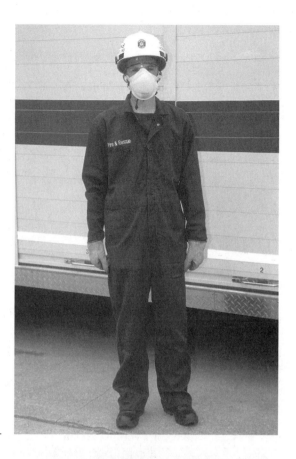

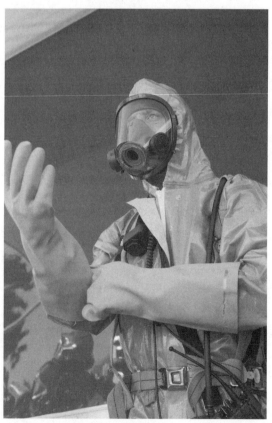

Level A:

_____

_____

Level B:

_____

_____

Level C:

_____

_____

Level D:

_____

_____

Ambulance Calls

The following case scenarios provide an opportunity to explore the concerns associated with patient management and paramedic care. Read each scenario, and then answer each question.

1. You are called to the infirmary of a local factory to see an employee who was injured in an unspecified "industrial accident." The plant manager who escorts you in explains, "There was a nasty accident. The valve on the tank of toluene wouldn't close. Jon was splashed in his face. I hope he's OK. He seems to have some trouble breathing. Our hazardous materials team had to go in and get him, and it took a few minutes for them to suit up and go in."

   Before initiating patient contact, you take out your _ERG_ and look up the chemical. The _ERG_ lists guide number 130. You look up guide 130. Under Protective Clothing, it lists:

   - Wear positive-pressure self-contained breathing apparatus (SCBA).
   - Structural fire fighters' protective clothing will provide only limited protection.

   Under Health, it states:

   - May cause toxic effects if inhaled or absorbed through skin.
   - Inhalation or contact with material may irritate or burn skin and eyes.
   - Fire will produce irritating, corrosive, and/or toxic gases.
   - Vapors may cause dizziness or suffocation.
   - Runoff from fire control or dilution water may cause pollution.

   a. Is the scene safe? List three considerations for your own immediate safety.

   (1) _____

   (2) _____

   (3) _____

2. You are called to the scene of a railway incident in which the last 5 cars of a 12-car freight train derailed and toppled onto a highway below, crushing motor vehicles beneath them. Before approaching the derailed freight cars and the injured motorists underneath them, you want to make sure those train cars were not carrying a hazardous cargo.

   a. List three potential sources of information regarding the nature of the train's cargo.

   (1) _____

   (2) _____

   (3) _____

b. You manage to determine that one of the derailed cars was carrying liquid chlorine, and as a matter of fact, you can already smell chlorine in the air. List the resources you would request at this point (assume that you are in the first public safety vehicle to reach the scene).

(1) _____

(2) _____

(3) _____

(4) _____

True/False

If you believe the statement to be more true than false, write the letter "T" in the space provided. If you believe the statement to be more false than true, write the letter "F."

1. You are called to the scene of a transportation crash in which a truck carrying radioactive waste (UN Class 7) overturned and caught fire. When you arrive, fire fighters have just extinguished the fire, but there is still a lot of smoke. The driver of the truck is pinned inside the crushed cabin. Indicate which of the following statements about handling this call are true and which are false.

_____ **a.** The ambulance should be parked upwind from the wrecked truck.

_____ **b.** The ambulance does not need to be prepared in a special fashion before the driver transports to the hospital.

_____ **c.** The acronym SLUDGEM will be important in the management of the driver of the truck in this situation.

_____ **d.** The MSDS are helpful in managing hazardous materials.

_____ **e.** The bill of lading describes the contents carried within a vehicle.

2. Indicate which of the following statements regarding hazardous materials incidents are true and which are false.

_____ **a.** If there are no unusual odors at the scene of a transportation crash, it is safe to assume that hazardous materials are not involved.

_____ **b.** EMS personnel at a hazardous materials incident may become contaminated with toxic materials by touching a patient who is contaminated.

_____ **c.** In decontaminating a patient exposed to hazardous materials, one should use a brush to scrub the skin briskly with strong soap and lots of water.

_____ **d.** When decontamination is carried out at the scene, it is unnecessary to notify the receiving hospital that you are bringing in a hazardous materials case.

_____ **e.** It is preferable that an ambulance team that was not involved in treating and decontaminating the patient be summoned to transport the patient to the hospital.

Short Answer

Complete this section with short written answers using the space provided.

1. The *Emergency Response Guidebook* (ERG) can provide responders with the following information:

a. _____

b. _____

c. _____

2. List other sources of information that may be useful to paramedics responding to a hazardous materials incident.

a. _____

b. _____

c. _____

d. _____

e. _____

3. Although it's axiomatic in EMS that you never know what you may find at a call until you reach the scene, there are nonetheless certain types of calls that should start red lights flashing in the back of your brain: ALERT! Possible hazardous materials call! Listed here are some calls to 9-1-1 during a busy month. Determine whether each case is apt to involve hazardous materials, and if so, indicate what sort of hazardous materials might be involved.

_____ **a.** Two-car collision downtown

_____

_____ **b.** Apartment-house fire

_____

_____ **c.** Three municipal workers collapsed in a sewer

_____

_____ **d.** Two police officers injured in a riot

_____

_____ **e.** Fire in a garden supply store warehouse

_____

_____ **f.** Semitrailer overturned on the interstate

_____

_____ **g.** Two "men down" on the maintenance staff of the municipal swimming pool

_____

_____ **h.** Freight train struck car on level crossing

_____

_____ **i.** Fire in a furniture factory

_____

Terrorism

Matching

Match each of the items in the right column to the appropriate definition in the left column.

_____ **1.** Type of energy that is emitted from a strong radiologic source; it is the least harmful penetrating type of radiation and cannot travel fast or through most objects.

_____ **2.** A commonly used industrial-grade fertilizer that is not in itself dangerous to handle or transport, but when mixed with fuel and other components, forms an extremely explosive compound.

_____ **3.** A deadly bacterium that lies dormant in a spore (protective shell); the germ is released from the spore when exposed to the optimal temperature and moisture. The route of entry is inhalation, cutaneous, or gastrointestinal.

_____ **4.** A type of violence sought by some terrorists, such as violent religious groups and doomsday cults, in which they wish to bring about the end of the world.

_____ **5.** A type of warfare in which groups wage war with unconventional weapons and covert tactics that are unequal—for example, when there are differences in military resources or capabilities.

_____ **6.** Microorganisms that reproduce by binary fission. These single-cell creatures reproduce rapidly. Some can form spores when environmental conditions are harsh.

_____ **7.** Type of energy that is emitted from a strong radiologic source; it is slightly more penetrating than alpha, and requires a layer of clothing to stop it.

_____ **8.** A very potent neurotoxin produced by bacteria; when introduced into the body, this neurotoxin affects the nervous system's ability to function and causes muscle paralysis.

_____ **9.** Enlarged lymph nodes (up to the size of tennis balls) that are characteristic of people infected with the bubonic plague.

_____ **10.** An epidemic that spread throughout Europe in the Middle Ages, causing over 25 million deaths, also called the Black Death; transmitted by infected fleas and characterized by acute malaise, fever, and the formation of tender, enlarged, inflamed lymph nodes that appear as lesions, called buboes.

_____ **11.** The first chemical agent ever used in warfare. It has a distinct odor of bleach and creates a green haze when released as a gas. Initially it produces upper airway irritation and a choking sensation.

_____ **12.** The ease with which a disease spreads from one human to another human.

A. Domestic terrorism

B. Ionizing radiation

C. Vesicants

D. Soman (GD)

E. Viruses

F. International terrorism

G. Alpha

H. Smallpox

I. MARK 1

J. Communicability

K. Guerilla warfare

L. Phosgene

_____ **13.** A hazardous agent that gives off little or no vapors; the skin is the primary route for this type of chemical to enter the body; also called a skin hazard.

_____ **14.** An adjective used to describe the ability of a person infected with a highly communicable disease to pass that disease to another person.

_____ **15.** Act in which the public safety community generally has no prior knowledge of the time, location, or nature of the attack.

_____ **16.** Occurs when a person is contaminated by an agent as a result of coming into contact with another contaminated person.

_____ **17.** Agent that affects the body's ability to use oxygen. It is a colorless gas that has an odor similar to almonds. The effects begin on the cellular level and are very rapidly seen at the organ system level.

_____ **18.** A natural process in which a material that is unstable attempts to stabilize itself by changing its structure.

_____ **19.** Name given to a bomb that is used as a radiologic dispersal device.

_____ **20.** An animal that, once infected, spreads a disease to another animal.

_____ **21.** The means by which a terrorist will spread a disease—for example, by poisoning the water supply or aerosolizing the agent into the air or ventilation system of a building.

_____ **22.** Terrorism that is carried out by native citizens against their own country.

_____ **23.** A nerve agent antidote kit that contains a single injection of both atropine (2 mg) and 2-PAM chloride (600 mg).

_____ **24.** A threat level in which a terrorist event is suspected, but there is no specific information about its timing or location.

_____ **25.** Early nerve agents that were developed by German scientists in the period after WWI and into WWII. There are three such agents: sarin, soman, and tabun.

_____ **26.** Type of energy that is emitted from a strong radiologic source that is far faster and stronger than alpha and beta rays. These rays easily penetrate through the human body and require either several inches of lead or concrete to prevent penetration.

_____ **27.** A form of warfare in which a small group that is not part of the official military engages in combat that uses the element of surprise, such as raids and ambushes; sometimes used by terrorists to protect their training camps and bases of operation.

_____ **28.** A threat level in which a terrorist event is known to be impending or will occur very soon.

_____ **29.** Describes the period of time from when a person is exposed to a disease to the time when symptoms begin.

_____ **30.** Terrorism that is carried out by those not of the host's country; also known as cross-border terrorism.

_____ **31.** Energy that is emitted in the form of rays, or particles.

_____ **32.** The amount of an agent or substance that will kill 50% of the people who are exposed to this level.

_____ **33.** A blistering agent that has a rapid onset of symptoms and produces immediate intense pain and discomfort on contact.

_____ **34.** A passive circulatory system that transports a plasma-like liquid called lymph, a thin fluid that bathes the tissues of the body.

M. Ammonium nitrate

N. Apocalyptic violence

O. Bacteria

P. Weaponization

Q. Weapon of mass destruction (WMD)

R. Phosgene oxime

S. Sarin

T. Ricin

U. Points of distribution

V. Suicide bombers

W. State-directed terrorism

X. National Terrorism Advisory System

Y. Viral hemorrhagic fevers

Z. Terrorism

AA. Tabun

BB. Sulfur mustard

CC. State-sponsored terrorism

DD. Beta

EE. Asymmetric warfare

FF. Anthrax

GG. Botulinum

HH. Bubonic plague

_____ **35.** Area of the lymphatic system where infection-fighting cells are housed.

_____ **36.** A nerve agent antidote kit containing two auto-injector medications, atropine and 2-PAM chloride.

_____ **37.** Bilateral pinpoint constricted pupils.

_____ **38.** A substance that mutates, damages, and changes the structure of DNA in the body's cells.

_____ **39.** The US system for informing citizens of a potential terrorist threat; it replaced the color-coded Homeland Security Advisory System.

_____ **40.** A class of chemicals called organophosphates; they function by blocking an essential enzyme in the nervous system, which causes the body's organs to become overstimulated and burn out.

_____ **41.** Biologic agents that are the most deadly substances known to humans; they include botulinum toxin and ricin.

_____ **42.** Type of energy that is emitted from a strong radiologic source; the fastest moving and most powerful form of radiation; the particles easily penetrate through lead, and require several feet of concrete to stop them.

_____ **43.** Terrorism that is either indigenous or transnational, and that does not receive direction or support from a government.

_____ **44.** The emitting of an agent after exposure—for example, from a person's clothes that have been exposed to the agent.

_____ **45.** A class of chemical found in many insecticides used in agriculture and in the home; nerve agents fall into this class of chemicals.

_____ **46.** Term used to describe how long a chemical agent will stay on a surface before it evaporates.

_____ **47.** A pulmonary agent that is a product of combustion, such as might be produced in a fire at a textile factory or house, or from metalwork or burning Freon; a very potent agent that has a delayed onset of symptoms, usually hours.

_____ **48.** A blistering agent that has a rapid onset of symptoms and produces immediate intense pain and discomfort on contact.

_____ **49.** A lung infection, also known as plague pneumonia, that is the result of inhalation of plague bacteria.

_____ **50.** Strategically placed facilities that have been preestablished for the mass distribution of antibiotics, antidotes, and vaccinations, along with other medications and supplies.

_____ **51.** Any material that emits radiation.

_____ **52.** Any container that is designed to disperse radioactive material.

_____ **53.** Neurotoxin derived from mash that is left from pressing oil from a castor bean; causes pulmonary edema and respiratory and circulatory failure, leading to death.

_____ **54.** Manner by which a toxic substance enters the body.

_____ **55.** A nerve agent that is one of the G agents; a highly volatile colorless and odorless liquid that turns from liquid to gas within seconds to minutes at room temperature.

_____ **56.** Additional explosives used by terrorists, which are set to explode after the initial bomb.

_____ **57.** A highly contagious disease; it is most contagious when blisters begin to form.

II. Contagious

JJ. Cross-contamination

KK. Decay

LL. Disease vector

MM. Elevated

NN. Gamma (x-rays)

OO. Persistency

PP. Off-gassing

QQ. Neutron radiation

RR. Nerve agents

SS. Chlorine

TT. Contact hazard

UU. Covert

VV. Cyanide

WW. Dissemination

XX. DuoDote

YY. G agents

ZZ. Organophosphates

AAA. Non-state-supported terrorism

BBB. Neurotoxins

CCC. Mutagen

DDD. Dirty bomb

EEE. Volatility

_____ **58.** A nerve agent that is one of the G agents; twice as persistent as sarin and five times as lethal; it has a fruity odor as a result of the type of alcohol used in the agent, and is both a contact and an inhalation hazard that can enter the body through skin absorption and through the respiratory tract.

_____ **59.** Small suitcase-sized nuclear weapons that were designed to destroy individual targets, such as important buildings, bridges, tunnels, or large ships.

_____ **60.** Terrorism directed by a government; the terrorists act as direct agents of the government.

_____ **61.** Terrorism that is funded or supported by nations that hold close ties with terrorist groups, but the terrorist group still acts independently.

_____ **62.** People who are terrorists who wear or carry a weapon, such as an explosive, and trigger its detonation, killing themselves in the process.

_____ **63.** A vesicant; it is a brownish-yellowish oily substance that is generally considered very persistent; has the distinct smell of garlic or mustard and, when released, it is quickly absorbed into the skin and/or mucous membranes and begins an irreversible process of damaging the cells.

_____ **64.** The monitoring, usually by local or state health departments, of patients presenting to emergency departments and alternative care facilities, the recording of EMS call volume, and the use of over-the-counter medications.

_____ **65.** A nerve agent that is one of the G agents; it is 36 times more persistent than sarin and approximately half as lethal; has a fruity smell and is unique because the components used to manufacture the agent are easy to acquire and the agent is easy to manufacture.

_____ **66.** A violent act dangerous to human life, in violation of the criminal laws of the United States or any segment to intimidate or coerce a government, the civilian population, or any segment thereof, in furtherance of political or social objectives.

_____ **67.** One of the G agents; it is a clear, oily agent that has no odor and looks like baby oil; over 100 times more lethal than sarin and is extremely persistent.

_____ **68.** An agent that enters the body through the respiratory tract.

_____ **69.** Blister agents; the primary route of entry is through the skin.

_____ **70.** A group of diseases that include the Ebola, Rift Valley, and yellow fever viruses, among others. This group of viruses causes the blood in the body to seep out from the tissues and blood vessels.

_____ **71.** Germs that require a living host to multiply and survive.

_____ **72.** Term used to describe how long a chemical agent will stay on a surface before it evaporates.

_____ **73.** Any agent designed to bring about mass death, casualties, and/or massive damage to property and infrastructure (eg, bridges, tunnels, airports, and seaports).

_____ **74.** The creation of a weapon from a biologic agent generally found in nature and that causes disease; the agent is cultivated, synthesized, and/or mutated to maximize the target population's exposure to the germ.

FFF. Vapor hazard

GGG. V agent

HHH. Syndromic surveillance

III. Special atomic demolition munitions

JJJ. Secondary device

KKK. Route of exposure

LLL. Radioactive material

MMM. Radiologic dispersal device

NNN. Pneumonic plague

OOO. Buboes

PPP. Imminent

QQQ. LD_{50}

RRR. Lymphatic system

SSS. Lymph nodes

TTT. Incubation

UUU. Miosis

VVV. Lewisite

Multiple Choice

Read each item carefully, and then select the best response.

1. A virus that has been added to the water supply is called a/an _____ weapon.
   - **A.** incendiary
   - **B.** chemical
   - **C.** biologic
   - **D.** explosive

2. The Department of Homeland Security rates the current terrorist threats using the NTAS. What does the term "imminent" mean?
   - **A.** This is a general risk of terrorist attack warning.
   - **B.** There is currently no specific information of terrorist attack.
   - **C.** There is currently no risk of a terrorist attack.
   - **D.** The threat is believed to be impending or expected soon.

3. A vesicant may produce all of the following, EXCEPT:
   - **A.** seizures.
   - **B.** large blisters.
   - **C.** stridor.
   - **D.** irritated eyes.

4. How long does it take for a patient to begin experiencing the signs and symptoms of sulfur mustard after being exposed?
   - **A.** Immediately
   - **B.** 2 to 4 hours
   - **C.** 4 to 6 hours
   - **D.** 6 to 8 hours

5. Which of the following agents causes chest tightness, severe cough, and shortness of breath?
   - **A.** Vesicant agent
   - **B.** Pulmonary agent
   - **C.** Nerve agent
   - **D.** All of the above

6. What does the "S" stand for in the medical mnemonic DUMBELS?
   - **A.** Salivation
   - **B.** Signs and symptoms
   - **C.** Stridor
   - **D.** Seizures

7. Which of the following statements correctly distinguishes a smallpox rash from other types of rashes?
   - **A.** The lesions will be in various stages of healing.
   - **B.** The lesions will all be identical in their development.
   - **C.** The lesions will start on the chest.
   - **D.** The lesions will be different sizes and shapes.

8. Which of the following is NOT a route of exposure for the bubonic plague?
   - **A.** Infected fleas
   - **B.** Infected rodents
   - **C.** Waste from infected rodents
   - **D.** Infected birds

9. What is the most deadly substance known to humans?
   - **A.** Anthrax
   - **B.** Smallpox
   - **C.** Neurotoxin
   - **D.** Vesicant

10. What is the least harmful form of radiation?
    - **A.** Alpha
    - **B.** Beta
    - **C.** Gamma
    - **D.** X-rays

ɔeling

el the three types of energy emitted from a strong radiologic source:

1. Alpha, Beta, and Gamma Radiation

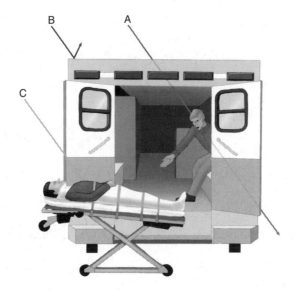

A. _____

B. _____

C. _____

Fill-in-the-Blank

Read each item carefully, and then complete the statement by filling in the missing word(s).

1. _____ _____ _____ _____ is any agent designed to bring about mass death, casualties, and massive damage to property.

2. Most of the terrorist acts are _____, meaning the public has no previous knowledge of the attack.

3. Additional explosives set at a site that are intended to injure responders are known as a/an _____ device.

4. _____ _____ _____ is how an agent most effectively enters the body.

5. _____ _____ are the most deadly chemicals developed.

6. G agents were developed by _____ scientists in the early to mid-1900s.

7. Bubonic plague infects the _____ system.

8. _____ is a deadly bacterium that lies dormant in a spore.

9. Ricin is made from _____ _____.

10. _____ _____ _____ are strategically placed stockpiles of antibiotics, vaccinations, and other medications.

Identify

For the following case study, list the chief complaint, vital signs, and pertinent negatives.

In your private vehicle, you respond to a vehicle crash about 2 miles from your home. Upon arriving at the scene, you see a truck that has rolled. The patient is outside of the truck and bystanders are trying to help him. He is covered in white powder that has spilled from the truck. You walk up and take C-spine precautions and start to assess the patient, knowing that your squad is about 3 minutes behind you. Jeff is 56 years old and is answering all your questions. You ask him what is in the truck because it is all over him and now you have some on you also. He says it is some kind of chemical he was taking to a local plant. Jeff has some cuts on his arms. As your squad arrives, you yell at everyone to get back and call for the fire department. Unfortunately, you forgot the first rule of scene safety and didn't look around well enough before entering the scene. The chemical is raw organophosphates. You and Jeff get a wonderful water bath from the fire department before anyone can come and help you. Finally, you get Jeff in the squad and find that he is bradycardic with a heart rate of 50 beats/min, and his blood pressure is 98/66 mm Hg. He begins to lose consciousness, respirations are dropping quickly to 9 breaths/min, oxygen saturation is 88%, and he is drooling terribly. You realize that atropine is indicated in organophosphate poisoning. After starting an IV, you give him 2 mg of atropine. You can give up to 5 mg, but you go with the lower dose because of his condition. You have your partner bagging him with 100% oxygen. After what seems like an eternity, he responds well with an increasing heart rate, blood pressure, and respiratory rate. You run Priority 1 (code 3) all the way to the hospital. You are evaluated as soon as you get there also to make sure you will be okay.

1. Chief complaint:

_____

_____

2. Vital signs:

_____

_____

3. Pertinent negatives:

_____

_____

omplete the Patient Care Report (PCR)

ad the case study in the preceding Identify exercise, and then complete the following PCR for the patient.

EMS Patient Care Report (PCR)					
Date:	**Incident No.:**	**Nature of Call:**		**Location:**	
Dispatched:	**En Route:**	**At Scene:**	**Transport:**	**At Hospital:**	**In Service:**

Patient Information	
Age:	**Allergies:**
Sex:	**Medications:**
Weight (in kg [lb]):	**Past Medical History:**
	Chief Complaint:

Vital Signs				
Time:	**BP:**	**Pulse:**	**Respirations:**	**SpO$_2$:**
Time:	**BP:**	**Pulse:**	**Respirations:**	**SpO$_2$:**
Time:	**BP:**	**Pulse:**	**Respirations:**	**SpO$_2$:**

EMS Treatment (circle all that apply)				
Oxygen @ _____ L/min via (circle one): NC NRM Bag-Mask Device		**Assisted Ventilation**	**Airway Adjunct**	**CPR**
Defibrillation	**Bleeding Control**	**Bandaging**	**Splinting**	**Other**

Narrative

Ambulance Calls

The following case scenarios provide an opportunity to explore the concerns associated with patient management and para-medic care. Read each scenario, and then answer each question.

1. You are among the first ambulance personnel to reach the scene of a train derailment involving at least 60 casualties. Authorities on the scene think that this could be an act of terrorism.

   a. As you recall, there are five categories of terrorist incidents. They are:

   (1) _____

   (2) _____

   (3) _____

   (4) _____

   (5) _____

   b. You are directed to begin triage of the people trying to get clear of the wreckage. There seem to be a lot of people who are ambulatory, but you are located in a bean field with nothing around you to send the walking wounded toward. There is only one road close by, and it is jammed up with emergency vehicles. What can you do with the ambulatory people?

   _____

   _____

2. You respond to the local swimming pool right before it is scheduled to open. Dispatch says there are several kids coughing and the lifeguards are having a hard time talking on the phone because of coughing spasms. As you arrive, you notice a green haze floating in the air around the pool house. There are about 50 kids standing around waiting for the pool to open.

   a. What is the cause of this green haze?

   _____

   _____

   b. Before you get out of the ambulance, what should you do?

   _____

   _____

   c. You have a total of seven kids who are coughing hard, and two lifeguards who are really struggling to breathe. After help arrives, you begin treatment on one of the lifeguards. What type of problems should you expect?

   _____

   _____

True/False

If you believe the statement to be more true than false, write the letter "T" in the space provided. If you believe the statement to be more false than true, write the letter "F."

_____ 1. There are suits made for paramedics to shield them from radiation.

_____ 2. Radiologic material can be found at hospitals, power plants, and colleges.

_____ 3. Antibiotics will not help with bacteria.

_____ 4. A virus can live and thrive outside the host body.

_____ 5. The period of time between being exposed and showing signs and symptoms is known as the incubation period.

_____ **6.** Ebola is a type of hemorrhagic fever.

_____ **7.** Sarin is a vesicant.

_____ **8.** A cyberterrorist's main goal is to scare masses of people through the Internet.

_____ **9.** The Oklahoma City Federal Building bombing was done by a domestic terrorist.

_____ **10.** The greatest threats to a paramedic during a weapons of mass destruction (WMDs) attack are contamination and cross-contamination.

Short Answer

Complete this section with short written answers using the space provided.

1. List three *reactions* sometimes seen in bystanders at a multiple-casualty incident (MCI).

a. _____

b. _____

c. _____

2. As care of the patients proceeds, it is important to fill in pertinent details on each casualty's triage tag. List the information that should be recorded if it can be obtained.

a. _____

b. _____

c. _____

d. _____

e. _____

f. _____

Fill-in-the-Table

Fill in the missing parts of the tables.

1. Nerve Agents

Nerve Agents						
Name	**Code Name**	**Odor**	**Special Features**	**Onset of symptoms**	**Volatility**	**Route of exposure**
_____	_____	Fruity	Easy to manufacture	Immediate	Low	Both contact and vapor hazard
_____	_____	None (if pure) or strong	Will off-gas while on victim's clothing	Immediate	High	Primarily respiratory vapor hazard; extremely lethal if skin contact is made
_____	_____	Fruity	Ages rapidly, making it difficult to treat	Immediate	Moderate	Contact with skin; minimal vapor hazard
_____	_____	None	Most lethal chemical agent; difficult to decontaminate	Immediate	Very low	Contact with skin; no vapor hazard (unless vaporized)

2. Chemical Agents

Class	Military Designation	Odor	Lethality	Onset of Symptoms	Volatility	Primary Route of Exposure
	Mustard (H) Lewisite (L) Phosgene oxime (CX)		Causes large blisters to form on victims; may severely damage upper airway if vapors are inhaled; severe intense pain and grayish skin discoloration (L, CX)		Very low (H, L) Moderate (CX)	Primarily contact; with some vapor hazard
	Chlorine (CL) Phosgene (CG)		Causes irritation; choking (CL); severe pulmonary edema (CG)		Very high	Vapor hazard
	Tabun (GA) Sarin (GB) Soman (GD) V agent (VX)		Most lethal chemical agents can kill within minutes; effects are reversible with antidotes		Moderate (GA, GD) Very high (GB) Low (VX)	Vapor hazard (GB) Both vapor and contact hazard (GA, GD) Contact hazard (VX)
	Hydrogen cyanide (AC) Cyanogen chloride (CK)		Highly lethal chemical gases; can kill within minutes; effects are reversible with antidotes		Very high	Vapor hazard

3. Symptoms of Persons Exposed to Nerve Agents

SLUDGEM and DUMBELS	
Military Mnemonic: SLUDGEM	
S	Salivation
L	
U	Urination
D	
G	GI distress
E	
M	Miosis
Medical Mnemonic: DUMBELS	
D	
U	Urination
M	
B	Bradycardia, Bronchorrhea
E	
L	Lacrimation
S	

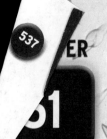

Disaster Response

Matching

Match each of the terms in the right column to the appropriate description in the left column.

_____ **1.** A guideline to follow regarding the distance to place between oneself and a person who sneezes or coughs, to avoid exposure to germs.

_____ **2.** The official internal report of the entire event, such as a disaster, which should contain the facts of the incident reflected in a chronologic, accurate manner.

_____ **3.** The act of conducting comprehensive preplanning that will apply to any disaster.

_____ **4.** The residue left behind from a volcanic eruption.

_____ **5.** Areas where slightly injured or noninjured displaced persons can be gathered together and transported by bus or truck for further treatment.

_____ **6.** A psychological condition that can develop in people who are exposed to cold weather for long periods of time, even if sheltered.

_____ **7.** The detailed plan describing the functioning of the agency in situations that disrupt normal operations.

_____ **8.** The external foundation in communities made up of structures and services critical in the day-to-day living activities of humans, including energy sources, fuel, water, sewage removal, food, hospitals, and transportation systems.

_____ **9.** An area away from the command post or emergency operations center, considered by engineering expertise to be a safe place to stage until directed otherwise.

_____ **10.** A widespread event that disrupts community resources and functions, in turn threatening public safety, lives, and property.

_____ **11.** A planned, coordinated response to a disaster that involves cooperation of multiple responders and agencies and enables effective triage and provision of care according to triage decisions.

_____ **12.** A phenomenon that can occur during an earthquake, in which particles of dust and debris are loosened and released into the air, producing a toxic and hypoxic atmosphere.

_____ **13.** A central command and control facility, found at all government levels, responsible for strategic overview; tactical decisions are left to incident commanders.

_____ **14.** Sickness that is larger than expected, area-wise and population-wise.

A. Thermals

B. Pandemic

C. Radio operators

D. Shelter-in-place

E. Emergency operations center (EOC)

F. Cold stress

G. 6-feet rule

H. All-hazards approach

I. Disaster management

J. Directed area

K. Critical infrastructure

L. Ashfall

M. Water buffalo trailers

N. Lister bags

_____ **15.** A team, usually staffed with physicians, nurses, and EMS providers, that performs minor surgical procedures and debridements in the field, taking some of the load from the hospital facility.

_____ **16.** A system implemented to manage disasters and multiple-casualty incidents in which section chiefs, including finance, logistics, operations, and planning, report to the incident commander.

_____ **17.** Heavy canvas bags that can be hung from trees containing water in amounts from 40 to 100 gallons.

_____ **18.** Documents that preplan how you will access help from other areas when needed.

_____ **19.** A situation in which a reservoir overflows its borders.

_____ **20.** An extensive epidemic.

_____ **21.** An area where medications or supplies can be administered on a temporary basis.

_____ **22.** Blasts from flowing or standing lava that can have a wide dispersal circumference, spewing ash and magma.

_____ **23.** Amateur radio operators who have a formal emergency communications set of SOPs. Most are licensed by the Federal Communications Commission (FCC).

_____ **24.** Depression that can affect persons in long periods of bad weather, usually winter.

_____ **25.** Securing one's position in the state found during an emergency; sometimes as simple as shutting the windows, going to the cellar, or turning off the heating and air conditioning systems.

_____ **26.** Debris from satellites and other man-made objects that reenter the earth's atmosphere.

_____ **27.** Rope or cord tied to a person who is entering a dangerous environment; used for quick retrieval, usually in conjunction with a harness.

_____ **28.** Differing temperatures and swirling patterns of moving air with changes in wind speed.

_____ **29.** A command system used in larger incidents in which there is a multiagency response or multiple jurisdictions are involved.

_____ **30.** Portable trailers that contain from 500 to 3,000 gallons of water.

O. Epidemic

P. Pyroclastic explosions

Q. Overtopping

R. Unified command system

S. Dust suffocation

T. Disaster

U. Continuity of operations plan (COOP)

V. Casualty collection points

W. After-action report

X. Forward surgical team

Y. Point of distribution

Z. Mutual aid agreements

AA. Incident command system (ICS)

BB. Seasonal affective disorder

CC. Space junk

DD. Tag lines

Multiple Choice

Read each item carefully, and then select the best response.

1. The critical infrastructure includes the food and hospitals as well as which of the following?
   A. Communications systems
   B. Electrical power grid
   C. Sewage removal
   D. All of the above

2. Disaster response preplanning includes assessing each of the following, EXCEPT:
   A. geography of response areas.
   B. number of paramedics on each ambulance.
   C. immunizations of personnel.
   D. training standards.

3. In planning for disasters, which nongovernmental organization should be included to assist with disaster relief?
   A. Homeland Security Agency
   B. The Red Cross
   C. FEMA
   D. NHTSA

4. When planning for sheltering, what will your plan need to consider?
   A. Adult supervision for children
   B. Access to ATMs
   C. Facilities for mass decontamination
   D. Housing for wild animals

5. Which of the following is NOT considered a high priority for after the event?
   A. Physical examination of personnel
   B. Stress reaction review
   C. Mobilization of personnel
   D. Finance and reimbursement

6. Each of the following is considered a natural disaster, EXCEPT:
   A. flooding.
   B. a tanker crash.
   C. a pandemic.
   D. a landslide or avalanche.

7. During an earthquake, the release of particles of debris into the air can cause:
   A. dust suffocation.
   B. a landslide.
   C. flooding.
   D. magma release.

8. Which of the following incidents should you consider sheltering-in-place?
   A. An earthquake nearby
   B. A drought in the valley this season
   C. A sandstorm or dust storm
   D. Prolonged cold weather and power outages

9. When people are exposed to cold weather for long periods of time, even though sheltered, they can develop a condition called:
   A. trench foot.
   B. frostbite.
   C. walking pneumonia.
   D. cold stress.

10. Which of the following is NOT a man-made disaster?
    A. A hazardous materials incident
    B. A pandemic
    C. A civil disturbance
    D. An IT (cyber) disruption

Fill-in-the-Blank

Read each item carefully, and then complete the statement by filling in the missing word(s).

1. The act of conducting comprehensive _____ for all types of disasters is called a/an _____-_____ approach.

2. EMS is normally accustomed to _____ _____ _____ that allow EMS agencies and fire departments in neighboring jurisdictions to cover emergency calls.

3. The _____ supervisor must maintain a/an _____ of all patients and the hospitals to which they are transported.

4. You must keep the _____ updated on field conditions so that they can _____ their priorities, if necessary.

5. Consider a press _____ location and provide prompt _____ so all the facts that you are allowed to release about the incident can be communicated through the _____.

6. The _____-_____ _____ is your official internal report of the entire event.

7. You may need to help set up field hospitals and first aid stations at _____ _____ _____.

8. EMS should be represented both in the _____ _____ _____ and in the unified command center.

9. During a heat wave, small, more frequent meals are better than large ones. Eat foods that are _____ in fluids, such as _____, fruits and salads.

10. A/an _____ is illness that affects a disproportionately large geographic area and number of people. A/an _____ is an extensive one.

Identify

For the following case study, list the chief complaint, vital signs, and pertinent negatives.

You have responded to a structure fire involving a strip mall with eight stores in a row. The suspected arsonist had a grudge against the owner of the Software Favorites store and pried open the rear door and started a fire with gasoline. It was around midnight and all the stores were closed, so aside from the potential danger to the fire fighters, there were no victims in the buildings. While you are standing by in the rehab sector, you are notified that the police found the suspected arsonist hiding in a nearby alleyway. They bring him to your EMS unit since most of the front of his clothing has been burned and he is disoriented and in a lot of pain. Your patient is a 22-year-old man who at first inspection has burns to his hands, arms, and the front of his chest, and his beard has been mostly burned off. Apparently the fire got out of control before he was able to exit the building and the gasoline had splashed the front of his clothing. He is conscious and alert, but you note he has a raspy voice and is in extreme pain. (He reports a 20 on the 10 scale!) He did remember the grade school lesson to "stop, drop, and roll," managing to put the fire on his clothing out by rolling around in a puddle in the alley.

Your partner starts the primary assessment and secondary assessment as you apply oxygen with a nonrebreathing mask. The rapid trauma exam shows only partial thickness burns on the hands and arms, but his chest is a full-thickness burn. You are most concerned with the potential for a respiratory burn and know this patient will end up in a burn bed this morning. As you remove his watch and rings and give them to the officer, your partner gets some vital signs. He is breathing 24 breaths/min and shallow, with an oxygen saturation of 96% and clear lung sounds. Pulse is 110 beats/min and regular, and blood pressure is 108/68 mm Hg. His pupils are PEARRL and fortunately were not burned. The patient rates his pain at a 10/10. His skin, in the noninjured areas, is pale, cool, and moist. You remove his remaining clothing and have him lie down on a burn sheet that was placed on your stretcher. The patient denies taking any medications and denies any allergies. He says he is normally as healthy as a horse. You get him in the unit, place him on the heart monitor (which shows sinus tachycardia with no ectopic beats), and then start a large-bore IV in a vein in an area that was not burned. You decide to administer plenty of fluids for the burns and fentanyl for pain due to his dropping blood pressure. After consultation with medical control, the decision is to transport him to the local high school soccer field where a landing zone has been set up for the Regional Medevac helicopter crew to pick him up and transport him to the burn center.

1. Chief complaint:

2. Vital signs:

3. Pertinent negatives:

Ambulance Calls

The following case scenario provides an opportunity to explore the concerns associated with patient management, paramedic care, and preparation for major incidents in your community. Read the scenario, and then answer each question.

1. It is a hot, stuffy day with high humidity in July in your community. You are on the medic unit today and state to your partner, "this makes 10 straight days of 90-degree temps." You have been running calls all morning, mostly patients with respiratory complaints. At 3:00 PM, you get a call for the Fairwood Nursing Home for an unconscious patient. On arrival you find a five-floor facility that normally houses 200 patients. It is extremely hot inside the lobby. As you are led to room 105 by a nursing aide, your partner notices that there are a number of patients in a community room who look unconscious on the couch with the TV blasting. The aide tells you that the air conditioner has been broken all week and the place only has two aides for each floor and one nurse in the office. Some doctors stop by in the mornings, but they are not there today. As you walk into the patient's room, you note it is a semi-private room and both occupants are restrained in a seated position in chairs. That sure makes it difficult for them to keep drinking fluids when then can't even get up out of their chairs. Further, they are wearing flannel night gowns! The aide, who has been very talkative, says he thinks there are a lot of patients getting sicker; he certainly is not feeling well. He also states that the windows have never opened. There is a large fan in the hallway, basically blowing hot air around the hallways.

As your partner begins to assess the patient in room 105, you decide to pick up the phone and discuss this situation with your supervisor, who promptly alerts dispatch to assign a group of ambulance, the police, the fire department (for ventilation), and the Special Operations Unit.

This story is based on an actual incident that occurred in the heat wave of 1978 in Queens, NY. It could happen in your community, too, if you live in a warmer climate.

a. List four problems and potential solutions to issues that occur during a heat wave.

(1) _____

_____

(2) _____

_____

(3) _____

_____

(4) _____

_____

b. What are five examples of the illnesses that you may be treating in a nursing home during a heat emergency similar to the one described in the scenario?

(1) _____

(2) _____

(3) _____

(4) _____

(5) _____

True/False

If you believe the statement to be more true than false, write the letter "T" in the space provided. If you believe the statement to be more false than true, write the letter "F."

_____ **1.** Woodland fires have a much higher death rate than structural fires.

_____ **2.** To avoid transmission of the germs from a sneeze, you should stay 3 feet away from the patient.

_____ **3.** When it is very cold out, you should dress in loose clothing and multiple layers.

_____ **4.** A hurricane usually requires emergency services personnel to notify the public to shelter-in-place.

_____ **5.** Tsunamis can come in a series.

_____ **6.** The biggest immediate danger from an earthquake is structural collapse.

_____ **7.** Cave-ins can release sewer and chemical gases.

_____ **8.** The media should not be a concern during a disaster.

_____ **9.** Your agency's designated infection control officer should be aware of each member's health status.

_____ **10.** If a crew is sent to another area, it may need to be self-sustaining for 48 to 72 hours.

Short Answer

Complete this section with short written answers using the space provided.

1. List the three phases of any plan of response to a disaster.

a. _____

b. _____

c. _____

2. List the considerations during a disaster.

_____

_____

_____

Fill-in-the-Table

Fill in the missing parts of the table.

1. Examples of Natural and Man-Made Disasters

Examples of Natural and Man-Made Disasters	
Natural Disasters	**Man-Made Disasters**
Forest and brush fires	_____
_____	Construction failures and building collapse
Tornadoes	_____
_____	Riots, civil disturbances, and stampedes
Tsunamis	_____
_____	Sniper, shooter, and hostage situations
Landslides, avalanches, mudslides	_____
_____	IT (cyber) disruptions
Volcanoes	_____
_____	Hazardous materials incidents
Sandstorms and dust storms	
_____	
Drought	
_____	
Meteors and space debris	
_____	

Crime Scene Awareness

Matching

Match each of the items in the right column to the appropriate definition in the left column.

_____ **1.** A gunman who has begun to fire on people and is still at large.

_____ **2.** Locations where illegal drugs such as methamphetamine, LSD, ecstacy, and PCP are manufactured.

_____ **3.** Protection from being seen.

_____ **4.** Technique that involves one paramedic making contact with the patient to provide care, while the second paramedic obtains patient information, gauges the level of tension, and warns his or her partner at the first sign of trouble.

_____ **5.** Obstacles that are difficult or impossible for bullets to penetrate.

_____ **6.** The evidence that ties a suspect or victim to a crime. It may include body materials, objects, or impressions.

_____ **7.** The main means of escape should violence erupt. This is usually the door you used to enter the building.

_____ **8.** Any other means of egress, including windows and doors.

_____ **9.** Knowing your surroundings, the people and groups in the environment, and the climate of violence or strife.

_____ **10.** Specially trained medics who provide care for SWAT team members conducting operations, barricaded patients, patients being held hostage, and other special operations.

_____ **11.** The oral documentation by a witness of the facts of a criminal act.

_____ **12.** Dangerous situation when a paramedic becomes so completely involved with patient care that he or she fails to see the possibility of physical harm to the patient or other care providers.

A. Contact and cover

B. Cover

C. Active shooter

D. Situational awareness

E. Primary exit

F. Physical evidence

G. Concealment

H. Testimonial evidence

I. Tunnel vision

J. Tactical paramedics

K. Clandestine drug laboratory

L. Secondary exit

Multiple Choice

Read each item carefully, and then select the best response.

1. For maximum safety when arriving at incidents with a single vehicle in which the potential danger is high, your vehicle should be positioned a minimum of how many feet behind the stopped vehicle?

A. 50

B. 15

C. 21

D. 10

2. When approaching a passenger vehicle (sedan), you should stop at which column (post) on the vehicle to look in the rear and side windows?

A. A

B. B

C. C

D. D

3. When announcing your arrival at the front door of a residence, where should you stand?
   A. To the doorknob side of the door
   B. To the hinged side of the door
   C. In front of the door
   D. Ten to 15 feet back from the door

4. When you enter a structure, the door you use to enter the building is referred to as the _____ exit.
   A. tertiary
   B. secondary
   C. primary
   D. general

5. Which of the following is considered concealment when you are confronted by violence?
   A. Curb
   B. Depression in the ground
   C. Utility pole
   D. Shrubbery

6. You are dispatched to a residence for a possible sick person. En route to the call, the dispatcher informs you that the caller hung up before all the information could be collected. When you are suspicious that something is not right, prior to announcing your arrival at the door, you should do all the following, EXCEPT:
   A. listen for loud noises.
   B. look for neighbors to talk with.
   C. look through a window for signs of a struggle.
   D. listen for threatening voices.

7. You have entered a residence that you initially thought was safe, but once inside you and your partner are suspicious that there might be trouble. You approach the patient to start the assessment, and your partner starts to look around to see if there is any immediate danger and gather information relevant to providing care. What is the technique called?
   A. Assess and act
   B. Contact and cover
   C. Respond and react
   D. Link and look

8. In a hostage situation, you should assume all of the following, EXCEPT:
   A. other hostages may look to you for guidance.
   B. your captors could kill you at any moment.
   C. your captors will be lenient on you because your uniform is an image of authority.
   D. removing your uniform may make you less threatening to the captors.

9. In all potentially violent situations, the paramedic's best (and often only) defense is:
   A. a hidden weapon.
   B. police backup.
   C. the portable radio.
   D. situational awareness.

10. You respond to a stabbing. While treating the patient and packaging for transport, you observe some footprints in the patient's blood and you try to work quickly with minimal disruption to the evidence. The footprints are considered _____ evidence.
   A. physical
   B. testimonial
   C. circumstantial
   D. substantiated

Fill-in-the-Blank

Read each item carefully, and then complete the statement by filling in the missing word(s).

1. Becoming completely involved with patient care and failing to see possible physical harm is called _____ _____.

2. For maximum safety when arriving at an incident with a single vehicle in which the potential for danger is high, position your vehicle at least _____ feet behind the stopped vehicle at a _____-degree angle.

3. When there are two or more paramedics in the unit and you come to the scene of a motor vehicle crash, the person riding in the right front seat of the ambulance is the _____ _____.

4. When you approach a van in a situation where safety is a concern, move 10 to 15 feet away from the passenger side, and then belly-in and walk parallel until you are approximately 45° forward of the _____ post.

5. When you enter a structure, pick a/an _____ exit and a/an _____ exit to keep one means of escape accessible at all times.

6. To enter a scene where violence is suspected, one technique is for one paramedic to start providing patient care and the other to obtain information and warn the partner at the first sign of trouble. This technique is called _____ and _____.

Identify

In the following case study, list the possible errors in handling scene safety, warning signs of danger, and potential evidence. You are assigned to respond to a call for an injured person in a residence in a middle-class neighborhood. You are provided no additional information by the dispatcher because the caller hung up before more questions could be asked. You approach the house and hear a loud conversation inside, and without announcing yourself, you stand in front of the door and knock. You enter through the front door (primary exit), and without looking around, you ask what is happening. You find a woman on the couch holding her right arm with bruising to the face. She appears to be in considerable pain. Both you and your partner go to the patient and do not pay much attention to the person on the other side of the room, who is still arguing with the patient. You see a ceramic object in pieces on the floor and brush it out of the way with your foot as you approach the patient. You start to assess the patient, and your partner cuts and rips through the bloody shirt sleeve to examine the arm. You decide the person standing on the other side of the room is a potential threat and realize that he is between you and the front door. You notice there are a number of tables with drawers and a fire poker in a stand next to the fireplace. Just as you and your partner become anxious about the potential threats, two police officers come through the front door.

1. Errors in handling scene safety:

   _____

   _____

   _____

   _____

2. Warning signs of danger:

   _____

   _____

   _____

   _____

3. Potential evidence:

   _____

   _____

   _____

   _____

Ambulance Calls

The following case scenarios provide an opportunity to explore the concerns associated with patient management and paramedic care. Read each scenario, and then answer each question.

1. You respond to a residence that has previously had calls for domestic violence, but the dispatcher informs you that the information provided was for a medical problem including severe difficulty breathing, and no information indicated danger or that responders would be at risk. You are told the police will not arrive for another 5 minutes after you are on the scene. When you arrive at the residence, you are suspicious. What precautions might you take to help ensure that there is no immediate violence that would place you at risk?

_____

_____

_____

_____

2. You and your paramedic partner, who is driving the ambulance, are the first emergency personnel to arrive at the scene where a car ran off the road into a guardrail. When you arrive on the scene, you see no activity around the vehicle, and you see only one person in the driver's seat of the car. You are initially suspicious.
   a. How should you park and approach the scene?

   _____

   _____

   b. What precautions should you take to identify the car?

   _____

   _____

   c. Who should be the incident commander, and how should that person proceed?

   _____

   _____

3. You receive a call for a sick child. You arrive on the scene of the call and someone is outside waiting for you. You are led into the house to find a wheezing pediatric patient who, you are told, is 7 years old. She is an asthmatic, and her family members report that they can't find her inhaler. You and your partner signal each other to use "contact and cover." You start to treat the patient, and your partner obtains information from the person who met the ambulance. Your partner's observations lead her to believe this residence is a clandestine drug laboratory.
   a. What does "contact and cover" mean?

   _____

   _____

   b. What actions should you and your partner take?

   _____

   _____

   c. What are your concerns?

   _____

   _____

4. Upon arrival at the scene of a shooting, you find a young patient shot in the leg and lying in a pool of blood. You and your partner do a rapid assessment and provide care quickly. The patient is prepared for transport, placed on the stretcher, and loaded into the ambulance. What are your primary concerns when trying to preserve evidence?

_____

_____

_____

_____

True/False

If you believe the statement to be more true than false, write the letter "T" in the space provided. If you believe the statement to be more false than true, write the letter "F."

_____ 1. Physical evidence is oral documentation by witnesses of facts.

_____ 2. Most hostage situations in the United States last 4.5 to 5 hours.

_____ 3. The secondary exit is the door that you use to enter the building.

_____ 4. When standing at the door to a residence, you should stand on the hinged side of the door.

_____ 5. When there are two paramedics in an ambulance and you arrive on the scene where a vehicle needs to be checked out, the incident commander is the driver of the ambulance.

_____ 6. Some agencies have developed standard operating procedures that guide how to handle potentially violent situations.

_____ 7. When checking out a vehicle where the back seat is occupied, do not pass the C column until you are sure that it is safe to do so.

_____ 8. When you arrive at the scene of a single-vehicle crash with potential danger, the ambulance should be parked at least 10 feet behind the vehicle.

_____ 9. To control an unexpected attack at a vehicle incident, use the interview stance in which you stand at approximately arm's length from the person with your body at a 45° angle.

_____ 10. Clandestine drug laboratories are not hazardous and present no danger to emergency medical services personnel.

Short Answer

Complete this section with short written answers using the space provided.

1. You are on the scene of a call that, because of unsafe circumstances, dictates your retreat to a safe area. After you have backed away from the danger zone and it is safe, what information would you want to provide to the dispatcher?

   a. _____

   b. _____

   c. _____

   d. _____

   e. _____

2. What three immediate hazards present dangers to emergency responders in regard to a clandestine drug laboratory?

   a. _____

   b. _____

   c. _____

3. When approaching a motor vehicle, a paramedic should always be attentive to impending danger. In which locations in a vehicle could a weapon be concealed?

a. _____

b. _____

c. _____

d. _____

e. _____

f. _____

g. _____

4. When you enter a structure, the primary exit is usually the door you used to enter. What is a secondary exit, and why should it be identified?

_____

_____

5. What is the difference between *cover* and *concealment*?

_____

_____

6. Give three examples each of cover and concealment that you can use when there is danger from a gun.

a. Cover

(1) _____

(2) _____

(3) _____

b. Concealment

(1) _____

(2) _____

(3) _____

7. If you are taken hostage by a subject with a gun, what should you assume during the capture stage?

_____

_____

8. There are two general classifications of evidence. Name and provide a brief description of each.

a. _____

b. _____

APPENDIX
A
Case Studies and Answers

Case Studies

Case Study 1

It is 9:00 AM and you have been dispatched to a Priority 1 (Charlie response) to a call for a serious injury. As you arrive at 9:08 AM, the police have just arrived and are calling you to come to the side of the house right away. The scene is safe, although there is a blood trail from a basement window to the spot where the patient is lying, holding his right leg and screaming out in pain. His airway is obviously open! You don appropriate personal protective equipment (PPE) and approach the patient to find a 20-year-old man who states he tried to kick open the basement window and managed to cut the back of his knee. He said it has continued to spurt bright red blood all over the place. Quickly you open the trauma kit and apply direct pressure with gauze to the large laceration to the artery behind the right knee. Meanwhile your partner determines the patient, who is screaming that he is in a lot of pain (10/10), is alert and restless. The patient reports no other injuries. His vitals are taken and are found to be as follows: respirations of 26 breaths/min, deep and full; pulse of 100 beats/min, thready and weak at the wrist. His skin is pale, cool, and clammy. The patient denies any other injuries and states he feels thirsty, weak, and dizzy at this point. You are busy trying to control the bleeding, following all the appropriate methods you learned in your paramedic training. Meanwhile, your partner applies a nonrebreathing mask with 100% oxygen to the patient as you prepare to load him on the stretcher. You both decide to do the secondary assessment en route to the hospital since the patient's condition is serious. As you load him into the ambulance, you note that the time is now 9:16 AM.

1. What is the appropriate order of initial management of this patient?

_____

_____

_____

_____

_____

_____

2. How will you manage the continued bleeding from the patient's injury?

_____

_____

_____

_____

_____

_____

_____

3. What is the appropriate intravenous (IV) fluid resuscitation regimen for this patient?

_____

_____

_____

_____

_____

_____

4. What is the difference between a crystalloid and a colloid solution?

_____

_____

_____

_____

_____

_____

5. What is the purpose of performing a secondary assessment?

_____

_____

_____

_____

_____

_____

6. Complete the PCR.

EMS Patient Care Report (PCR)

Date:	Incident No.:	Nature of Call:	Location:

Dispatched:	En Route:	At Scene:	Transport:	At Hospital:	In Service:

Patient Information

Age:	Allergies:
Sex:	Medications:
Weight (in kg [lb]):	Past Medical History:
	Chief Complaint:

Vital Signs

Time:	BP:	Pulse:	Respirations:	SpO$_2$:
Time:	BP:	Pulse:	Respirations:	SpO$_2$:
Time:	BP:	Pulse:	Respirations:	SpO$_2$:

EMS Treatment (circle all that apply)

Oxygen @ _____ L/min via (circle one): NC NRM Bag-Mask Device	Assisted Ventilation	Airway Adjunct	CPR
Defibrillation	Bleeding Control	Bandaging	Splinting	Other

Narrative

Case Study 2

It is 5:00 PM and you have been dispatched to a Priority 1 (Charlie response) to a call for an elderly woman with breathing difficulty. As you arrive, at 5:07 PM, the fire department is just pulling up in front of the house. There is a family member, most likely the patient's daughter, who meets you at the front door of the residence. The scene is safe and you have enough help. You don your PPE as you enter the bedroom in the rear of the second floor. The patient is sitting in bed, propped with about four pillows, and is in obvious respiratory distress. She is pale with blue lips, and her skin is warm and clammy to touch. She is confused but tries to talk to you in two-word sentences. Her level of consciousness (LOC), which is altered, is a "V." Her daughter begins to fill you in as your partner determines her airway is open and clear and tries to assess her respirations. The daughter states that her mother, Millie, is 72 years old and has a long history of smoking two packs a day until she was diagnosed with emphysema a few years ago. She is on a long list of medications, which do not seem to be working today, and she has had a fever of 101.5°F all day. She called you because Millie's breathing has continued to get worse and now she is acting very confused. The last time she was this bad she spent 2 weeks in a critical care unit on a respirator. Your partner reports that Millie's respirations are 28 breaths/min, labored and shallow; her pulse is about 120 beats/min and irregular; her blood oxygen saturation (SpO_2) is 88%; and she does feel like she is burning up.

As you begin to set up for a nebulizer treatment, you ask the daughter whether Millie has any allergies. Your partner applies the electrodes for an electrocardiogram (ECG), which reveals an atrial rhythm that is irregulary irregular. Next her lung sounds are found to be wheezes on expiration in all lung fields. She looks like she is tiring out, so you decide to assist her breathing and "bag in the treatment" with a bag-valve mask (BVM) as your partner starts an IV. Once the IV is in place and the first treatment is on board, the next decision will likely involve a nasal intubation, or better yet, perhaps continuous positive airway pressure (CPAP) and transportation. You both decide to do the rest of the secondary assessment en route to the hospital because the patient's condition is serious. The daughter hands you a long list of medications to take along to the hospital, which includes albuterol (Ventolin), digoxin (Lanoxin), methyldopa (Aldomet), and warfarin (Coumadin). As you load Millie into the ambulance, you note that the time is now 5:20 PM.

1. What initial management is indicated for this patient?

   _____

   _____

   _____

   _____

   _____

   _____

2. What is your interpretation of this cardiac rhythm?

   _____

   _____

   _____

   _____

   _____

   _____

3. What is your field impression of this patient?

_____

_____

_____

_____

_____

_____

4. Are the patient's vital signs and SAMPLE history consistent with your field impression?

_____

_____

_____

_____

_____

_____

5. What specific treatment is required for this patient's condition?

_____

_____

_____

_____

_____

_____

6. Is further treatment required for this patient?

_____

_____

_____

_____

_____

_____

7. Are there any special considerations for this patient?

_____

_____

_____

_____

8. Complete the PCR.

EMS Patient Care Report (PCR)

Date:	Incident No.:	Nature of Call:		Location:

Dispatched:	En Route:	At Scene:	Transport:	At Hospital:	In Service:

Patient Information

Age:	Allergies:
Sex:	Medications:
Weight (in kg [lb]):	Past Medical History:
	Chief Complaint:

Vital Signs

Time:	BP:	Pulse:	Respirations:	SpO$_2$:
Time:	BP:	Pulse:	Respirations:	SpO$_2$:
Time:	BP:	Pulse:	Respirations:	SpO$_2$:

EMS Treatment
(circle all that apply)

Oxygen @ _____ L/min via (circle one): NC NRM Bag-Mask Device	Assisted Ventilation	Airway Adjunct	CPR
Defibrillation	Bleeding Control	Bandaging	Splinting	Other

Narrative

Case Study 3

It is 7:00 PM and you have been dispatched to a Priority 1 (Charlie response) to a call for an elderly woman who fell in the hallway of the nursing home. As you arrive at 7:08 PM, an aide meets you to escort you to the location where the patient was found. Apparently Mrs. Smith wandered out of her room and was found on the floor in the hallway near the dining room. A family member has been called and will be meeting you at the local hospital ED. The scene is safe and you have enough help. You don your PPE as you approach the patient, who is lying on her back on the floor and looking very uncomfortable. The patient's right leg seems to be twisted laterally, which leads you to suspect she may have injured her hip when she fell. She is a bit confused but glad that help has arrived at her side. According to the aide, Mrs. Smith is 68 years old and has a history of diabetes and osteoarthritis. She takes medications for both conditions and has no known allergies. You ask her a few questions and determine she is verbally responsive and note she has an open airway and is breathing adequately. She is pale and clammy, and her radial pulse is fast and irregular. Your partner provides manual stabilization of the cervical spine as you do a quick head-to-toe exam on the patient. Moments later your supervisor arrives on the scene and assists in placing the C-collar and then securing the patient on the long backboard.

Vitals reveal the following: Respirations are 24 breaths/min and regular, her pulse is about 100 beats/min and irregular, blood pressure is 110/70 mm Hg, and her SpO_2 is 98%. You decide to place a board between the legs to secure the possible fractured hip, and then do a quick test of her blood glucose because the aide says she is usually alert and very talkative. Your partner places ECG electrodes and confirms sinus tachycardia with occasional premature ventricular contractions (PVCs) as well as a blood glucose of 70. You have decided that she be immobilized in a supine position, which has been a bit difficult due to the kyphosis of her spine, so giving sugar by mouth might be difficult. You therefore start an IV and quickly administer 10% dextrose (D_{10}). Once you document another set of vitals and note her mental status is now alert, you decide that hypoglycemia was part of the cause of the fall. Now it is time to get rolling to the hospital because there is a potential for internal bleeding from the hip fracture, which you realize elderly patients do not compensate well for. You will be reassessing the blood glucose, monitoring vitals, listening to her lungs, carefully administering fluid, and acquiring a 12-lead ECG on the way to the hospital. As you load Mrs. Smith into the ambulance, you note that the time is now 7:20 PM.

1. What are common contributing factors to falls in the elderly?

_____

_____

_____

_____

_____

_____

2. What are some common causes of altered mental status in the elderly?

_____

_____

_____

_____

_____

_____

3. What is kyphosis? How will you immobilize this patient's spine and hip?

_____

_____

_____

_____

_____

_____

4. How does aging affect the body's ability to compensate for shock?

_____

_____

_____

_____

_____

_____

5. Complete the PCR.

EMS Patient Care Report (PCR)

Date:	Incident No.:	Nature of Call:		Location:

Dispatched:	En Route:	At Scene:	Transport:	At Hospital:	In Service:

Patient Information

Age:	Allergies:
Sex:	Medications:
Weight (in kg [lb]):	Past Medical History:
	Chief Complaint:

Vital Signs

Time:	BP:	Pulse:	Respirations:	SpO$_2$:
Time:	BP:	Pulse:	Respirations:	SpO$_2$:
Time:	BP:	Pulse:	Respirations:	SpO$_2$:

EMS Treatment
(circle all that apply)

Oxygen @ _____ L/min via (circle one): NC NRM Bag-Mask Device		Assisted Ventilation	Airway Adjunct	CPR
Defibrillation	Bleeding Control	Bandaging	Splinting	Other

Narrative

Case Study 4

It is 10:00 PM and you have been dispatched to a Priority 1 (Charlie response) to a call for a serious injury from a bar fight. The police are already on the scene and they are looking for you to respond directly to the alleyway behind the tavern. As you arrive at 10:06 PM, the police are assisting a 23-year-old man to your ambulance. You barely open the doors to get your equipment out when the patient is already passing out on the ground just behind the ambulance. A fire fighter begins to hold the head and neck while you note the patient has a slash wound to his face and lots of bleeding on the front of his shirt. You note the patient has an airway, but he is having difficulty breathing. You assign a rescuer to deal with the bleeding to the face while you remove the patient's shirt and listen to his lungs. He has equal lung sounds, but you note a stab wound in the anterior chest on the left side, way too close to the heart. You seal the wound with an occlusive dressing and note that he has jugular venous distention (JVD). Your partner states he has a barely palpable radial pulse, so the decision is to put him on a backboard, begin assisting his ventilations, and do the rest while en route to the trauma center.

Once in the ambulance, a full set of vital signs reveals the following: weak pulse of 108 beats/min, respirations of 26 breaths/min and shallow, blood pressure of 90/60 mm Hg, and SpO$_2$ of 96%. You are assisting his ventilations with a BVM and 100% oxygen while a large-bore IV is inserted. A reassessment of vital signs shows a barely palpable radial pulse, and the blood pressure is now 78/64 mm Hg. You make a quick call to the ED and tell them you suspect his heart was nicked by the knife because his pulse pressure is narrowing, his neck veins are distended, and the location of the wound is close to the heart. There is too much noise with the siren blaring to listen for muffled heart sounds. The ED appreciates the early warning so they can be prepared to crack his chest upon your arrival. As you pull up at the ED, you note that the time is now 10:22 PM.

1. What immediate care is required for this patient?

_____

_____

_____

_____

_____

_____

2. What does JVD in this patient suggest?

_____

_____

_____

_____

_____

_____

3. What additional signs may accompany JVD in a patient with penetrating chest trauma?

_____

_____

_____

_____

_____

_____

4. What specific treatment is required to treat this patient's condition?

_____

_____

_____

_____

_____

_____

5. Complete the PCR.

EMS Patient Care Report (PCR)					
Date:	**Incident No.:**	**Nature of Call:**		**Location:**	
Dispatched:	**En Route:**	**At Scene:**	**Transport:**	**At Hospital:**	**In Service:**
Patient Information					
Age:			**Allergies:**		
Sex:			**Medications:**		
Weight (in kg [lb]):			**Past Medical History:**		
			Chief Complaint:		
Vital Signs					
Time:	**BP:**	**Pulse:**	**Respirations:**		**SpO$_2$:**
Time:	**BP:**	**Pulse:**	**Respirations:**		**SpO$_2$:**
Time:	**BP:**	**Pulse:**	**Respirations:**		**SpO$_2$:**
EMS Treatment (circle all that apply)					
Oxygen @ _____ L/min via (circle one): NC NRM Bag-Mask Device		**Assisted Ventilation**	**Airway Adjunct**		**CPR**
Defibrillation	**Bleeding Control**	**Bandaging**	**Splinting**		**Other**
Narrative					

Case Study 5

It is 6:30 AM and you have been dispatched to a Priority 2 (Bravo response) to a call for a sick child. As you arrive at 6:40 AM, the father is waiting at the front door of the residence. He leads you to the nursery where their 18-month-old daughter sleeps. She has not been sleeping all night and the father states that her mom has been up with her because she was so irritable and crying. The scene is safe and you decide to don PPE once entering the room since the mother states her daughter is running a fever and has been vomiting. She believes she has a headache and a neck ache and she has never seen her so irritable before. You decide that because there is no obvious immediate life threat, the child can stay in her mom's lap during your assessment.

The airway is open and clear. The breathing is slightly elevated, but skin color is good and the tidal volume seems adequate. It is obvious the child, whose name is Jessica, has a fever, and you decide that masks and eye shields are appropriate in addition to the gloves. As you examine the child, you see some petechiae on the extremities, but no purpura is present and there is no obvious trauma. Jessica is alert according to the mom but still very irritable. You decide that oxygen would be helpful but do not want to get the child any more agitated than she is already, so you let mom administer blow-by with a pediatric nonrebreathing mask. Your partner gets a full set of vitals, and you compare them to the vitals in the pocket guide in your pediatric kit. The pulse is fast, blood pressure is slightly low, and respirations are on the high side of the normal range. After talking with the mother, you find this is a normally healthy child who has been sick for the last day and unable to keep any food down. The child takes no medications and has no allergies.

After consulting with your partner and the family, the plan is to wrap the child up so she is warm and to transport to the local pediatric ED. If the respirations become depressed, you will switch to BVM, and if the mental status changes or pulse further increases, you will consider venous access by IV or intraosseous (IO) line and then administer 20-mg/kg boluses to improve the perfusion. As you load Jessica into the ambulance, you note that the time is now 6:50 AM.

1. What is your initial treatment for this child?

_____

_____

_____

_____

_____

_____

2. What is your field impression of this child?

_____

_____

_____

_____

_____

_____

3. What are petechiae and purpura? What do they indicate?

_____

_____

_____

_____

_____

_____

4. What treatment will you provide to this child en route to the hospital?

_____

_____

_____

_____

_____

_____

5. Complete the PCR.

EMS Patient Care Report (PCR)				
Date:	Incident No.:	Nature of Call:		Location:
Dispatched:	En Route:	At Scene:	Transport:	At Hospital:	In Service:

Patient Information	
Age: Sex: Weight (in kg [lb]):	Allergies: Medications: Past Medical History: Chief Complaint:

Vital Signs				
Time:	BP:	Pulse:	Respirations:	SpO$_2$:
Time:	BP:	Pulse:	Respirations:	SpO$_2$:
Time:	BP:	Pulse:	Respirations:	SpO$_2$:

EMS Treatment (circle all that apply)				
Oxygen @ _____ L/min via (circle one): NC NRM Bag-Mask Device	Assisted Ventilation	Airway Adjunct	CPR
Defibrillation	Bleeding Control	Bandaging	Splinting	Other

Narrative

Answers and Summary

Case Study 1

1. What is the appropriate order of initial management for this patient?

Management for the critically injured patient is based on what is going to kill the patient first. In most cases, airway management takes priority over all else; however, this is not always the case. The following represents the appropriate order of initial management for *this* patient:

- **Bleeding control**
  - The bright red blood spurting from the injury behind the patient's knee suggests a severed or partially severed popliteal artery. If not immediately controlled, severe arterial bleeding can result in death within a matter of minutes.
  - In the case of *this particular patient*, bleeding control takes priority over airway management. Because the patient is screaming in pain, he obviously has a patent airway.
- **100% supplemental oxygen**
  - The patient's respirations, although increased, are producing adequate tidal volume. Therefore, 100% oxygen via nonrebreathing mask is appropriate.
  - This patient is displaying signs of shock (ie, restlessness, tachycardia, diaphoresis). Therefore, 100% supplemental oxygen should be administered as soon as possible.
  - Monitor the patient for signs of inadequate breathing (eg, shallow depth, decreased mental status), and be prepared to provide ventilatory assistance.
- **Shock management**
  - Elevate the patient's legs 6 to 12 inches (unless not in your local protocol).
  - Elevation of the legs will not only help control bleeding from the lower extremity wound, but will facilitate venous return to the right side of the heart (increased preload), increasing cardiac output and maintaining perfusion to the vital organs of the body.
- **Thermal management**
  - Place a blanket on the patient to help maintain body temperature. Patients in shock do not have the amount of oxygen needed to produce energy and maintain body temperature.
  - Hypothermia interferes with the body's clotting mechanisms and may worsen the patient's bleeding.

2. How will you manage the continued bleeding from the patient's injury?

Initial management for severe bleeding involves applying direct pressure to the wound. Elevating the extremity above the level of the heart may also be helpful. Direct pressure and elevation are typically performed simultaneously and, in the majority of cases, adequately control the bleeding. A pressure dressing should then be applied over the wound to maintain constant pressure. If bleeding continues, place additional dressings over the pressure dressing. The site should be closely monitored for signs of continued bleeding, as evidenced by blood soaking through the pressure dressing. The popliteal fossa is a difficult place to secure an adequate pressure dressing. Be prepared to proceed to the next step in bleeding control should direct pressure fail.

There are occasions when, despite the application of direct pressure and elevation, the wound continues to bleed. This is common when large arteries (eg, femoral, radial, popliteal) are damaged or in areas of the body where maintenance of adequate pressure is difficult (eg, popliteal fossa). If, despite initial bleeding control measures, the wound continues to bleed, consider the use of a hemostatic dressing or an arterial tourniquet.

It should be noted that continuing to apply additional dressings to a severely bleeding wound will prove ineffective. Although the blood is contained within the additional dressings, the patient is still losing blood externally. If the wound continues to bleed uncontrollably, apply a tourniquet to the extremity proximal to the site of bleeding. This may not be possible if the bleeding is coming from the proximal humerus or proximal thigh—two locations where application of a tourniquet proximal will not be feasible because of the shoulder and hip, respectively. However, for bleeding at the level of the elbow or distal in the upper extremity or at the level of the knee and distal in the lower extremity (as in the current situation), correct tourniquet application is almost always an effective means of controlling bleeding.

Another method for controlling severe bleeding if initial methods fail is to remove all dressings, locate the site of the bleeding, and apply a hemostatic dressing directly to the site.

In the worst-case scenario, when all attempts to control bleeding fail, immediately transport the patient to the closest hospital while continuing bleeding control efforts en route.

IV therapy would clearly be of no benefit to the patient with severe, uncontrolled bleeding. Remember to focus your efforts on treating what will kill the patient *first*.

3. What is the appropriate IV fluid resuscitation regimen for this patient?

The goal of IV therapy in the shock trauma patient is to maintain adequate perfusion, regardless of whether the patient is bleeding internally or externally. Optimally, lost blood should be replaced with blood. However, because blood must be refrigerated, typed, and cross-matched, and because it has a short shelf life, it is not practical for use in the prehospital setting.

Crystalloid solutions, such as normal saline or lactated Ringer's, are more practical for use in the prehospital setting than blood is. They are well-balanced solutions that closely resemble the electrolyte concentration of plasma. Additionally, they are less expensive and have a longer shelf life than blood does.

As previously discussed in other case studies within this book, IV therapy for the patient with internal bleeding should be somewhat conservative, infusing just enough IV fluid to maintain adequate perfusion (eg, good mental status, systolic blood pressure of 90 mm Hg). Because internal bleeding cannot be controlled in the prehospital setting, rapid IV fluid infusions may interfere with the body's hemostatic processes, thus resulting in increased internal hemorrhage and deterioration of the patient's condition.

External bleeding, however, can be controlled in the prehospital setting; therefore, IV fluid resuscitation in the hypotensive patient should be more aggressive. After you have controlled all external bleeding and you have no reason to suspect internal hemorrhage, infuse 1,000 mL of a crystalloid solution and then reassess the patient. Continue to administer fluid boluses as needed until you have stabilized the patient's blood pressure at 90 mm Hg and/or systemic perfusion has improved (eg, improved mental status, stronger peripheral pulses).

Because two thirds of crystalloid solutions leave the intravascular space within 1 hour of administration, you must administer 3 mL of crystalloid solution for every 1 mL of estimated blood loss.

Crystalloid solutions improve tissue perfusion by increasing circulating volume and facilitating the transport of oxygen-carrying red blood cells that remain in the vascular space; however, they do not carry oxygen themselves. Additionally, because excessive crystalloid administration may result in hemodilution of the blood, administration of more than 3 liters in the prehospital setting should be reserved for situations where perfusion cannot be maintained by any other means.

The paramedic should follow locally established protocols or contact medical control as needed regarding IV fluid resuscitation for the shock patient.

4. What is the difference between crystalloid and colloid solutions?

Crystalloid solutions, which are the primary solutions used for prehospital fluid resuscitation, contain electrolytes and water. However, because crystalloids lack proteins and larger molecules, their presence in the vascular space, once administered, is of relatively short duration. Furthermore, crystalloids, unlike whole blood, do not have the ability to carry oxygen.

The three main types of crystalloid solutions are classified by their tonicity (number of particles per unit volume) relative to that of blood plasma:

- **Isotonic crystalloids**
  - Tonicity is equal to that of blood plasma; therefore, in a normally hydrated patient, they will not cause a significant shift in fluids or electrolytes.
  - 0.9% sodium chloride (normal saline) and lactated Ringer's are examples of isotonic crystalloids.
- **Hypertonic crystalloids**
  - These have a higher solute concentration than that of the cells; therefore, when administered to a normally hydrated patient, they cause fluid to shift out of the intracellular space and into the extracellular space.
  - 50% dextrose in water ($D_{50}W$) is an example of a hypertonic crystalloid.
- **Hypotonic crystalloids**
  - These have a lower solute concentration than that of the cells; therefore, when administered to a normally hydrated patient, they cause fluid to shift from the extracellular space and into the intracellular space.
  - 0.45% sodium chloride (half normal saline) and 5% dextrose in water (D_5W) are examples of hypotonic crystalloids.

As previously discussed, normal saline and lactated Ringer's are the most commonly used IV crystalloids in the prehospital setting because of their ability to expand circulating volume immediately and rapidly.

Colloid solutions contain large proteins and molecules that cannot pass through the capillary membrane; therefore, relative to crystalloids, they remain in the vascular space for a longer period of time. Additionally, the osmotic properties of colloids attract water into the vascular space; therefore, a small amount of colloid can significantly increase intravascular volume. The following are examples of colloid solutions:

- **Plasmanate (plasma protein fraction).** The principal protein in Plasmanate is albumin, which is suspended in a saline solution.
- **Dextran.** Not a protein; however, it contains large sugar molecules with osmotic properties similar to that of albumin.
- **Hetastarch (Hespan).** Similar to dextran in that it contains large sugar molecules with osmotic properties similar to those of proteins.
- **Salt-poor albumin.** Contains only human albumin. Each gram of albumin administered causes retention of approximately 18 mL of water in the vascular space.

Although colloids maintain vascular volume better than crystalloids, their use in the prehospital setting is not practical. Colloids have a short shelf life, are costly, and have specific storage requirements—attributes that make them more suitable for the hospital setting. Like crystalloids, the colloids listed do not have the ability to carry oxygen.

5. What is the purpose of performing a secondary assessment?

The secondary assessment is a comprehensive head-to-toe examination that is performed on patients who are either critically injured or unconscious. It encompasses all of the components of the primary assessment; however, it is more in-depth and methodical, and takes more time to perform.

The purpose of the secondary assessment is to detect injuries or conditions that were either not evident during earlier assessments or did not require immediate emergency care.

With critically ill or injured patients, you will seldom have time to perform this time-consuming examination on the scene because you will often be preoccupied performing reassessments and rendering emergency treatment. If, while en route to the hospital, the patient's condition deteriorates, you should immediately repeat a primary assessment and address any newly developed life-threatening conditions. Because this may occur several times throughout transport, you will likely not have time to perform a secondary assessment.

If, however, your transport time to the hospital is lengthy and you have addressed all life-threatening injuries or conditions, a secondary assessment should be performed.

It is most appropriate to perform a secondary assessment of your patient in the back of the ambulance while en route to the hospital. Remaining at the scene to perform a thorough examination on a critically ill or injured patient would clearly delay definitive care and increase the possibility of a poor patient outcome.

Summary

During the primary assessment of your patient, all airway, breathing, and circulation problems must be corrected immediately. Invasive procedures, such as IV therapy or intubation, are of no value to the patient if there is uncontrolled bleeding or a non-patent airway.

The patient in this case study had an obviously patent airway; however, he had an uncontrolled arterial hemorrhage. Therefore, controlling the bleeding had priority over applying oxygen. If, however, sufficient help were available (eg, EMR, law enforcement), then bleeding control and oxygen therapy could have been accomplished simultaneously. Remember that the order in which you manage your patient's injuries or condition is based on what will be the *most rapidly* fatal. A severe, uncontrolled arterial hemorrhage will kill the patient before you can even prefill the reservoir of a nonrebreathing mask!

Once a patent airway has been established and all external bleeding has been controlled, the patient should be rapidly assessed for signs of shock. If signs of shock are present, immediately transport the patient and perform all interventions, such as IV therapy and cardiac monitoring, en route to the hospital.

In addition to 100% oxygen and thermal management, shock caused by external blood loss should be treated with aggressive IV infusions of an isotonic crystalloid solution (eg, normal saline, lactated Ringer's). The goal of IV therapy is to maintain adequate perfusion (eg, systolic blood pressure of 90 mm Hg, improved mental status). Because crystalloid solutions quickly leave the vascular space, you must infuse 3 mL for each 1 mL of estimated blood loss. Because excessive crystalloids may hemodilute the blood, more than 3 liters should not be administered in the prehospital setting unless absolutely necessary to maintain perfusion.

Continually monitor the patient en route to the hospital, and be prepared to infuse additional IV fluids for blood pressure maintenance, assist ventilations for inadequate breathing, or perform CPR if the patient develops cardiac arrest.

Show the PCR to your instructor and ask for some feedback!

Case Study 2

1. What initial management is indicated for this patient?

Positive-pressure ventilations (BVM device or pocket-mask device) are indicated. This patient has multiple signs of inadequate breathing, including confusion, rapid and labored respirations, inability to speak in full sentences, and perioral cyanosis.

Tidal volume is needed and can be provided only with the use of positive-pressure ventilatory support.

Consider placing a nasopharyngeal airway if the patient's LOC further decreases.

2. What is your interpretation of this cardiac rhythm?

The cardiac rhythm described is *atrial fibrillation*, which is characterized by an irregularly irregular rhythm and the absence of discernible P waves.

Atrial fibrillation is caused by multiple ectopic foci in the atria that discharge in a chaotic fashion. Many of the impulses are blocked at the AV junction, whereas others are allowed to pass through. This randomized impulse passage through the AV junction causes the ventricular rhythm in atrial fibrillation to be irregularly irregular.

Atrial fibrillation is often seen with conditions such as congestive heart failure and COPD (eg, emphysema) and is commonly caused by pulmonary hypertension with subsequent atrial dilation.

3. What is your field impression of this patient?

This patient is suffering from an *acute exacerbation of emphysema* and is quickly approaching complete respiratory failure. The following assessment findings support this field impression:

- History of emphysema, no doubt attributed to her history of cigarette smoking.
- Recent flu-like symptoms, which indicate a possible respiratory tract infection, the most common precursor to acute exacerbation of COPD.
- Temperature of 101.5°F, which confirms the presence of an infection.
- Acute worsening of her shortness of breath, which is classic in COPD exacerbation following an acute respiratory tract infection.

Emphysema falls within a myriad of conditions collectively called COPD. Other forms of COPD include chronic bronchitis and, to a lesser degree, asthma, which is more of an episodic disease than a chronic one.

Emphysema is a progressive, irreversible pulmonary disease that is most often attributed to a history of long-term cigarette smoking or repeated exposure to other toxic substances. The incidence of emphysema is much higher in men than in women.

Emphysema results in gradual destruction of the alveolar walls due to a loss of pulmonary surfactant, which decreases the surface area of the alveolar membrane and interferes with gas exchange in the lungs. Additionally, the number of pulmonary capillaries decreases, which increases the resistance to pulmonary blood flow. This process ultimately causes pulmonary hypertension, which may lead to right-sided heart failure (cor pulmonale). Because the right side of the heart must pump against a high-pressure gradient, atrial dilation may occur, thus resulting in atrial fibrillation.

Emphysema also weakens the walls of the small bronchioles, which, in combination with alveolar wall destruction, decreases the ability of the lungs to recoil effectively during exhalation. This causes air to become trapped in the lungs, giving the person's chest a characteristic barrel-shaped appearance. Frequent pulmonary infections further the degree of air trapping because of inflammation and mucous production within the bronchioles.

The destruction of lung tissue causes the alveoli to collapse (atelectasis). The patient attempts to compensate for this by breathing through pursed lips, thus creating an effect similar to that of positive-end expiratory pressure (PEEP).

As the degenerative process of emphysema continues, the partial pressure of oxygen in the arterial blood (Pa_{O_2}) decreases and remains chronically low. This stimulates red blood cell production, perhaps even to excessive levels (polycythemia), which would explain why the patient's skin remains pink (pink puffer) despite inadequate pulmonary gas exchange. The presence of cyanosis, therefore, would indicate severe hypoxia in patients with emphysema, more so than if it were present in an otherwise healthy person.

Patients with COPD tend to retain carbon dioxide and, therefore, have a chronically elevated partial pressure of arterial carbon dioxide (Pa_{CO_2}). Chemoreceptors that monitor the levels of oxygen in carbon dioxide in the body eventually become accustomed to this, and the respiratory center in the brain (medulla oblongata) stops using increased Pa_{CO_2} levels to regulate breathing, as it does in an otherwise healthy person. This activates a mechanism called the hypoxic drive, which increases breathing stimulation when Pa_{O_2} levels fall and inhibits breathing stimulation when Pa_{O_2} levels increase. In rare cases, the administration of high-concentration oxygen, which can quickly increase Pa_{O_2} levels, may cause the chemoreceptors to stop stimulating the respiratory centers, resulting in hypoventilation or even apnea. If this occurs, simply assist the patient's ventilations. Never withhold oxygen from a hypoxic patient, even in the face of this potential—although highly uncommon—threat.

Patients with emphysema are predisposed to lower respiratory tract infections such as pneumonia because of their diminished ability to expel secretions from the lungs effectively. In addition, hypoxia-related cardiac dysrhythmias may occur.

Patients with emphysema and COPD in general learn to live with their chronic illness on a daily basis and grow accustomed to the normal respiratory distress and physical limitations that accompany it. When they call EMS, something has changed for the worse.

4. Are the patient's vital signs and SAMPLE history consistent with your field impression?

The patient's vital signs do not reinforce a field impression of COPD exacerbation as much as her medical history does. In particular, the recent flu-like symptoms that preceded an acute exacerbation of her respiratory distress make this a classic case.

Because this patient takes numerous medications, each of which is used to treat different conditions, it would be worthwhile to review each of them briefly.

- **Albuterol (Ventolin, Proventil).** Selective beta 2-agonist that dilates the bronchioles and is thus used to treat diseases associated with bronchiole constriction and/or inflammation, such as asthma, emphysema, and bronchitis
- **Digoxin (Lanoxin, digitalis).** A cardiac glycoside that is used for, among other conditions, ventricular rate control in patients with chronic atrial fibrillation
- **Warfarin (Coumadin).** An anticoagulant commonly prescribed as prophylactic therapy to patients with atrial fibrillation who are prone to developing microemboli (small clots) when blood stagnates in the poorly contracting atria
- **Methyldopa (Aldomet).** A centrally acting antiadrenergic used in the treatment of hypertension. Its active metabolite, alpha-methylnorepinephrine, lowers the blood pressure by stimulating central inhibitory alpha-adrenergic receptors and reducing plasma levels of renin. Renin is a proteolytic enzyme of the kidney that plays a major role in the release of angiotensin, a potent vasoconstrictor.

5. What specific treatment is required for this patient's condition?

- **Endotracheal intubation.** If the paramedic has difficulty providing effective ventilations utilizing basic means (BVM device, pocket-mask device), endotracheal intubation should be performed to facilitate administration of 100% oxygen directly into the patient's lungs and more definitively protect the patient's airway.

  As evidenced by the patient's falling oxygen saturation level and markedly diminished LOC, it is clear that BVM ventilation is not providing adequate oxygenation.

  Because of the patient's already diminished LOC, a hypnotic-sedative drug (Versed, etomidate) may be all that is required to facilitate intubation. If sedation alone is not effective, however, a neuromuscular blocker (paralytic) may be needed to perform rapid sequence intubation (RSI).

  When inducing paralysis with medications, succinylcholine (Anectine) is the preferred initial agent to use. Succinylcholine has a duration of action of only 3 to 5 minutes, which means that if intubation is unsuccessful, you will not have to ventilate the patient with a BVM device for a prolonged period of time. Succinylcholine does, however, depolarize potassium ions, which produces muscular fasciculations (generalized muscle twitching). Therefore, use of a nondepolarizing paralytic, such as vecuronium (Norcuron) in a premedication (priming) dose prior to inducing full neuromuscular blockade with succinylcholine is advisable. Once intubation is *successfully performed and confirmed*, neuromuscular blockade can be maintained with a longer-acting paralytic, especially if your transport time will be prolonged. Again, vecuronium, which has a 45-minute duration of action, would be an appropriate drug to use.

  Follow locally established protocols regarding the use and doses of neuromuscular blockers for RSI.

- **Pharmacologic interventions.**
  - *Aerosolized bronchodilators* can be administered endotracheally with a small-volume inline nebulizer. The following medications can be given alone, or in combination:
    - Selective beta 2-adrenergic agonists, such as albuterol (Ventolin, Proventil), metaproterenol (Alupent), or isoetharine (Bronkosol)
    - Anticholinergic bronchodilators such as ipratropium (Atrovent)

  When used in combination with beta agonists, the beta agonist must be administered first, followed by a 5-minute interval prior to administering Atrovent.

Aerosolized bronchodilators, because of their rapid onset of action (3 to 5 minutes), would be the preferred initial pharmacologic intervention because of the severity of the patient's condition. The significant bronchoconstriction, which is impairing effective positive-pressure ventilation in this patient, must be reversed as soon as possible. Follow locally established protocols regarding the dose of endotracheally administered bronchodilators.

- *IV glucosteroids*:
  - Methylprednisolone (Solu-Medrol): Reduces acute and chronic inflammation and potentiates the relaxation of bronchiole smooth muscle caused by beta-adrenergic agonists.
  - Solu-Medrol has an onset of action of approximately 1 to 2 hours. The adult dose varies, usually ranging from 40 to 125 mg IV.

The goal in treating patients with acute COPD decompensation—or any lower airway disorder for that matter—is to correct hypoxemia and to relieve the bronchoconstriction that is causing the hypoxemia. These actions will prevent respiratory failure and subsequent cardiac arrest.

Administration of 100% supplemental oxygen is the first and most important intervention. Oxygen may be given with a nonrebreathing mask or via positive-pressure ventilatory support if the patient's respiratory effort is inadequate.

Medications, administered by aerosol or IV or both, are needed to relax the smooth muscles of the lower airways, thus improving ventilation and facilitating oxygenation.

6. Is further treatment required for this patient?

By improving this patient's oxygenation status, her LOC may improve. The patient may fight the endotracheal tube, making it safer to consider removal. Because of the potential for vomiting and aspiration following removal of the endotracheal tube and the possibility that her condition could worsen, she should remain intubated. Extubation in the field (unless done by the patient) is not commonly performed. For patient comfort and to prevent field extubation by the patient, consider administering additional doses of a long-acting paralytic (eg, Norcuron) and/or keeping the patient sedated with the appropriate medications (Versed, Valium).

Although her oxygen saturation of 88% was low, it may not come up to 98% due to her chronic condition. An improvement from 88% to 92% might be as good as she gets in the field. Continue to monitor her ventilatory status, oxygen saturation, and ECG. She is still prone to cardiac dysrhythmias.

7. Are there any special considerations for this patient?

As previously mentioned, patients with COPD have chronically low Pao_2 levels and are stimulated to breathe based on these levels (hypoxic drive).

If high concentrations of oxygen are administered, the respiratory centers in the brain may be fooled into thinking that the patient is adequately oxygenated and will therefore send messages to the respiratory muscles to decrease the rate and strength of breathing. Oxygen-induced hypoventilation or apnea occurs in less than 3% to 5% of patients with COPD. Should this rare event occur, simply provide positive-pressure ventilatory support. Never withhold oxygen from a hypoxic patient!

Summary

When patients with chronic respiratory disease call EMS, a significant change has occurred in their condition. Otherwise your assistance would not have been requested.

Due to the nature of their illness, patients with COPD typically have a baseline respiratory distress; however, they cannot live with *severe* hypoxia any better than a healthy person could.

An acute lower respiratory tract infection, such as pneumonia, in which the patient cannot effectively expel secretions from the lungs, is the most common precursor to exacerbation of COPD. The mucous production and bronchiole inflammation that accompany many respiratory infections only worsen the patient's hypoxia.

You must perform a careful, systematic assessment of the patient and provide the appropriate treatment in a timely manner. It is critical that you recognize the difference between an adequately and an inadequately breathing patient.

Prehospital care focuses on ensuring adequate oxygenation and ventilation and pharmacologically reversing bronchoconstriction. Definitive care includes treating the underlying cause of the exacerbation, which usually involves antibiotics to treat the underlying infection. If the patient begins to show signs of respiratory failure, such as a rapidly falling oxygen saturation level or decreasing LOC, use sedating agents and neuromuscular blocking medications to intubate the patient without delay.

Show the PCR to your instructor and ask for some feedback!

Case Study 3

1. What are common contributing factors to falls in the elderly?

Falls are a common cause of injury in elderly patients and can result in serious problems. According to the American Geriatric Society, fall-related injuries are a leading cause of accidental death in the elderly. Additionally, 50% of falls result in lesser injuries (eg, soft-tissue trauma), which may not be life threatening, but can have a profound impact on the patient's quality of life. Children and young adults have a higher incidence of falls than the elderly; however, unlike the elderly, their injuries are not associated with a high mortality rate.

Falls in the elderly are caused by intrinsic (patient-related) factors, extrinsic (environmental) factors, or a combination of both (multifactorial). Extrinsic factors include torn or loose rugs, poor lighting, furniture obstructions, wet floors, and high steps on stairways.

Intrinsic factors may be age related or the result of an acute or prior medical condition. Age-related changes include impaired balance and coordination (gait impairment), decreased muscle and bone strength, impaired vision and depth perception, and decreased proprioception (perception of body position and movement).

Common acute medical conditions include myocardial infarction, stroke, hypoglycemia, and infection with associated dehydration. Prior medical illnesses—such as stroke, cataracts, and Parkinson disease—can impair the elderly patient's balance and coordination, leading to falls.

The use of certain medications can also predispose the elderly patient to falls. These medications include anxiolytics such as temazepam (Restoril) and diazepam (Valium), antidepressants such as amitriptyline (Elavil) and paroxetine (Paxil), and antihypertensives such as propranolol (Inderal) and metoprolol (Lopressor). Medication-related falls are often the result of nervous system impairment, drug-to-drug interaction, or inadvertent overdose. Many elderly patients take multiple medications (polypharmacy) for different medical conditions, and it is often impossible to determine how one drug will interact with another.

The cause of falls in the elderly is often multifactorial. An overmedicated patient may trip on a loose rug or fall down steps, or the patient may experience a syncopal episode and strike his or her head on an end table while falling.

Through a careful and systematic assessment of the patient, the paramedic must attempt to determine the cause of the patient's fall. In many cases, a fall may be the only presenting sign of an acute illness. Unfortunately, the patient's fall may be the result of physical abuse, which should be suspected when the injury sustained does not coincide with the mechanism described.

2. What are some common causes of altered mental status in the elderly?

You should assume that any alteration in mental status is abnormal until proven otherwise, regardless of the patient's age. Advanced age does not automatically equate to an altered mental status. Elderly patients are frequently capable of highly creative and productive thought processes.

By the time a person reaches the age of 80 years, brain size has decreased by approximately 10%; however, this decrease in brain size does not affect the person's intelligence. The following slight changes, which are not present in all patients, are commonly associated with the aging process:

- Forgetfulness
- Psychomotor slowing
- Decreased reaction time
- Difficulty remembering recent events

When assessing an elderly patient with altered mental status, you must first determine the patient's baseline mental status. According to the aide, your patient is normally well oriented. This confirms the presence of a new onset in altered mentation.

Elderly patients are predisposed to several neurologic disorders that can produce alterations in mentation. It may not be possible to determine the exact cause in the prehospital setting, which is why these patients should be evaluated in the ED.

Approximately 15% of Americans over the age of 65 years experience varying degrees of dementia. Dementia is defined as a progressive impairment of cognitive function. Alzheimer disease, a common cause of dementia, is a degenerative disease of the brain that results in impaired memory, thinking, and behavior. Approximately 5.4 million Americans are affected by Alzheimer disease. Brain tumors, which typically grow slowly, are another possible cause of dementia.

In the prehospital setting, dementia is often difficult to differentiate from delirium, especially in the absence of a friend or family member who is familiar with the patient's normal mental state. Unlike dementia, delirium is characterized by an acute onset of cognitive impairment and is frequently caused by a life-threatening medical condition. Delirium can be reversed if the underlying cause is rapidly identified and promptly treated.

Once it has been established that the altered mental status is a new onset, the paramedic should carefully and systematically assess the patient in an attempt to identify and treat the underlying cause. Routine actions include evaluating for signs of trauma, obtaining a blood glucose reading, and considering the administration of naloxone (Narcan) if a drug overdose is suspected.

Again, do not become complacent and assume that an altered mental status in the elderly patient is simply the result of advanced age.

3. What is kyphosis? How will you immobilize this patient's spine and hip?

Kyphosis is an exaggerated curvature (concave ventral) of the spine that results in a rounded or hunched back. Kyphosis can occur for many reasons and at any age; however, in the elderly, it is most commonly caused by osteoporosis. As the bones of the spine weaken and thin, they begin to deteriorate and compress. This results in deformation of the spine, most commonly in the upper thoracic region.

Because of the age-related deterioration of bone structure (eg, osteoporosis), fractures of the spine can occur with even minor mechanisms of injury. Therefore, spinal immobilization of this patient is clearly necessary.

Immobilizing this patient's kyphotic spine will require modification of the spinal immobilization technique. Additionally, as evidenced by the lateral rotation and shortening of her left leg, you should suspect and treat this patient for a hip fracture.

When immobilizing the spine of kyphotic patients, several pillows or blankets may be required to provide support to the head and upper back. Padding of these areas is necessary to provide support, because the kyphotic patient's back will not completely conform to the spine board.

Hip fractures are actually fractures of the proximal portion of the femur near or at the site of articulation with the acetabulum. Commonly, fractures of the proximal femur can occur between the femoral head and the trochanteric region (femoral neck fractures), between the greater and lesser trochanters (intertrochanteric), or below the lesser trochanter (subtrochanteric).

Hip fractures are commonly splinted by placing pillows or other padding under the injured extremity to support the fracture site in the deformed position. Splinting the extremity in the position in which it was found will minimize the risk of further injury as well as reduce the patient's pain.

A long spine board or an orthopedic (scoop) stretcher can be used to immobilize a fractured hip. These devices will allow the patient and the splinting material to be properly secured. Traction splints are not recommended for immobilizing hip fractures. Because it is not possible to determine the exact location of the fracture in the prehospital setting, it is not possible to assess the integrity of the pelvis accurately. If the fracture involves the pelvis, applying a traction splint could actually be detrimental and result in further displacement and potential injury. Furthermore, the risk of injury to the skin and other soft tissues with the application of traction splints in the elderly is potentially higher. Thus, the use of these devices in elderly hip fracture patients should be avoided unless alternatives are inadequate or otherwise inappropriate.

4. How does aging affect the body's ability to compensate for shock?

Even at rest, the aging body's physiologic functions are diminished. Therefore, the ability of the elderly person to compensate for a low cardiac output, hypoxia, and shock effectively is markedly diminished. The respiratory, nervous, and cardiovascular systems are the key body systems that compensate during shock; therefore, age-related changes that occur with each of these systems will be discussed.

The aging process adversely affects ventilatory function, thus impairing the elderly person's ability to compensate for hypoxia. Smooth muscles of the lower airway weaken with age. When increases in tidal volume are needed (eg, hypoxia, shock), the patient attempts to breathe deeply; however, the walls of the lower airway collapse. This reduces tidal volume.

Loss of respiratory muscle mass, increases in the stiffness of the thoracic cage, and a decreased surface area available for air exchange contribute to a decrease in vital capacity (volume of air exchanged after maximal inhalation and exhalation) of up to 50%. Decreased vital capacity causes an increase in residual volume, which is the amount of air remaining in the lungs following a maximal exhalation. This leaves more stagnant air in the alveoli, which impairs effective gas exchange.

With aging, the body's chemoreceptors become less sensitive. Chemoreceptors, which are located in the aortic arch, sense changes in arterial oxygen and carbon dioxide and send signals to the brainstem to regulate breathing accordingly. Additionally, nerve impulse transmission from the brainstem to the diaphragm and the nerves of the intercostal muscles is decreased. The net effect is a decreased ability to increase respirations quickly in response to conditions that cause hypoxia (ie, shock).

The cardiovascular system undergoes, to varying degrees, age-related deterioration that decreases its ability to compensate for shock. The vasculature loses its elasticity, which causes an increase in systolic blood pressure and afterload (the force against which the heart must pump). As a result, the wall of the left ventricle becomes enlarged (hypertrophy) and thickens. The myocardium also loses its ability to stretch effectively (Frank-Starling effect), thus decreasing ventricular filling and contractility. Hypertrophy of the mitral and tricuspid valves also occurs, which impedes blood flow into and out of the heart. These myocardial changes cause a natural decrease in stroke volume and cardiac output. Furthermore, the ability to increase cardiac output to meet increased demands of the body is decreased.

Baroreceptors, which are located in the aortic arch and carotid sinus, become less sensitive to changes in blood volume with age. These receptors, which sense changes in arterial blood pressure, send messages to the adrenal glands, causing them to secrete the hormones epinephrine and norepinephrine, which causes increases in heart rate, myocardial contractility, and blood pressure. The heart's response to epinephrine and norepinephrine decreases with age; therefore, the elderly person is less able to compensate for blood loss and decreases in blood volume quickly and effectively.

Due to age-related decreases in elastin and collagen in the vascular walls, blood vessel elasticity can be reduced by as much as 70% in the elderly person. Therefore, compensation in shock is significantly reduced because the peripheral vasculature must be able to constrict and dilate accordingly to maintain blood pressure and adequate perfusion.

Summary

Falls are a leading cause of accidental death in patients over the age of 65 years. Contributing factors to falls in the elderly can be intrinsic (eg, age-related changes, acute or prior illness), extrinsic (eg, loose rugs, poor lighting), or a combination of both. When assessing the elderly patient who has fallen, the paramedic must attempt to determine the cause of the fall. Because of osteoporosis, spinal fractures can occur with even minor mechanisms of injury; therefore, the elderly patient who has fallen should be immobilized, with modifications made as needed for the patient with a kyphotic spine.

Hip fractures account for nearly 30% of orthopedic hospital admissions each year. Approximately 80% of hip fractures occur in women, and they are most frequently seen in the elderly. The elderly are prone to fractures because of osteoporosis, which makes the bones very fragile. Approximately 20% of patients over the age of 65 who are hospitalized for a hip fracture die within the first 6 months following the injury. In the acute setting, death following a hip fracture is usually caused by pneumonia, myocardial infarction, or pulmonary embolus. Long-term, common causes of death include pulmonary embolus and sepsis.

Mental status changes do not occur in all patients with age. Many elderly patients maintain effective cognitive processes. Any change in mentation must be assumed to be abnormal until proven otherwise. The paramedic should determine, by talking with friends or family members, whether the patient's mental status has changed and, if so, to what degree. Common causes of altered mental status in the elderly include hypoglycemia, medication-related issues, and stroke. Any patient with an altered mental status should be given supplemental oxygen or assisted ventilations as needed.

Age-related changes reduce the elderly person's ability to compensate for hemodynamic compromise (eg, blood loss) quickly and effectively. The muscles of the respiratory system weaken, and the chemoreceptors become less sensitive to changes in oxygen and carbon dioxide levels in the blood. Due to hypertrophy and thickening of the ventricular myocardium, stroke volume decreases, resulting in a decreased cardiac output, both at rest and in times of increased demand. Blood vessel elasticity decreases, making the peripheral vasculature less able to constrict and dilate in response to the body's demands.

Show the PCR to your instructor and ask for some feedback!

Case Study 4

1. What immediate care is required for this patient?

This patient has multiple significant mechanisms of injury. Each one must be addressed based on severity (ie, what will kill the patient first). Continue to have the fire fighter maintain manual stabilization of the patient's head while you and your partner perform the following interventions:

- **Control of external hemorrhage**
  - All external bleeding must be stopped immediately. Your partner can accomplish this while you tend to the patient's airway.
  - The stab wound to the left anterior chest should be covered with an occlusive dressing. Any open wound to the chest could indicate underlying pulmonary injury and an open pneumothorax (sucking chest wound).
- **100% supplemental oxygen**
  - Although increased, this patient's respiratory effort is adequate (good tidal volume); therefore, 100% supplemental oxygen via a nonrebreathing mask should be applied.
  - Monitor this patient's respiratory effort carefully and be prepared to initiate positive-pressure ventilatory support if his breathing becomes inadequate (eg, reduced tidal volume, profoundly labored).

Teamwork between you and your partner is critical to providing effective patient care. Had the fire fighters not been present to assist with spinal immobilization (meaning that your partner would have to), your first priority would have been to control the external bleeding. Only after the external bleeding is controlled would you apply oxygen. You must treat injuries in the order in which they would kill the patient. Severe external bleeding can cause death within a few seconds if not immediately controlled. Delaying oxygen therapy for the 1 or 2 minutes that it takes to control the severe bleeding will not kill the patient.

2. What does JVD in this patient suggest?

The stab wound to the left side of the chest and JVD should make you suspicious of a *pericardial tamponade*. The presence of bilaterally equal breath sounds rules out a tension pneumothorax, another potential cause of JVD.

The heart is encased in a fibrous, inelastic membrane called the pericardium. The pericardial space, which is actually a potential space that normally contains 20 to 30 mL of lubricating fluid, exists between the pericardium and the heart. Blood can enter the pericardial space if small myocardial blood vessels (eg, coronary arteries) are torn or if direct penetration of the myocardium occurs. As a result, a condition called hemopericardium occurs. As more blood enters the pericardial space, a pericardial tamponade can develop.

Pericardial tamponade is most commonly associated with stab wounds to the chest. Larger penetrating injuries, such as gunshot wounds, often create a large enough hole in the pericardium for blood to exit the pericardial space and are typically associated with exsanguination into the thoracic cavity rather than pericardial tamponade.

Because the tough, fibrous pericardium does not stretch, accumulating blood puts pressure on the heart, affecting both the systolic and the diastolic phases of the cardiac cycle. Pressure on the heart impairs venous return to the heart (preload) and limits right ventricular filling. As venous pressure increases, the jugular veins become distended.

3. What additional signs may accompany JVD in a patient with penetrating chest trauma?

In the adult patient, the pericardial space can hold 200 to 300 mL of blood before signs of a pericardial tamponade become evident; however, smaller volumes of blood can still significantly reduce cardiac output. Progression of a pericardial tamponade depends on how fast blood is filling the pericardial space.

As previously discussed, pericardial tamponade causes an increase in venous pressure and JVD. In addition, right ventricular expansion (and filling) is impaired, which compromises output through the pulmonary arteries and subsequent venous return to the left side of the heart. This causes a *decreased cardiac output and systemic hypotension*. A *reflex tachycardia* attempts to (but cannot) compensate for the low cardiac output.

Because myocardial contractility is compromised, the patient's systolic blood pressure decreases. Additionally, decreased ability of the myocardium to relax fully causes an increase in the diastolic blood pressure. These factors result in a *narrowed pulse pressure* (the difference between the systolic and diastolic blood pressure).

Pulsus paradoxus, which is characterized by a drop in systolic blood pressure of greater than 10 mm Hg during inspiration, may also occur and is caused when the expanding lungs literally stop the heart in animation by putting additional pressure on the already compressed myocardium. Pulsus paradoxus can be determined clinically by noting a diminished or even disappearing radial pulse upon inspiration.

Increasing amounts of blood in the pericardium may also cause *muffled or distant heart sounds*; however, this is often difficult to hear, especially in a loud environment such as the back of a moving ambulance.

Beck's triad, a classic finding in pericardial tamponade, is characterized by three clinical signs: (1) JVD, (2) muffled heart sounds, and (3) a narrowing pulse pressure. However, all three of these clinical signs may not be present, especially if the patient is hypovolemic from other injuries (eg, pelvic fracture).

4. What specific treatment is required to treat this patient's condition?

Patients with pericardial tamponade require rapid transport to a trauma center with continuous monitoring of airway, breathing, and circulation en route. As with any critical trauma patient, unnecessary delays must not occur in the field. Treatment for patients with pericardial tamponade includes removing blood from the pericardium by a procedure called *pericardiocentesis*. This procedure, however, is almost exclusively performed in the ED and is only a temporizing intervention until bleeding control and surgical repair of the injury can occur in the operating room. Refer to locally established protocols in regard to performing pericardiocentesis in the prehospital setting.

Prehospital management begins by ensuring airway patency and administering 100% supplemental oxygen. If the patient's respiratory effort is inadequate (eg, reduced tidal volume), assisted ventilations with 100% oxygen will be necessary.

Perform spinal immobilization if the mechanism of injury suggests spinal trauma. Because this patient was pushed out of a moving vehicle, he will clearly require immobilization.

Crystalloid IV fluids should be administered to increase venous return to the right atrium (preload). By increasing preload, the full and vigorously contracting atrium will force blood into the ventricles, thus stretching its walls. Stretching of the ventricular wall enhances contractility and the force with which it ejects blood out to the body. Increased cardiac contractility due to stretching of the myocardial wall is called the *Frank-Starling mechanism*; by administering IV fluids, the Frank-Starling mechanism will be enhanced and can maintain cardiac output until a pericardiocentesis can be performed.

Continuous cardiac monitoring is essential in the management of a patient with pericardial tamponade. Decreased cardiac output and hypoperfusion can result in life-threatening dysrhythmias. Pericardial tamponade is also associated with pulseless electrical activity (PEA), a condition in which a cardiac rhythm is present on the cardiac monitor but a palpable pulse is not present.

Summary

Pericardial tamponade is a condition in which blood accumulates in the pericardium and causes hemodynamic compromise. It is most often the result of penetrating trauma, specifically stab wounds to the chest. A small tear in a myocardial blood vessel or direct penetrating trauma to the myocardium causes blood to seep into the myocardium, which puts pressure on the heart and impairs its performance. The progression of a pericardial tamponade depends on the rate at which blood is accumulating within the pericardium.

Patients with pericardial tamponade typically present with signs of shock (eg, tachycardia, hypotension, diaphoresis) as well as JVD, muffled heart sounds, and a narrowing pulse pressure (Beck's triad). If the patient is severely hypovolemic from other injuries, however, JVD may not be present.

Complications associated with pericardial tamponade include cardiac dysrhythmias, such as ventricular fibrillation or ventricular tachycardia, or cardiac arrest with PEA.

A careful, systematic assessment of the patient is required to identify the signs of pericardial tamponade and to initiate the most appropriate treatment. Prehospital management consists of ensuring a patent airway, administering 100% oxygen (or ventilatory support if needed), immobilizing the spine if the mechanism of injury suggests spinal trauma, infusing IV crystalloids to increase venous return, and rapidly transporting the patient to a trauma center. Cardiac monitoring en route is essential in being able to identify and treat life-threatening cardiac dysrhythmias.

A pericardiocentesis is required to remove blood from the pericardium, thus improving cardiac output. However, this is almost exclusively performed in the ED by a physician and is only a temporizing intervention until the injury can be repaired surgically.

Show the PCR to your instructor and ask for some feedback!

Case Study 5

1. What is your initial treatment for this child?

- **Minimize the child's anxiety.** Although the child is clearly ill, your findings in the primary assessment do not warrant immediate separation of her from her mother. If possible, continue your assessment of the child while her mother is holding her. This will minimize the child's anxiety and may facilitate a more accurate assessment.
- **Administer 100% supplemental oxygen.** Use a pediatric nonrebreathing mask or the blow-by technique.

Although the child's respirations are increased, they are unlabored and are producing adequate tidal volume; therefore, ventilatory assistance is not indicated at this point. Administer passive oxygenation in a nonthreatening manner to avoid increasing the child's anxiety. If she becomes more irritable after applying a nonrebreathing mask, have the mother hold oxygen tubing near her nose and mouth.

Continue to monitor the child's respiratory effort and closely observe for signs of inadequate ventilation, such as a shallow depth of breathing (reduced tidal volume) or a decreasing mental status. Be prepared to assist ventilations with a BVM device if signs of inadequate breathing are observed.

2. What is your field impression of this child?

This child's clinical presentation is highly suggestive of meningitis. The following signs, symptoms, and historic findings support this field impression:

- **Fever**
- **Headache.** Young children will often grab the sides of their head or place their hand on their head when they are experiencing a headache. Older children are usually able to tell you that their head hurts.
- **Irritability.** Irritability is a very common sign of meningitis in smaller children. You should be especially suspicious if the child tends to become more irritable when she is picked up (paradoxical irritability); this indicates increased pain as traction is pulled on the inflamed meninges surrounding the spinal cord.
- **Apparent nuchal rigidity (neck stiffness).** The fact that the child will not move her head suggests that she is experiencing nuchal rigidity—a classic sign of meningitis. Nuchal rigidity may not be a reliable sign in children less than 18 to 24 months of age.

Meningitis, also referred to as spinal meningitis, is an inflammation of the meningeal layers that surround and protect the brain and spinal cord. The infection can be bacterial, viral, or even fungal in origin. In many cases, meningitis is preceded by upper respiratory infection (URI) symptoms. In the prehospital setting, it is not possible to determine the etiologic pathogen causing the disease (eg, bacterial, viral, fungal); therefore, you should assume the disease to be bacterial in origin (the most life threatening) until proven otherwise.

Bacterial meningitis remains a significant cause of mortality and morbidity in children. According to the Centers for Disease Control and Prevention (CDC), 3% to 6% of cases of meningitis in children are fatal; 20% of the patients who survive experience hearing loss or other long-term sequelae (eg, neurologic impairment).

Relative to viral (aseptic) meningitis, which typically does not pose the risk of permanent neurologic damage, bacterial meningitis is a potentially life-threatening infection. It is often associated with an altered mental status, seizures, and increased intracranial pressure (ICP). If left untreated, bacterial meningitis can result in severe sepsis, permanent neurologic damage, and even death.

Prior to 1990, *Haemophilus influenzae* type b (Hib) was the most common cause of bacterial meningitis; however, because a vaccine for Hib is now administered to children as part of their routine immunizations, the occurrence of *H. influenzae* has decreased. According to the CDC, the incidence of Hib-related meningitis between 1980 and 1990 was approximately 40 to 100 per 100,000 children under 5 years of age. Since vaccinations against Hib began, the incidence has decreased to 1.3 per 100,000 children in that same age group. *Neisseria meningitidis* (also called meningococcal meningitis) and *Streptococcus pneumoniae* (also called pneumococcal meningitis) are currently the leading causes of bacterial meningitis in children greater than 1 month of age. In neonates (birth to 1 month of age), meningitis is usually caused by *Escherichia coli* (*E. coli*), group B streptococcus, or *Listeria monocytogenes*.

Classic signs and symptoms of bacterial meningitis include high fever, headache, and nuchal rigidity. In infants, the clinical presentation is commonly that of increased irritability, poor feeding, vomiting, a bulging fontanelle (sign of increased ICP), and inconsolability. Because infants and children less than 18 to 24 months of age often lack adequately developed neck musculature, nuchal rigidity may not manifest; therefore, it is an unreliable sign in this age group. Only in children older than 18 to 24 months are headache and nuchal rigidity reliable manifestations of meningitis.

The signs and symptoms of meningitis can develop over several hours or a few days and may vary depending on the child's age. For example, infants may present with increased irritability, poor feeding, and difficulty in being consoled; older children are often unable to maintain a comfortable position secondary to muscle stiffness.

In older children, the inability to extend the legs with the hips flexed (Kernig sign) and/or involuntary flexion of the hip, knee, or ankle when the neck is passively flexed (Brudzinski sign) are suggestive of meningeal irritation. However, the absence of these clinical findings does not rule out meningitis.

Bacterial meningitis is a contagious disease. The primary mode of transmission is via the airborne droplet route, such as the exchange of respiratory secretions (eg, coughing, sneezing, kissing). Unlike the common cold or flu, however, the bacteria are not spread via casual contact with an infected person. Nonetheless, the appropriate standard precautions—gloves and facial protection—must be strictly followed when caring for a patient with suspected meningitis.

3. What are petechiae and purpura? What do they indicate?
Petechiae are small (< 0.05 cm) circumscribed areas of superficial bleeding into the skin. Initially, they appear as red pinpoint-sized spots and then turn purple or dark blue. A petechial rash is not a disease itself, but a manifestation of an underlying problem. The presence of petechiae indicates a low platelet count (thrombocytopenia) and is associated with a severe systemic infection (sepsis).

Approximately 25% of children with meningococcal meningitis develop an erythematous (red) maculopapular rash followed by petechiae or purpura, most commonly located on the extremities. Purpura, also a manifestation of thrombocytopenia, appears as purple circumscribed skin lesions greater than 0.5 cm in size.

Although petechiae and purpura are classically seen in children with meningococcal meningitis, they can also occur in conjunction with other infectious diseases, viral or bacterial.

4. What treatment will you provide to this child en route to the hospital?
Children with suspected meningitis must be closely monitored for the presence of increased ICP, seizures, and signs of septic shock. Because infants and small children have relatively immature immune systems, they are particularly vulnerable to sepsis.

If respiratory depression develops (suggestive of increased ICP), assist the child's ventilations with a BVM device and 100% oxygen. Endotracheal intubation may be necessary if you are unable to provide effective BVM ventilations or your transport time to the hospital will be lengthy.

Provided the child remains hemodynamically stable, allow him or her to remain with the caregiver. Continue oxygen therapy as tolerated and promptly transport the child to the hospital. If signs and symptoms of septic shock are present, obtain IV or IO access and administer 20-mL/kg boluses of normal saline or lactated Ringer's as needed to maintain adequate perfusion. If the child is hemodynamically stable, consider deferring IV therapy until the child is in the ED. Remember, you should avoid any unnecessary procedures; these will likely increase the child's anxiety and could cause acute deterioration of his or her clinical condition.

If the child experiences a seizure, administer a benzodiazepine drug such as diazepam (Valium) or midazolam (Versed). If IV or IO access is not available, diazepam can be given via the rectal route; midazolam can be given intramuscularly if needed. Follow locally established protocols or contact medical control as needed regarding the pediatric doses of these drugs.

If, despite two or three crystalloid fluid boluses, the child remains hypotensive, medical control may order an infusion of one of the following vasoactive drugs, both of which should be titrated as necessary to improve perfusion:

- Epinephrine: 0.1 to 1 μg/kg/min
- Dopamine: 2 to 20 μg/kg/min (Usual starting dose is 5 to 10 μg/kg/min.)

Definitive treatment for a child with meningitis and septic shock involves the administration of antibiotics—an intervention that cannot be provided in the prehospital setting. Therefore, rapid transport to an appropriate medical facility is essential.

Summary

Meningitis remains a significant cause of mortality and morbidity in children. *Neisseria meningitidis* (also called meningococcal meningitis) and *Streptococcus pneumoniae* (also called pneumococcal meningitis) are the most common causes of bacterial meningitis in children older than 1 month of age. *Haemophilus influenzae* type b (Hib) has been virtually eradicated as a cause of bacterial meningitis in children due to Hib vaccinations that began in the late 1980s. If left untreated, bacterial meningitis may result in septic shock, permanent neurologic impairment, or death.

Meningitis should be suspected in any child who presents with fever, headache, and nuchal rigidity; however, headache and nuchal rigidity are most reliably assessed in children older than 18 to 24 months of age. Other signs and symptoms include nausea and vomiting, irritability, photophobia, signs of increased ICP, seizures, and a petechial or purpuric rash. In infants, common signs include paradoxical irritability, poor feeding, a bulging fontanelle, and inconsolability.

Prehospital care for a child with meningitis begins by taking the appropriate standard precautions, including gloves and facial protection; bacterial meningitis is a contagious disease that is spread by the airborne droplet route. Obtain and maintain the child's airway and provide supplemental oxygen or assisted ventilation as needed. If signs of hypoperfusion are present, 20-mL/kg IV or IO crystalloid fluid boluses should be given. Vasopressor therapy (eg, epinephrine, dopamine) may be required for fluid-refractory hypoperfusion. If the child is hemodynamically stable, consider deferring IV therapy to avoid causing unnecessary anxiety. Promptly transport the child to an appropriate medical facility, while closely monitoring his or her ABCs en route. Meningitis is diagnosed in the ED with a lumbar puncture (spinal tap) and is treated definitively with antibiotic therapy.

Show the PCR to your instructor and ask for some feedback!

National Registry Skill Sheets

Skill Evaluation Sheets

Bleeding Control/Shock Management

Alternative Airway Device (Supraglottic Airway)

Dynamic Cardiology

Intravenous Therapy

Intravenous Bolus Medications

Patient Assessment—Medical

Oral Station

Patient Assessment—Trauma

Pediatric Intraosseous Infusion

Pediatric (< 2 yr) Ventilatory Management

Spinal Immobilization (Seated Patient)

Spinal Immobilization (Supine Patient)

Static Cardiology

Ventilatory Management—Adult

NOTE: At the time of printing of this Student Workbook these were the most up to date skill sheets. Since testing standards do change from time to time it is always a good idea to check the NREMT website for updates.

Candidate: _____ Examiner: _____

Date: _____ Signature: _____

Bleeding Control/Shock Management

Time Start: _____

	Possible Points	Points Awarded
Takes or verbalizes body substance isolation precautions	1	
Applies direct pressure to the wound	1	
NOTE: The examiner must now inform the candidate that the wound continues to bleed		
Applies tourniquet	1	
NOTE: The examiner must now inform the candidate that the patient is exhibiting signs and symptoms of hypoperfusion		
Properly positions the patient	1	
Administers high concentration oxygen	1	
Initiates steps to prevent heat loss from the patient	1	
Indicates the need for immediate transportation	1	
TOTAL:	7	

Time End: _____

CRITICAL CRITERIA

_____ Did not take or verbalize body substance isolation precautions

_____ Did not apply high concentration of oxygen

_____ Did not control hemorrhage using correct procedures in a timely manner

_____ Did not indicate the need for immediate transportation

You must factually document your rationale for checking any of the above critical items on the reverse side of this form.

Candidate: _____ Examiner: _____

Date: _____ Signature: _____

Device: _____

Alternative Airway Device (Supraglottic Airway)

NOTE: If candidate elects to initially ventilate with BVM attached to reservoir and oxygen, full credit must be awarded for steps denoted by "**" so long as first ventilation is delivered within 30 seconds.

Time Start: _____

	Possible Points	Points Awarded
Takes or verbalizes body substance isolation precautions	1	
Opens the airway manually	1	
Elevates tongue, inserts simple adjunct [oropharyngeal or nasopharyngeal airway]	1	
NOTE: Examiner now informs candidate no gag reflex is present and patient accepts adjunct		
**Ventilates patient immediately with bag-valve-mask device unattached to oxygen	1	
**Ventilates patient with room air	1	
NOTE: Examiner now informs candidate that ventilation is being performed without difficulty and that pulse oximetry indicates the patient's blood oxygen saturation is 85%		
Attaches oxygen reservoir to bag-valve-mask device and connects to high-flow oxygen regulator [12–15 L/minute]	1	
Ventilates patient at a rate of 10–12/minute with appropriate volumes	1	
NOTE: After 30 seconds, examiner auscultates and reports breath sounds are present and equal bilaterally and medical direction has ordered insertion of a supraglottic airway. The examiner must now take over ventilation		
Directs assistant to pre-oxygenate patient	1	
Checks/prepares supraglottic airway device	1	
Lubricates distal tip of the device [may be verbalized]	1	
NOTE: Examiner to remove OPA and move out of the way when candidate is prepared to insert device		
Positions head properly	1	
Performs a tongue-jaw lift	1	
Inserts device to proper depth	1	
Secures device in patient [inflates cuffs with proper volumes and immediately removes syringe or secures strap]	1	
Ventilates patient and confirms proper ventilation [correct lumen and proper insertion depth] by auscultation bilaterally over lungs and over epigastrium	1	

(continues)

Alternative Airway Device (Supraglottic Airway) (continued)

Adjusts ventilation as necessary [ventilates through additional lumen or slightly withdraws tube until ventilation is optimized]	1	
Verifies proper tube placement by secondary confirmation such as capnography, capnometry, EDD or colorimetric device	1	
NOTE: The examiner must now ask the candidate, "How would you know if you are delivering appropriate volumes with each ventilation?"		
Secures device or confirms that the device remains properly secured	1	
Ventilates patient at proper rate and volume while observing capnography/capnometry and pulse oximeter	1	
TOTAL:	19	

Time End: _____

CRITICAL CRITERIA

_____ Failure to initiate ventilations within 30 seconds after taking body substance isolation precautions or interrupts ventilations for greater than 30 seconds at any time

_____ Failure to take or verbalize body substance isolation precautions

_____ Failure to voice and ultimately provide high oxygen concentration [at least 85%]

_____ Failure to ventilate the patient at a rate of 10-12/minute

_____ Failure to provide adequate volumes per breath [maximum two errors/minute permissible]

_____ Failure to pre-oxygenate patient prior to insertion of the supraglottic airway device

_____ Failure to insert the supraglottic airway device at a proper depth or location within three attempts

_____ Failure to inflate cuffs properly and immediately remove the syringe

_____ Failure to secure the strap (if present) prior to cuff inflation

_____ Failure to confirm that patient is being ventilated properly (correct lumen and proper insertion depth) by auscultation bilaterally over lungs and over epigastrium

_____ Insertion or use of any adjunct in a manner dangerous to the patient

_____ Failure to manage the patient as a competent EMT

_____ Exhibits unacceptable affect with patient or other personnel

_____ Uses or orders a dangerous or inappropriate intervention

You must factually document your rationale for checking any of the above critical items on the reverse side of this form.

Candidate: _____   Examiner: _____

Date: _____   Signature: _____

SET #: _____

Dynamic Cardiology

Time Start: _____

	Possible Points	Points Awarded
Takes or verbalizes infection control precautions	1	
Checks patient responsiveness	1	
Checks ABCs (responsive patient) or checks breathing and pulse (unresponsive patient)	1	
Initiates CPR if appropriate [verbally]	1	
Attaches ECG monitor in a timely fashion [patches, pads, or paddles]	1	
Correctly interprets initial rhythm	1	
Appropriately manages initial rhythm	2	
Notes change in rhythm	1	
Checks patient condition to include pulse and, if appropriate, BP	1	
Correctly interprets second rhythm	1	
Appropriately manages second rhythm	2	
Notes change in rhythm	1	
Checks patient condition to include pulse and, if appropriate, BP	1	
Correctly interprets third rhythm	1	
Appropriately manages third rhythm	2	
Notes change in rhythm	1	
Checks patient condition to include pulse and, if appropriate, BP	1	
Correctly interprets fourth rhythm	1	
Appropriately manages fourth rhythm	2	
Orders high percentages of supplemental oxygen at proper times	1	
TOTAL:	24	

Time End: _____   (continues)

Dynamic Cardiology (continued)

CRITICAL CRITERIA

_____ Failure to deliver first shock in a timely manner

_____ Failure to verify rhythm before delivering each shock

_____ Failure to ensure the safety of self and others [verbalizes "all clear" and observes]

_____ Inability to deliver DC shock [does not use machine properly]

_____ Failure to demonstrate acceptable shock sequence

_____ Failure to immediately order initiation or resumption of CPR when appropriate

_____ Failure to order correct management of airway [ET when appropriate]

_____ Failure to order administration of appropriate oxygen at proper time

_____ Failure to diagnose or treat two or more rhythms correctly

_____ Orders administration of an inappropriate drug or lethal dosage

_____ Failure to correctly diagnose or adequately treat V-fib, V-tach, or asystole

_____ Failure to manage the patient as a competent EMT

_____ Exhibits unacceptable affect with patient or other personnel

_____ Uses or orders a dangerous or inappropriate intervention

You must factually document your rationale for checking any of the above critical items on the reverse side of this form.

Candidate: _____ Examiner: _____

Date: _____ Signature: _____

Intravenous Therapy

Time Start: _____

	Possible Points	Points Awarded

Checks selected IV fluid for:
  -Proper fluid (1 point)
  -Clarity (1 point)
  -Expiration Date (1 point)
	3	

Selects appropriate catheter	1	
Selects proper administration set	1	
Connects IV tubing to the IV bag	1	
Prepares administration set [fills drip chamber and flushes tubing]	1	
Cuts or tears tape [at any time before venipuncture]	1	
Takes/verbalizes body substance isolation precautions [prior to venipuncture]	1	
Applies tourniquet	1	
Palpates suitable vein	1	
Cleanses site appropriately	1	

Performs venipuncture
  -Inserts stylette (1 point)
  -Notes or verbalizes flashback (1 point)
  -Occludes vein proximal to catheter (1 point)
  -Removes stylette (1 point)
  -Connects IV tubing to catheter (1 point)
	5	

Disposes/verbalizes disposal of needle in proper container	1	
Releases tourniquet	1	
Runs IV for a brief period to assure patent line	1	
Secures catheter [tapes securely or verbalizes]	1	
Adjusts flow rate as appropriate	1	
TOTAL:	22	

Time End: _____

(continues)

Intravenous Therapy (continued)

NOTE: Check here (_____) if candidate did not establish a patent IV within three attempts in 6 minutes. Do _not_ evaluate the candidate in IV Bolus Medications.

CRITICAL CRITERIA

_____ Failure to establish a patent and properly adjusted IV within 6 minute time limit

_____ Failure to take or verbalize body substance isolation precautions prior to performing venipuncture

_____ Contaminates equipment or site without appropriately correcting situation

_____ Performs any improper technique resulting in the potential for uncontrolled hemorrhage, catheter shear, or air embolism

_____ Failure to successfully establish IV within three attempts during 6 minute time limit

_____ Failure to dispose/verbalize disposal of blood-contaminated sharps immediately in a proper container at the point of use

_____ Failure to manage the patient as a competent EMT

_____ Exhibits unacceptable affect with patient or other personnel

_____ Uses or orders a dangerous or inappropriate intervention

You must factually document your rationale for checking any of the above critical items on the reverse side of this form.

Intravenous Bolus Medications

Time Start: _____

	Possible Points	Points Awarded
Asks patient for known allergies	1	
Selects correct medication	1	
Assures correct concentration of drug	1	
Assembles prefilled syringe correctly and dispels air	1	
Continues to take or verbalize body substance isolation precautions	1	
Identifies and cleanses injection site [Y-port or hub]	1	
Reaffirms medication	1	
Stops IV flow	1	
Administers correct dose at proper push rate	1	
Disposes/verbalizes proper disposal of syringe and needle in proper container	1	
Turns IV on and adjusts drip rate to TKO/KVO	1	
Verbalizes need to observe patient for desired effect/adverse side effects	1	
TOTAL:	**12**	

Time End: _____   (continues)

Intravenous Bolus Medications (continued)

CRITICAL CRITERIA

_____ Failure to continue to take or verbalize appropriate body substance isolation precautions

_____ Failure to begin administration of medication within 3 minute time limit

_____ Contaminates equipment or site without appropriately correcting situation

_____ Failure to adequately dispel air resulting in potential for air embolism

_____ Injects improper medication or dosage [wrong medication, incorrect amount, or pushes at inappropriate rate]

_____ Failure to turn on IV after injecting medication

_____ Recaps needle or failure to dispose/verbalize disposal of syringe and needle in proper container

_____ Failure to manage the patient as a competent EMT

_____ Exhibits unacceptable affect with patient or other personnel

_____ Uses or orders a dangerous or inappropriate intervention

You must factually document your rationale for checking any of the above critical items on the reverse side of this form.

Candidate: _____   Examiner: _____

Date: _____   Signature: _____

Scenario: _____

Patient Assessment—Medical

Time Start: _____

	Possible Points	Points Awarded
Takes or verbalizes body substance isolation precautions	1	
SCENE SIZE-UP		
Determines the scene/situation is safe	1	
Determines the mechanism of injury/nature of illness	1	
Determines the number of patients	1	
Requests additional help if necessary	1	
Considers stabilization of spine	1	
PRIMARY SURVEY		
Verbalizes general impression of the patient	1	
Determines responsiveness/level of consciousness	1	
Determines chief complaint/apparent life-threats	1	

Assesses airway and breathing
    -Assessment (1 point)
    -Assures adequate ventilation (1 point)
    -Initiates appropriate oxygen therapy (1 point)
	3	

Assesses circulation
    -Assesses/controls major bleeding (1 point)
    -Assesses skin [either skin color, temperature, or condition] (1 point)
    -Assesses pulse (1 point)
	3	

Identifies priority patients/makes transport decision	1	
HISTORY TAKING AND SECONDARY ASSESSMENT		

History of present illness
    -Onset (1 point)   -Severity (1 point)
    -Provocation (1 point)   -Time (1 point)
    -Quality (1 point)   -Clarifying questions of associated signs and symptoms as
    -Radiation (1 point)   related to OPQRST (2 points)
	8	

Past medical history
    -Allergies (1 point)   -Past pertinent history (1 point)   -Events leading to
    -Medications (1 point)   -Last oral intake (1 point)   present illness (1 point)
	5	

(continues)

Patient Assessment—Medical (continued)

Performs secondary assessment [assess affected body part/system or, if indicated, completes rapid assessment] 　-Cardiovascular　　-Neurological　　-Integumentary　　-Reproductive 　-Pulmonary　　　-Musculoskeletal　-GI/GU　　　　-Psychological/Social	5	
Vital signs 　-Pulse (1 point)　　　　-Respiratory rate and quality (1 point each) 　-Blood pressure (1 point)　-AVPU (1 point)	5	
Diagnostics [must include application of ECG monitor for dyspnea and chest pain]	2	
States field impression of patient	1	
Verbalizes treatment plan for patient and calls for appropriate intervention(s)	1	
Transport decision re-evaluated	1	
REASSESSMENT		
Repeats primary survey	1	
Repeats vital signs	1	
Evaluates response to treatments	1	
Repeats secondary assessment regarding patient complaint or injuries	1	
TOTAL:	48	

Time End: _____

CRITICAL CRITERIA

_____ Failure to initiate or call for transport of the patient within 15 minute time limit

_____ Failure to take or verbalize body substance isolation precautions

_____ Failure to determine scene safety before approaching patient

_____ Failure to voice and ultimately provide appropriate oxygen therapy

_____ Failure to assess/provide adequate ventilation

_____ Failure to find or appropriately manage problems associated with airway, breathing, hemorrhage or shock [hypoperfusion]

_____ Failure to differentiate patient's need for immediate transportation versus continued assessment and treatment at the scene

_____ Does other detailed history or physical examination before assessing and treating threats to airway, breathing, and circulation

_____ Failure to determine the patient's primary problem

_____ Orders a dangerous or inappropriate intervention

_____ Failure to provide for spinal protection when indicated

You must factually document your rationale for checking any of the above critical items on the reverse side of this form.

Candidate: _____   Examiner: _____

Date: _____   Signature: _____

Scenario: _____

Oral Station

Time Start: _____

	Possible Points	Points Awarded
SCENE MANAGEMENT		
Thoroughly assessed and took deliberate actions to control the scene	3	
Assessed the scene, identified potential hazards, did not put anyone in danger	2	
Incompletely assessed or managed the scene	1	
Did not assess or manage the scene	0	
PATIENT ASSESSMENT		
Completed an organized assessment and integrated findings to expand further assessment	3	
Completed primary survey and secondary assessment	2	
Performed an incomplete or disorganized assessment	1	
Did not complete a primary survey	0	
PATIENT MANAGEMENT		
Managed all aspects of the patient's condition and anticipated further needs	3	
Appropriately managed the patient's presenting condition	2	
Performed an incomplete or disorganized management	1	
Did not manage life-threatening conditions	0	
INTERPERSONAL RELATIONS		
Established rapport and interacted in an organized, therapeutic manner	3	
Interacted and responded appropriately with patient, crew, and bystanders	2	
Used inappropriate communication techniques	1	
Demonstrated intolerance for patient, bystanders, and crew	0	
INTEGRATION (VERBAL REPORT, FIELD IMPRESSION, AND TRANSPORT DECISION)		
Stated correct field impression and pathophysiological basis, provided succinct and accurate verbal report including social/psychological concerns, and considered alternate transport destinations	3	

(continues)

Oral Station (continued)

Stated correct field impression, provided succinct and accurate verbal report, and appropriately stated transport decision	2	
Stated correct field impression, provided inappropriate verbal report or transport decision	1	
Stated incorrect field impression or did not provide verbal report	0	
TOTAL:	15	

Time End: _____

CRITICAL CRITERIA

_____ Failure to appropriately address any of the scenario's "Mandatory Actions"

_____ Failure to manage the patient as a competent EMT

_____ Exhibits unacceptable affect with patient or other personnel

_____ Uses or orders a dangerous or inappropriate intervention

You must factually document your rationale for checking any of the above critical items on the reverse side of this form.

Candidate: _____   Examiner: _____

Date: _____   Signature: _____

Scenario: _____

Patient Assessment—Trauma

NOTE: Areas denoted by "**" may be integrated within sequence of primary survey.

Time Start: _____	Possible Points	Points Awarded
Takes or verbalizes body substance isolation precautions	1	
SCENE SIZE-UP		
Determines the scene/situation is safe	1	
Determines the mechanism of injury/nature of illness	1	
Determines the number of patients	1	
Requests additional help if necessary	1	
Considers stabilization of spine	1	
PRIMARY SURVEY/RESUSCITATION		
Verbalizes general impression of the patient	1	
Determines responsiveness/level of consciousness	1	
Determines chief complaint/apparent life-threats	1	
Airway -Opens and assesses airway (1 point) -Inserts adjunct as indicated (1 point)	2	
Breathing -Assesses breathing (1 point) -Assures adequate ventilation (1 point) -Initiates appropriate oxygen therapy (1 point) -Manages any injury which may compromise breathing/ventilation (1 point)	4	
Circulation -Checks pulse (1 point) -Assesses skin [either skin color, temperature, or condition] (1 point) -Assesses for and controls major bleeding if present (1 point) -Initiates shock management (1 point)	4	
Identifies priority patients/makes transport decision based on calculated ACS	1	

(continues)

Patient Assessment—Trauma (continued)

HISTORY TAKING		
Obtains, or directs assistant to obtain, baseline vital signs	1	
Attempts to obtain SAMPLE history	1	
SECONDARY ASSESSMENT		
Head -Inspects mouth**, nose**, and assesses facial area (1 point) -Inspects and palpates scalp and ears (1 point) -Assesses eyes for PERRL** (1 point)	3	
Neck** -Checks position of trachea (1 point) -Checks jugular veins (1 point) -Palpates cervical spine (1 point)	3	
Chest** -Inspects chest (1 point) -Palpates chest (1 point) -Auscultates chest (1 point)	3	
Abdomen/pelvis** -Inspects and palpates abdomen (1 point) -Assesses pelvis (1 point) -Verbalizes assessment of genitalia/perineum as needed (1 point)	3	
Lower extremities** -Inspects, palpates, and assesses motor, sensory, and distal circulatory functions (1 point/leg)	2	
Upper extremities -Inspects, palpates, and assesses motor, sensory, and distal circulatory functions (1 point/arm)	2	
Posterior thorax, lumbar, and buttocks** -Inspects and palpates posterior thorax (1 point) -Inspects and palpates lumbar and buttocks area (1 point)	2	
Manages secondary injuries and wounds appropriately	1	
Reassesses patient	1	
TOTAL:	42	

Time End: _____

(continues)

Patient Assessment—Trauma (continued)

CRITICAL CRITERIA

____ Failure to initiate or call for transport of the patient within 10 minute time limit

____ Failure to take or verbalize body substance isolation precautions

____ Failure to determine scene safety

____ Failure to assess for and provide spinal protection when indicated

____ Failure to voice and ultimately provide high concentration of oxygen

____ Failure to assess/provide adequate ventilation

____ Failure to find or appropriately manage problems associated with airway, breathing, hemorrhage or shock [hypoperfusion]

____ Failure to differentiate patient's need for immediate transportation versus continued assessment/treatment at the scene

____ Does other detailed history or physical exam before assessing/treating threats to airway, breathing, and circulation

____ Failure to manage the patient as a competent EMT

____ Exhibits unacceptable affect with patient or other personnel

____ Orders a dangerous or inappropriate intervention

You must factually document your rationale for checking any of the above critical items on the reverse side of this form.

Candidate: _____ Examiner: _____

Date: _____ Signature: _____

Pediatric Intraosseous Infusion

Time Start: _____

	Possible Points	Points Awarded
Checks selected IV fluid for: -Proper fluid (1 point) -Clarity (1 point) -Expiration date (1 point)	3	
Selects appropriate equipment to include: -IO needle (1 point) -Syringe (1 point) -Saline (1 point) -Extension set or 3-way stopcock (1 point)	4	
Selects proper administration set	1	
Connects administration set to bag	1	
Prepares administration set [fills drip chamber and flushes tubing]	1	
Prepares syringe and extension tubing or 3-way stopcock	1	
Cuts or tears tape [at any time before IO puncture]	1	
Takes or verbalizes body substance isolation precautions [prior to IO puncture]	1	
Identifies proper anatomical site for IO puncture	1	
Cleanses site appropriately		
Performs IO puncture: -Stabilizes tibia without placing hand under puncture site and "cupping" leg (1 point) -Inserts needle at proper angle (1 point) -Advances needle with twisting motion until "pop" is felt or notices lack of resistence (1 point) -Removes stylette (1 point)	4	
Disposes/verbalizes proper disposal of needle in proper container	1	
Attaches syringe and extension set to IO needle and aspirates; or attaches 3-way stopcock between administration set and IO needle and aspirates; or attaches extension set to IO needle [aspiration is not required for any of these as many IO sticks are "dry" sticks]	1	
Slowly injects saline to assure proper placement of needle	1	
Adjusts flow rate/bolus as appropriate	1	
Secures needle and supports with bulky dressing [tapes securely or verbalizes]	1	
TOTAL:	24	

Time End: _____

(continues)

Pediatric Intraosseous Infusion (continued)

CRITICAL CRITERIA

_____ Failure to establish a patent and properly adjusted IO line within the 6 minute time limit

_____ Failure to take or verbalize body substance isolation precautions prior to performing IO puncture

_____ Contaminates equipment or site without appropriately correcting situation

_____ Performs any improper technique resulting in the potential for air embolism

_____ Failure to assure correct needle placement [must aspirate or watch closely for early signs of infiltration]

_____ Failure to successfully establish IO infusion within two attempts during 6 minute time limit

_____ Performing IO puncture in an unacceptable manner [improper site, incorrect needle angle, holds leg in palm and performs IO puncture directly above hand, etc.]

_____ Failure to properly dispose/verbalize disposal of blood-contaminated sharps immediately in proper container at the point of use

_____ Failure to manage the patient as a competent EMT

_____ Exhibits unacceptable affect with patient or other personnel

_____ Uses or orders a dangerous or inappropriate intervention

You must factually document your rationale for checking any of the above critical items on the reverse side of this form.

Candidate: _____   Examiner: _____

Date: _____   Signature: _____

Pediatric (< 2 yr) Ventilatory Management

NOTE: If candidate elects to ventilate initially with BVM attached to reservoir and oxygen, full credit must be awarded for steps denoted by "" so long as first ventilation is delivered within 30 seconds.**

Time Start: _____

	Possible Points	Points Awarded
Takes or verbalizes body substance isolation precautions	1	
Opens the airway manually	1	
Elevates tongue, inserts simple adjunct [oropharyngeal or nasopharyngeal airway]	1	
NOTE: Examiner now informs candidate no gag reflex is present and patient accepts adjunct		
**Ventilates patient immediately with bag-valve-mask device unattached to oxygen	1	
**Ventilates patient with room air	1	
NOTE: Examiner now informs candidate that ventilation is being performed without difficulty and that pulse oximetry indicates the patient's blood oxygen saturation is 85%		
Attaches oxygen reservoir to bag-valve-mask device and connects to oxygen regulator [12-15 L/minute]	1	
Ventilates patient at a rate of 12–15/minute and assures visible chest rise	1	
NOTE: After 30 seconds, examiner auscultates and reports breath sounds are present, equal bilaterally and medical direction has ordered intubation. The examiner must now take over ventilation.		
Directs assistant to pre-oxygenate patient	1	
Identifies/selects proper equipment for intubation	1	
Checks laryngoscope to assure operational with bulb tight	1	
NOTE: Examiner to remove OPA and move out of the way when candidate is prepared to intubate		
Places patient in neutral or sniffing position	1	
Inserts blade while displacing tongue	1	
Elevates mandible with laryngoscope	1	
Introduces ET tube and advances to proper depth	1	
Directs ventilation of patient	1	
Confirms proper placement by auscultation bilaterally over each lung and over epigastrium	1	
NOTE: Examiner to ask, "If you had proper placement, what should you expect to hear?"		
Secures ET tube [may be verbalized]	1	
TOTAL:	**17**	

Time End: _____

(continues)

Pediatric (< 2 yr) Ventilatory Management (continued)

CRITICAL CRITERIA

_____ Failure to initiate ventilations within 30 seconds after applying gloves or interrupts ventilations for greater than 30 seconds at any time

_____ Failure to take or verbalize body substance isolation precautions

_____ Failure to pad under the torso to allow neutral head position or sniffing position

_____ Failure to voice and ultimately provide high oxygen concentrations [at least 85%]

_____ Failure to ventilate patient at a rate of 12–15/min

_____ Failure to provide adequate volumes per breath [maximum two errors/min permissible]

_____ Failure to pre-oxygenate patient prior to intubation

_____ Failure to successfully intubate within three attempts

_____ Uses gums as a fulcrum

_____ Failure to assure proper tube placement by auscultation bilaterally **and** over the epigastrium

_____ Inserts any adjunct in a manner dangerous to the patient

_____ Attempts to use any equipment not appropriate for the pediatric patient

_____ Failure to manage the patient as a competent EMT

_____ Exhibits unacceptable affect with patient or other personnel

_____ Uses or orders a dangerous or inappropriate intervention

You must factually document your rationale for checking any of the above critical items on the reverse side of this form.

Candidate: _____   Examiner: _____

Date: _____   Signature: _____

Spinal Immobilization (Seated Patient)

Time Start: _____

	Possible Points	Points Awarded
Takes or verbalizes body substance isolation precautions	1	
Directs assistant to place/maintain head in the neutral, in-line position	1	
Directs assistant to maintain manual immobilization of the head	1	
Reassesses motor, sensory, and circulatory function in each extremity	1	
Applies appropriately sized extrication collar	1	
Positions the immobilization device behind the patient	1	
Secures the device to the patient's torso	1	
Evaluates torso fixation and adjusts as necessary	1	
Evaluates and pads behind the patient's head as necessary	1	
Secures the patient's head to the device	1	
Verbalizes moving the patient to a long backboard	1	
Reassesses motor, sensory, and circulatory function in each extremity	1	
TOTAL:	12	

Time End: _____

CRITICAL CRITERIA

_____ Did not immediately direct or take manual immobilization of the head

_____ Did not properly apply appropriately sized cervical collar before ordering release of manual immobilization

_____ Released or ordered release of manual immobilization before it was maintained mechanically

_____ Manipulated or moved patient excessively causing potential spinal compromise

_____ Head immobilized to the device before device sufficiently secured to torso

_____ Device moves excessively up, down, left, or right on the patient's torso

_____ Head immobilization allows for excessive movement

_____ Torso fixation inhibits chest rise, resulting in respiratory compromise

_____ Upon completion of immobilization, head is not in a neutral, in-line position

_____ Did not reassess motor, sensory, and circulatory functions in each extremity after voicing immobilization to the long backboard

_____ Failure to manage the patient as a competent EMT

_____ Exhibits unacceptable affect with patient or other personnel

_____ Uses or orders a dangerous or inappropriate intervention

You must factually document your rationale for checking any of the above critical items on the reverse side of this form.

Candidate: _____   Examiner: _____

Date: _____   Signature: _____

Spinal Immobilization (Supine Patient)

Time Start: _____

	Possible Points	Points Awarded
Takes or verbalizes body substance isolation precautions	1	
Directs assistant to place/maintain head in the neutral, in-line position	1	
Directs assistant to maintain manual immobilization of the head	1	
Reassesses motor, sensory, and circulatory function in each extremity	1	
Applies appropriately sized extrication collar	1	
Positions the immobilization device appropriately	1	
Directs movement of the patient onto the device without compromising the integrity of the spine	1	
Applies padding to voids between the torso and the device as necessary	1	
Immobilizes the patient's torso to the device	1	
Evaluates and pads behind the patient's head as necessary	1	
Immobilizes the patient's head to the device	1	
Secures the patient's legs to the device	1	
Secures the patient's arms to the device	1	
Reassesses motor, sensory, and circulatory function in each extremity	1	
TOTAL:	14	

Time End: _____

CRITICAL CRITERIA

_____ Did not immediately direct or take manual immobilization of the head

_____ Did not properly apply appropriately sized cervical collar before ordering release of manual immobilization

_____ Released or ordered release of manual immobilization before it was maintained mechanically

_____ Manipulated or moved patient excessively causing potential spinal compromise

_____ Head immobilized to the device **before** device sufficiently secured to torso

_____ Patient moves excessively up, down, left, or right on the device

_____ Head immobilization allows for excessive movement

_____ Upon completion of immobilization, head is not in a neutral, in-line position

(continues)

Spinal Immobilization (Supine Patient) (continued)

_____ Did not reassess motor, sensory, and circulatory functions in each extremity after voicing immobilization to the device

_____ Failure to manage the patient as a competent EMT

_____ Exhibits unacceptable affect with patient or other personnel

_____ Uses or orders a dangerous or inappropriate intervention

You must factually document your rationale for checking any of the above critical items on the reverse side of this form.

Candidate: _____   Examiner: _____

Date: _____   Signature: _____

SET #: _____

Static Cardiology

NOTE: No points for treatment may be awarded if the diagnosis is incorrect. Only document incorrect responses in spaces provided.

Time Start: _____

	Possible Points	Points Awarded
STRIP #1 Diagnosis:	1	
Treatment:	2	
STRIP #2 Diagnosis:	1	
Treatment:	2	
STRIP #3 Diagnosis:	1	
Treatment:	2	

(continues)

Static Cardiology (continued)

STRIP #4 Diagnosis:	1	
Treatment:	2	
TOTAL:	12	

Time End: _____

Candidate: _____   Examiner: _____

Date: _____   Signature: _____

Ventilatory Management—Adult

NOTE: If candidate elects to ventilate initially with BVM attached to reservoir and oxygen, full credit must be awarded for steps denoted by "**" so long as first ventilation is delivered within 30 seconds.

Time Start: _____

	Possible Points	Points Awarded
Takes or verbalizes body substance isolation precautions	1	
Opens the airway manually	1	
Elevates tongue, inserts simple adjunct [oropharyngeal or nasopharyngeal airway]	1	
NOTE: Examiner now informs candidate no gag reflex is present and patient accepts adjunct		
**Ventilates patient immediately with bag-valve-mask device unattached to oxygen	1	
**Ventilates patient with room air	1	
NOTE: Examiner now informs candidate that ventilation is being performed without difficulty and that pulse oximetry indicates the patient's blood oxygen saturation is 85%		
Attaches oxygen reservoir to bag-valve-mask device and connects to oxygen regulator [12-15 L/minute]	1	
Ventilates patient at a rate of 10-12/minute with appropriate volumes	1	
NOTE: After 30 seconds, examiner auscultates and reports breath sounds are present, equal bilaterally and medical direction has ordered intubation. The examiner must now take over ventilation.		
Directs assistant to pre-oxygenate patient	1	
Identifies/selects proper equipment for intubation	1	
Checks equipment for: -Cuff leaks (1 point) -Laryngoscope operational with bulb tight (1 point)	2	
NOTE: Examiner to remove OPA and move out of the way when candidate is prepared to intubate		
Positions head properly	1	
Inserts blade while displacing tongue	1	
Elevates mandible with laryngoscope	1	
Introduces ET tube and advances to proper depth	1	
Inflates cuff to proper pressure and disconnects syringe	1	
Directs ventilation of patient	1	
Confirms proper placement by auscultation bilaterally over each lung and over epigastrium	1	
NOTE: Examiner to ask, "If you had proper placement, what should you expect to hear?"		
Secures ET tube [may be verbalized]	1	

(continues)

Ventilatory Management—Adult (continued)

NOTE: Examiner now asks candidate, "Please demonstrate one additional method of verifying proper tube placement in this patient."		
Identifies/selects proper equipment	1	
Verbalizes findings and interpretations [checks end-tidal CO_2, colorimetric device, EDD recoil, etc.]	1	
NOTE: Examiner now states, "You see secretions in the tube and hear gurgling sounds with the patient's exhalation."		
Identifies/selects a flexible suction catheter	1	
Pre-oxygenates patient	1	
Marks maximum insertion length with thumb and forefinger	1	
Inserts catheter into the ET tube leaving catheter port open	1	
At proper insertion depth, covers catheter port and applies suction while withdrawing catheter	1	
Ventilates/directs ventilation of patient as catheter is flushed with sterile water	1	
TOTAL:	**27**	

Time End: _____

CRITICAL CRITERIA

_____ Failure to initiate ventilations within 30 seconds after applying gloves or interrupts ventilations for greater than 30 seconds at any time

_____ Failure to take or verbalize body substance isolation precautions

_____ Failure to voice and ultimately provide high oxygen concentrations [at least 85%]

_____ Failure to ventilate patient at a rate of 10–12/min

_____ Failure to provide adequate volumes per breath [maximum two errors/minute permissible]

_____ Failure to pre-oxygenate patient prior to intubation and suctioning

_____ Failure to successfully intubate within three attempts

_____ Failure to disconnect syringe **immediately** after inflating cuff of ET tube

_____ Uses teeth as a fulcrum

_____ Failure to assure proper tube placement by auscultation bilaterally **and** over the epigastrium

_____ If used, stylette extends beyond end of ET tube

(continues)

Ventilatory Management—Adult (continued)

_____ Inserts any adjunct in a manner dangerous to the patient

_____ Suctions the patient excessively

_____ Does not suction the patient

_____ Failure to manage the patient as a competent EMT

_____ Exhibits unacceptable affect with patient or other personnel

_____ Uses or orders a dangerous or inappropriate intervention

You must factually document your rationale for checking any of the above critical items on the reverse side of this form.

Answer Key

Section 1: Preparatory
Chapter 1: EMS Systems

Matching

1. C (page 30)   **2.** D (page 29)   **3.** A (page 30)   **4.** F (page 30)   **5.** G (page 29)

6. B (page 30)   **7.** I (page 29)   **8.** H (page 30)   **9.** E (page 29)   **10.** J (page 30)

Multiple Choice

1. A (page 6)   **2.** C (page 7)   **3.** D (page 11)   **4.** B (page 19)   **5.** B (page 23)

6. D (page 16)   **7.** C (page 21)   **8.** B (page 6)   **9.** C (page 10)   **10.** C (pages 11–12)

Fill-in-the-Blank

1. mobile intensive care units (page 6)

2. dispatcher (EMD) (page 11)

3. reciprocity (pages 9–10)

4. empathy (page 16)

5. first priority (page 18)

6. continuous quality improvement (CQI) (page 19)

7. Prospective (page 23)

Ambulance Calls

1. a. When your spouse is calling for the ambulance, she should give the name and the location of the theater, and possibly the theater number if it is a large multiplex. Always give the patient's chief complaint and current status of the patient (eg, alert and oriented), and tell whether the patient is breathing. Your spouse should also tell the EMD that there is a paramedic on the scene.

b. Any patient who experiences syncope needs to be seen by a physician in the ED. Syncopal episodes can be caused by problems involving the heart (eg, life-threatening dysrhythmia), problems involving the brain (eg, a stroke or TIA), shock (eg, orthostatic hypotension, vasovagal syncope, dehydration, or blood loss), or a number of other problems. In this scenario, the patient could have also hurt herself when she fell.

2. a. You should always ensure scene safety for yourself, your crew, bystanders, and the patient. This is your number-one priority. Make sure the driver has moved the vehicle far enough away from the patient so care can be given. You should also make sure the vehicle is in park and the engine is turned off, with the parking brake set. You can also control the scene by having bystanders block traffic to the area until law enforcement arrives.

b. You should begin treatment by having the EMT hold cervical spine immobilization on this patient. You should start with your primary assessment (ABCs) and move to the secondary assessment. After completing the trauma exam, if you determine that the patient has a broken femur, you should apply manual traction to the leg to help stabilize it and control the pain and bleeding until the ambulance arrives.

True/False

1. T (page 5)   **2.** F (page 6)   **3.** T (page 11)   **4.** F (page 11)   **5.** F (page 12)

6. F (page 18)   **7.** T (page 20)   **8.** T (page 23)   **9.** F (page 18)   **10.** T (page 16)

Short Answer

1.
  a. Integrity—Be open, honest, and truthful with the patients. (page 16)
  b. Empathy—Understand and identify the feelings of the patients and their families. (page 16)
  c. Self-motivation—Be driven to keep yourself competent in your skills and your professional manners. (page 16)
  d. Confidence—Instill confidence in your patients and colleagues by showing that you are confident in your abilities and skills. (page 16)
  e. Communications—Express and exchange your ideas, thoughts, and findings on the scene. (page 16)
  f. Teamwork and respect—All involved must work together to achieve a common goal to provide the best possible prehospital care to ensure the overall well-being of the patient. (page 16)
  g. Patient advocacy—Always act in the best interest of your patient. (page 16)
  h. Injury prevention—Help on the scene by pointing out dangerous situations for the patient in his or her home or surroundings. (page 16)
  i. Careful delivery of service—Follow protocols and procedures, and continuously evaluate your performance. (page 16)
  j. Time management—Use your time wisely; for example, prioritize your patient's needs. (page 16)

2.
  a. Preparation—Physical; mental; emotional; knowledge, skills, and abilities; equipment that is appropriate and in working order. (page 17)
  b. Response—Timely and safe. (page 18)
  c. Scene management—Safety of yourself and your team, safety of the patient and bystanders, assessing the situation, use of PPE. (page 18)
  d. Patient assessment and care—Appropriate, organized assessment; recognize and prioritize patient's needs. (page 18)
  e. Management and disposition—Follow protocols or radio medical director; know capabilities of receiving facilities. (page 18)
  f. Patient transfer and report—Give brief, concise hand-off report; protect the patient's privacy. (page 18)
  g. Documentation—Fill out patient care report. (page 18)
  h. Return to service—Restock and prepare unit. (page 18)

3. Medical control is set up by law as a supervisor for the paramedic. The roles of the medical director are as follows: educating and training personnel (ensuring their competency in the field), participating in selection of new personnel, helping with equipment selection for the field, developing clinical protocols, ensuring a CQI program is in place, providing input on patient care, interfacing with the EMS systems and other health care agencies, acting as an EMS advocate in the community, and serving as the "medical conscience" of the EMS system. (page 19)

4.
  a. Online medical control—Allows the paramedic immediate patient care resources. It allows the paramedic to transfer data immediately to the receiving facility for better patient care. (page 19)
  b. Protocols—Treatment plans for a specific illness or injury (eg, the patient with chest pain usually gets oxygen, ASA, nitroglycerin, and sometimes morphine and Lopressor). (page 19)
  c. Standing orders—Protocols that are written and signed by the medical director and outline specific directions, permissions, and sometimes publications (eg, the BLS care given to a patient with an allergic reaction, such as oxygen and epinephrine). (page 19)

Chapter 2: Workforce Safety and Wellness

Matching

Part I

1. A (page 39)   **2.** B (page 39)   **3.** B (page 39)   **4.** A (page 39)

5. B (page 39)   **6.** A (page 39)   **7.** B (page 39)

Part II

1. B (page 41)   **2.** C (page 41)   **3.** A (page 41)

Part III

1. D (page 57)   **2.** F (page 57)   **3.** H (page 57)   **4.** J (page 57)   **5.** A (page 57)

6. C (page 57)   **7.** G (page 57)   **8.** I (page 57)   **9.** E (page 57)   **10.** B (page 57)

Multiple Choice

1. C (page 41)   **2.** D (page 42)   **3.** A (page 43)   **4.** C (page 50)   **5.** B (page 48)

6. D (pages 41–42)   **7.** D (page 41)   **8.** C (page 41)   **9.** A (page 41)   **10.** B (page 43)

Fill-in-the-Blank

1. **a.** projection (page 41)
b. denial (page 41)
c. conversion hysteria (page 42)
d. displacement (page 41)

2. **a.** Take care of your own health: (page 44)
Get enough rest.
Eat a balanced diet.
Get regular exercise.
Treat your body with respect (avoid cigarettes, drugs).
b. Give yourself some "me" time every day.
c. Learn how to relax.
d. Do not make unreasonable demands on yourself.
e. Do not make unreasonable demands on others.
f. Stay in touch with your feelings.
g. Learn techniques for shedding stress while on duty.
h. Debrief after tough calls.

Identify

1. Pertinent Negatives (pages 42–44)
a. Not sleeping
b. Too much caffeine
c. Not exercising
d. Smoking
e. Eating too much of the wrong foods
f. Projecting his negative attitude

2. Stress Reactions (pages 40–41)
a. Projection
b. Anger

Ambulance Calls

1. **a.** This is a critical incident for all members of the team. This death of a child is particularly hard on John because of the fact that he also has an infant boy about the same age. He is probably feeling that he is a bad paramedic because the child died, even though every effort was made during the resuscitation. This also might affect his feelings about being a father. (page 46)

b. Paramedics are often under a lot of stress at their job. They can do several things to reduce stress and avoid burnout, such as get enough sleep, eat a balanced diet, and do 30 minutes of aerobic activity three to four times a week. Avoid caffeine, smoking, and recreational drugs. Limit alcohol intake. Make sure you can devote some time during each day to yourself, and learn to relax with hobbies and social activities. Don't make unreasonable demands on yourself or others. Share your stress by talking or crying. Always debrief after a rough call. (page 44)

2. a. You never want to just blurt out that you think the patient isn't going to make it. Tell the patient that his condition is serious, but that you and the hospital team are going to do everything you can for him. Let him talk, and be sympathetic to anything he says. Remember, you might be the last to speak to him, so if he has dying words for his family, make sure to write them down. Make sure the doctor at the hospital has these words to give to the family when he breaks the news that their loved one has died. (page 45)

b. First, remember that not all dying people will experience all five stages. They may not experience them in "order" either. Encourage the patient to talk about these feelings if possible. (pages 44–45)

(1) Denial. The patient might say things like, "This can't happen to me."

(2) Anger. Anger might appear as blaming the paramedic, family, or even God. Anger can come in the form of yelling or physical outbursts.

(3) Bargaining. This can be a patient's way of praying: "Please just let me live long enough to see my family again." They may bargain with you, the doctor, and God.

(4) Depression. This is characterized by quiet time by the patient, crying, or may be physical contact with anyone close to them, including you.

(5) Acceptance. The patient may leave the sorrow behind and reflect on his or her life. The patient might want to leave words for his or her family and to let them know that things will be okay. Usually, this is the hardest time for the family. The patient doesn't appear to be fighting for life, and that sometimes angers family members. Once again, anger is a stage of grief, and the family members will exhibit these feelings also.

True/False

1. F (pages 33–34)   **2.** T (page 37)   **3.** F (pages 36–37)   **4.** F (page 39)   **5.** T (page 42)

6. F (page 41)   **7.** F (page 42)   **8.** T (page 43)   **9.** F (page 44)   **10.** T (page 49)

11. F (pages 48–49)   **12.** T (page 49)   **13.** F (page 35–36)   **14.** T (page 41)

Short Answer

1. a. Cold sweat
   b. Pounding heart
   c. Dry mouth
   d. Feeling "energized" (pages 39–40)

2. a. Let the family see the body.
   b. Use the word *dead* instead of euphemisms for the word.
   c. Let the family see your resuscitation efforts.
   d. Give the family some time with the body.
   e. Try to arrange for further support (eg, neighbors, clergy).
   f. Accept the family's right to experience a variety of feelings. (pages 45–46)

3. a. Anxiety
   b. Blind panic
   c. Depression
   d. Overreaction
   e. Conversion hysteria (page 42)

Problem Solving

a. 76
b. $220 - 46 = 174$
c. $174 - 76 = 98 \times 0.7 = 69$
d. $69 + 76 = 145$ (pages 35–36)

Chapter 3: Public Health

Matching
(pages 68–69)

1. C   **2.** A   **3.** D   **4.** D   **5.** A

6. B   **7.** C   **8.** A   **9.** B   **10.** D

Multiple Choice

1. B (page 61)   **2.** B (page 61)   **3.** C (page 74)   **4.** A (page 77)   **5.** C (page 76)

6. D (page 75)   **7.** C (page 73)   **8.** B (pages 67–68)   **9.** C (pages 66–68)   **10.** D (page 62)

Fill-in-the-Blank

1. intervention (page 66)

2. intentional (page 61)

3. education; enforcement; engineering/environment; economic incentives (pages 68–69)

4. passive intervention (page 69)

5. tobacco; sexually transmitted diseases; unwanted pregnancies; physical inactivity (page 74)

6. process objective (pages 75–76)

7. teachable moment (page 77)

Identify

1. Pertinent Negatives: (page 77)
  a. Bath water still standing
  b. Boiling water on stove
  c. Trampoline with no safety net
  d. Knitting needles and scissors left out

Ambulance Calls

1. a. Any time you are entering a home with the unknown, it is wise to call for law enforcement. As a result of not being able to gain entry, the officer has provided probable cause for breaking the window. This covers the paramedic for unlawful entry. This could also be a potential crime scene, so law enforcement is a must.

    b. When entering a home, you should always carry a radio to contact your team on the outside. A flashlight is also important because finding a light switch in the dark can be difficult. Pay attention to the broken glass from the window to prevent an injury to the person entering the home. An old blanket or tarp should be laid inside the window to prevent being cut by broken glass.

    c. The teachable moment here is done after they determine the patient is okay and does not need to be transported. While waiting for the neighbor, Missy and Jake could talk to the patient about how and where to hide an outside key to the home and give the location to the lifeline personnel. Lifeline services could then let dispatch know where the key is hidden. Also they could construct a list of neighbors with the key to the home. Finally, they could talk to the patient about always taking the cordless phone, or cell phone, with him into the bathroom or anytime he is away from a wall phone. (page 77)

2. a. S: Simple. This display needs to be simple for the children to understand it.
    M: Measurable. They need to have a play cell phone for the children to practice calling. That way they can see if their demo has helped the children understand.
    A: Accurate. All of the information given on the demo and during the practice session should be clear and accurate.
    R: Reportable. During the next year, the dispatch center will keep records on the children that use the 9-1-1 system. This allows the following years' programs to change if there is a need.
    T: Trackable. After the call, it is evident that the video helped Ryan. Once again this should be reported and the case kept on file. (page 74)

b. This video took the scariness away for Ryan. He was able to realize that his mother would not wake up. When he was unable to arouse her, he remembered the 9-1-1 number to call for help. Good job, Larry and Courtney! Part of your job as a paramedic is to help the community help themselves.

True/False

1. F (page 67) **2.** T (page 62) **3.** F (page 70) **4.** T (pages 70–71) **5.** F (pages 72–73)

6. T (page 74) **7.** T (page 74) **8.** F (page 74) **9.** T (page 76) **10.** F (pages 77–78)

Short Answer

1. *Primary injury prevention* is defined as keeping an injury from ever occurring. Example: Removal of small choking hazards such as buttons from a stuffed animal.

Secondary injury prevention is defined as reducing the effects of an injury that has already happened. Example: Air bags reduce the impact on the person with the steering wheel during a motor vehicle crash. (page 67)

2. *Students should list three of the following:*
  a. EMS providers are widely distributed in a population.
  b. EMS providers reflect the composition of the community.
  c. In rural communities, EMS providers are sometimes the highest medically trained persons.
  d. EMS providers can reduce overall injuries as a result of intervention.
  e. EMS providers are high-profile role models.
  f. EMS providers are perceived as champions of their patients.
  g. EMS providers are welcomed to school and organizations for preventive programs.
  h. EMS providers are perceived as authorities on injuries and illness. (pages 67–68)

3. **a.** Education: Education for the public to reduce injuries and illness (page 68)
  b. Enforcement: Laws to help curb destructive behaviors (page 69)
  c. Engineering/Environment: Changing design of products or spaces to reduce injuries (page 69)
  d. Economic Incentives: Provides monetary incentives to reinforce safe behavior (page 69)

4. **a.** Host: Child that drowns (page 71)
  b. Agent: Drowning (page 71)
  c. Environment: The swimming pool (page 71)

5. *Students should list three of the following:*
  a. Being male
  b. Access to firearms
  c. Alcohol abuse
  d. History of childhood abuse
  e. Mental illness
  f. Poverty (page 73)

Fill-in-the-Table

Top 10 Causes of Death in 2007
1. Heart disease
2. Cancer
3. Stroke
4. Chronic, lower respiratory disease
5. Unintentional injuries
6. Alzheimer disease
7. Diabetes
8. Influenza and pneumonia
9. Kidney disease
10. Septicemia

Chapter 4: Medical, Legal, and Ethical Issues

Matching

1. A (page 96)
2. A (page 96)
3. B (page 96)
4. A (page 96)
5. A (page 96)
6. B (page 96)
7. B (page 116)
8. C (page 116)
9. A (page 117)
10. D (page 116)
11. M (pages 86–88)
12. E (pages 86–88)
13. UE (pages 86–88)
14. E (pages 86–88)
15. UE (pages 86–88)
16. M (pages 86–88)
17. UE (pages 86–88)
18. UE (pages 86–88)
19. M (pages 86–88)
20. UE (pages 86–88)

Multiple Choice

1. B (page 90)
2. C (page 90)
3. D (page 93)
4. A (pages 100–101)
5. D (page 103)
6. B (page 96)
7. C (page 96)
8. A (page 90)
9. C (pages 95–96)
10. A (page 91)
11. B (page 91)
12. C (pages 106–107)
13. C (page 105)
14. A (pages 105–106)
15. D (page 86)

Fill-in-the-Blank

1. **a.** informed (page 96)
   b. custodial parent; legal guardian (page 96)
2. plaintiff; defendant (page 89)
3. scope of practice (page 93)
4. advance directive (page 105)
5. emancipated (page 99)
6. person; place; day (page 98)

Identify

1. Chief complaints: Low blood glucose and unconsciousness. Blood glucose levels should be between 80 and 120 mg/dL. This patient's level was 42 mg/dL. He became unconscious at the scene, which gave us implied consent to treat him.
2. Vitals signs: Oxygen saturation of 97%, respirations of 20 breaths/min, blood glucose 42 mg/dL, blood pressure 132/70 mm Hg, pulse 96 beats/min, lung sounds clear, skin cool, and pupils sluggish. After IV and D_{50}, the scenario says vitals were within normal limits and blood glucose returned to a level of 118 mg/dL.
3. Pertinent negatives: What is NOT wrong with the patient? We look for why the patient became unresponsive. He did not choke, he is not hypoxic, and the medic cannot see any obvious trauma to his head. He has a strong pulse, so we know that he is not in cardiac arrest. He also wakes back up as soon as the D_{50} is given to him. This tells us that the most likely problem was the blood glucose levels. However, the medic should always look into a person becoming unconscious with a very good SAMPLE history before being done and letting the patient sign off.

Ambulance Calls

1. **a.** Actions to take: The boy's injury is not life threatening; nor is it likely to be appreciably aggravated by waiting another hour or so. Tell the school authorities to keep trying to reach the boy's parents and call you back when they have gotten permission to have the boy treated.
   b. Provide treatment: This is a classic case of implied consent.
   c. Actions to take: Some people would argue that any person who attempts suicide is, by definition, not mentally competent and therefore not able to give informed consent (or informed refusal). But you cannot depend on that argument to protect you from a charge of technical assault and battery if you touch the patient or false imprisonment if you take her to the hospital against her will. Ask the boyfriend if the patient is under psychiatric care; if so, perhaps her psychiatrist can be enlisted to help. In states where suicide is a felony, you can call the police for help. In any event, contact medical command for advice.
   d. Actions to take: The best thing to do in this situation is to call for police backup. In all probability, this patient will have to be forcibly restrained, and the police are the only ones permitted to authorize that action.
   e. Provide treatment: This is a classic case of implied consent.
   f. Actions to take: This patient is probably having a heart attack and definitely needs to be in the hospital—but the only legal way to get him there is through patient, sympathetic persuasion. You will need to spend time talking with him, trying to understand his fears, and explaining to him the possible consequence of ignoring

his symptoms. If despite your best efforts at persuasion he still refuses treatment and transport, you may not transport him against his will. But be sure to "leave the door open" so that he feels free to call you back later if he should change his mind. (pages 96–100)

2. *Students should list three of the following:*
   a. Orientation to person, place, and day
   b. Responds to questions appropriately
   c. Absence of signs of mental impairment from alcohol, drugs, head injury, and so on
   d. Evidence that the patient understands the nature of his condition
   e. Evidence that the patient can describe a reasonable plan for follow-up care
   f. Oxygen saturation levels are within normal levels
   g. Blood glucose levels are within normal limits (page 98)

True/False

1. F (page 90)	**2.** T (page 91)	**3.** T (pages 91–92)	**4.** T (page 93)	**5.** F (pages 108–109)
6. T (pages 100–101)	**7.** F (page 106)	**8.** T (page 96)	**9.** F (page 99)	**10.** T (page 91)
11. F (page 85)	**12.** T (page 86)	**13.** T (page 87)	**14.** F (page 103)	**15.** T (page 106)
16. F (page 105)	**17.** T (page 105)	**18.** F (page 107)	**19.** T (page 88)	**20.** F (page 107)

Short Answer

1. *Students should list three of the following:*
   a. Obvious or suspected homicide (page 96)
   b. Obvious or suspected suicide (page 96)
   c. Any other violent or sudden, unexpected death (page 96)
   d. Death of a prison inmate (page 96)

2. Good Samaritan laws were written to provide immunity from liability to anyone who stops to help at the scene of an emergency. The care provided is free of charge. Paramedics now have a legal duty to act, which is not covered by the Good Samaritan laws. (pages 108–109)

3. a. That harm resulted (pages 100–101)
   b. That the paramedic had a duty to act (pages 100–101)
   c. That there was a breach of that duty (pages 100–101)
   d. That the failure to act appropriately was the proximate cause of the plaintiff's injury (pages 100–101)

4. *Students should list four of the following:*
   a. Child abuse
   b. Elder abuse
   c. Injury sustained during commission of a felony
   d. Drug-related injuries
   e. Childbirth occurring outside a medical facility
   f. Rape
   g. Animal bites
   h. Certain communicable diseases
   i. Domestic violence (pages 95–96)

5. a. MOLST stands for Medical Orders for Life-Sustaining Treatment. Although similar to a DNR, the MOLST is more expansive and designed for both prehospital providers and health care providers. (page 107)
   b. Check with your instructor or medical director to see whether MOLST is used in your state. (page 107)

6. Clearly, each person will have a private code of right and wrong. The paramedic's guiding principle, however it is worded, should be based on overriding concern for the welfare of the patient. (page 86)

7. This is a very hard situation to handle. The first thing that should be done is to speak directly to the senior paramedic about how offending his or her remarks are. If the remarks continue, it would be time to address this with the chain of command. (pages 86–87)

8. When responding to code and presented with a DNR order, you must begin to verify the order quickly. Your local protocols will tell you everything you should look for. These are a few of the things that should be on every order: name of patient (confirm with ID that this is the right patient), original signatures of patient and doctor, and dates. Your online medical director will also be able to help you with any questions. (page 106)

Chapter 5: EMS Communications

Matching

Part I
(pages 134–135)

1. O	**2.** C	**3.** C	**4.** C	**5.** O
6. C	**7.** C	**8.** O	**9.** C	**10.** C

Part II
(pages 122–124)

1. UHF	**2.** VHF	**3.** Cellular	**4.** Cellular
5. VHF	**6.** UHF	**7.** Cellular, VHF, and UHF	

Part III

1. (pages 129–130)

(1) F: The patient is a 60-year-old woman who collapsed in the bathroom while sitting on the toilet.

(2) J: She was apparently well until this morning.

(3) D: Her daughter says that the patient complained of a severe headache before she collapsed.

(4) B: The patient has a history of high blood pressure. (In fact, this is really part of the history of the present illness, if you know what the patient's problem is! She seems to have had a hemorrhagic stroke, so her high blood pressure is one of the predisposing factors.)

(5) L: She was hospitalized 6 years ago for an AMI.

(6) H: The patient's medications include nitroglycerin and Aldomet (methyldopa).

(7) E: The patient was still conscious when we arrived, but she rapidly lost consciousness.

(8) A: Pulse is 50 beats/min and regular, respirations are 36 breaths/min and deep, and blood pressure is 180/126 mm Hg.

(9) I: Her left pupil is larger than the right and does not react to light.

(10) K: Her neck is somewhat stiff.

(11) C: The deep tendon reflexes are hyperactive.

(12) G: We are administering oxygen at 4 L/min by nasal cannula.

Multiple Choice

1. C (page 128)	**2.** C (page 132)	**3.** D (page 121)	**4.** C (page 125)	**5.** C (page 123)
6. D (pages 132–134)	**7.** A (pages 133–134)	**8.** C (page 135)	**9.** B (page 137)	**10.** D (page 134)
11. C (page 136)	**12.** A (page 134)	**13.** B (page 135)	**14.** D (page 141)	**15.** B (pages 140–141)

Fill-in-the-Blank

The order of answers given will vary for 1-6.

1. The **person calling for help** needs to be able to talk with **the dispatcher**. The best technical means of establishing that link is **landline (telephone)**. (page 131)

2. The **dispatcher** needs to be able to talk with **the paramedics or other rescuers**. The best technical means of establishing that link is **a two-way radio (although a pager will suffice for dispatch)**. (page 132)

3. The **dispatcher** needs to be able to talk with **other agencies, such as police, fire, utility companies, and civil defense**. The best technical means of establishing that link is **landline (telephone)**. (page 132)

4. The **paramedic** needs to be able to talk with **medical command**. The best technical means of establishing that link is **radio or cellular telephone**. (page 129)

5. The **paramedic** needs to be able to talk with **the receiving hospital**. The best technical means of establishing that link is **radio or cellular telephone**. (page 129)

6. The **area hospital** needs to be able to talk with **one another**. The best technical means of establishing that link is **landline with radio backup**. (page 129)

7. communication (page 134)

8. calm (page 134)

9. inflection (page 134)

10. open-ended question (p 134)

11. neutral (page 139)

12. police (page 138)

13. toys (page 138)

14. respect (page 139)

Identify

1. Chief complaint: Chest pain

2. History of the present illness: The pain was "squeezing" in character, radiated to the left shoulder and jaw, and had been present for 2 hours. The pain was accompanied by increasing difficulty in breathing.

3. Other medical history: He is known to be a heart patient.

4. General appearance: The patient was sitting bolt upright; he appeared alert and apprehensive and was in moderate respiratory distress, breathing shallowly at 30 breaths/min.

5. Vital signs: Respiratory rate 30 breaths/min; pulse 130 beats/min, weak and regular; and blood pressure 200/90 mm Hg.

6. Head-to-toe exam: His neck veins were distended to the angle of the jaw at 45°. Wet crackles were heard at both lung bases, and auscultation of the heart revealed a gallop rhythm. The abdomen was not distended. There was a 1+ presacral and ankle edema.

7. Treatment given: The patient was given oxygen by nonrebreathing mask at 12 L/min, had a 12-lead ECG taken, had an IV of normal saline, and was transported to Mount Fiore Hospital in a semi-Fowler's position.

8. Pertinent negatives: The abdomen was not distended; the patient denied nausea, vomiting, sweating, or palpitations.

Ambulance Calls

Part I

1. Just about everything was wrong with the transmission quoted!
   a. The unit being called should be mentioned first. So, it should have been, "County Hospital, Medic 12."
   b. It was unnecessarily wordy, wasting a lot of time. ("Be advised that . . ." or "Please 10-9 your message.")
   c. The patient's name was mentioned on the air, along with an abbreviation that a layperson could easily misunderstand. To compound the offense, the paramedic spelled out the initials of the chief complaint in nonstandard phonetic alphabet, using insulting words to do so.
   d. The paramedic was apparently trying to be funny. He may have thought the whole thing was a laugh a minute, but Maggie Jones might be forgiven if she didn't think so. Making insulting references to the patient ("well endowed with adipose tissue") or to the other party on the radio ("Are you deaf or something?") is highly unprofessional and simply reflects on the immaturity of the speaker.
   e. The report of the patient's findings was not given in any sort of standard format. As a result, the people at County Hospital had to waste a lot of time trying to drag the important information out of the paramedics.
   f. Words that are poorly heard by radio, such as "yes," were used.
   g. The paramedic did not repeat back the medication orders to make sure he had received them correctly.
   h. The radio was used for nonmedical communications. ("Pop a few doughnuts into the microwave.")

2. The best way to find out just how difficult the dispatcher's job can be is to step into that job for a few hours. The information you need to try to obtain from the hysterical caller reporting a crash is as follows:
   • What is the exact location of the incident?
   • What is the telephone number from which the caller is phoning?
   • At this point, dispatch the (first) ambulance. ("Unspecified accident at such-and-such address. Details will follow.")
   • What is the nature of the incident (eg, explosion, road crash, train derailment, building collapse)?
   • How many victims are there?
   • Are there any hazards at the scene, specifically:
     (a) Traffic hazards
     (b) Fire

(c) Spills

(d) Downed electrical wires

- If it is a *transport* collision (motor vehicles, train):

  (a) How many vehicles are involved?

  (b) Is it possible to determine what cargoes the vehicles are carrying?

  Contact the responding vehicle with additional information. Dispatch additional vehicles and contact other agencies as needed.

Part II

1. There is no single correct answer to the dilemma posed in this question: How do you reply to a patient when he asks, "Am I going to die?" However, there are some general guidelines:

   - Do not try to minimize the seriousness of the patient's situation. Most patients who are near death *know* at least that they are in serious condition. If you are merrily chirping, "There, there, everything is going to be fine," the patient will simply assume that (a) you don't understand the situation, or (b) it is forbidden for him to speak to you honestly about his fears. Those are *not* the messages you want to convey!

   - Do not, on the other hand, take away all hope. As long as the patient is alive, there is hope for him.

   - In the situation described, therefore, you might say something like this: "Sir, your situation is very serious, but we have an excellent rescue team here, with the best medical backup, and we're going to do everything we can to save your life." Also let the patient know that you are willing to listen to what he has to say, to transmit any messages he has for other people, and so forth. (pages 133–135)

2. In the case of the diabetic patient, you have to remember the patient can become violent. You should begin to talk calmly to the patient. Tell her your name and reassure her you are there to help her. Take a nonaggressive stance, but be wary of the patient. Explain to the patient that you want to test her blood glucose level, start an IV, and give her glucose through the IV. If the patient is fighting you, you may need to use law enforcement to subdue the patient. As soon as you get the patient's glucose levels to normal, she will calm down and thank you. (page 138)

3. **a.** You should have asked if there is anybody able to translate for the patient and the family in the area.
   b. Explain to the translator why the candles must be blown out before using the oxygen. You may ask for permission first; if it is not granted, move the woman before applying the oxygen.
   c. The student's "rock out" sign has made her feel that the devil has just arrived in her bedroom. Along with you using the red pen to write her name, she now feels you are both associated with the devil.
   d. Your translator can help keep the woman and her family calm and make your transition to her caregiver much easier. You should have the translator explain *everything* that you are doing *before* you do it. Most important is to take the translator to the hospital with you to continue care and keep the patient calm on the way to the hospital. (pages 139–140)

True/False

1. T (page 123)	**2.** T (page 123)	**3.** F (page 121)	**4.** T (page 126)	**5.** F (page 128)
6. T (page 130)	**7.** F (page 132)	**8.** T (page 136)	**9.** T (page 136)	**10.** F (page 137)
11. F (page 134)	**12.** T (page 133)	**13.** T (page 137)	**14.** F (page137)	**15.** T (page 139)

Short Answer

1. Most radio communications systems require a basic minimum of components. (pages 121–122)

Component	Function
Base station	Dispatch and coordination area
Mobile transceiver	Communications with ambulances
Portable transceiver	Communications with paramedics when they are out of their vehicle
Repeater	To extend the range of low-power transceivers
Remote consoles in hospitals	To allow communications with receiving hospitals
Landline/cellular backup	To extend the user network

2. The job of the dispatcher (EMD) includes the following duties. *Students should list four of the following:*
   a. Extracting information from panicky callers.
   b. Directing the right emergency vehicle to the right address.
   c. Giving advice and first-aid instructions by telephone to distraught people.
   d. Coordinating the response of different agencies to an emergency.
   e. Monitoring field communications to determine if help is needed.
   f. Keeping written records of data such as response times. (pages 131–132)

3. An EMS communications system has to provide for at least the following linkages (*students will draw a diagram*):
   a. Citizen to dispatch center
   b. Dispatch center to ambulances
   c. Dispatch center to hospitals
   d. Dispatch center to medical control
   e. Dispatch center to other services
   f. Ambulance to hospitals
   g. Paramedic to medical control (pages 131–132)

4. Telemetry dispatcher: Go ahead, Medic 785, you are clear to transmit with MD 802 from Saint Peter's Hospital on Med channel 2.

Medic 785: MD 802, this is Medic 785 on med 2. How do you read?

MD 802: Medic 785, this is MD 802. You are loud and clear; proceed with your transmission.

Medic 785: I am treating a 58-year-old man who is in moderate distress with a chief complaint of chest pain. He states it came on suddenly while shoveling snow. He describes the pain as crushing under his breastbone and radiating down his left arm. The pain is a 10 on 10, and he has had the pain for about 15 minutes. The patient states he has no prior history and denies any shortness of breath. He has an allergy to Novocain and takes three aspirins daily as well as 10 mg of Lipitor. He states he has a history of hypertension and high cholesterol with CAD in his family. His last oral intake was lunch 3 hours ago and the 162 mg of chewable aspirin the dispatcher advised him to take prior to our arrival. The events leading up to the incident involved shoveling heavy snow.

Physical exam reveals some crackles at the bases of both lungs, not JVD or pedal edema. His vital signs are respirations of 20 breaths/min and regular, pulse of 110 beats/min, strong and regular, and a blood pressure of 146/82 mm Hg. His oxygen saturation is 96% on a nonrebreathing mask, and his ECG is sinus tachycardia with no ectopy, but the 12-lead shows ST-segment elevation in V3 and V4 (possible anterior wall MI).

We are treating him as a rule-out MI and have administered morphine and oxygen. Nitroglycerin and aspirin were self-administered. We are currently transporting and our plan is to continue monitoring him and go through the rest of the fibrinolytic checklist. What's your pleasure on 5 mg of metoprolol?

MD 802: Medic 785, go ahead with the metoprolol, and I will alert the cath lab staff right away.

Medic 785: Received. Our ETA is 20 minutes.

Fill-in-the-Table

(page 127)

A	Alpha	J	Juliette	S	Sierra
B	Bravo	K	Kilo	T	Tango
C	Charlie	L	Lima	U	Uniform
D	Delta	M	Mike	V	Victor
E	Echo	N	November	W	Whiskey
F	Foxtrot	O	Oscar	X	X-ray
G	Golf	P	Papa	Y	Yankee
H	Hotel	Q	Quebec	Z	Zebra
I	India	R	Romeo		

Chapter 6: Documentation

Matching

Part I
(pages 159–161)

1. F	**2.** C	**3.** B	**4.** E	**5.** G	**6.** A	**7.** F	**8.** D	**9.** H	**10.** B
11. E	**12.** F	**13.** F	**14.** C	**15.** B	**16.** F	**17.** E	**18.** D	**19.** C	**20.** D
21. B	**22.** G	**23.** B	**24.** H	**25.** B	**26.** F				

27. In rearranging the sentences into the correct sequence for presentation, there may be some variation in the order of sentences within a given category (eg, the sentences that make up the "history of the present illness," which you labeled B); but all sentences from category B should precede those from category C, which should precede those from category D, and so forth. (page 160)

HISTORY

A. Chief Complaint

    (1) 6: The patient is a 51-year-old man with chest pain.

B. History of the Present Illness

    (2) 3: The pain came on while he was watching television.

    (3) 25: He describes the pain as squeezing.

    (4) 23: The pain radiates down his left arm.

    (5) 10: Nothing seemed to make the pain better or worse.

    (6) 15: He also felt nauseated.

    (7) 21: He denies any shortness of breath.

C. Other Medical History

    (8) 19: He is under the care of Dr. Tums for an ulcer.

    (9) 14: The patient takes Maalox (alumina/magnesia) and cimetidine (Tagamet) regularly.

    (10) 2: The patient is allergic to penicillin.

PHYSICAL ASSESSMENT

D. General Appearance

    (11) 18: He was sitting in a chair and appeared to be frightened.

    (12) 20: He was alert and oriented to person, place, and day.

    (13) 8: His skin was pale, cold, and sweaty (diaphoretic).

E. Vital Signs

    (14) 11: The pulse was 52 beats/min and full, with an occasional premature beat.

    (15) 17: His respirations were 20 breaths/min and unlabored.

    (16) 4: The blood pressure was 190/110 mm Hg.

F. Head-to-Toe Examination

    (17) 13: There was no cyanosis of the lips.

    (18) 12: The neck veins were not distended.

    (19) 7: The chest was clear.

    (20) 26: Lung sounds were clear.

    (21) 16: His abdomen was soft and nontender.

    (22) 1: There was no pedal edema.

TREATMENT

    (23) 5: He was given supplemental oxygen by nonrebreathing mask at 12 L/min.

    (24) 2: An IV was started with normal saline to a KVO rate.

CONDITION DURING TRANSPORT

    (25) 9: The patient was transported in a semi-Fowler's position.

    (26) 24: The blood pressure came down to 170/90 mm Hg during transport.

Part II
Question: What do you think is wrong with this patient? Should anything else have been done that was not done?
Now that you've had some practice, this second exercise should be a little easier than the first.

1. F   2. E   3. B   4. C, B   5. F   6. D   7. G   8. A   9. E   10. D

11. G   12. B   13. F   14. G   15. F   16. H   17. F   18. F   19. F

20. The following shows the sentences rearranged into the correct sequence for documentation on the PCR:
HISTORY
A. Chief Complaint

(1) 35: The patient is a middle-aged man who was struck by a car while crossing the street.

B. History of the Present Illness

(2) 39: He apparently staggered into the street without looking, as if he were drunk.

(3) 30: Bystanders say that the car that hit him was traveling very fast.

(4) 31: He has a medical identification bracelet that says he is a diabetic.

C. Other Medical History

(Apparently none is available; the medical identification bracelet could have been listed here, as previously noted.)
PHYSICAL ASSESSMENT
D. General Appearance

(5) 37: The patient was unconscious and did not withdraw from painful stimuli.

(6) 33: His skin is pale, cool, and moist.

E. Vital Signs

(7) 29: The pulse was 92 beats/min, somewhat weak, and regular.

(8) 36: Respirations were 30 breaths/min, deep, and noisy; blood pressure was 160/110 mm Hg.

F. Head-to-Toe Examination

(9) 32: There is a bruise on the left forehead.

(10) 44: There was no blood or fluid draining from his nose or ears.

(11) 42: The pupils were equal, midposition, and reactive to light.

(12) 40: The chest wall was stable, and breath sounds were equal bilaterally.

(13) 45: His abdomen was soft.

(14) 28: The right leg was severely angulated at the mid-femur.

(15) 46: The dorsalis pedis pulses were equal.

G. Treatment

(16) 38: An oropharyngeal airway was inserted, and supplemental oxygen was given by nonrebreathing mask at 12 L/min.

(17) 41: We put the right leg in a traction splint.

(18) 34: He was secured to a long backboard.

H. Condition During Transport

(19) 43: There was no change in his condition during transport.

Part III

1. In taking a history and carrying out a physical examination, you go to a lot of trouble to obtain important information about the patient. It would be a shame if that information were lost because you could not document it in an order that other health care providers could easily process. (page 160)
AGE, SEX, AND CHIEF COMPLAINT

(1) F: The patient is a 60-year-old woman who collapsed in the bathroom while sitting on the toilet.

A. History of the Present Illness

(2) J: She was apparently well until this morning.

(3) D: Her daughter says the patient complained of a severe headache before she collapsed.

B. Past Medical History

(4) B: The patient has a history of high blood pressure. (In fact, this is really part of the history of the present illness, if you know what the patient's problem is! She seems to have had a hemorrhagic stroke, so her high blood pressure is one of the predisposing factors.)

(5) L: She was hospitalized 6 years ago for an AMI.

(6) H: The patient's medications include nitroglycerin and Aldomet (methyldopa).

PHYSICAL ASSESSMENT

C. State of Consciousness

(7) E: The patient was still conscious when we arrived, but she rapidly lost consciousness.

D. Vital Signs

(8) A: Pulse is 50 beats/min and regular, respirations are 36 breaths/min and deep, and blood pressure is 180/126 mm Hg.

E. Head-to-Toe Survey

(9) I: Her left pupil is larger than the right and does not react to light.

(10) K: Her neck is somewhat stiff.

(11) C: The deep tendon reflexes are hyperactive.

TREATMENT GIVEN SO FAR

(12) G: We are administering oxygen at 12 L/min by nonrebreathing mask.

Multiple Choice

1. C (page 151) **2.** B (page 153) **3.** A (page 157) **4.** C (pages 157–158) **5.** B (page 158)

6. B (page 149) **7.** A (pages 150–151) **8.** C (page 158) **9.** C (pages 154–155) **10.** C (page 162)

Fill-in-the-Blank

Part I

1. Abd = abdomen (page 168)

2. ADL = activity of daily living (page 168)

3. AICD = automated implanted cardiac defibrillator (page 168)

4. BM = bowel movement (page 168)

5. BS = blood sugar, breath sounds, bowel sounds, bachelor of science (degree) (page 168)

6. as soon as possible = ASAP (page 168)

7. central venous pressure = CVP (page 169)

8. deep venous thrombosis = DVT (page 169)

9. chronic obstructive pulmonary disease = COPD (page 169)

10. history of present illness = HPI (page 170)

Part II

1. cyst(o)- = pertaining to the bladder or any fluid-containing sac (page 165)

2. dermat(o)- = pertaining to the skin (page 165)

3. ortho- = straight or normal (page 165)

4. brady- = slow (page 165)

5. hydr(o)- = water (page 165)

6. cephal(o)- = pertaining to the head (page 165)

7. cerebr(o)- = pertaining to the cerebrum, a part of the brain (page 165)

8. rhin(o)- = pertaining to the nose (page 166)

9. tri- = three (page 166)

10. supra- = above (page 166)

11. -lysis = decline, disintegration, or destruction (page 166)

12. -scope = instrument for examination (page 166)

13. -uria = pertaining to a substance in the urine or the condition so indicated (page 166)

14. -megaly = enlargement of (page 166)

15. -otomy = surgical incision (page 166)

Identify

1. Chief complaint: Chest pain
2. History of the present illness: The pain was described as a "pressure in the center of the chest with left arm numbness," and had been present for 30 minutes. The pain was accompanied by difficulty in breathing.
3. Other medical history: She is known to have a history of angina and asthma.
4. General appearance: The patient was sitting bolt upright; she appeared alert and apprehensive and was in moderate respiratory distress, breathing shallowly at 32 breaths/min.
5. Vital signs: Respiratory rate 32 breaths/min; pulse 136 beats/min, weak and regular; and blood pressure 180/80 mm Hg.
6. Head-to-toe exam: Her neck veins were distended to the angle of the jaw at 45°. Rales were heard at both lung bases, and auscultation of the heart revealed a gallop rhythm. The abdomen was not distended.
7. Treatment given: The patient was given oxygen by nonrebreathing mask at 12 L/min; a 12-lead ECG was acquiredand transmitted and shows a STEMI; an IV of normal saline was started at KVO rate; and morphine, ASA and nitroglycerin have been administered. She was transported to St. Joseph's Hospital cath lab in a semi-Fowler's position.
8. Pertinent negatives: The abdomen was not distended; the patient denied vomiting.

True/False

1. F (page 163)   2. F (page 163)   3. T (page 163)   4. T (page 172)   5. T (page 172)
6. F (page 174)   7. T (page 174)   8. T (page 174)   9. T (pages 149–150)   10. F (pages 149–150)

Short Answer

1. a. Besides the standard information regarding the patient's medical history and physical findings, the trip sheet (PCR) should contain a record of the times (time the call was received, time the ambulance departed, time the ambulance reached the scene, and so on). (page 159)
   b. Such a record is important to enable evaluation of such things as response times or how much time is being spent at the scene. (page 159)
2. Two reasons for making sure that your trip sheets (PCRs) are accurate and complete are:
   a. For the benefit of the patient, whose subsequent care may depend on the information that you have (or have not) provided.
   b. For your own benefit, if the case should ever become a subject for court proceedings. The trip sheet reflects on the person who wrote it. If your trip sheet (PCR) is sloppy and incomplete, a court would not be unjustified in wondering whether the care you gave the patient was also sloppy and incomplete. (page 159)
3. a. Number of patients: Record only when more than one patient is present. "This is patient 2 of 3."
   b. Standard precautions: Were standard precautions initiated? If so, state which precautions you used and why.
   c. MOI/NOI: Simply state. For example, "motor vehicle crash" or "difficulty breathing."
   d. Oxygen: Record if oxygen was used, how it was applied, and how much was administered. (page 159)

Complete the Patient Care Report (PCR)

Show your completed PCR to your paramedic instructor and ask for feedback on how well you recorded the case you were given.

Section 2: The Human Body and Human Systems
Chapter 7: Anatomy and Physiology

Matching

Part I
(page 184)

1. J	**2.** I	**3.** B	**4.** A	**5.** G
6. F	**7.** C	**8.** H	**9.** D	**10.** E

Part II
(page 202)

1. H	**2.** D	**3.** I	**4.** G	**5.** B
6. C	**7.** E	**8.** A	**9.** F	

Multiple Choice

1. D (page 197)	**2.** B (page 198)	**3.** C (page 211)	**4.** C (page 216)	**5.** B (page 221)
6. D (page 228)	**7.** C (page 232)	**8.** A (page 232)	**9.** C (page 241)	**10.** B (page 241)
11. B (page 247)	**12.** A (page 251)	**13.** D (page 252)	**14.** B (page 252)	**15.** B (page 266)
16. D (page 266)	**17.** D (page 269)	**18.** B (page 269)	**19.** B (page 269)	**20.** B (page 274)

Fill-in-the-Blank

1. liver; gallbladder; bile (page 280)
2. small intestine; large intestine; colon (page 280)
3. endocrine; hormones; endocrine; exocrine (page 281)
4. growth; thyroid; luteinizing; oxytocin; contract (page 284)
5. ovaries; fallopian tubes; placenta; vagina; labia majora; labia minora; vestibule (page 301)

Labeling

1. (page 217, Figure 38)
   A. frontal bone
   B. orbit
   C. nasal bone
   D. zygoma
   E. maxilla
   F. mandible
   G. parietal bone
   H. temporal bone
   I. external auditory meatus
   J. mastoid process
   K. temporomandibular joint
   L. cervical vertebrae
2. (page 224, Figure 53)
   A. pelvis
   B. femoral head
   C. greater trochanter
   D. lesser trochanter
   E. femur
   F. patella
   G. fibula

    H. tibia
    I. tarsals
    J. metatarsals
    K. phalanges
3. (page 233, Figure 64)
    A. nasopharynx
    B. nasal air passage
    C. pharynx
    D. oropharynx
    E. mouth
    F. epiglottis
    G. larynx
    H. apex of the lung
    I. carina
    J. base of the lung
    K. diaphragm
    L. trachea
    M. alveoli
    N. bronchioles
    O. main bronchi

True/False

(page 268, Figure 105)

1. T	**2.** T	**3.** T	**4.** F	**5.** F
6. F	**7.** F	**8.** T	**9.** T	**10.** F

Chapter 8: Pathophysiology

Matching

Part I
(page 340)

1. D   **2.** B   **3.** A   **4.** E   **5.** C

Part II

1. F (page 369)   **2.** B (page 367)   **3.** G (page 369)   **4.** E (page 368)

5. A (page 367)   **6.** D (page 368)   **7.** C (page 368)

Multiple Choice

1. C (page 336)   **2.** A (page 340)   **3.** D (page 341)   **4.** B (page 357)   **5.** D (page 341)

6. D (page 359)   **7.** D (page 362)   **8.** B (page 365)   **9.** C (page 367)   **10.** A (page 373)

Fill-in-the-Blank

1. homeostasis (page 337)

2. Adipose tissue (page 337)

3. Hyperplasia (page 340)

4. Baroreceptors (page 337)

5. oliguria (page 344)

6. Hyperkalemia (page 344)

7. buffers (page 347)

8. apoptosis (page 356)

9. Multiple organ dysfunction syndrome (pages 369–370)

10. Endotoxins (page 354)

Labeling

1. (page 336, Figure 1)

A. Nucleus

B. Ribosomes

C. Golgi complex

D. Rough endoplasmic reticulum

E. Smooth endoplasmic reticulum

F. Cytoplasm

G. Plasma membrane

H. Mitochondrion

I. Centriole

J. Vacuole

K. Lysosome

2. (page 385, Figure 37)

A. allergen

B. Plasma

C. antibodies

D. mast cells

E. IgE

F. histamine

G. dilation

H. mucus

I. contraction

J. smooth

Identify

1. Chief complaint: Can't breathe
2. Vital signs: Respirations are 28 breaths/min and shallow. Pulse is 90 beats/min with occasional irregular beats. Blood pressure is 160/90 mm Hg. Oxygen saturation is 90%, and skin is warm and moist.
3. Pertinent patient history: Chronic obstructive pulmonary disease (COPD), fever, coughing with bloody sputum
4. Presumptive diagnosis: Acute exacerbation of COPD

Ambulance Calls

1. **a.** Based on the angiotensin-converting enzyme (ACE) inhibitor and the peaked T wave, this patient is likely hyperkalemic, having an elevated potassium level.
   b. The immediate treatment is to contact medical control to discuss administering calcium chloride.
2. **a.** Crohn disease affects the gastrointestinal system. It is a chronic inflammatory condition that affects the colon and/or the terminal part of the small intestine.
   b. Symptoms include diarrhea, abdominal pain, nausea, fever, weakness, and weight loss. (page 364)
3. Alzheimer patients might have memory loss and be disorientated to time and day in the early stages. In later stages, they may exhibit restlessness and agitation, and in the final stages of the disease, they may be unable to communicate, may experience urinary and fecal incontinence, and possibly may have seizures. (page 365)

True/False

1. T (page 336)　　**2.** T (page 337)　　**3.** F (page 340)　　**4.** T (page 344)　　**5.** F (page 347)
6. F (page 358)　　**7.** F (page 368)　　**8.** T (page 374)　　**9.** T (page 385)　　**10.** T (page 386)

Short Answer

1. **a.** Urine (60%)
   b. Lungs (via respiration) and the skin (28%)
   c. Feces (6%)
   d. Sweat (6%) (page 340)
2. **a.** Capillary hydrostatic pressure
   b. Capillary colloidal osmotic pressure
   c. Tissue hydrostatic pressure
   d. Tissue colloidal osmotic pressure (pages 341–342)
3. *Students should provide four of the following:*
   a. Lactic acidosis
   b. Ketoacidosis
   c. Aspirin (acetylsalicylic acid) overdose
   d. Alcohol ingestion (and also gastrointestinal losses)
   e. Gastrointestinal losses (page 351)
4. *Students should provide five of the following:*
   a. Hypoxic injury (page 352)
   b. Chemical injury (page 353)
   c. Infectious injury (pages 354–355)
   d. Immunologic and inflammatory injury (page 355)
   e. Injurious genetic factors (page 356)
   f. Injurious nutritional imbalances (page 356)
   g. Injurious physical agents or conditions (page 356)
5. **a.** Emphysema
   b. Chronic bronchitis
   c. Acute bronchitis
   d. Sinusitis
   e. Laryngitis
   f. Pneumonia
   g. Asthma (page 358)

6. **a.** Exercise-induced syncope
   b. Syncope associated with chest pain
   c. History of syncope in a close family member (ie, parent, sibling, child)
   d. Syncope associated with startle, such as the response to a loud noise (page 362)

7. **a.** Stage 1 (early): Memory loss, lack of spontaneity, subtle personality changes, and disorientation to time and date
   b. Stage 2: Impaired cognition and abstract thinking, restlessness and agitation, wandering, inability to carry out daily living activities, impaired judgment, and inappropriate social behavior
   c. Stage 3 (advanced): Indifference to food, inability to communicate, urinary and fecal incontinence, and seizures (page 365)

8. **a.** Basophil
   b. Eosinophil
   c. Neutrophil
   d. Monocyte
   e. Lymphocyte (page 373)

9. **a.** Margination
   b. Activation
   c. Adhesion
   d. Transmigration (diapedesis)
   e. Chemotaxis (pages 380–381)

10. **a.** Alarm
    b. Resistance
    c. Exhaustion (pages 387–389)

Fill-in-the-Table

Signs and Symptoms of Compensated and Decompensated Hypoperfusion	
Compensated	**Decompensated**
Agitation, anxiety, restlessness	Altered mental status (verbal to unresponsive)
Sense of impending doom	**Hypotension**
Weak, rapid (thready) pulse	**Labored or irregular breathing**
Clammy (cool, moist) skin	Thready or absent peripheral pulses
Pallor with cyanotic lips	Ashen, mottled, or cyanotic skin
Shortness of breath	**Dilated pupils**
Nausea, vomiting	**Diminished urine output (oliguria)**
Delayed capillary refill time in infants and children	Impending cardiac arrest
Thirst	
Normal blood pressure	

Chapter 9: Life Span Development

Matching

(page 401)

1. C	**2.** I	**3.** F	**4.** B	**5.** E
6. J	**7.** A	**8.** D	**9.** G	**10.** H

Multiple Choice

1. D (page 403)	**2.** B (page 401)	**3.** D (page 403)	**4.** B (page 404)	**5.** C (page 412)
6. D (page 412)	**7.** A (page 413)	**8.** A (page 411)	**9.** B (page 411)	**10.** C (page 408)

Fill-in-the-Blank

1. 6; 8; 5%; 10%; fluid (page 402)
2. palmar grasp (page 403)
3. fontanelles (page 403)
4. Growth plates (page 403)
5. Bonding (page 404)
6. Trust; mistrust; routine (page 404)
7. aneurysm (page 411)
8. mesentery (page 412)
9. terminal drop hypothesis (page 413)
10. increases; decreases (page 411)

Labeling

(page 403)

- **A.** anterior
- **B.** posterior
- **C.** mastoid
- **D.** sphenoidal

Identify

1. Chief complaint: Fell and hip hurts a great deal
2. Vital signs: Pulse 90 beats/min and thready; respirations 24 breaths/min and shallow; and blood pressure 100/70 mm Hg
3. SAMPLE history:
   Signs/symptoms: Externally rotated foot, discoloration, and a great deal of pain
   Allergies: None
   Medications: Medications for congestive heart failure
   Pertinent medical history: Congestive heart failure, past smoker, and heart attack last year
   Last oral intake: Ate breakfast a few hours ago
   Event: Tripped and fell (page 413)

Ambulance Calls

1. (pages 402–403)

Reflex	How to Test	Appropriate Response
Moro reflex	Startle the infant (clap your hands once near child).	Infant opens arms wide and spreads fingers; Seems to grab at things.
Palmar grasp	Place an object–a finger–in the infant's palm.	The infant should grasp your finger.
Rooting reflex	Touch the infant's cheek.	The infant should turn his or her head toward the touch.
Sucking reflex	Stroke the infant's lips.	The infant should respond as if preparing to feed.

2. a. The patient is considered a late adult. It is not uncommon to have visual issues that make it difficult for her to get around and that may also contribute to trauma such as a low fall. She may not be able to read small print such as that found on a prescription medical container, and she may not be focusing well.
In addition, she may have some hearing loss that makes it difficult for her to hold a conversation and be understood, potentially leading to confusion and inaccurate responses to questions. (pages 410–413)

   b. While going through body systems, be concerned about cardiac-related issues and aneurysms when addressing cardiovascular issues. She may have a cardiac history and diminished cardiac output as a result of her age. Her body may not be able to compensate with rapid blood pressure changes, so vital signs are important and you must consider asking if she gets dizzy when she sits up or stands. A cardiac event is always a consideration even if there are no overt signs present. When considering respiratory issues, be aware of an elderly person's diminished ability to clear secretions and the fact that she may have diminished lung capacity, which can mean low air exchange. Ask yourself whether there are any signs of respiratory distress in this patient. Because stagnant air can remain in the lungs, hypercarbia is a concern. When considering renal and gastric issues, ask about pain and discomfort as well as bowel and urinary habits. The renal and gastrointestinal systems become less efficient with age, causing an inability to process fluids, nutrients, and electrolytes properly. The nervous system should be addressed. Elderly people have slower motor and sensory responses, which can place them at risk for injury. Slow bleeds into the brain may initially appear with subtle signs. If there is a concern, perform a stroke assessment. (pages 412–413)

3. a. Privacy is an issue among adolescents. Therefore, with both her mother and girlfriend in the room, asking if she is pregnant is inappropriate. Your partner should have waited until no family or friends were present before asking this question. If the opportunity does present itself before reaching the emergency department, let the staff know.

   b. Palpation of the abdomen must be done in a way that respects the patient's privacy and, if possible, by a paramedic of the same gender as the patient. It may have been appropriate to wait until the patient was loaded into the ambulance to perform this assessment. (pages 408–409)

True/False

1. T (page 402)   **2.** F (page 403)   **3.** F (page 403)   **4.** T (page 404)   **5.** F (page 408)

6. T (page 410)   **7.** T (page 411)   **8.** F (page 413)   **9.** T (page 413)   **10.** F (page 412)

Short Answer

1. a. Moro reflex
   b. Palmar grasp
   c. Rooting reflex
   d. Sucking reflex (pages 402–403)

2. a. Cholesterol
   b. Calcium (pages 410–411)

3. a. Decreased ability to clear secretions
   b. Decreased cough reflex
   c. Decreased gag reflex
   d. Cilia diminish with age
   e. Innervation of airway structures decreases, resulting in decreasing sensation. (page 411)

4. **a.** Diminished visual acuity
   b. Visual distortions
   c. Harder for the eye to focus
   d. Narrower peripheral field
   e. Greater sensitivity to glare
   f. Hearing loss
   g. Loss of taste bud sensation (page 413)

5. **a.** Gastrointestinal distress
   b. Upper respiratory tract infection (page 405)

6. **a.** Control
   b. Following rules
   c. Competitiveness (page 406)

7. **a.** Loss of respiratory muscle mass
   b. Increased stiffness of the thoracic cage
   c. Decreased surface area available for air exchange (page 411)

Fill-in-the-Table

1. (page 408)

Male Characteristics	Female Characteristics
External organs enlarge.	Breasts and thighs increase in size.
Pubic and ancillary hair begins to appear.	Menstruation begins (can begin younger than teenage years).
Voice changes.	Acne occurs.
Acne occurs.	Follicle-stimulating hormone and luteinizing hormone (both of which increase estrogen and progesterone production) is released.

2. (page 401)

Vital Signs at Various Ages				
Age	Pulse Rate (beats/min)	Respirations (breaths/min)	Blood Pressure (mm Hg, systolic)	Temperature (°F)
Newborn (0 to 1 mo)	**100 to 180**	**30 to 60**	50 to 70	98 to 100
Infant (1 month to 1 y)	**100 to 160**	25 to 50	**70 to 95**	96.8 to 99.6
Toddler (1 to 3 y)	90 to 150	20 to 30	**80 to 100**	96.8 to 99.6
Preschool age (3 to 5 y)	80 to 140	**20 to 25**	80 to 100	**98.6**
School age **(6 to 12 y)**	70 to 120	15 to 20	**80 to 100**	98.6
Adolescent **(13 to 17 y)**	**60 to 100**	**12 to 20**	**90 to 110**	98.6
Early adult (18 to 40 y)	**60 to 100**	12 to 20	90 to 140	98.6
Middle adult (41 to 60 y)	60 to 100	12 to 20	90 to 140	98.6
Late adult (61 y and older)	Depends on health	Depends on health	**Depends on health**	98.6

Section 3: Pharmacology
Chapter 10: Principles of Pharmacology

Matching

A number of the medications administered by paramedics or medications patients may have overdosed on are considered controlled substances. (page 424)

1. III **2.** V **3.** I **4.** II **5.** IV

6. IV **7.** I **8.** II **9.** II **10.** III

Multiple Choice

1. B (page 425) **2.** C (page 423) **3.** A (page 423) **4.** C (page 437) **5.** B (page 425)

6. D (page 425) **7.** B (page 425) **8.** B (page 429) **9.** C (page 435) **10.** A (page 430)

Fill-in-the-Blank

1. indications (page 433)
2. neutralization (page 437)
3. antagonist (page 459)
4. potentiation (page 437)
5. alpha-1 (page 429)
6. beta-2 (page 429)
7. Diuretic (page 455)
8. beta-blocking (page 446)
9. Cardiac glycosides (page 446)
10. corticosteroids (page 446)

Identify

1. Chief complaint: Heart palpitations
2. Vital signs: Pulse is 60 beats/min, regular and weak; respirations are slightly labored at 22 breaths/min; blood pressure is 90/60 mm Hg; and skin is pale.
3. Pertinent negatives: No pain (it should be noted that she may be having a "silent MI," which is a myocardial infarction [MI] without pain or discomfort), no nausea, and relatively good health.
Note: The fact that the patient she started a new medication might be a significant finding because she may be having an adverse effect. (page 434)

Ambulance Calls

1. a. Right patient—Does this patient meet the criteria and based on the assessment, vital signs, and SAMPLE history?
   b. Right medication—Is morphine the correct medication for this patient?
   c. Right dose—Based on the patient's weight and your protocols, are you giving the right amount?
   d. Right route—Is the drug being given in the optimal way?
   e. Right time—Is this drug given when it should be and has the patient already taken or been given any other drugs that could interact?
   f. Right documentation and reporting—What time was the medication administered, exactly what amount was administered, and by what route? Because this is a controlled substance, are there any other legal requirements for documentation? (page 444)

2. a. An inactive substance can be active, capable of producing desired or unwanted clinical effects (active metabolite).

   b. An active medication can be changed into another active medication (active metabolite).

   c. An active medication can be completely or partially inactivated (inactive metabolite).

   d. A medication can be transformed into a substance (active or inactive metabolite) that is easier for the body to eliminate. (page 442)

3. a. Age

   b. Weight (the doses for many drugs administered are calculated based on the weight of the patient)

   c. Environment

   d. Genetic factors

   e. Pregnancy

   f. Psychosocial factors (pages 430–432)

True/False

1. F (page 425)   **2.** F (page 424)   **3.** T (page 430)   **4.** T (page 443)   **5.** T (page 430)

6. F (page 431)   **7.** T (page 450)   **8.** T (page 434)   **9.** F (page 435)   **10.** F (page 445)

Short Answer

1. a. Chemical name

   b. Generic name

   c. Trade or brand name (page 425)

2. a. Drug names

   b. Category or class of medication

   c. Uses/indications

   d. Mechanism of action (pharmacodynamics)

   e. Pregnancy risk factors

   f. Contraindications

   g. Available forms

   h. Dosages (often differentiated based on age indication)

   i. Administration and monitoring considerations

   j. Potential incompatibility

   k. Adverse effects

   l. Pharmacokinetics (page 426)

3. a. No leading zero before decimal point; for example, .8 mg can be interpreted as 8 mg, so use a zero before the decimal point: 0.8 mg.

   b. MSO can be misinterpreted as magnesium sulfate, so write out morphine sulfate.

   c. $MgSO_4$ can be misinterpreted as morphine sulfate, so write out magnesium sulfate.

   d. SC may be interpreted as SL, so write out as subcutaneous.

   e. IN can be interpreted as IV or IM, so write out intranasal. (page 444)

4. *Students should provide eight of these common adverse effects:*

   a. nausea

   b. vomiting

   c. sedation

   d. palpitations

   e. hypotension

   f. hypertension

   g. bradycardia

   h. tachycardia

   i. respiratory depression

   j. endocrine abnormalities

   k. dizziness (page 434)

5. **a.** Antiemetics
   b. Antidiarrheals
   c. Antibiotics
   d. Antacids
   e. Antihistamines
   f. Beta-blocking agents
   g. Benzodiazepines
   h. Corticosteroids
   i. Fibrinolytics
   j. Hormone replacement drugs
   k. Narcotic analgesics
   l. Sympathomimetics (pages 445–447)

Fill-in-the-Table

1. (page 439)

Veins Used During IO Infusion	
Intraosseous Site	**Vein**
Proximal tibia	**Popliteal vein**
Femur	**Femoral vein**
Distal tibia (medial malleolus)	Great saphenous vein
Proximal humerus	Axillary vein
Manubrium (sternum)	**Internal mammary and azygos veins**

2. (page 438)

GI Medication Absorption	
Factor	**Medication Absorption**
GI motility	Ability of medication to pass through the GI tract into the bloodstream
GI pH	Perfusion of the GI system (may be decreased during systemic trauma or shock)
Presence of food, liquids, or chemicals in the stomach	Injury or bleeding in the GI system (both can alter GI motility, decreasing the time that oral medications can be absorbed)

3. (page 424)

Sources of Medication	
Source	**Example**
Plant	Atropine, aspirin, digoxin, morphine
Animal	Heparin, antivenom, thyroid preparations, insulin
Microorganism	Streptokinase, numerous antibiotics
Minerals	Iron, magnesium sulfate, lithium, phosphorus, calcium

Chapter 11: Medication Administration

Matching

Part I
(page 536)

1. D   **2.** C   **3.** B   **4.** A   **5.** C   **6.** B   **7.** A

Part II
(page 473)

1. C   **2.** B   **3.** D   **4.** A

Multiple Choice

1. C (page 473)   **2.** A (page 474)   **3.** D (page 477)   **4.** B (page 480)   **5.** B (page 484)

6. C (page 486)   **7.** A (page 493)   **8.** C (page 494)   **9.** B (page 496)   **10.** B (page 472)

11. D (page 511)   **12.** B (page 512)   **13.** C (page 519)   **14.** C (page 528)   **15.** B (page 510)

Fill-in-the-Blank

1. colloid (page 540)

2. crystalloid; saline (page 540)

3. hypertonic; hypotonic; isotonic; hypertonic; isotonic; hypotonic (page 541)

4. lower; higher; osmosis (page 541)

5. dyspnea; hypertension (page 495)

Labeling

Common Sites for Intramuscular Injections (page 519)

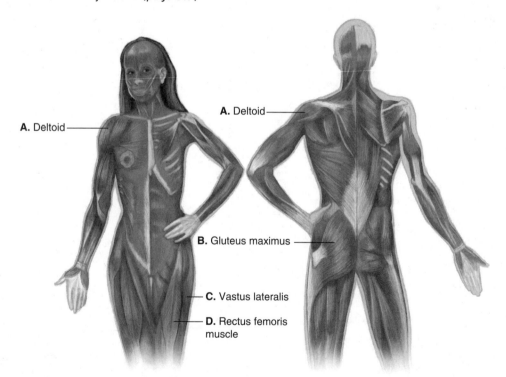

A. Deltoid

A. Deltoid

B. Gluteus maximus

C. Vastus lateralis

D. Rectus femoris muscle

Ambulance Calls

Intravenous lines are supposed to help save lives, but they may cause problems (most of which can be prevented!).

1. a. You are the patient's problem! You weren't keeping an eye on the IV. The 59-year-old man who is suddenly short of breath has most probably developed circulatory overload because his "keep-open" IV became a "runaway IV" and poured an extra liter of fluid into his vascular space in a very short period of time.

   b. What you need to do is slow the IV to keep-open, sit the patient up with his legs dangling, and radio your physician for further instructions. (page 495)

2. a. The frail old woman probably has very frail veins, and your IV has apparently ruptured the wall of one of those veins and infiltrated.

   b. What you have to do is discontinue the IV and start a new one at another site, if she really needs it. If not, wait until you reach the ED, where a new IV can be inserted under more controlled conditions.

   c. Other problems that might cause an IV to slow down include tightening of the clamp, a kink in the tubing, the tip of the catheter resting against the wall of the vein, flexion at a joint causing the vein to kink, and the IV bag hung too low. (page 494)

3. a. When bright red blood comes spurting back in your face, it is a pretty good indication that you have accidentally cannulated an artery.

   b. What you need to do is immediately withdraw the catheter and hold firm pressure over the puncture site for at least 5 minutes. (page 494)

4. a. A painful, red, swollen venipuncture site is a sign of thrombophlebitis.

   b. The treatment is to discontinue the IV and put a warm compress (hot pack) over the puncture site.

   c. The likelihood of thrombophlebitis can be minimized by:

   (1) Adequately disinfecting the skin before venipuncture

   (2) Wearing sterile gloves to start an IV

   (3) Covering the puncture site with a sterile dressing

   (4) Securing the catheter firmly so it cannot wobble around inside the vein (page 493)

5. a. Yes, he is probably seriously injured. The reason for that conclusion is the signs of shock already evident: restlessness; cold, clammy skin; and the thirst itself.

   b. You decide to start an IV with lactated Ringer's, which is a **crystalloid** solution. To calculate the IV rate, you need to recall the equation:

$$\frac{\text{Volume to be infused} \times \text{gtt/mL}}{\text{Time of infusion (in minutes)}} = \frac{200 \text{ mL} \times 10 \text{ gtt/mL}}{60 \text{ min}}$$

2,000 gtt ÷ 60 min = 33.3 gtt/min

(for practical purposes, that is 30 gtt/min) (page 506)

   c. The steps in troubleshooting an IV are as follows:

   (1) Check the IV fluid.

   (2) Check the administration set.

   (3) Check the height of the IV bag.

   (4) Check the type of catheter used.

   (5) Check the constricting band. (page 492)

True/False

1. F (page 540) **2.** T (pages 473–474) **3.** F (page 474) **4.** F (page 474) **5.** T (page 474)

6. F (pages 475–476) **7.** F (page 476) **8.** T (page 477) **9.** F (page 477) **10.** T (page 480)

11. F (page 482) **12.** F (page 483) **13.** F (page 484) **14.** F (page 487) **15.** T (page 492)

16. T (page 494) **17.** F (page 495) **18.** T (page 496) **19.** F (page 497) **20.** F (page 497)

21. T (page 502) **22.** F (page 504) **23.** T (page 505) **24.** T (page 507) **25.** T (page 469)

Short Answer

1. **a.** Allow the arm to hang off the stretcher.
   b. Pat or rub the area.
   c. Apply chemical heat packs for at least 60 seconds (page 486)

2. **a.** The gauge of the needle
   b. The IV attempts versus successes
   c. The site (eg, left forearm, left external jugular)
   d. The type of fluid that you are administering
   e. The rate at which the fluid is running (page 486)

3. *Students should list three of the following:*
   a. Infiltration: Signs and symptoms are local edema around the site, continued IV flow after occlusion of the vein above the insertion site, and patient complaints of tightness and pain around the IV site. (page 492)
   b. Occlusion: Signs and symptoms are decreasing drip rate or the presence of blood in the tubing or a positional IV. Also, if the bag of fluids is empty, it can cause an occlusion by clotting around the site of the IV. (page 493)
   c. Vein irritation: Signs and symptoms include the solution tingling, stinging, itching, or burning. If redness develops at the IV site, discontinue the IV and start a new IV with all new equipment and fluids. (page 493)
   d. Thrombophlebitis: Signs and symptoms are tenderness and pain along the vein, as well as redness and edema at the site of the enipuncture. (page 493)
   e. Hematoma: Signs and symptoms are rapid blood pooling below the skin around the IV site, leading to tenderness and pain. Use direct pressure to stop the hematoma. Evaluate the site to see if the IV is good and can be used. If not, pull out the IV and apply direct pressure. (page 494)
   f. Nerve, tendon, or ligament damage: Signs and symptoms are numbness, tingling, and sudden shooting pain. Remove the IV and select a different site. (page 494)
   g. Arterial puncture: Signs and symptoms are bright red spurting blood with a much faster flow. Discontinue the site and apply direct pressure to the IV site until the bleeding stops. (page 494)

4. **a.** Name of the drug
   b. The dose of the drug
   c. Time you administered the drug
   d. Route of administration (eg, IV, IM)
   e. Name of the paramedic who administered the drug
   f. The patient's response to the medication, whether positive or negative (page 471)

Fill-in-the-Table

Route of Administration	Where on the Body the Medication Goes
Enteral	1. Gastrointestinal tract (page 540)
Oral	2. By the mouth (page 508)
Intradermal	3. Injection into the dermis (page 541)
Percutaneous	4. Through the skin and mucous membranes (page 542)
Sublingual	5. Under the tongue (page 542)
Endotracheal	6. Bagged in through the ET tube (page 531)
Buccal	7. Between the cheek and gums (page 527)
Transdermal	8. Applied topically (page 526)
Intramuscular	9. Injection into the muscle (page 518)
Rectal	10. Into the rectal mucosa (page 510)
Parenteral	11. Any route other than the gastrointestinal tract (page 542)
Subcutaneous	12. Injection between dermis and muscle (page 517)
Intravascular	13. Directly into a vein (page 541)
Ocular	14. Drop or ointment into the eye (page 527)
Aural	15. Into the ear canal (page 528)
Inhalation	16. Inhaled into the lungs (page 541)
Intranasal	17. Within the nose (page 541)

Problem Solving

1. To give the baker 200 mL per hour with a macrodrop set (page 507):

$$\frac{\text{Volume to be infused} \times \text{gtt/mL of administration set}}{\text{Total time of infusion in minutes}} = \text{gtt/min}$$

$$\frac{200 \text{ mL/h} \times 10 \text{ gtt/mL}}{60 \text{ min}} = \text{approximately } 33.3 \text{ gtt/min}$$

2. For the patient who needs only a keep-open line (page 507):

$$\frac{30 \text{ mL} \times 60 \text{ gtt/mL}}{60 \text{ min}} = 30 \text{ gtt/min}$$

3. This problem, which involves calculating concentrations and flow rates, is not merely a theoretical exercise; it is typical of the calculations you will be making every day in your work as a paramedic, and a slip of the decimal point could kill someone!

   a. Your vial of lidocaine contains 50 mL of 4% lidocaine, so by definition it contains (pages 506–507):

   $$\frac{4 \text{ g of lidocaine}}{100 \text{ mL}} = \frac{2 \text{ g of lidocaine}}{50 \text{ mL}}$$

   b. When you add that 2 g of lidocaine to a volume of 500 mL:

   $$\frac{2 \text{ g} = 2{,}000 \text{ mg}}{500 \text{ mL} \quad 500 \text{ mL}} = 4 \text{ mg/mL} = .0004$$

   (Ignore the volume in which the lidocaine was suspended.)

   c. If the patient is to receive 2 mg per minute, he must receive:

   $$\frac{2 \text{ mg/min}}{4 \text{ mg/mL}} = 0.5 \text{ mL/min}$$

   d. Thus, the number of drops per minute at which you have to set the infusion is:
   0.5 mL/min × 60 gtt/mL = 30 gtt/min

4. 12 g × 1,000 mg/g = 12,000 mg (pages 504)

5. $\dfrac{156 \text{ lb}}{2.2 \text{ lb/kg}} = 70.9 \text{ kg}$

   Round up to 71 kg (page 504)

6. Step 1: 135 ÷ 2 = 67.5
   Step 2: 67.5 × 0.10 = 6.75
   Round 6.75 to 7
   Step 3: 67.5 – 7 = 60.5
   Round up to 61
   Patient's weight in kilograms for field purposes is 61 kg. (page 504)

7. $\dfrac{6 \text{ mg}}{10 \text{ mg/mL}} = 0.6 \text{ mL}$

   (page 505)

8. Concentration on hand (pages 505–506):

$$\frac{20 \text{ mg}}{10 \text{ mL}} = 2 \text{ mg/mL}$$

Volume you will give:

$$\frac{2 \text{ mg}}{2 \text{ mg/mL}} = 1 \text{ mL}$$

9. (page 507)

   a. 10 µg/kg/min × 80 kg = 800 µg/min (desired dose)

   b. $\dfrac{800 \text{ mg (or } 800{,}000 \text{ µg)}}{500 \text{ mL}} = 1.6 \text{ mg/mL}$

   c. 1.6 mg/mL × 1,000 µg/mg = 1,600 µg/mL (page 507)

   d. $\dfrac{800 \text{ µg/min}}{1{,}600 \text{ µg/mL}} = 0.5 \text{ mL/min}$

   e. 0.5 mL/min × 60 gtt/mL = 30 gtt/min

10. (page 502)

Microgram (µg)	Milligram (mg)	Gram (g)	Kilogram (kg)
500.0	0.5	0.0005	0.0000005
1,000,000.0	1,000.0	1.0	0.001
1,000,000,000.0	1,000,000.0	1,000	1.0
1,000.0	1.0	0.001	0.000001
1.0	0.001	0.000001	0.000000001
800,000.0	800.0	0.8	0.0008
15.0	0.015	0.000015	0.000000015

Milliliter (mL)	Deciliter (dL)	Liter (L)
5,000.0	50.0	5.0
1.0	0.01	0.001
10.0	0.1	0.01
1,000.0	10.0	1.0
250.0	2.5	0.25

11. (page 504)

Patient's weight (lb)	Patient's weight (lb) ÷ 2	Weight (lb) ÷ 2 × 10%	Subtract your 10% from the weight ÷ 2	Patient's weight in kilograms (kg)	Patient's weight in lb ÷ 2.2 = patient's weight in kilograms (kg)
60	60 ÷ 2 = 30	30 × 10% = 3	30 - 3 = 27	27	27.27
16	8	0.8 (≈ 1)	8 - 1 = 7	7	7.27
138	69	6.9 (≈ 7)	69 - 7 = 62	62	62.72
8	4	0.4 (≈ 0.5)	4 - 0.5 = 3.5	3.5	3.64
250	125	12.5	125 - 12.5 = 112.5	112.5	113.64
36	18	1.8 (≈ 2)	18 - 2 = 16	16	16.36
82	41	4.1 (≈ 4)	41 - 4 = 37	37	37.27
180	90	9.0	90 - 9 = 81	81	81.82
330	165	16.5 (≈ 17)	165 - 17 = 148	148	150

12. (page 503) Volume conversions

1,000 mL NS	500 mL NS	250 mL NS	100 mL NS	50 mL NS
100 g	50 g	25 g	10 g	5 g
1,600 g	800 g	**400 g**	**160 g**	**80 g**
1,000 g	**500 g**	250 g	100 g	50 g
40 g	**20 g**	**10 g**	4 g	**2 g**
100 g	50 g	**25 g**	**10 g**	**5 g**

13. (page 503)
   a. $120 \div 60 = 2$ mL/min
   b. $120 \div 15 = 8$ mL/min
   c. $120 \div 30 = 4$ mL/min

14. (page 504) This table is based on the formula: $(F - 32) \times 0.555 = C$.

Temperature in degrees F	Degrees F - 32	Degrees F - 32 × 0.555	Temperature in degrees C
32	0	0	0
95.0	**95 - 32 = 63**	**63 × 0.555 = 34.97**	**34.97 (approx 35)**
98.6	98.6 - 32 = 66.6	66.6 × 0.555 = 36.96	36.96 (approx 37)
101.0	**101 - 32 = 69**	**69 × 0.555 = 38.3**	**38.3 (approx 38)**
104.0	**104 - 32 = 72**	**72 × 0.555 = 39.96**	**39.96 (approx 40)**

15. (page 504) Determine how much medication is prescribed for your patient by body weight by filling in the following table.

Desired dose	Patient's weight in pounds (lb)	Patient's weight in kilograms (kg)	Medication administered
1 mg/kg lidocaine	90	90 ÷ 2.2 = 40.9 kg (≈ 41 kg)	41 kg × 1 mg lidocaine = 41 mg lidocaine to administer
0.2 mg/kg atropine	30	**30 ÷ 2.2 = 13.6**	**13.6 kg × 0.2 mg atropine = 2.72 mg atropine to administer**
0.05 mg/kg lorezapam	180	**180 ÷ 2.2 = 81.8**	**81.8 kg × 0.5 mg = 4.09 mg lorezapam to administer**
30 mg/kg methylpred-nisolone	220	**220 ÷ 2.2 = 100**	**100 kg × 30 mg = 3,000 mg = 3 g methylpred-nisolone to administer**
15 mg/kg phenobarbital	12	**12 ÷ 2.2 = 5.5**	**5.5 kg × 15 mg = 82.5 mg phenobarbitol to administer**

16. (page 505) Base your calculations on volumes replaced at 20 mL/kg of patient body weight.

Patient's weight in pounds (lb)	Patient's weight in kilograms: weight in lb ÷ 2.2 = wt in kg (or use the "10% trick")	Volume to be infused with first bolus @ 20 mL/kg
60	60 lb ÷ 2.2 = 27 kg	27 kg × 20 mL/kg = 540 mL
80	80 lb ÷ 2.2 = 36 kg	36 kg × 20 mL/kg = 720 mL
100	100 lb ÷ 2.2 = 45 kg	45 kg × 20 mL/kg = 900 mL
125	125 lb ÷ 2.2 = 57 kg	57 kg × 20 mL/kg = 1,140 mL
150	150 lb ÷ 2.2 = 68 kg	68 kg × 20 mL/kg = 1,360 mL
175	175 lb ÷ 2.2 = 80 kg	80 kg × 20 mL/kg = 1,600 mL
190	190 lb ÷ 2.2 = 86 kg	86 kg × 20 mL/kg = 1,720 mL
220	220 lb ÷ 2.2 = 100 kg	100 kg × 20 mL/kg = 2,000 mL (= 2 L)
300	300 lb ÷ 2.2 = 136 kg	136 kg × 20 mL/kg = 2,720 mL

17. (page 505) Find the weight of the following medications in 1 mL of solution:
- **a.** 100 mg/10 mL lidocaine = 10 mg/1 mL lidocaine
- **b.** 1 mg/10 mL epinephrine = 0.1 mg/1 mL epinephrine
- **c.** 40 mg/14 mL furosemide = 2.9 mg/1 mL furosemide
- **d.** 6 mg/2 mL adenosine = 3 mg/1 mL adenosine
- **e.** 20 mg/5 mL diazepam = 4 mg/1 mL diazepam
- **f.** 10 mg/5 mL naloxone = 2 mg/1 mL naloxone
- **g.** 2 mg/5 mL albuterol = 0.4 mg/1 mL albuterol
- **h.** 150 mg/3 mL amiodarone = 50 mg/1 mL amiodarone
- **i.** 25 g/125 mL activated charcoal = 0.2 g/1 mL activated charcoal = 200 mg/1 mL activated charcoal

18. (page 505) Find the weight of the following medications in 1 mL of solution. Follow this example: 50% dextrose = 50 g/100 mL = 0.5g/1 mL.
- **a.** 1 % xylocaine = 1 g/100 mL = 0.01 g/1 mL (or 10 mg/mL)
- **b.** 10% dextrose = 10 g/100 mL = 0.1 g/1 mL (or 100 mg/mL)
- **c.** 0.5% albuterol = 0.5 g/100 mL = 0.005 g/1 mL (or 5 mg/mL)
- **d.** 10% calcium chloride = 10 g/100 mL = 0.1 g/1 mL (or 100 mg/mL)
- **e.** 50% magnesium sulfate = 50 g/100 mL = 0.5 g/1 mL (or 500 mg/mL)
- **f.** 5% alupent = 5 g/100 mL = 0.05 g/1 mL (or 50 mg/mL)
- **g.** 0.9% sodium chloride = 0.9 g/100 mL = 0.009 g/1 mL (or 9 mg/mL)

19. (page 507) Determine the amount of dopamine in micrograms (μg) per milliliter when 800 milligrams (mg) of dopamine are added to the following bags of normal saline (NS): (note: 1 mg = 1,000 μg)
- **a.** 800 mg/500 mL = 1.6 mg/1 mL = 1,600 μg/1 mL
- **b.** 800 mg/250 mL = 3.2 mg/1 mL = 3,200 μg/mL
- **c.** 800 mg/1,000 mL = 0.8 mg/1 mL = 800 μg/mL
- **d.** 800 mg/100 mL = 8.0 mg/1 mL = 8,000 μg/mL

20. (page 507) Desired dose in mg ÷ concentration in mg/1 mL = volume to administer (concentration = the "dose on hand")
- **a.** Desired dose = 15 mg labetalol

  Concentration = 100 mg/20 mL = 5 mg/1 mL

  15 mg ÷ 5 mg/mL = 3 mL of medication will be administered
- **b.** Desired dose = 3 mg haloperidol

  Concentration = 5 mg haloperidol/1 mL

  3 mg ÷ 5 mg/mL = 0.6 mL of haloperidol will be administered
- **c.** Desired dose = 750 mg calcium chloride

  Concentration = 1,000 mg calcium chloride/10 mL = 100 mg calcium chloride/1 mL

  750 mg ÷ 100 mg/mL = 7.5 mL of calcium chloride will be administered

Skill Drills

Part I

1. Drawing Medications From an Ampule (pages 513–514)

Step 1: Gently tap the stem of the ampule to shake medication into the base.

Step 2: Grip the neck of the ampule using a 4" × 4" gauze pad, and snap the neck off.

Step 3: Without touching the outer sides of the ampule, insert the needle into the medication in the ampule, and draw the solution into the syringe.

Step 4: Holding the syringe with the needle pointing up, gently tap the barrel to loosen air trapped inside.

Step 5: Gently press on the plunger to dispel any air bubbles, and recap the needle using the one-handed method.

2. Administering a Medication via Small-Volume Nebulizer (page 532)

Step 1: Check the medication and the expiration date.

Step 2: Add premixed medication to the bowl of the nebulizer.

Step 3: Connect the T piece with the mouthpiece to the top of the bowl, connect it to the oxygen tubing, and set the flowmeter at 6 L/min.

Step 4: Instruct the patient to breathe as deeply as possible and hold his or her breath for 3 to 5 seconds before exhaling. Monitor the patient for effects.

Part II

1. Drawing Medication From a Vial (page 515)

Step 1: Check the medication and its **expiration** date.

Step 2: Wipe the vial rubber top with an alcohol prep before touching it with the needle. Determine the amount of medication needed, and draw that amount of **air** into the syringe.

Step 3: Invert the **vial**, and insert the needle through the rubber stopper. Expel the air in the syringe to the vial, and then withdraw the amount of medication needed.

Step 4: Withdraw the **needle**, and expel any air in the syringe.

Step 5: Recap the needle using the **one-handed** method. Label the syringe if the medication is not immediately given to the patient.

Chapter 12: Emergency Medications

Matching

(page 546)

1. C	**2.** D	**3.** B	**4.** G	**5.** A
6. E	**7.** I	**8.** F	**9.** H	**10.** J

Multiple Choice

1. C (page 548)	**2.** D (page 545)	**3.** C (page 545)	**4.** B (page 545)	**5.** B (page 546)
6. B (page 547)	**7.** A (page 547)	**8.** C (page 547)	**9.** D (page 548)	**10.** C (pages 550–554)
11. D (page 555)	**12.** B (pages 559–560)	**13.** C (page 563)	**14.** A (page 564)	**15.** B (page 566)

Ambulance Calls

1. The 50-year-old man with severe chest pain should get morphine, oxygen, nitrates, and aspirin.
2. The 22-year-old man who is having bronchoconstriction due to his asthma should get albuterol, atrovent, and oxygen.
3. The 19-year-old woman who has severe pain from a severely angulated right forearm should get morphine and oxygen.
4. The 40-year-old man who has just had his second seizure in a row without regaining consciousness should get valium, or Ativan, and oxygen.
5. The 62-year-old woman who is in cardiac arrest with asystole on the ECG should get epinephrine and oxygen.

True/False

1. T (page 550)	**2.** F (page 551)	**3.** T (page 552)	**4.** T (page 553)	**5.** F (page 553)
6. F (page 554)	**7.** T (page 555)	**8.** T (page 556)	**9.** F (page 558)	**10.** T (page 559)
11. T (page 559)	**12.** T (page 560)	**13.** F (page 561)	**14.** T (page 562)	**15.** F (page 563)

Short Answer

1. *Students should include three of the following:*
   a. hypersensitivity
   b. second- or third-degree AV block in the absence of an artificial pacemaker
   c. Stokes-Adams syndrome
   d. prophylactic use in AMI
   e. wide complex ventricular escape beats with bradycardia (page 563)

2. *Students should include three of the following:*
   a. seizures of eclampsia (toxemia of pregnancy)
   b. torsades de pointes
   c. hypomagnesemia
   d. ventricular fibrillation/pulseless ventricular tachycardia that is refractory to amiodarone
   e. life-threatening dysrhythmias due to digitalis toxicity (page 564)

3. *Students should include three of the following:*
   a. head injury
   b. exacerbated COPD
   c. depressed respiratory drive
   d. hypotension
   e. undiagnosed abdominal pain
   f. decreased level of consciousness
   g. suspected hypovolemia
   h. patients who have taken MAOIs within 14 days (page 566)

Fill-in-the-Table

(page 546)

Common Metric Conversions	
Weight	
1 kilogram (kg)	**2.2 pounds (lb)**
1 kilogram (kg)	1,000 grams (g or gm)
1 gram (g or gr)	**1,000 milligrams (mg)**
1 milligram (mg)	1,000 micrograms (µg or mcg)
Volume	
1 liter (L)	1,000 milliliters or cubic centimeters (mL or cc)
Temperature	
37° Celsius (°C)	**98.6° Fahrenheit (°F)**
Length	
1 centimeter (cm)	10 millimeters (mm)
100 centimeters (cm)	1 meter (m)

Section 4: Patient Assessment
Chapter 13: Patient Assessment

Matching

Part I

1. A (page 607) **2.** A (page 607) **3.** B (page 616) **4.** A (page 616) **5.** A (page 616)

6. B (page 616) **7.** B (page 616) **8.** A (page 616) **9.** A (page 607) **10.** A (pages 607–608)

11. A (page 608) **12.** A (page 608) **13.** A (pages 615–616)

Part II

Spotting abnormal physical signs is only part of physical assessment; the other part is drawing the correct conclusions from those signs.

1. I **2.** J, M **3.** D, O, U **4.** A, G, V **5.** T **6.** J, L

7. N, C **8.** K, L **9.** B **10.** S **11.** O **12.** C

13. R **14.** F **15.** Q **16.** H **17.** E **18.** P

Part III

1. S (pages 598–599) **2.** NS (pages 597–601) **3.** S (pages 598–600) **4.** NS (pages 598–600)

5. NS (pages 597–601) **6.** S (pages 597–598) **7.** S (pages 597–600) **8.** NS (pages 597–600)

Multiple Choice

1. B (page 605) **2.** C (page 615) **3.** A (page 615) **4.** D (page 618) **5.** B (page 619)

6. D (page 619) **7.** C (page 620) **8.** B (page 622) **9.** A (page 621) **10.** C (pages 622–623)

11. D (page 627) **12.** B (page 630) **13.** A (page 629) **14.** C (page 597) **15.** C (page 639)

16. A (page 663) **17.** B (page 670) **18.** C (page 656) **19.** D (page 672) **20.** C (page 638)

21. A (page 592) **22.** C (page 597) **23.** D (page 595) **24.** A (page 620) **25.** A (page 597)

26. C (page 603) **27.** D (page 610) **28.** D (page 601) **29.** C (page 632) **30.** A (page 597)

Labeling

1. Nine Regions of the Abdomen (page 658)
   A. Right hypochondrial region
   B. Epigastric region
   C. Left hypochondrial region
   D. Right lumbar region
   E. Umbilical region
   F. Left lumbar region
   G. Right iliac region
   H. Hypogastric region
   I. Left iliac region

Fill-in-the-Blank

1. field impression (page 589)

2. introduce yourself (page 605)

3. present illness (page 607)

4. medical terms (page 622)

5. face-to-face (page 622)

6. Empathy (page 614)

7. reflection (page 615)

8. HIPAA (page 606)

9. medical history (pages 607–608)

10. age-appropriate; education-appropriate (page 605)

Ambulance Calls

1. Accident scenes like the one pictured in this question are fairly characteristic of those you will encounter in your work. You can learn a lot from the scene and the people there if you know what to look for and what to ask.

  a. The potential sources of information about what happened to the patient at the scene are:

    (1) The scene itself

    (2) The patient

    (3) The bystanders at the bus stop and perhaps in the diner

    (4) Any medical identification devices the patient might be carrying

  b. From observing the scene, you can tell that:

    (1) The driver was driving somewhat erratically.

    (2) Something caused him to swerve off the road (perhaps he saw something in the road or thought he saw something).

    (3) The driver was conscious when he went off the road (he was able to apply the brakes).

    (4) Massive forces were involved in the accident (enough to break the telephone pole).

    (5) The driver struck his head against the windshield.

  c. It is necessary to take a history:

    (1) To find out what happened. Why did he swerve off the road? Did something cross his path? Did he suddenly feel ill?

    (2) To find out what hurts—that is, to start searching for his most serious injuries.

    (3) To find out whether he has any underlying medical problems that might complicate his care. If, for example, he is taking anticoagulant drugs (drugs that interfere with blood clotting) after a previous heart attack, he could lose a great deal of blood from what might otherwise be a fairly minor wound.

    (4) To gather information that might otherwise be unavailable to the hospital staff, such as data on the mechanisms of injury.

  d. Before you start taking the history, you need to:

    (1) Clear your mind of any preconceived ideas about the patient (eg, "He must have been drunk.").

    (2) Introduce yourself, and explain your role.

    (3) Find out the patient's name.

    (4) Try to position yourself at the patient's level; to do so, lean over or crouch down near the car window.

    (5) Initiate some physical contact; for example, put a hand on the patient's shoulder and instruct him not to move until you have examined him.

True/False

1. T (page 589)   **2.** F (page 618)   **3.** F (page 617)   **4.** T (page 619)   **5.** T (page 620)

6. T (page 682)   **7.** T (page 608)   **8.** F (page 589)   **9.** F (page 606)   **10.** T (page 615)

11. F (page 679)   **12.** T (page 677)   **13.** T (page 677)   **14.** F (page 673)   **15.** T (page 656)

16. F (page 628)   **17.** F (pages 663–665)   **18.** T (page 662)   **19.** T (page 656)   **20.** F (page 629)

Short Answer

1. a. In eliciting the history of the present illness from a patient whose chief complaint is "pain in my gut," one would want to know at least the following:

    (1) Did anything in particular provoke the pain? What brought it on? Does anything make it worse? Does anything make it better?

    (2) What is the quality of the pain? What is it like?

    (3) Does the pain radiate anywhere? Where is it precisely?

    (4) How severe is the pain?

(5) What was the timing of the pain; that is, when did it come on? Has it been there constantly since, or does it come and go?

(6) Are there any associated symptoms, such as nausea, vomiting, diarrhea, constipation? (pages 606–607)

  b. In inquiring about the patient's other medical history, you need to find out the following:

(1) Does he have any major underlying medical problems? One way to find out is to ask, "Are you presently under a doctor's care for any condition?"

(2) Does he take any medications regularly?

(3) Does he have any allergies?

(4) Does he have a family doctor, or does he go regularly to a particular hospital? (pages 607–609)

2. In taking the history of a head-injured patient, you need to find out the following. *Students should provide five of the following:*

  a. The circumstances of the accident: How did the injury occur? What were the mechanisms of injury?

  b. Whether the patient lost consciousness at any point. If so, when? For how long?

  c. Whether the patient vomited.

  d. What the patient's current symptoms are (assuming he is conscious and can tell you).

  e. Whether the patient has ingested drugs or alcohol within the past few hours.

  f. Whether the patient has any significant underlying illnesses. (page 610)

3. The four questions you need to answer in making your survey of the scene are the following:

  a. Is it safe for me to approach the victim(s)?

  b. Is there any hazard to the patient?

  c. Will I need any help?

  d. Do I need any special equipment to reach the patient?

If you do not ask and answer those questions at every incident scene, your career as a paramedic may be very short indeed, for you will not notice the downed high-tension line draped over the car, or the little trail of fire creeping toward the vehicle, or the bus about to plow into the disabled vehicle that is still in the middle of the road. (page 592)

4. Possible sources of information about what happened to the patient include the following:

  a. The patient himself or herself (the most important source if the patient is conscious)

  b. Bystanders or family

  c. The scene (mechanisms of injury)

  d. Medical identification devices (page 597)

Fill-in-the-Table

Tests for Disability in Cranial Nerves	
Cranial Nerve	**Test**
I	Check smell
II	Check visual acuity
III	Check pupil size, shape, symmetry, response to light, eye movements
IV	Check eye movements
V	Check jaw clench; touch both sides of face at forehead, cheeks, and jaw
VI	Check eye movements
VII	Check facial symmetry; look for abnormal movements; raise eyebrows, grin broadly, frown, shut eyes tightly, puff out cheeks; note any asymmetry
VIII	Check hearing and balance
IX, X	Check swallowing; perform general physical exam
XI	Check shoulder shrug; turn head from left to right and back
XII	Check swallowing; turn head from left to right and back

1. When you assess an injured patient from head to toe, it helps to know what you are looking for. (pages 601–602)

Body Region	What I Will Be Looking for in Particular (in addition to DCAP-BTLS)
Head	**Deformity, lacerations, CSF leak, Battle's sign, maxillofacial injury**
Neck	**Open wounds, subcutaneous emphysema, tracheal deviation, jugular distention, bruises over cervical spine**
Chest	**Bruises, open wounds, instability, inequality of breath sounds, dullness or hyperresonance**
Abdomen	**Contusions, open wounds, evisceration, distention, rigidity, cough rebound**
Extremities	**Deformity, swelling, ecchymosis, pulses, movement, sensation**
Back/buttocks	**Just DCAP-BTLS**

Skill Drill

1. Examining the Nervous System
   1. Evaluate cranial nerve function.
   2. Evaluate the patient's neuromuscular status by checking muscle strength against resistance.
   3. Evaluate the patient's coordination by performing the finger-to-nose test using alternating hands.
   4. If appropriate, test the patient's gait and balance by having the patient walk heel-to-toe or perform the heel-to-shin stance.
   5. Perform the pronator drift test by asking the patient to close his or her eyes and hold both arms out in front of the body. (page 674)
2. Examining the Chest
   1. Inspect the chest for any obvious DCAP-BTLS.
   2. Note the shape of the chest and symmetry of movement.
   3. Auscultate the lung fields, noting any abnormal lung sounds.
   4. Percuss the chest to detect any abnormalities. (page 650)

Chapter 14: Critical Thinking and Clinical Decision Making

Matching

1. A (page 697) **2.** B (page 697) **3.** A (pages 695–697) **4.** A (pages 695–697) **5.** B (pages 695–697)

6. B (pages 695–697) **7.** A (pages 695–697) **8.** B (pages 695–697) **9.** A (pages 695–697) **10.** B (pages 695–697)

Multiple Choice

1. C (page 695) **2.** B (pages 698–699) **3.** D (page 699) **4.** A (page 699) **5.** B (pages 702–704)

6. D (pages 702–703) **7.** C (pages 701–702) **8.** B (pages 695–696) **9.** A (page 698) **10.** C (page 697)

Fill-in-the-Blank

1. gathering (page 695)
2. protocols (page 696)
3. think; work (page 697)
4. concept formation (page 698)
5. critical life threats (page 698)
6. working diagnosis (page 699)
7. reading; scene (page 702)
8. trends (page 703)

Identify

1. Chief complaint: General malaise
2. Vital signs: Blood glucose is 110 mg/dL; blood pressure is 160/100 mm Hg. The ECG is normal sinus rhythm with some slight ST-segment depression, with a pulse of 92 beats/min and regular. Oxygen saturation is 97%, lungs are clear, and respirations are 18 breaths/min. Skin is warm and dry, and she is PEARRL and alert.
3. Pertinent negatives: After the intervention of the IV at TKO and the nitroglycerin paste, the blood pressure drops to 120/70 mm Hg.

Ambulance Call

1. a. The little girl in this scenario is unable to tell you her name or where she is. This tells you that she is only a V, or verbal response, using the AVPU scale. She will respond but is not oriented to person, place, or day. She is classified as having an altered mental status and is a priority patient from the start.

b. You can treat this child under implied consent. Because she has a severe life threat, you can assume the parents would want lifesaving treatment to be provided for their daughter.

c. The vital signs are suggesting that the intracranial pressure is rising. Blood pressure is high for this child's age, and the pulse and respirations are dropping. This tells the paramedics they better be moving toward a regional trauma center as fast and as safely as they can.

d. The major concern here is to keep a patent airway and provide supplemental oxygen for this patient. Because the patient is breathing under 8 breaths/min and her oxygen saturation is 88%, you know that she is hypoxic. She needs an advanced airway to be inserted as soon as possible, and she may be a candidate for RSI if she continues to have a gag reflex.

2. a. Use the highest point or even stand on a car hood (not the one that crashed) and have someone honk the horn until you get the attention of the people around you. Identify yourself and ask the crowd if anyone has medical training. Then, identify a bystander for crowd control. Also designate someone to move down the line of cars and have the person move to the road's shoulder so that emergency vehicles can get through.

b. Everything the locals have is needed! Gain use of a cell phone to communicate with dispatch. Identify yourself and the fact that you are incident command until someone arrives to take over for you. Jaws of Life will be needed and any medical helicopters and ALS units around. Try to get the number of injured patients to the dispatcher as soon as possible. When using the Jaws of Life, a fire truck should be present, so try to get the area cleared of vehicles that were not involved in the collision.

c. You will start to triage the occupants of the two vehicles. That way, when help arrives you can direct them to the most critical of patients. Always remember that your safety and the bystanders' safety come first.

True/False

1. T (page 695)   **2.** T (page 695)   **3.** F (page 696)   **4.** F (page 698)

5. F (page 698)   **6.** T (pages 699–700)   **7.** F (page 701)   **8.** T (page 702)

Short Answer

1. **a.** Read the scene: As a paramedic, you must ensure your safety and the safety of your crew, patient, and bystanders. Scene safety is first! You will also use your scene to give you clues to the patient's condition. Weather and mechanism of injury (MOI) are also something to look for when reading your scene. (page 702)

   b. Read the patient: In this phase, you decide if your patient is sick or not sick. You will observe, talk to, and touch your patient in this phase. You will also look for any life threats and take baseline vital signs. (pages 702–703)

   c. React: Always address any life threats first and handle them as they come up in your assessment. At this time, you will begin to think about your working diagnosis. (page 703)

   d. Reevaluate: Always check your interventions to make sure they are helping your patient. You will also check to make sure you have gathered all the information on your patient at this time and will watch for any other problems to pop up. (page 703)

   e. Revise the plan: Once you have begun your treatment, you may realize that your "drunken" patient is really a patient who is having a diabetic emergency. So your treatment plan will have to be revised at this time to treat your patient correctly. (pages 703–704)

   f. Review your performance: After your call is over, you should do an informal review to see where you can improve your patient care. Sometimes this can be a formal process. It always helps to talk to your team members about each call and learn something from every call you run. (page 704)

2. When gathering information, start by asking all the questions you are taught to ask. Start with the chief complaint, SAMPLE history, OPQRST, and all the mnemonics you have been taught to use. The good paramedic will be able to use open- and closed-ended questions. Frequently, there will be circumstances that will make it hard to gather a good history. Your patient may be unconscious with no family members present to answer questions. There may be a language barrier, or the patient may be unable to speak clearly or hear your questions clearly. You will need to look at the scene around you to help gather information about your patient. You will often need to look at the patient's body position or facial expression. These clues will help you gather information about your patient quickly.

When evaluating the information that you have gathered, you must begin to ask whether your information is pertinent to the patient's current condition. This is the point where you begin to formulate and enact your treatment plan for the patient. Remember, you must constantly reevaluate your patient and your treatments.

Synthesizing your information goes hand in hand with the evaluation process. This process takes you a little deeper into understanding the disease process or what organ systems have been affected by trauma. This helps you prepare for any upcoming problems the patient may face. A thinking paramedic will be able to put all the information together and treat the patient in the best way possible. (page 704)

Section 5: Airway Management
Chapter 15: Airway Management and Ventilation

Matching

Part I
(page 738)

1. B   **2.** A   **3.** A   **4.** B

Part II

1. T (pages 787–788)   **2.** C (page 824)   **3.** T (pages 787–788)   **4.** N (page 786)

5. N (pages 791–792)   **6.** T (pages 787–788)   **7.** T (pages 787–788)   **8.** C (pages 824–825)

Part III

1. E, F (pages 761–763)   **2.** B (page 754)   **3.** C (page 759)   **4.** A (pages 754–755)

5. D, E (pages 760–762)   **6.** B (page 754)   **7.** C, D (pages 759–760)   **8.** B (page 754)

Multiple Choice

1. C (page 715)   **2.** A (page 746)   **3.** D (page 754)   **4.** B (page 776)   **5.** B (page 815)

6. D (page 812)   **7.** A (page 830)   **8.** B (pages 719–720)   **9.** C (page 730)   **10.** D (page 731)

11. C (page 814)   **12.** D (pages 814–815)   **13.** C (page 815)   **14.** A (page 817)   **15.** C (page 817)

Fill-in-the-Blank

1. hypoxia; preoxygenation (page 780)

2. sniffing (page 780)

3. 30 (page 783)

4. rise; carbon dioxide; fall; oxygen (page 721)

5. stroke (pages 747–748)

6. French; whistle-tip; tonsil-tip (page 740)

7. roof; mouth (pages 744–745)

8. preoxygenate (page 780)

9. intact gag reflex; esophageal disease; caustic substance (page 820)

10. partially exposed; Mallampati (page 776)

Labeling

1. Parts of the Larynx (page 714)
  A. Hyoid bone
  B. Thyrohyoid ligament
  C. Laryngeal prominence (Adam's apple)
  D. Cricothyroid membrane
  E. Trachea
  F. Corniculate cartilage (behind larynx)
  G. Thyroid cartilage
  H. Aryteroid cartilage (behind larynx)
  I. Cricoid cartilage
2. The Child's Epiglottis and Surrounding Structures (page 718)
  A. Soft palate
  B. Tongue
  C. Epiglottis
  D. Vallecula
  E. Hyoid bone
  F. Trachea
  G. Esophagus

Identify

1. Chief complaint: Choking

2. Vital signs: Respirations are 28 breaths/min and shallow. Decreased right-side lung sounds. Pulse is 98 beats/min and regular. Blood pressure is 128/86 mm Hg. Skin is cyanotic and cool. Oxygen saturation is 88% and the patient is confused.

3. Pertinent negatives: The patient has clear lung sounds on the left, which suggest to the paramedic that the cap has gone down the right mainstem. Because there are sounds on the right, you know that only a portion of the right lung has been blocked and the cap must be stuck in the bronchial tree.

   There is nothing other than oxygen and a fast but safe ride that you can give this patient! He needs to get to surgery as soon as possible.

Complete the Patient Care Report (PCR)

Show your completed PCR to your paramedic instructor and ask for feedback on how well you recorded the case you were given.

Ambulance Calls

1. **a.** 2. The patient described in this question is showing classic signs of choking. He gives the universal distress sign for choking (clutches his neck), staggers, and falls—all without making a sound. The reason he isn't making a sound is because no air is moving past his vocal cords, which means his upper airway is completely obstructed—and that means he is going to die if you don't act immediately. (page 749)

   b. 2. The most urgent priority is to try to expel the foreign body from his airway, which means giving him manual thrusts. There is no reason to pump his stomach (answer 1) because his problem is what didn't make it into his stomach, not what did. Clearly, he is not in any shape to gargle with saltwater (answer 3); nor would it help him if he could. At the moment, he doesn't need epinephrine (answer 4), although he may need it very soon, if his airway obstruction is not relieved and he suffers cardiac arrest as a consequence. And he certainly doesn't need a sedative such as diazepam (Valium) (answer 5); he is already sedated quite enough by his hypoxemia. (What's hypoxemia? Check the glossary if you don't remember.) Both this question and the one preceding illustrate why it is not a good idea to try to grab a quick dinner while you're on duty. Caroline's Law of Dining on Duty states: If you are going to get called to a cardiac arrest during your shift, the call will come at the precise moment that the pizza you ordered comes out of the oven. (page 749)

2. **a.** 5. When your friend starts to choke on his hot dog, as evidenced by his paroxysm of violent coughing, the first thing you should do is encourage him to keep coughing (answer 5). A cough generates airflows of gale-force velocity—far more powerful than anything you could generate artificially by, for example, using manual thrusts (answer 3). Sticking your finger in the mouth of a panicky, choking person (answer 2) is a good way to lose a finger; and reaching blindly into the throat with any instrument, let alone barbecue tongs (answer 4), is as likely to produce a rather messy tonsillectomy as it is to snare a wayward hot dog. There's no point in trying to ventilate your friend artificially (answer 1); he still has some air exchange by his own efforts, and blowing into his mouth may just force the hot dog farther down his airway. (page 749)

   b. 3. When coughing fails to expel the foreign object and your friend becomes completely obstructed (as evidenced by his aphonia), that is the time to give the Heimlich maneuver (abdominal thrust) (answer 3). He is still conscious, so the finger sweep (answer 2) and head tilt (answer 1) are still inappropriate. The barbecue tongs (answer 4) are always inappropriate. And there's no point now in encouraging him to keep coughing (answer 5); if he could cough, he would. (page 749)

   c. When the Heimlich maneuver (abdominal thrust) does not work and your friend becomes unconscious, your next steps should be as follows:

   (1) Carefully position him on the ground.

   (2) Begin 30 chest compressions.

   (3) Open the airway and look in the mouth. Attempt to remove the foreign body only if you actually see it, and then attempt to ventilate the patient.

   (4) If you cannot force air past the obstruction, give chest compressions until the foreign body is expelled from the victim's airway. (page 749)

   d. When the paramedics arrive with all their gear, you finally have the means to take definitive action. At that point, you should take the following steps:

   (1) With the patient's head in the sniffing position, open the patient's mouth and insert the laryngoscope blade.

(2) Visualize the obstruction, and retrieve the object with the Magill forceps.

(3) Remove the object with the Magill forceps.

(4) Attempt to ventilate the patient. (page 750)

3. Probably this bodybuilder has a short, very muscular neck, which is a classic situation for a difficult intubation.

   a. When the cords will not come into view, ask your partner to apply the **BURP maneuver**, which is **backward, upward, rightward** pressure on the larynx. (page 783)

   b. gum elastic bougie (page 783)

   c. When you finally have the tube in and have confirmed its position, you need to secure it. Be sure to document the following on the PCR:

     (1) You visualized it going through the vocal cords.

     (2) You auscultated both lungs and the stomach.

     (3) The end-tidal waveform capnography reading.

     (4) The depth of the tube as noted by the centimeter marking at the teeth. (page 786)

4. Nasotracheal intubation does not always go smoothly, and one needs to be prepared to spend a little time getting it right.

   a. You can tell that the tip is moving toward the glottis by:

     (1) Putting your ear over the tube and hearing and feeling the movement of air through the tube. This can also be done using a stethoscope. (page 798)

     (2) Seeing misting inside the tube (from condensation of the patient's breath). (page 790)

     (3) Using a BAAM device and listening for the sounds of breathing. (page 790)

   b. When the bleeps from the monitor start getting further and further apart, it means that the patient's heart is slowing down (ie, she is developing bradycardia). (page 790)

   c. You must immediately:

     (1) Stop advancing the tube.

     (2) Attach the tube to an oxygen source and consider ventilating.

     (3) Consider using a BLS airway until the patient is no longer hypoxic. (page 790)

5. **a.** 33 minutes.

   b. The oxygen will run out before you get back.

$$\text{Duration of flow} = \frac{(\text{Tank pressure in psi} - 200 \text{ psi}) \times \text{Cylinder constant}}{\text{Flow rate in L/min}}$$

$$\frac{(800 \text{ psi} - 200 \text{ psi}) \times 0.28}{5 \text{ L/min}} = 33.6$$

Only if you let the cylinder run down all the way to zero will you manage to squeeze 40 minutes' worth of oxygen out of it, but you will have to make sure you keep up your pace as you trudge through the woods carrying the stretcher. If you are starting to drag, you'd better decrease the flow rate to the nasal cannula to about 4 L/min. And next time, make sure you take a full oxygen cylinder with you. (pages 750–751)

6. (1) Seeing the patient's chest rise and fall with each breath you give

   (2) Feeling the compliance of the patient's lungs in your own lungs

   (3) Hearing and feeling air escape through the patient's mouth during his passive exhalation (page 758)

7. **a.** To minimize gastric distention during artificial ventilation, you need to:

     (1) Reposition and reassess the airway to keep it fully open.

     (2) Observe the chest for adequate rise and fall, avoiding excessive ventilation volumes. Blow in only that volume of air needed to obtain visible chest rise.

     (3) Limit ventilation times to 1 second. (page 766)

   b. If the patient's gastric distention begins to interfere seriously with your ability to get any air into his lungs, you will have to attempt to decompress the stomach. It will not be a pleasant job. Follow the steps for insertion of an orogastric tube or nasogastric tube.

If you answered either of those "What should you do?" questions with the phrase, "Call an ambulance!" give yourself an extra point. Unless you want to spend the night doing CPR all by yourself in the movie theater, you should send someone for help at the very outset. (page 766)

8. The advantages of the pocket mask over other devices for giving artificial ventilation include:

   (1) Its immediate availability (assuming you remember to carry it in your pocket).

   (2) Its adaptability; it can be deployed with or without supplemental oxygen.

   (3) Its potential to be used as a simple face mask if the patient resumes breathing.

   (4) Its effectiveness; it is much easier to maintain a good seal with a pocket mask (and therefore deliver good volumes) than it is with a bag-mask device as a single rescuer. (page 758)

9. The patient in congestive heart failure has fluid in his alveoli, and for that reason a portion of his cardiac output is not picking up any oxygen as it passes through the lungs (a situation called shunt). It is not surprising, therefore, that his oxygen saturation is reduced.

   a. 3. The SaO_2 reading of 86% is abnormally low. A normal reading would be between 97% and 99% on room air. There's no reason to suspect an artifact (erroneous reading) because the reading is consistent with the patient's clinical presentation. (page 733)

   b. The measure you need to take immediately when you see a reading like that (or, even without a pulse oximeter, when you see a patient in respiratory distress) is to administer oxygen. (What would be the best device for administering supplemental oxygen to this patient?) (page 733)

   c. Possible sources of an erroneous reading in this patient include the following. *Students should list three of the following:*

   (1) Bright ambient light may be interfering with the reading. Cover the sensor with a towel or aluminum foil if you suspect that is the problem.

   (2) Check whether the patient is moving. The oximeter may confuse patient motion for a pulse.

   (3) The sensor may be picking up venous pulsations. Move it to a different finger or to the earlobe and recheck.

   (4) If it is cold in the ambulance and the patient's peripheral blood vessels constrict as a consequence, the resulting poor perfusion of the extremities may lead to false oximetry readings. (page 734)

10. Probably the primary indication for using an end-tidal carbon dioxide monitor is to confirm and monitor the placement of an endotracheal tube.

    a. In the case described, you can conclude that the tracheal tube is in the esophagus. If the tube were in the trachea, as it is supposed to be, the carbon dioxide concentration of the exhaled gas ought to be at least 2%, translating into a tan or yellow color on the sensor. (page 736)

    b. The action you should take right away is to deflate the cuff and remove the tracheal tube. Preoxygenate the patient before you make another attempt to intubate. (pages 735–736)

11. a. The person breathing quietly at 12 breaths/min with a tidal volume of approximately 500 mL has a minute volume as follows:

$$\text{Minute volume} = \text{Respiratory rate} \times \text{Tidal volume}$$
$$= 12 \text{ breaths/min} \times 500 \text{ mL/breath}$$
$$= 6,000 \text{ mL/min (6 L) (page 720)}$$

    b. After the crash, when paralysis of the respiratory muscles prevents the person from taking deep breaths (and respiratory distress and fear prompt him to increase his respiratory rate), the minute volume changes as follows:

$$\text{Minute volume} = \text{Respiratory rate} \times \text{Tidal volume}$$
$$= 20 \text{ breaths/min} \times 200 \text{ mL/breath}$$
$$= 4,000 \text{ mL/min (page 720)}$$

    c. The situation is much more serious than it might seem from a 33% reduction in minute volume. A person whose tidal volume is so small is doing little more than moving his dead space back and forth (do you remember what dead space is?), so there is little true alveolar ventilation and therefore little carbon dioxide removal.

    Because carbon dioxide will not be removed efficiently, the level of carbon dioxide in the blood will rise, and the arterial PCO_2 will rise, by definition a situation of hypoventilation. (page 720)

    d. As a result, the patient's pH will **fall**, reflecting the increased acidity of his blood. (page 723)

e. The resulting derangement in his acid–base balance is called a respiratory acidosis—"acidosis" because the pH is lower than normal, "respiratory" because the source of the problem is in the respiratory system (the failure to breathe deeply enough). (page 723)

f. The treatment required in the acute situation is to assist the patient's ventilations to improve the tidal volume and flush out some of that excess carbon dioxide. (page 728)

12. Next time you have to go up four flights of steps, you will probably remember to take a full E cylinder, not a half-empty D cylinder.

$$\text{Duration of flow} = \frac{(\text{Tank pressure} - 200\ \text{psi}) \times C}{\text{Flow rate}}$$

$$\frac{(900\ \text{psi} - 200\ \text{psi}) \times 0.16\ \text{L/psi}}{10\ \text{L/min}} = \text{about 11 (11.2) minutes (page 751)}$$

13. In this question about a head-injured patient, you had to review both some respiratory physiology and the pathophysiology of head injury.

a. If the patient's respiratory rate is 8 per minute and his tidal volume is 500 mL, his minute volume is calculated as follows:

$$\text{Minute Volume} = \text{Tidal volume} \times \text{Respiratory rate}$$
$$= 500\ \text{mL/breath} \times 8\ \text{breaths/min}$$
$$= 4{,}000\ \text{mL/min (4 L/min) (page 720)}$$

b. That minute volume is smaller than normal. (Normal is around 6 L/min.) (page 720)

c. Therefore, you can conclude that the patient's arterial PCO_2 will tend to **increase**, so his pH will **decrease**. The net effect will be an acid–base disorder called a **respiratory acidosis**. The way you can help correct that abnormality is to **assist the patient's ventilations. This will thereby increase his minute volume (which will blow off more carbon dioxide)**. (pages 722–723)

14. Hypercarbia occurs when a person is not moving enough air in and out of the lungs to remove the carbon dioxide being produced by metabolism.

a. Hypercarbia can be caused by:

(1) Conditions that increase CO_2 production (eg, diabetic ketoacidosis, hypoventilation from a head injury)

(2) Narcotic overdose (decreased respiratory rate)

(3) Spine injury (decreased tidal volume)

(4) Rib fracture (decreased tidal volume—because it hurts to take breaths of normal volume)

b. The way to help normalize the PCO_2 of a hypercarbic patient is to increase his minute volume; that is, assist his ventilations so that his tidal volume is larger (and perhaps give an extra breath here and there, to increase his respiratory rate as well). (page 727)

15. a. *Students will list six of the following conditions that can cause respiratory distress and inadequate ventilation:*

(1) Severe infection

(2) Trauma

(3) Brainstem insult

(4) A noxious or oxygen-poor environment

(5) Upper or lower airway obstruction

(6) Respiratory muscle impairment (eg, spinal injury)

(7) A central nervous system impairment (eg, head trauma) (page 729)

b. The treatment for hypoxia/hypoxemia is to give supplemental oxygen. That may sound obvious, but it is truly remarkable how many hypoxemic patients arrive at the emergency room by ambulance without oxygen being administered. Don't be stingy with oxygen. (page 729)

True/False

One of the most important things to remember about suctioning is that suctioning removes air as well as liquids.

1. T (pages 740–741)   **2.** T (page 741)   **3.** F (page 741)   **4.** T (page 742)

5. F (page 803)   **6.** F (page 725)   **7.** F (page 725)   **8.** T (page 725)

Short Answer

1. *Students should list four of the following:*
   a. The tongue
   b. A foreign body*
   c. Swelling (edema)
   d. Trauma to the face or neck
   e. Aspirated vomitus (pages 746–749)

2. a. Provides a secure airway
   b. Protects the airway from aspiration
   c. Enables delivery of aerosolized drugs directly into the lung for rapid absorption into the bloodstream (page 776)

3. *Students should list three of the following:*
   a. Airway control needed as a result of coma, respiratory arrest, and/or cardiac arrest
   b. Ventilatory support before impending respiratory failure
   c. Prolonged ventilator support required
   d. Absence of a gag reflex
   e. Traumatic brain injury
   f. Unresponsiveness
   g. Impending airway compromise (as in burns or trauma)
   h. Medication administration (as a last resort) (page 778)

4. a. Accidental intubation of the esophagus (page 784)
   b. This complication can be avoided by:
      (1) Positioning the patient correctly for intubation
      (2) Seeing the tube pass through the vocal cords
      (3) Checking for breath sounds over both lungs after intubation and epigastrium
      (4) Always using end-tidal waveform capnography to confirm and monitor the tube (page 784)
   c. If it does occur, intubation of the esophagus can be detected by:
      (1) Gurgling noises over the epigastrium during ventilation
      (2) Absence of breath sounds over the lungs during ventilation
      (3) Failure of the patient to "pink up" on ventilation

   Once detected, accidental intubation of the esophagus can be corrected by immediately withdrawing the tracheal tube and ventilating the patient with a bag-mask device. No further attempt to intubate the patient should be made until the patient has been reoxygenated for at least 3 minutes. (page 784)
   d. Accidental intubation of a bronchus (usually the right main bronchus) (page 784)
   e. Can be avoided by stopping as soon as the cuff passes the vocal cords (page 784)
   f. If it does occur, bronchial intubation can be detected by absence of breath sounds over one lung (usually the left).

   Once detected, bronchial intubation can be corrected by deflating the cuff, and then slowly drawing the tube back until breath sounds become audible in both lungs. Then, reinflate the cuff and mark the tube at the teeth. (page 784)

5. The principal hazard of using a neuromuscular blocker is that it converts a breathing patient with some sort of airway into a nonbreathing patient without any airway; therefore, if you are unable to intubate within 30 seconds and you have trouble maintaining an airway manually, the patient will need a surgical airway urgently. (page 811)

6. a. Minute volume = Tidal volume × Respiratory rate
         = 500 mL/breath × 12 breaths/min = 6,000 mL (6 L)

   (page 720)
   b. The minute volume will decrease if:
      (1) The tidal volume is decreased (shallow breaths, as in spinal cord injury), or
      (2) The respiratory rate slows (as in heroin overdose) (page 720)
   c. If the minute volume does decrease, the arterial blood gases will show a rise in PCO_2 because carbon dioxide will not be removed efficiently and will therefore accumulate in the blood. (Unless a person stops breathing altogether, or very nearly so, decreases in minute volume do not affect the oxygenation of the blood as dramatically.) (page 727)

7. *Students should list six of the following:*
   a. Pulmonary edema
   b. Pneumonia

    c. Drowning

    d. Chest trauma

    e. Airway obstruction

    f. Pneumothorax

    g. Inhalation of smoke or toxic fumes

    h. Respiratory arrest (page 750)

8. *Students should list four of the following:*

    a. Tachypnea (rapid breathing)

    b. Hyperpnea (abnormally deep breathing)

    c. Use of accessory muscles to breathe

    d. Nasal flaring

    e. Cyanosis (bluish tinge to the lips and nail beds)

    f. If you mentioned dyspnea—a feeling of shortness of breath—that's all right, but technically speaking, dyspnea is a symptom, not a sign. (page 729)

9. *Students should list six of the following:*

    a. No smoking!

    b. No grease.

    c. Keep out of extreme heat.

    d. Use the right valve.

    e. Keep all valves closed when not in use.

    f. Keep cylinders firmly secured.

    g. Keep your face and body to the side of the cylinder.

    h. Have the cylinder tested every 10 years. (pages 751–752)

10. *Students should list six of the following:*

    a. Airway obstruction by the tongue in an unconscious person

    b. Choking

    c. Laryngeal edema

    d. Respiratory center depression (drugs, head injury)

    e. Stroke

    f. Electric shock

    g. Primary cardiac arrest (page 758)

11. **a.** LOOK at the chest to see if it rises and falls. For a respiratory complaint, we do a visual observation.

    b. LISTEN over the nose and mouth for the sound of airflow. For a respiratory complaint, we listen (auscultate) lungs for air movement.

    c. FEEL with your cheek over the nose and mouth for the movement of air. For a respiratory complaint, we palpate the chest for equal movement. (page 729)

12. A person who has suffered respiratory arrest will need **artificial** ventilation. (page 758)

13. In artificial ventilation, the rescuer has to breathe for the patient. In assisted ventilation, by contrast, the patient is breathing spontaneously, and the rescuer simply boosts the tidal volume. (page 758)

14. With any form of artificial ventilation, the primary objective is to normalize the PCO_2 by moving air in and out of the lungs. Controlled ventilation also aims to supply oxygen to the alveoli. (pages 726–727)

15. In general, any time you have a patient whose state of oxygenation may be in jeopardy, the pulse oximeter can help you keep tabs on things. *Students should list three situations.* (pages 733–734)

    a. A patient with trauma to the chest, in whom pneumothorax or hemothorax (or both) may interfere with oxygenation

    b. A patient in pulmonary edema, who has a large shunt because of fluid in his or her alveoli

    c. A patient undergoing tracheal intubation

    d. A patient undergoing suctioning

    e. A patient having a severe asthma attack or deterioration of chronic lung disease

    f. A drowning victim

16. The spine-injured patient with weakness or partial paralysis of the respiratory muscles does not have the strength to inhale deeply. Thus, his tidal volume will be smaller than normal, so his minute volume will also **decrease**, leading to an **increase** in his arterial PCO_2. (page 725)

Fill-in-the-Table

1. Knowing when to deploy a piece of equipment is just as important as knowing how to deploy it.

	Oropharyngeal Airway	**Nasopharyngeal Airway**
Use for:	Deeply unconscious patient who has no gag reflex, especially if being ventilated by bag-mask device Bite block for intubated patient	Patient with an altered mental status
Do not use for:	Patient with intact gag reflex	Patient with trauma to the nose Suspected basilar skull fracture (blood or clear fluid draining from nose)

(pages 744–746)

2. Oxygen-Delivery Devices

Device	**Flow Rate (L/min)**	**Oxygen Delivered (%)**
Nasal cannula	1-6 L/min	24-44%
Nonrebreathing mask	15 L/min	90-100%
Bag-mask device with reservoir	15 L/min flush	Nearly 100%

(page 755)

3. Every piece of equipment in the ambulance has its indications and sometimes contraindications. You need to be aware of both.

Adjunct	**Indicated for:**	**Do not use in:**
Oropharyngeal airway	Airway maintenance in deeply unconscious, breathing patient To improve effectiveness of bag-mask ventilation	Patient who is not deeply unconscious Severe trauma in the mouth Any patient with intact gag reflex
Combitube	Cardiac arrest when it is not feasible to intubate the trachea Patient who has swallowed corrosives	Patient who is not deeply unconscious
LMA	Cardiac arrest when it is not feasible to intubate the trachea	Patient who has food in his stomach and may aspirate
Endotracheal intubation	Cardiac arrest Deep coma Absent gag reflex Imminent danger of upper airway obstruction (eg, respiratory burns)	Patients with intact gag reflex or likelihood of laryngospasm

(pages 744, 778, 814, 817)

Skill Drills

1. Nasogastric Tube Insertion in a Responsive Patient (page 767)

   Step 1: Explain the procedure to the patient, and oxygenate the patient if necessary. Ensure the patient's head is in a neutral position, and suppress the gag reflex with a topical anesthetic spray.

   Step 2: Constrict the blood vessels in the nares with a topical alpha-agonist if available.

   Step 3: Measure the tube for the correct depth of insertion (nose to ear to xiphoid process.)

   Step 4: Lubricate the tube with a water-soluble gel.

   Step 5: Advance the tube gently along the nasal floor.

   Step 6: Encourage the patient to swallow or drink to facilitate passage of the tube.

   Step 7: Advance the tube into the stomach.

   Step 8: Confirm proper placement: Auscultate over the epigastrium while injecting 30 to 50 mL of air and/or observe for gastric contents in the tube. There should be no reflux around the tube.

   Step 9: Apply suction to the tube to aspirate the gastric contents, and secure the tube in place.

Section 6: Medical
Chapter 16: Respiratory Emergencies

Matching

1. F (page 905) **2.** J (page 905) **3.** C (page 906) **4.** H (page 905) **5.** A (page 905)

6. E (page 905) **7.** B (page 904) **8.** I (page 904) **9.** G (page 904) **10.** D (page 904)

Multiple Choice

1. B (page 854) **2.** C (page 896) **3.** D (page 872) **4.** C (page 891) **5.** A (page 868)

6. C (page 867) **7.** C (page 868) **8.** B (page 861) **9.** D (page 890) **10.** A (page 887)

Fill-in-the-Blank

1. atelectasis (page 893)

2. cilia (page 856)

3. polycythemia (page 859)

4. flail chest (page 862)

5. orthopnea; cyanosis (pages 869, 881)

6. paroxysmal nocturnal dyspnea (page 863)

7. Tactile fremitus (page 873)

8. three; two (page 865)

9. end-tidal (page 876)

10. pursed-lip breathing (page 888)

Labeling

1. The Upper Airway (page 855)
   A. Frontal sinus
   B. Nasal conchae
   C. Nasal vestibule
   D. External nares
   E. Hard palate
   F. Oral cavity
   G. Tongue
   H. Mandible
   I. Hyoid bone
   J. Arytenoid cartilage
   K. Thyroid cartilage
   L. Cricoid cartilage
   M. Esophagus
   N. Trachea
   O. Internal nares
   P. Nasopharynx
   Q. Pharyngeal tonsil
   R. Entrance to auditory tube
   S. Soft palate
   T. Palatine tonsil
   U. Oropharynx
   V. Epiglottis
   W. Glottis
   X. Laryngopharynx
   Y. Vocal cord

2. Anatomy of the Larynx (page 856)
   A. Vellecula
   B. Arytenoid cartilage
   C. Thyroid cartilage
   D. Cricoid cartilage
   E. Epiglottis
   F. Cricothyroid membrane
   G. Trachea
   H. Esophagus

3. Respiratory Patterns (page 870)
   A. Cheyne-Stokes breathing
   B. Central neurogenic hyperventilation
   C. Apneustic respiration
   D. Biot respiration
   E. Ataxic respiration
   F. Agonal gasps

Identify

1. Chief complaint: Unresponsive, not breathing
2. Vital signs: Heart rate 46 beats/min; oxygen saturation 64%
3. Pertinent negatives: No chest rise and fall

Tommy was unconscious and not breathing. He had no chest rise and fall upon trying to ventilate him. He did have a faint brachial pulse, which identified that compressions were not needed yet because his airway had not been blocked for very long. Oxygen saturation was 64%, heart rate was 46 beats/min, and there were no spontaneous respirations. Blood pressure was unattainable. After the airway is opened, Tommy quickly returns to normal with 100% supplemental oxygen.

Ambulance Calls

1. **a.** Although it is possible for a 22-year-old to suffer a heart attack, it is not very likely; so, when you are confronted with a patient of that age complaining of chest pain, you need to think about other possibilities—such as a pulmonary embolism, a spontaneous pneumothorax, or, as this case turns out to be, hyperventilation syndrome. The tip-offs are the paresthesia around the mouth, the carpopedal spasm, and, incidentally, the increased respiratory rate. That last is significant because, strangely enough, often tachypnea and hyperpnea are not the most prominent features of hyperventilation syndrome, and, as in this case, other signs or symptoms may predominate. (page 853)

   b. The steps in management are:

   (1) Calm and reassure the patient.

   (2) Help her to take conscious control of her breathing by telling her to breathe as you slowly count (about one number every 5 seconds).

   (3) If the acute episode does not pass, the patient needs to be evaluated in the ED. (pages 853–854)

   c. This woman's arterial PCO_2 is probably **lower** than normal because **her minute ventilation is increased; that is, she is blowing off more carbon dioxide than usual.** (page 853)

2. The 985,500 cigarettes (give or take a few) that Mr. Koff has smoked over the past 45 years seem to be catching up with him. You can do the arithmetic yourself: 3 packs/day × 20 cigarettes/pack × 365 days/year × 45 years.

   a. Now you find him in respiratory distress. Signs of respiratory distress (increased work of breathing) include the following:

   (1) Bony retractions

   (2) Soft-tissue retractions

   (3) Nasal flaring

   (4) Tracheal tugging

   (5) Paradoxical respiratory movement

   (6) Pulsus paradoxus

   (7) Pursed-lip breathing

   (8) Grunting (page 865)

b. What needs to be done immediately on encountering a patient in this condition is to administer supplemental oxygen before you ask any more questions or proceed any further with your examination. It is also a good idea to attach the patient to a cardiac monitor and to obtain a 12-lead ECG at this stage because a hypoxic patient is a patient who is very likely to develop serious, possibly life-threatening cardiac dysrhythmias—and you would like to have some warning that they are coming. (pages 864–865)

c. In taking the history, the following are the pieces of information you would like to know (pages 871–872):

Regarding the dyspnea, the OPQRST questions are, in order:

(1) O: Onset—When it did start?

(2) P: We already have a general idea of what provoked the symptoms (probably it was being in the recumbent position for several hours); but it would be useful to know what palliates them. Is there a position in which the patient is more comfortable? Has he taken anything to try to relieve his symptoms? If so, did it help?

(3) Q: What is the quality of the dyspnea? Is it the same as his usual shortness of breath or qualitatively different?

(4) R: Radiates—Does pain go anywhere else?

(5) S: How severe is the dyspnea? Ask the patient to rate it on a 1 to 10 scale, with 1 being nothing and 10 being the worst, against his usual dyspnea, in terms of ability to do specific things (eg, walk up a flight of stairs).

(6) T: What was the timing of this particular attack? When specifically did it come on? What symptom came first, and what came next?

(7) Take a SAMPLE history.

d. In conducting the physical assessment, you are looking for some very specific signs. (pages 873–874)

Part of the Body	What I Am Looking for in Particular
General appearance	Position; level of consciousness (to indicate cerebral oxygenation); degree of distress; skin—sweating cyanosis
Vital signs	Tachycardia; abnormal respiratory rate, depth, or pattern; noisy breathing
Head	Cyanosis of mucous membranes; nasal flaring
Neck	Tracheal tugging or deviation; use of neck muscles to breathe; distended neck veins
Chest	Barred chest; abnormal or unequal breath sounds; inadequate air exchange
Abdomen	Paradoxical respiratory movement; painful, palpable liver in right upper quadrant
Extremities	Cigarette stains; clubbing of the fingers; pedal edema

e. (1) (answer b) This patient is most likely suffering from an acute decompensation of chronic obstructive pulmonary disease (COPD). (page 891)

(2) The steps of management should include the following: (page 892)

- Administer supplemental oxygen. (You should have done that already.)
- Keep the patient sitting up. (He probably won't allow you to do otherwise).
- Start IV fluids at TKO rate.
- Monitor cardiac rhythm.

If you chose to withhold oxygen from this patient, or even to give it in a stingy fashion, you flunk—because the patient may die. Go back and reread the section in your textbook on COPD. No, oxygen should not be withheld from this patient; nor should it be given in very low flows. The treatment of choice for COPD in decompensation is oxygen, oxygen, oxygen. That is the only drug that can save the patient's life.

The doctor has ordered a breathing treatment for the patient as well. You will see in a moment whether that was a judicious choice, but meanwhile it gives you an opportunity to review the pharmacology of albuterol (Proventil, Ventolin). (page 882)

3. a. The 56-year-old man with the sudden onset of dyspnea and pleuritic chest pain has most probably suffered a pulmonary embolism (answer 1), to which his chronic heart disease predisposed him. (pages 896–897)

    b. Prehospital management of the case includes the following steps:

      (1) Administer 100% supplemental oxygen.

      (2) Start an IV large bore with fluid to keep a vein open.

      (3) Monitor cardiac rhythm.

      (4) Transport without delay. (pages 896–897)

True/False

1. T (page 859)	**2.** F (page 860)	**3.** T (page 861)	**4.** T (page 869)	**5.** F (page 864)
6. T (page 868)	**7.** T (page 864)	**8.** T (page 873)	**9.** T (page 875)	**10.** T (page 875)
11. T (page 868)	**12.** F (page 895)	**13.** F (page 892)	**14.** T (page 889)	**15.** T (page 878)
16. F (page 878)	**17.** F (page 882)	**18.** F (page 883)	**19.** F (page 883)	**20.** F (pages 883–884)

Short Answer

1. Four things that can cause a pulmonary embolism are the following (pages 896–897):

    a. Fat embolism from a broken bone

    b. Amniotic fluid leakage

    c. Air embolism from trauma or IV

    d. Blood clot caused by heart rhythms or lifestyle

2. Diagnosis of a pulmonary embolism is cyanosis that does not resolve with the administration of supplemental oxygen. A good history, finding out about such events as a recent surgery or broken bone, also helps with the diagnosis. Cardiac history and your patient's current heart rhythm also help. The patient may have a history of deep vein thrombus. Also, the patient may present with an acute pain centered in the chest that does not radiate. Lung sounds are generally good with maybe a small area of diminished sounds. (pages 896–897)

3. There are no contraindications to oxygen in the prehospital setting. (page 881)

4. Not everything that wheezes is an acute asthmatic attack. Other causes of wheezing include the following:

    a. Left-sided heart failure (page 891)

    b. Smoke inhalation or inhalation of toxic fumes

    c. Chronic bronchitis (page 889)

    d. Foreign body obstruction of a major airway (eg, the patient who has a peanut lodged in a bronchus or a tumor compressing a bronchus) (page 891)

5. Signs that should alert you to the seriousness of an asthmatic attack in a child include the following (page 889):

    a. Sleepiness

    b. Pulsus paradoxus

    c. Cyanosis

    d. Hyperinflation of the chest

    e. A silent chest

Fill-in-the-Table

1. Breathing Patterns

Pattern	Comments
Agonal	**Irregular gasps** that are widely spaced; usually represent **stray neurologic impulses** in a dying patient; occasional agonal gasp not unusual in patients with no pulse; not actually considered a form of breathing
Apneustic	Characterized by a **prolonged inspiratory hold** (sometimes called "**fish** breathing"); follows damage to the **pneumotaxic center** in the brain; an ominous sign of severe **brain injury**
Ataxic	Chaotically irregular respirations that indicate **severe** brain injury or **brainstem herniation**

(continues)

Pattern	Comments
Biot respirations	Irregular pattern, **rate**, and depth of respirations, characterized by intermittent patterns of **apnea**; indicates severe brain injury or **brainstem** herniation
Bradypnea	Unusually **slow** respirations
Central neurogenic hyperventilation	Tachypneic **hyperpnea**; rapid and deep respirations caused by **increased intracranial pressure** or direct **brain injury**; drives **carbon dioxide** level down and **pH** up, resulting in respiratory **alkalosis**
Cheyne-Stokes respirations	**Crescendo-decrescendo** breathing with a period of **apnea** between cycles; not considered ominous unless grossly **exaggerated** or occurs in a patient with brain **trauma**
Cough	Forced exhalation against a closed **glottis**; an airway-clearing maneuver; also seen when **foreign substances** irritate the airways; controlled by the cough center in the brain (**Antitussive** medications work on the cough center to reduce this sometimes annoying physiologic response.)
Eupnea	**Normal** breathing
Hiccup	Spasmodic contraction of the **diaphragm**, causing short **exhalations** with a characteristic sound; sometimes seen in cases of diaphragmatic (or **phrenic**) nerve irritation from **acute myocardial infarction**, ulcer disease, or **endotracheal intubation**
Hyperpnea	Abnormally **increased** rate and depth of breathing; seen in various **neurologic** or chemical disorders, including overdose with certain drugs
Hypopnea	Abnormally **decreased** rate and depth of breathing
Kussmaul respirations	The same pattern as in **central neurogenic hyperventilation**, but caused by the body's response to metabolic **acidosis**, attempting to rid itself of blood **acetone** via the lungs; seen in diabetic **ketoacidosis**; accompanied by a **fruity** (acetone) breath odor and, usually, **cracked** and dry mouth and lips
Sighing	Periodically taking a very deep breath of about **twice** the normal volume; forces open **alveoli** that routinely close from time to time
Tachypnea	Unusually **rapid** breathing; does not reflect **depth** of respiration and does not mean a patient is **hyperventilating** (breathing too rapidly and deeply, resulting in a lowered **carbon dioxide** level); often involves moving only small volumes of air, or **hypoventilation** (much like a panting dog)
Yawning	Seems beneficial in the same manner as **sighing**

Problem Solving

1. **a.** 200 mL

   (page 860)

   b. 700 – 200 = 500

   500 – 150 = 350 mL

   (page 860)

2. **a.** 120 mL

   (page 860)

   b. 600 – 120 = 480 mL

   480 – 150 = 330 mL

   (page 860)

Complete the Patient Care Report (PCR)

Show your completed PCR to your paramedic instructor and ask for feedback on how you recorded the case you were given.

Chapter 17: Cardiovascular Emergencies

Part 1: Cardiac Function

Matching

1. D (page 1031) **2.** J (page 1029) **3.** I (page 1033) **4.** E (page 1030) **5.** B (page 1030)

6. A (page 1034) **7.** C (page 1031) **8.** F (page 1033) **9.** H (page 1032) **10.** G (page 1029)

Multiple Choice

1. B (page 911) **2.** B (page 911) **3.** D (page 918) **4.** B (page 942) **5.** C (page 935)

6. C (page 936) **7.** D (page 1011) **8.** C (page 1024) **9.** A (page 1014) **10.** B (page 1015)

Fill-in-the-Blank

1. collateral circulation (page 911)
2. aortic (pages 911–912)
3. diastole; systole (page 912)
4. pulmonary circulation (page 913)
5. arteriole; aorta (page 914)
6. Stroke volume (page 915)
7. gatekeeper (page 918)
8. depolarize (page 919)
9. absolute refractory period (page 920)
10. T wave (page 921)

Labeling

1. Coronary Arteries (page 913)
   - **A.** Superior vena cava
   - **B.** Right atrium
   - **C.** Right coronary artery in coronary sulcus
   - **D.** Inferior vena cava
   - **E.** Aorta
   - **F.** Pulmonary artery
   - **G.** Left coronary artery
   - **H.** Left atrium
   - **I.** Circumflex branch of left coronary artery
   - **J.** Anterior descending branch of left coronary artery
   - **K.** Coronary vein
   - **L.** Aorta
   - **M.** Left pulmonary artery
   - **N.** Pulmonary veins
   - **O.** Left atrium
   - **P.** Coronary sinus
   - **Q.** Left ventricle
   - **R.** Superior vena cava
   - **S.** Right pulmonary artery
   - **T.** Pulmonary veins
   - **U.** Right atrium
   - **V.** Inferior vena cava
   - **W.** Right ventricle
   - **X.** Posterior descending coronary artery in posterior interventricular groove

2. Structure of a Blood Vessel (page 915)
    A. Lumen
    B. Epithelium
    C. Tunica intima
    D. Tunica media
    E. Tunica adventitia

3. Major Arteries and Veins (page 916)
    A. Internal carotid
    B. External carotid
    C. Common carotid
    D. Subclavian
    E. Innominate
    F. Axillary
    G. Pulmonary
    H. Ascending aorta
    I. Brachial
    J. Descending aorta
    K. Common iliac
    L. Ulnar
    M. Radial
    N. Palmar arches
    O. Digital
    P. Deep femoral
    Q. Superficial femoral
    R. Popliteal
    S. Anterior tibial
    T. Posterior tibial
    U. Peroneal
    V. Dorsal pedis
    W. Arcuate
    X. Internal jugular
    Y. External jugular
    Z. Innominate
    AA. Subclavian
    BB. Axillary
    CC. Superior vena cava
    DD. Pulmonary
    EE. Cephalic
    FF. Brachial
    GG. Antecubital
    HH. Inferior vena cava
    II. Common iliac
    JJ. Volar digital
    KK. Great saphenous
    LL. Femoral
    MM. Popliteal
    NN. Anterior tibial
    OO. Peroneal
    PP. Posterior tibial
    QQ. Dorsal venous arch

True/False

1. T (pages 930–932)   **2.** F (pages 1022–1023)   **3.** F (page 1021)   **4.** T (page 1019)   **5.** T (page 1020)

6. T (pages 1017–1018)   **7.** F (page 1017)   **8.** F (page 1014)   **9.** T (page 1014)   **10.** T (page 1012)

Fill-in-the-Table

1. (page 920)

Role of Electrolytes in Cardiac Function	
Electrolyte	**Role in Cardiac Function**
Sodium (Na+)	Flows into the cell to initiate depolarization
Potassium (K+)	Flows out of the cell to initiate **repolarization** Decreased or increased levels of potassium result in the following: • *Hypokalemia* → increased myocardial irritability • *Hyperkalemia* → decreased automaticity/conduction
Calcium (Ca++)	Has a major role in the depolarization of **pacemaker** cells (maintains depolarization) and in myocardial contractility (involved in contraction of heart muscle tissue) Decreased or increased levels of calcium result in the following: • *Hypocalcemia* → decreased contractility and increased myocardial irritability • *Hypercalcemia* → increased contractility
Magnesium (Mg++)	Stabilizes the cell membrane; acts in concert with **potassium**, and opposes the actions of calcium Decreased or increased levels of magnesium result in the following: • *Hypomagnesemia* → decreased conduction • *Hypermagnesemia* → increased myocardial irritability

2. (page 921)

Components of the ECG	
ECG Representation	**Cardiac Event**
P wave	Depolarization of the atria
PR interval	Depolarization of the atria and delay at the AV junction
QRS complex	Depolarization of the ventricles
ST segment	Period between ventricular depolarization and beginning of repolarization
T wave	Repolarization of the ventricles
R-R interval	Time between two ventricular depolarizations

Part 2: Heart Rhythms and the ECG

Matching

1. G (page 938)   **2.** C (page 938)   **3.** I (page 942)   **4.** D (page 943)   **5.** B (page 947)

6. F (page 948)   **7.** E (page 951)   **8.** A (page 957)   **9.** J (page 959)   **10.** H (page 974)

Multiple Choice

1. B (page 985)   **2.** D (pages 937–939)   **3.** C (page 977)   **4.** A (page 967)   **5.** B (page 1008)

6. C (page 950)   **7.** D (page 992)   **8.** A (page 997)   **9.** B (page 1019)   **10.** A (page 944)

Fill-in-the-Blank

1. Sinus arrest (page 950)

2. supraventricular tachycardia (page 952)

3. accelerated junctional rhythm (page 955)

4. third-degree heart block (page 958)

5. Ventricular fibrillation (page 962)

6. bigeminy; trigeminy (pages 961–962)

7. Asystole (page 962)

8. delta wave (page 974)

9. unifocal; multifocal (page 960)

10. sinus bradycardia (page 947)

True/False

1. T (page 938)   **2.** F (page 942)   **3.** F (pages 945–946)   **4.** T (page 948)   **5.** F (page 953)

6. F (page 952)   **7.** T (page 957)   **8.** F (page 960)   **9.** T (page 960)   **10.** F (page 963)

Short Answer

1. Shave body hair to prevent movement and facilitate skin contact. Wipe chest area with an alcohol swab to remove oil and dead tissue. Wait for alcohol to dry before application. Always attach electrodes to the cable before applying them to the chest area. Confirm the proper placement of all electrodes. (pages 937–938)

2. The P wave is the depolarization of the SA node. P-R interval occurs while the impulse is delayed at the AV node. This delay allows the ventricles to fill fully. QRS complex is the depolarization of both the ventricles. The T wave represents the repolarization of both ventricles. (pages 942–943)

3. A 12-lead ECG "looks" at the heart as a whole. It gives views of the heart different from the standard three leads. It helps in localizing the site of injury in the heart. (page 937)

4. Always start with scene safety and standard precautions. Check for responsiveness, open the airway and assess breathing, and if the patient is not breathing, give two breaths. Check pulse and start compressions if needed. Ready your defibrillator and check the patient's rhythm. After the rhythm is established, follow advanced cardiac life support (ACLS) and/or your local protocol. (pages 1004–1006)

5. You and the medical director should practice different scenarios in preparation for having to deliver any bad news. You should role-play and discuss the correct way to break the news of the patient's death to the family. You must feel comfortable and develop strategies in advance for dealing with these situations. (pages 1010–1011)

Part 3: Putting It All Together and Practice ECG Strips

Matching

1. I (page 932)   **2.** B (page 931)   **3.** E (page 932)   **4.** F (page 926)   **5.** A (page 931)

6. C (page 927)   **7.** H (page 931)   **8.** D (page 926)   **9.** J (page 927)   **10.** G (page 926)

Labeling

1. Electrical Conduction System (page 918)
   A. Anterior internodal pathway
   B. SA node
   C. Wenckebach tract
   D. Thorel tract
   E. Right bundle branch
   F. AV node
   G. Bundle of His
   H. Bachmann bundle
   I. Left bundle branch
   J. Left posterior fascicle
   K. Left anterior fascicle
   L. Purkinje fibers

2. Schematic Representation of a 12-Lead ECG (page 970)
   A. LCx
   B. Inferior wall LV
   C. aVL

    D. aVF

    E. LAD

    F. LAD

    G. Anterior wall LV

    H. V_6

Ambulance Calls

1. a. Chief complaint: Severe chest pain

Vital signs: Skin is pale and cool, pulse is 82 beats/min and thready, respirations are 32 breaths/min and shallow, blood pressure is 90/62 mm Hg, and oxygen saturation is 91% on room air.

    b. (1) Apply high-flow supplemental oxygen.

        (2) Listen to lung sounds.

        (3) Apply heart monitor.

        (4) Start an IV medication line.

He is not a candidate for nitroglycerin at this point, but having the patient chew 325 mg of aspirin would be appropriate. (page 1015)

    c. (1) Yes

        (2) About 135 beats/min

        (3) Hidden in QRS; some are seen as inverted after QRS

        (4) Not present

        (5) Not present

        (6) 0.12 seconds

        (7) Present and upright

        (8) Junctional tachycardia (pages 955–956)

    d. Without a 12-lead ECG, you cannot confirm an AMI. However, because the patient has chest pain, AMI and chest pain protocols should be followed. (pages 928–929)

    e. Treatment should consist of ACLS guidelines. Nitrates would not be good for this patient because of the low blood pressure. (pages 1005–1006)

2. a. Chief complaint: Severe dyspnea

Vital signs: Skin is cyanotic, pulse is 102 beats/min and irregular, respirations are 60 breaths/min and labored, blood pressure is 170/94 mm Hg, lungs have crackles, and oxygen saturation is 86%.

    b. (1) Provide high-flow supplemental oxygen.

        (2) Monitor the ECG.

        (3) Obtain a 12-lead ECG if possible.

        (4) Start an IV. Keep the patient sitting up. (page 1019)

    c. Right-sided heart failure (pages 1020–1021)

    d. Provide oxygen to help bring up saturations. Follow ACLS guidelines for pulmonary edema, and drop the patient's blood pressure with a nitrate after an IV has been started. (page 1020)

3. a. Chief complaint: Syncope/low heart rate

Vital signs: Skin is cool, pulse is 44 beats/min and regular, respirations are 22 breaths/min, blood pressure is 82/40 mm Hg, and oxygen saturation is 94%. Chest pain is not measurable. Lungs are clear. (page 1002)

    b. (1) Decreased cerebral perfusion

        (2) Dysrhythmias

        (3) Increased vagal tones

        (4) Heart lesions (page 929)

    c. (1) Provide high-flow oxygen.

        (2) Start an IV. Atropine 0.5 mg can be used to speed up the heart rate. An epinephrine drip or a bolus of epinephrine can also be used. Consult your protocols. (page 1002)

    d. Transcutaneous pacing (TCP) (page 999)

4. a. Chief complaint: Feeling poorly

Vital signs: Skin is cool, pulse is 76 beats/min and irregular, blood pressure is 110/74 mm Hg, and oxygen saturation is 97%. Lungs are clear.

b. (1) No (irregular)

(2) 76 beats/min (approx.)

(3) Absent

(4) Not present

(5) n/a (P waves not present)

(6) None

(7) QRS complex is normal.

(8) Atrial fibrillation

(9) Treatment is supportive. Monitor the patient. Do not convert A-fib in the field unless absolutely necessary. (page 951)

5. a. Accelerated idioventricular rhythm (page 960)
b. Sinus dysrrhythmia (page 950)
c. Atrial flutter (page 951)
d. Second-degree heart block, Mobitz type II (page 958)
e. Polymorphic ventricular tachycardia (page 961)
f. Third-degree heart block (page 959)
g. Accelerated junctional rhythm (page 955)
h. Junctional rhythm (page 955)
i. Idioventricular rhythm (page 959)
j. Sinus arrest (page 950)
k. Multifocal atrial tachycardia (page 954)
l. Second-degree heart block, Mobitz type I (page 957)
m. Monomorphic ventricular tachycardia (page 961)
n. First-degree heart block (page 957)
o. Wandering atrial pacemaker (page 953)
p. Supraventricular tachycardia (page 952)
q. Sinus bradycardia (page 948)
r. Ventricular fibrillation (page 963)

6. a. Premature junctional complexes (page 956)
b. Premature ventricular complex (page 961)
c. Premature atrial complex (page 953)

Short Answer

1. 0.04 seconds (page 944)

2. 5 (page 944)

3. a. Altered level of consciousness (LOC) and mental status
b. Chest pain
c. Hypotension
d. Other signs of shock
e. Heart rate above 150 beats/min (page 1005)

4. Adenosine (page 1005)

5. Amiodarone (page 1005)

6. Begin transcutaneous pacing (TCP) (if the patient is conscious, consider analgesic if that can be accomplished rapidly) (page 1002)

7. a. Epinephrine 1 mg (page 1008)
b. Vasopressin 40 units (as a replacement for the first or second epinephrine, but not both) (page 1007)
c. Dopamine 2 to 10 mcg/kg/min drip (page 1001)
d. Atropine 0.5 mg (page 1001)
e. Epinephrine 2–10 µg/min (page 1001)
f. Adenosine 6 mg (page 1003)
g. Amiodarone 150 mg/10 min (page 1003)

8. Hypovolemia

Hypoxemia

Hydrogen ion (acidosis)

Hypo-/hyperkalemia

Hypoglycemia

Hypothermia

Toxins

Tamponade, cardiac

Tension pneumothorax

Thrombosis (coronary or pulmonary)

Trauma (hypovolemia) (page 1008)

Problem Solving

1. 75 mL/min × 72 mL = 5,400 mL/min (page 918)
2. 100 beats/min × 90 mL = 9,000 mL/min (page 918)
3. **a.** L
   b. R
   c. R
   d. L
   e. R
   f. R
   g. L (pages 1018–1020)
4. MAP = DBP + 1/3 (SBP − DBP) (page 1025)
   a. 116 (approx.)
   b. 151 (approx.)
   c. 105 (approx.)

ECG Practice Strips

1. Rate: 75

   Rhythm: Regular

   Significant findings: Anteroseptal AMI with elevated ST and flat ST segments in V_1 to V_4

2. Rate: 75

   Rhythm: Regular

   Significant findings: Anteroseptal AMI with elevated ST in V_1 to V_4 and Q waves in V_2 to V_4

3. Rate: 70

   Rhythm: Regular

   Significant findings: Anteroseptal AMI with lateral extension and ST changes in V_1 to V_5 and I and aVL

4. Rate: 150

   Rhythm: Regular

   Significant findings: Anteroseptal AMI with lateral extension and elevated ST in V_1 to V_5, I, and aVL and reciprocal changes in the inferior leads

5. Rate: 60

   Rhythm: Regular

   Significant findings: High lateral AMI with flat ST segments and elevation in I and aVL and reciprocal changes in the inferior leads

6. Rate: 60 to 70

   Rhythm: Regular

   Significant findings: Inferolateral AMI with ST elevation in II, III, and aVF; reciprocal changes of ST depression in I and aVL; and ST elevation in V_3 to V_6

7. Rate: 120 to 130

   Rhythm: Regular

   Significant findings: Inferolateral AMI with ST segment elevations in II, III, aVF, and V_3 to V_6 and reciprocal changes in I and aVL

8. Rate: 150

 Rhythm: Regular

 Significant findings: Inferolateral (apical) AMI with ST elevation in I, II, III, aVF, and V_2 to V_6

9. Rate: 100

 Rhythm: Regular

 Significant findings: Inferolateral (apical) AMI with ST segment elevation in I, II, III, aVF, and V_2 to V_6 and Q waves in the inferior leads

10. Rate: 75 to 100

 Rhythm: Irregular with aberrantly conducted APCs and/or JPCs

 Significant findings: Oh my! Take it piece by piece. Let's rule out wandering pacemaker and multifocal atrial tachycardia and notice the ST elevation in I, II, aVL, aVF, and V_2 to V_6

11. Rate: 90

 Rhythm: Regular

 Significant findings: Inferior wall AMI with ST elevations and Q waves in II, III, and aVF; reciprocal changes in I and aVL; and ST elevation in V_1 to V_3

12. Rate: 80

 Rhythm: Regular

 Significant findings: Inferior wall AMI with right ventricular involvement and ST elevation in II, III, and aVF; reciprocal changes in the inferior leads; and ST elevation in lead III

13. Rate: 60 or less

 Rhythm: Irregular

 Significant findings: Inferoposterior AMI with lateral extension and ST elevation in II, III, and aVF; reciprocal ST depression in aVL; and ST elevation in V_5 and V_6

14. Rate: 120

 Rhythm: Regular

 Significant findings: Inferior posterior lateral AMI with ST elevations in II, III, aVF, and V_4 to V_6: reciprocal ST depression in aVL; and ST depression in V_1 and V_2

15. Rate: 75

 Rhythm: Regular

 Significant findings: Inferior right ventricular posterior AMI with elevations in limb leads and reciprocal changes in lateral, ST elevation in III that are taller than II, and positive ST elevation in V_4R

16. Rate: 60 to 75

 Rhythm: Irregular

 Significant findings: Inferior right ventricular posterior AMI with lateral extension and ST elevation in II, III, and aVF and reciprocal changes in I, V_1, V_2, V_3, and V_4

17. Rate: 100

 Rhythm: Regular

 Significant findings: Hyperkalemia, massive peaked T waves in leads V_2 to V_4 and tall T waves in III and aVF

18. Rate: 75

 Rhythm: Regular

 Significant findings: Hyperkalemia, very tall symmetrical T waves in leads I, II, III, aVF, and V_2 to V_6

19. Rate: 60

 Rhythm: Regular

 Significant findings: Wide ventricular complex with no P waves and hyperkalemia with peaked T waves

20. Rate: Not for long

 Rhythm: Irregular

 Significant findings: Oh no! Start CPR and hope the defibrillator is handy. Get an IV or IO for some ʳ and magnesium! This patient has a long QT with frequent aberrant beats leading to torsades and ʼ fully with high-quality CPR and quick actions, back to normal sinus rhythm

Chapter 18: Neurologic Emergencies

Matching

(pages 1086–1087)

1. F **2.** E **3.** I **4.** D **5.** G

6. C **7.** H **8.** B **9.** J **10.** A

Multiple Choice

1. D (page 1043) **2.** C (page 1043) **3.** A (page 1042) **4.** B (page 1061) **5.** C (page 1050)

6. C (pages 1052–1053) **7.** A (page 1056) **8.** D (page 1057) **9.** D (page 1073) **10.** B (page 1076)

Labeling

1. Areas of the Brain (page 1041)
   A. Midbrain
   B. Pituitary gland
   C. Pons
   D. Medulla
   E. Hypothalamus
   F. Thalamus
   G. Meninges
   H. Corpus callosum
   I. Skull

2. Parts of a Neuron (page 1042)
   A. Neuron
   B. Dendrite
   C. Axon
   D. Synapse
   E. Nucleus
   F. Axon terminal

3. Pupil Responses (page 1053)

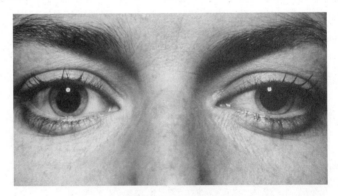

   C. Dilated

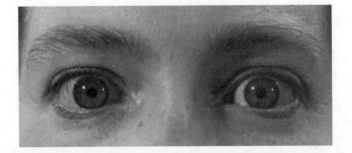

A. Normal

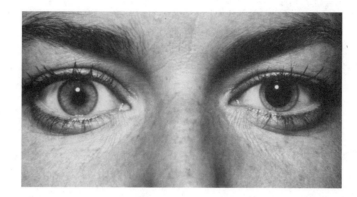

D. Unequal

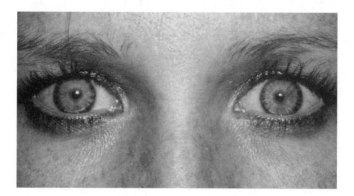

B. Constricted (pinpoint)

Fill-in-the-Blank

1. pons (page 1041)
2. neurotransmitters (page 1042)
3. endotoxin (page 1078)
4. brain; blood; cerebrospinal fluid (page 1060)
5. decrease; increase (pages 1060–1061)
6. 15; 3 (page 1051)
7. expressive aphasia (page 1054)
8. Glucose; 60–120 (page 1056)
9. ischemic; hemorrhagic (pages 1058–1059)
10. febrile; generalized; partial (page 1067)

Identify

1. Chief complaint: General weakness, visual disturbance
2. Vital signs: Blood pressure is 128/76 mm Hg, pulse is 84 beats/min, oxygen saturation is 98%
3. Pertinent negatives: No pain, vital signs in normal ranges, no facial droop, no trauma, normal temperature

   Wow, what a tricky patient! Vital signs are all pretty normal, blood pressure is 128/76 mm Hg, pulse is 84 beats/min and regular, and oxygen saturation is 98%. The patient is alert and has a patent airway. He is breathing regularly. His blood glucose level is 112 mg/dL. The vital signs are telling you that nothing is wrong, but the negatives are telling you more. The patient has no signs of trauma, infection, or illness. He is not in any pain. His symptoms and signs are very vague, and supportive care and transport are all that are required.

Complete the Patient Care Report (PCR)

Show your completed PCR to your paramedic instructor and ask for feedback on how you recorded the case you were given.

Ambulance Calls

1. This is a case of status epilepticus.
   a. When you get around to doing a rapid medical assessment, you will want to be particularly alert for the following causes of seizures (page 1067). *Students should list 10 of the following:*
      (1) abscess
      (2) alcohol
      (3) birth anomaly
      (4) brain infections (meningitis, encephalitis)
      (5) brain trauma
      (6) diabetes mellitus
      (7) febrile
      (8) idiopathic (no known cause)
      (9) inappropriate medication dosage
      (10) organic brain syndromes
      (11) recreational drug use
      (12) stroke or TIA
      (13) systemic infection
      (14) tumor
      (15) uremia (kidney failure)
   b. The steps in treating a patient in status epilepticus are (page 1069):
      (1) Protect the patient from injury.
      (2) Ensure an open airway, which may mean inserting an endotracheal tube the first chance you get once the seizure activity subsides. It will be difficult to impossible during the actual seizure. After the tube is in, insert an oropharyngeal airway as well to prevent the patient from biting down on the endotracheal tube, and secure them both in place. (Patients having seizures have been known to bite an endotracheal tube in half!)
      (3) Administer supplemental oxygen. Remember: Deaths from seizures are hypoxic deaths.
      (4) Start an IV with a large-bore catheter and secure it very well.
   c. The medication most commonly used in the field for status epilepticus is diazepam (Valium) (page 1069).
      (1) The contraindications to giving diazepam are in patients who are pregnant and those who have already taken other sedative drugs or alcohol.
      (2) The correct dosage is 5.0 mg slowly via IV given after you have measured a baseline blood pressure. Then, wait a few minutes and recheck the blood pressure. You may repeat diazepam every 10 to 15 minutes with 5.0 mg (total dosage should not exceed 30 mg). You may also use lorazepam 0.05 mg/kg (maximum dose at one time is 4 mg). Repeat the lorazepam in 10 to 15 minutes with a maximum dose of 8 mg in a 12-hour period. (page 1069)
      (3) The possible side effects of IV diazepam include hypotension and even respiratory or cardiac arrest (those more serious complications are more likely to occur in elderly patients). (You may need to refer to the *Principles of Pharmacology* chapter for more details on the drug.)

2. The person calling 9-1-1 got it right: The woman with a "possible stroke" has almost certainly had a stroke.
   a. She is most likely right-handed, remember the left side of the brain controls the right side of the body and vice versa. You know that the stroke involves the left side of her brain because the right side of her body is paralyzed. You suspect that the left side of her brain is the dominant side because the stroke has robbed her of speech. Most right-handed people are "left-dominant"; that is, the left side of the brain is the dominant side in terms of speech and several other functions. (page 1060)
   b. The steps in treating this woman are as follows (pages 1061–1063):
      (1) Protect her airway because she cannot (she has no gag reflex). Suction secretions as needed, and keep her in the stable side position.
      (2) Administer supplemental oxygen.

(3) Monitor cardiac rhythm, and be prepared to deal with dysrhythmias.

(4) Start an IV with a microdrip infusion set, and hang normal saline at a keep-open rate.

(5) Protect the paralyzed extremities. The patient should be lying on her nonparalyzed (left) side so that she can feel if she is putting too much pressure on an arm or leg.

(6) Maintain a running conversation with the patient, and provide honest reassurance.

3. Here you have a patient in coma of unknown cause.

   a. The easiest way to remember the possible causes of coma is through the mnemonic AEIOU-TIPS (page 1066):

      (1) A   Alcohol/acidosis

      (2) E   Epilepsy/electrolyte imbalance/endocrine

      (3) I   Insulin (hypoglycemia)

      (4) O   Overdose/poisoning

      (5) U   Uremia

      (6) T   Trauma

      (7) I   Infection

      (8) P   Psychosis

      (9) S   Stroke

   b. (1) Establish an airway (consider holding off intubation, though, until you can assess the results of dextrose and naloxone).

      (2) Administer supplemental oxygen.

      (3) Establish an IV in a large vein.

      (4) Give thiamine, 100 mg slowly IV.

      (5) Give 50% dextrose, 50 mL slowly IV, preferably after checking the blood glucose level.

      (6) If the patient does not wake in response to dextrose and there is reason to suspect narcotic overdose (eg, pinpoint pupils), give naloxone, 0.4 to 2 mg slowly IV; if there is no response after 2 to 3 minutes, repeat the dose.

      (7) If there is no response to two doses of naloxone, intubate the trachea.

      (8) Monitor cardiac rhythm.

Other steps include: Keep a flow sheet of neurologic and vital signs; protect the patient's eyes (tape them shut); and transport the patient to the hospital (page 1066).

True/False

  1. T (page 1043)   **2.** F (page 1043)   **3.** F (page 1045)   **4.** T (page 1071)   **5.** T (page 1045)

  6. F (page 1060)   **7.** T (page 1044)   **8.** T (page 1048)   **9.** F (page 1053)   **10.** F (page 1060)

  11. T (page 1056)   **12.** F (page 1057)   **13.** F (page 1064)   **14.** T (page 1064)   **15.** T (page 1067)

Short Answer

  1. Vocabulary

    a. Hemiparesis: Weakness of one half (side) of the body (*hemi-* + *-paresis*) (page 1054)

    b. Neuropathy: Disease of nerves (*neuro-* + *-pathy*) (page 1079)

  2. a. Seizure disorders (page 1067)

    b. Diabetes

    c. Atrial fib/blood clots

Fill-in-the-Table

1. (page 1051)

Glasgow Coma Scale		
	Adult	**Pediatric (<5 y)**
Eye opening	**4. Spontaneous** 3. Voice 2. Pain stimulation 1. None	**4. Spontaneous** **3. To shout/voice** 2. Pain stimulation 1. None
Verbal	**5. Oriented** 4. Disoriented **3. Inappropriate words** **2. Incomprehensible** 1. None	5. Cry, smile, coo, words correct for age **4. Cries, inappropriate words for age** **3. Inappropriate scream or cry** **2. Grunts** 1. None
Motor	**6. Obeys** 5. Localizes pain **4. Withdraws from pain** **3. Decorticate** 2. Decerebrate 1. None	**6. Spontaneous** 5. Localizes pain **4. Withdraws from pain** 3. Decorticate **2. Decerebrate** 1. None

2. (page 1067)

Common Causes of Seizures	
A	Abscess, alcohol
B	Birth anomaly, brain infections (meningitis, encephalitis), brain trauma
D	Diabetes mellitus
F	Fever
I	Idiopathic, inappropriate medication dosage
O	Organic brain syndromes
R	Recreational drugs
S	Stroke, systemic infection
T	Tumor, transient ischemic attack (TIA)
U	Uremia

Problem Solving

1. Cincinnati Prehospital Stroke Scale (page 1064)
   a. Smile is not equal.
   b. She has difficulty saying, "You can't teach an old dog new tricks."
   c. She closes her eyes and right arm drifts down.
2. Los Angeles Prehospital Stroke Screen (page 1064)
   a. Age is greater than 45.
   b. Smile is unequal.
   c. Blood glucose is normal.
   d. Her grip strength is not equal.
   e. Right arm drifts.
   f. Patient is not bedridden.
   g. Symptom onset is less than 24 hours.
   h. She has no history of seizures or epilepsy.

Chapter 19: Diseases of the Eyes, Ears, Nose, and Throat

Matching

1. G (page 1091)   **2.** E (page 1091)   **3.** K (page 1091)   **4.** I (page 1092)   **5.** C (page 1092)

6. O (page 1097)   **7.** H (page 1098)   **8.** A (page 1100)   **9.** D (page 1101)   **10.** F (page 1104)

11. N (page 1105)   **12.** M (page 1106)   **13.** B (page 1107)   **14.** L (page 1108)   **15.** J (page 1111)

Multiple Choice

1. B (page 1091)   **2.** B (page 1092)   **3.** C (page 1092)   **4.** A (page 1093)   **5.** C (page 1100)

6. A (page 1101)   **7.** C (pages 1102–1103)   **8.** D (page 1104)   **9.** A (page 1105)   **10.** B (page 1114)

Labeling

1. Structures of the Eye (page 1092)
   A. Iris
   B. Cornea
   C. Pupil
   D. Lens
   E. Optic nerve
   F. Retina
   G. Choroid
   H. Sclera

2. Structures of the Ear (page 1103)
   A. Pinna
   B. External auditory canal
   C. Tympanic membrane
   D. Semicircular canals
   E. Cochlea
   F. Eustachian tube
   G. Stapes
   H. Incus
   I. Malleus

Fill-in-the-Blank

1. tough; maintain (page 1091)

2. cornea; anterior; iris; pupil (page 1091)

3. conjunctiva; sclera (page 1091)

4. iris; pupil (page 1092)

5. circular; iris (page 1092)

6. **A.** auricle
   B. pinna
   C. external auditory canal
   D. tympanic membrane
   E. ossicles
   F. cochlear duct
   G. oval window
   H. cochlea
   I. organ of Corti (page 1102)

7. **A.** crown
   B. cusps

    C. pulp

    D. Dentin

    E. alveoli

    F. alveolar ridges (page 1109)

Identify

1. **a.** Chief complaint: Dizziness
   b. Vital signs: Respiratory rate of 20 breaths/min and regular, pulse of 118 beats/min and regular, blood pressure of 98/P mm Hg, and SpO_2 of 89%
   c. Pertinent negatives: Denies LOC; denies pain to head, chest, or abdomen

2. **a.** Chief complaint: Nosebleed and headache
   b. Vital signs: Respiratory rate of 20 breaths/min and regular, pulse of 108 beats/min and irregular, blood pressure of 170/102 mm Hg, and SpO_2 of 95%
   c. Pertinent negatives: No LOC, no trauma

Ambulance Calls

1. **a.** Very serious, potentially vision-threatening injury, such as a hyphema (page 1100)
   b. Lightly cover the eye, apply cold to the swelling of the orbit bone, and transport to the most appropriate ED.
   c. Prepare for a vomiting patient with an emesis basin, suction, and towel. Consider administering an antiemetic medication.

2. **a.** Flush with plenty of saline or sterile water. (page 1095)
   b. The Morgan lens (page 1095)
   c. Administer a topical anesthetic such as tetracaine (Pontocaine, Dicaine). (page 1095)

True/False

1. T (pages 1095–1096)	**2.** T (page 1093)	**3.** F (page 1092)	**4.** F (page 1092)	**5.** T (page 1105)
6. T (page 1106)	**7.** T (page 1109)	**8.** F (page 1110)	**9.** T (page 1111)	**10.** F (page 1113)

Chapter 20: Abdominal and Gastrointestinal Emergencies

Matching

1. F (page 1157) **2.** G (page 1157) **3.** J (page 1158) **4.** K (page 1158) **5.** C (page 1157)

6. L (page 1157) **7.** H (page 1157) **8.** N (page 1158) **9.** M (page 1157) **10.** O (page 1158)

11. B (page 1158) **12.** A (page 1158) **13.** E (page 1158) **14.** I (page 1157) **15.** D (page 1158)

Multiple Choice

1. A (page 1140) **2.** C (page 1142) **3.** B (page 1151) **4.** C (page 1146) **5.** A (page 1134)

6. D (page 1140) **7.** C (pages 1139–1140) **8.** B (page 1134) **9.** D (page 1143) **10.** B (page 1149)

Fill-in-the-Blank

1. liver disease; longer (page 1149)

2. alcohol; smoking; mucosal (page 1140)

3. portal; venous; absorbed (page 1126)

4. duodenum; jejunum; ileum (page 1129)

5. immunocompromised; food-borne (page 1147)

6. *Helicobacter pylori*; nonsteroidal (page 1140)

7. Biliary tract disorders (pages 1142–1143)

8. colitis (page 1145)

9. Ulcerative colitis; hereditary (page 1145)

10. early; ripe; rupture (page 1143)

Labeling

1. Abdominal Organs (page 1127)
   A. Liver
   B. Gallbladder
   C. Chyme
   D. Small intestine
   E. Pancreas

2. The Stomach (page 1126)
   A. Lower esophageal sphincter
   B. Esophagus
   C. Cardiac opening
   D. Pyloric sphincter
   E. Duodenum
   F. Mucosa
   G. Submucosa

Identify

1. a. Chief complaint: GI bleed, hypovolemic shock, and near syncope
   b. Vital signs: Skin is diaphoretic, ashen, cool; blood pressure is 88/P mm Hg by palpation; heart rate is 118 beats/min; oxygen saturation is 89%
   c. Pertinent negatives: None indicated for this call

2. a. Chief complaint: Per law enforcement, "man down"; per the patient, abdominal pain
   b. Vital signs: Skin is jaundiced, cool, dry; capillary refill is delayed; ECG shows sinus tachycardia; oxygen saturation is 94%; blood pressure is 142/86 mm Hg; blood glucose level is 110 mg/dL
   c. Pertinent negatives: Patient denies any injuries or falls (page 1148)

3. a. Chief complaint: Severe abdominal pain
  b. Vital signs: ECG shows sinus rhythm; bilateral radial pulses are equal; capillary refill is normal; pulse is 92 beats/min, strong and regular; oxygen saturation is 99%; skin color is normal, and skin is warm and diaphoretic.
  c. Pertinent negatives: No recent injury or trauma

Ambulance Calls

1. a. The patient in this ambulance call has a classical presentation of appendicitis. (page 1143)
  b. (1) Oxygen

    (2) IV access

    (3) Volume resuscitation as necessary

    (4) Dopamine for septicemia, if indicated

    (5) Pain management

    (6) Nausea management (page 1143)
  c. (1) Ondansetron (Zofran): 0.4 mg IV/IO/IM. This medication should be administered slowly over at least 2 minutes.

    (2) Diphenhydramine (Benadryl): 10 to 50 mg IV/IO/IM. This medication is typically used for allergic reactions, but also has antiemetic properties. Be cautious when using this medication because it can cause drowsiness and a drop in blood pressure.

    (3) Hydroxyzine (Vistaril): 25 to 100 mg IM. Be cautious when administering this medication to patients who have taken any medication that has CNS depressive effects. Hydroxyzine (Vistaril) increases the CNS depressive effects of other medications.

    (4) Promethazine (Phenergan): 12.5 to 25 mg IV/IO/IM. Be cautious when administering this medication to patients who have taken any medication that has CNS effects. Like hydroxyzine, promethazine increases the CNS depressive effects of other medications. Also, this medication tends to cause a marked burning sensation during injection. Administer slowly. (page 1136)

2. a. Aggressive management of ABCs, including positioning to facilitate drainage and suctioning
  b. Rapid but safe immediate transport
  c. Fluid resuscitation
  d. Pharmacologic management of nausea and vomiting (pages 1139–1140)

3. a. Standard precautions
  b. Effective positioning of the patient to ensure adequate drainage of material out of the mouth
  c. Oxygen
  d. Listen to lung sounds.
  e. Administer hypotonic solution.
  f. Consider pain management.
  g. Consider medications that may be administered for management of nausea. (pages 1136–1137)

True/False

1. T (page 1136) **2.** F (pages 1145–1146) **3.** T (page 1148) **4.** T (pages 1140–1141) **5.** F (page 1134)

6. F (page 1134) **7.** T (page 1138) **8.** T (page 1133) **9.** T (page 1131) **10.** F (page 1135)

Short Answer

1. a. Borborygmi: A bowel sound characterized by increased activity within the bowel. (page 1133)
  b. Cholecystitis: Inflammation of the gallbladder. (page 1142)
  c. Scaphoid: A concave shape of the abdomen. This can be caused by evisceration. (page 1132)
  d. Mallory-Weiss syndrome: A condition in which the junction between the esophagus and the stomach tears. (page 1140)

2. a. Somatic (page 1134)
  b. Appendicitis (page 1143)
  c. Irritation or injury to tissue, causing activation of peripheral nerve tracts (page 1143)

3. a. Somatic (page 1134)
   b. Usually occurs after an initial visceral, parietal, or somatic pain; similar nerve tracts cause "pain" in distant locations. (page 1134)

Fill-in-the-Table

1. The patient's symptoms and signs can tell you a lot.

Finding	What the Finding Tells Me
Coffee-ground vomitus	The patient is bleeding into his stomach, and the blood has been there for some time.
Severe bradycardia	This may be a cardiac and not an abdominal problem.
Melena	The patient is bleeding somewhere in the GI tract.
Tenting of the skin	The patient is severely dehydrated.
Patient very still	The patient probably has peritonitis.
Pulsatile abdominal mass	Likely abdominal aortic aneurysm.
Rigid abdomen	Almost certainly peritonitis.

Chapter 21: Genitourinary and Renal Emergencies

Matching

1. D (page 1180)   **2.** A (page 1181)   **3.** K (page 1180)   **4.** E (page 1181)

5. B (page 1180)   **6.** H (page 1182)   **7.** J (page 1182)   **8.** F (page 1182)

9. G (page 1181)   **10.** I (page 1181)   **11.** C (page 1182)   **12.** M (page 1182)

13. N (page 1181)   **14.** P (page 1181)   **15.** L (page 1182)   **16.** O (page 1181)

Multiple Choice

1. C (page 1161)   **2.** B (page 1161)   **3.** B (page 1162)   **4.** D (page 1162)   **5.** A (page 1170)

6. B (page 1170)   **7.** C (page 1170)   **8.** A (page 1176)   **9.** B (page 1176)   **10.** A (page 1170)

Labeling

1. The Urinary System (page 1161, Figure 1A)
 A. Kidneys
 B. Ureters
 C. Urinary bladder
 D. Urethra

2. The Glomerulus of the Kidneys (page 1163, Figure 3)
 A. Afferent arteriole
 B. Efferent arteriole
 C. Glomerular capillaries
 D. Bowman's capsule
 E. *Glomerular filtration*
 F. Peritubular capillary
 G. *Tubular reabsorption*
 H. *Tubular secretion*
 I. Renal tubule

3. Male Urethra (page 1165, Figure 4A)
 A. Prostate gland
 B. Cowper's gland
 C. External urethral orifice
 D. Ureter
 E. Smooth muscle
 F. Ureteral opening
 G. Internal sphincter
 H. Pelvic diaphragm
 I. External sphincter
 J. Urethra

4. Female Urethra (page 1165, Figure 4B)
 A. Ureter
 B. Smooth muscle
 C. Ureteral opening
 D. Internal sphincter
 E. Pelvic diaphragm
 F. External sphincter
 G. Urethra
 H. External urethral orifice

Fill-in-the-Blank

1. comfort; support (page 1170)

2. cortex; medulla; pelvis (page 1162)

3. Antidiuretic hormone (page 1163)
4. hemodialysis (page 1174)
5. Disequilibrium syndrome (page 1175)
6. priapism (page 1176)
7. Visceral (page 1168)
8. cardiovascular (page 1173)
9. pain relief (page 1170)
10. lower (page 1169)

Identify

1. Chief complaint: Kidney stone, abdominal pain
2. Vital signs: Patient is alert; oxygen saturation is 98%; respirations are 18 breaths/min; lungs are clear; pulse is 96 beats/min; ECG shows sinus tachycardia; blood pressure is 148/94 mm Hg; blood glucose is 96 mg/dL; skin is warm and dry; temperature is 98.6°F. Pain is 10/10.
3. Pertinent negatives: History of salty food and drink with no water consumption.

Ambulance Calls

1. The first patient with abdominal pain you had to deal with is a 42-year-old man.
   a. Poorly localized, crampy pain associated with other autonomic symptoms such as nausea is called visceral pain. (page 1168)
   b. Visceral pain usually comes about because of obstruction of a hollow organ that causes distention and stretching of the organ wall.
   c. Visceral pain is characteristic of conditions such as bowel obstruction, urethral stone, or a stone in the bile duct. (page 1168)
2. E. The patient is in obvious pain and is probably bleeding internally as a result of the trauma to the kidneys. Remember that kidneys are solid organs that filter the blood, and they hold a lot of blood. Rapid assessment of this patient with IV support should be established quickly, and then he should be transported to the regional trauma center.
3. With more and more patients being maintained on chronic renal dialysis, paramedics will find themselves dealing more often with the problems to which dialysis patients are prone.
   a. (1) The patient who feels too weak to move and has peaked T waves on his ECG is most likely suffering from hyperkalemia. (page 1176)
      (2) The steps to take are as follows:
      (a) Continue to monitor his cardiac rhythm carefully.
      (b) Give atropine, 0.5 mg rapidly IV.
      (c) Contact medical control to consider giving 10 mL of a 10% solution of calcium chloride IV.
      (d) Make sure the calcium chloride has infused. Then contact medical control to consider giving 50 mEq of sodium bicarbonate IV.
      (e) Transport without delay, and be prepared to deal with a cardiac arrest en route. (page 1175)
   b. (1) The patient with paroxysmal nocturnal dyspnea has classic signs of congestive heart failure (CHF).
      (2) The treatment is very nearly the same as for any other patient with CHF except that some of the medications usually given in CHF will probably be useless.
      (a) Keep the patient sitting up with legs dangling.
      (b) Administer supplemental oxygen with positive pressure.
      (c) You can try giving sublingual nitroglycerin, but it is not likely to work. Don't bother trying diuretics such as furosemide (Lasix)—for certain, those will not work.
      (d) Transport without delay, and notify the receiving facility that the patient will require emergency dialysis, which is the treatment of choice for his CHF. If the receiving hospital does not have the means to carry out an emergency dialysis, ED physicians may have to perform a phlebotomy of about a unit of blood as a temporizing measure until the patient can reach a dialysis unit.
   c. (1) The patient with a post-dialysis headache and signs of increased intracranial pressure is probably suffering from disequilibrium syndrome as a consequence of the dialysis, but at that point you cannot rule out a subdural hematoma. (page 1175)

(2) You have to assume the worst and treat him for a possible subdural hematoma (page 1176):

    (a) Ensure an open airway, be alert for vomiting, and be prepared to suction.

    (b) Administer supplemental oxygen.

    (c) Monitor cardiac rhythm.

    (d) Transport without delay.

True/False

1. T (page 1172)   **2.** F (page 1176)   **3.** F (page 1161)   **4.** T (page 1162)   **5.** F (page 1162)

6. F (page 1163)   **7.** T (page 1164)   **8.** T (page 1165)   **9.** F (page 1169)   **10.** T (page 1170)

Short Answer

1. **a.** Oliguria: Very small urine output. (page 1181)

    b. Diuretics: Chemicals that increase urinary output. (page 1181)

    c. Paraphimosis: A condition that results when the foreskin is retracted over the glans penis and becomes entrapped; constriction of the glans causes it to swell even further. (page 1181)

    d. Azotemia: Increased nitrogenous wastes in blood. (page 1180)

    e. Phimosis: Inability to retract the distal foreskin over the glans penis. (page 1182)

    f. Renal pyramids: Parallel cone-shaped bundles of urine-collecting tubules that are located in the medulla of the kidneys. (page 1182)

    g. Efferent arteriole: the structure in the kidney where blood drains from the glomerulus. (page 1181)

    h. Uremia: The presence of excessive amounts of urea and other waste products in the blood. (page 1182)

2. We scarcely ever think about our kidneys and how much they do for us. It is only when the kidneys are not working that we can begin to appreciate all the things they do when they are functioning. And when they aren't working, a whole lot of other things start going wrong as well. Thus, patients with chronic renal failure, who have dialysis treatments, are much more vulnerable to the following conditions (page 1176):

    a. Congestive heart failure

    b. Hypertension

    c. Myocardial infarction

    d. Pericardial tamponade

    e. Uremic pericarditis

Fill-in-the-Table

(page 1171, Table 2)

Signs and Symptoms of Acute Renal Failure	
Type of Acute Renal Failure	**Signs and Symptoms**
Prerenal	Hypotension Tachycardia Dizziness Thirst
Intrarenal	Flank pain Joint pain Oliguria Hypertension Headache Confusion Seizure
Postrenal	Pain in lower flank, abdomen, groin, and genitalia Oliguria Distended bladder Hematuria Peripheral edema

Chapter 22: Gynecologic Emergencies

Matching

1. H (page 1208)　　**2.** C (page 1207)　　**3.** E (page 1208)　　**4.** J (page 1208)

5. A (page 1208)　　**6.** K (page 1208)　　**7.** N (page 1207)　　**8.** F (page 1208)

9. I (page 1208)　　**10.** B (page 1208)　　**11.** P (page 1207)　　**12.** O (page 1207)

13. G (page 1208)　　**14.** M (page 1208)　　**15.** L (page 1208)　　**16.** D (page 1208)

Multiple Choice

1. C (page 1186)　　**2.** D (page 1187)　　**3.** B (page 1193)　　**4.** B (page 1199)　　**5.** B (page 1194)

6. A (page 1197)　　**7.** C (page 1201)　　**8.** D (page 1193)　　**9.** B (page 1201)　　**10.** C (page 1202)

Labeling

1. Anatomy of the Female Reproductive System (page 1186, Figure 2)
   - **A.** Ovary
   - **B.** Uterine (fallopian) tube
   - **C.** Uterus
   - **D.** Cervix
   - **E.** Vagina
2. Reproductive System With an Ectopic Pregnancy (page 1193, Figure 7)
   - **A.** Fallopian tube
   - **B.** Fertilized oocyte
   - **C.** Uterus
   - **D.** Ovary

Fill-in-the-Blank

1. vagina (page 1185)
2. imperforate hymen (page 1186)
3. amenorrhea (page 1188)
4. Menopause (page 1187)
5. endometriosis (pages 1194–1195)
6. Toxic shock syndrome (page 1198)
7. Scene safety (page 1188)
8. modesty (page 1188)
9. Cullen; Grey Turner (page 1191)
10. Ketamine hydrochloride (page 1202)

Identify

1. Chief complaint: Severe abdominal pain.
2. Vital signs: Patient is alert, pain is 10 out of 10, pulse is 120 beats/min, blood pressure is 140/92 mm Hg, ECG shows sinus tachycardia, oxygen saturation is 99%, respirations are 20 breaths/min, the temperature is 102°F, pupils are PEARRL, and lungs are clear.
3. Pertinent negatives: No illness, no trauma, and no sexual activity yet.

   What is wrong? She has a ruptured ovarian cyst. The lack of sexual activity takes out the possibility of ectopic pregnancy. She is running a fever with no other signs of illness. The rebound tenderness, abdominal distention, and vomiting tell you that this patient is very ill, and because of her vitals, she appears to be in septic shock. Rapid transport is indicated for her.

Ambulance Calls

1. **a.** The 25-year-old woman with fever and abdominal pain that began not long after her menstrual period is most likely suffering from pelvic inflammatory disease (answer E).
   b. (1) The prehospital management is gentle transport.
   (2) In view of the woman's tachycardia, fever, and history of vomiting, she is probably dehydrated, so it is a good idea to start an IV with crystalloid and run in fluids en route to the hospital. (page 1196)
2. **a.** The 24-year-old woman who thinks she has appendicitis more likely has an embryo developing in her right fallopian tube—that is, an ectopic pregnancy (answer D). Crampy, unilateral abdominal pain followed by spotting and signs of early shock are good enough evidence to start treatment.
   b. Treatment is as follows:
   (1) Administer supplemental oxygen.
   (2) Keep the patient recumbent.
   (3) Start a large-bore IV and run it wide open (or per local protocol).
   (4) Allow nothing by mouth.
   (5) Keep the patient warm.
   (6) Monitor ECG rhythm and vital signs.
   (7) Notify the receiving hospital.
   (8) Transport without delay. (page 1194)

True/False

1. F (page 1200)   **2.** F (page 1201)   **3.** T (page 1201)   **4.** F (page 1200)   **5.** T (page 1201)
6. T (page 1196)   **7.** F (page 1192)   **8.** F (page 1194)   **9.** F (page 1190)   **10.** T (page 1191)

Short Answer

1. In evaluating a woman of childbearing age whose chief complaint is abdominal pain, you will want to know more about the pain, about associated symptoms, and about her obstetric and gynecologic history. (pages 1190–1191)
   a. Among the questions you should ask in taking the history, therefore, are the following. (*Students should list 10.*)
   (1) What provoked the pain? Does anything make it better or worse?
   (2) What is the pain like? Sharp? Dull? Crampy?
   (3) Where is the pain? Does it radiate anywhere else?
   (4) How severe is the pain? Compare it to prior experience, or rate it on a scale of 1 to 10.
   (5) When did the pain start? What is the temporal relationship between the pain and other symptoms?
   (6) What other symptoms has the patient noticed? Has she had vaginal bleeding? Has she felt dizzy or faint?
   (7) When was her last normal menstrual period?
   (8) Has she noticed any breast tenderness, urinary frequency, or nausea in the mornings?
   (9) What, if any, type of contraception does the woman use?
   (10) Has she had any vaginal discharge?
   (11) How many previous pregnancies has she had? How many deliveries?
   (12) What gynecologic problems has she had in the past?
   (13) Does she have any serious underlying illnesses?
   b. On physical examination, what you want to look for in particular are the following:
   (1) Signs of hypovolemia, such as anxiety, restlessness, cold and clammy skin, tachycardia, and postural changes in vital signs
   (2) Signs of peritoneal irritation, such as abdominal rigidity or pain on movement (page 1191)
2. Risk factors for ectopic pregnancy include the following. (*Students should list two.*)
   a. Previous pelvic inflammatory disease
   b. Previous ectopic pregnancy
   c. Using an IUD for contraception
   d. Previous pelvic surgery (page 1190)

3. The classic triad of findings in ectopic pregnancy is:
a. Abdominal pain
b. Amenorrhea
c. Vaginal bleeding (page 1194)

Fill-in-the-Table

1. (pages 1202–1203, Table 1)

Drugs Used to Facilitate Rape				
Drug	Street Names	General Information	Symptoms	Emergency Care
Gammahy-droxybutyric acid (GHB)	• Georgia home boy • Grievous bodily harm • Easy lay • G • Scoop • Liquid X • Soap • Salty water	• Depressant, has amnestic properties • Common in the "rave" and "club" crowds • Colorless liquid • Generally has a salty taste that is disguised when mixed in a drink	• Range from sleepiness, loss of muscle tone, and forgetfulness to seizurelike activity • Respirations and pulse rate are depressed, progressing to a comalike state that generally lasts about 2 hours	• **Supportive** • **Make sure that adequate ventilator support is initiated for patients in respiratory depression.** • **There is no current antidote for GHB ingestion.** • **Naloxone (Narcan) and flumazenil (Romazicon, a benzodiazepine agonist) are of no benefit.**
Ketamine hydrochloride (Ketalar, Ketaset)	• Special K • Vitamin K • Cat Valium • Fort Dodge	• Predominantly marketed in the United States as a veterinary anesthetic • Blocks pain pathways • May produce frightening hallucinations • Available in liquid and powder form • Can be inhaled, injected, or mixed into a drink	• Loss of coordination • Muscle rigidity • Slurred speech • Catatonic or blank stare • General sense of numbness • Can lead to aggressive and violent behavior and an exaggerated sense of strength • Symptoms of overdose include nausea and vomiting, hypertension, and respiratory impairment leading to oxygen deprivation of the brain	• **There is no field antidote for ketamine; transport**
Ecstasy (methylene-dioxy methamphetamine [MDMA])	• XTC • Adam • X • Lover's speed • Clarity	• Methamphetamine derivative with hallucinogenic properties; a stimulant • Generally sold in capsule or tablet form • Can also be found as a powder • Can be injected, inhaled, ingested, or smoked • Regular users may use paraphernalia such a rubber or candy pacifiers to ease the effects • A surgical mask smeared with Vicks VapoRub is also a clue of ecstasy use because the vapors reportedly increase the effect of the "rush" • Logos that may appear on tablets: Superman, Batman, Nike, Mercedes, Rolls Royce	• Similar to those of cocaine and speed • Rapid pulse rate • Rapid increase of body temperature, often to deadly levels • Anxiety • Hypertension • Blurred vision • Mental confusion • Nausea • Excessive sweating, leading to dangerous levels of dehydration • Rapid eye movement • Tremors • Bruxism (teeth clenching)	• **Transport**

(continues)

Drugs Used to Facilitate Rape				
Drug	Street Names	General Information	Symptoms	Emergency Care
Rohypnol	• Roofies • Roof • Roachies • Rocha • Mexican Valium	• Has sedative-hypnotic, amnestic, and anesthetic properties • Legally marketed outside the United States by Roche Pharmaceuticals as a sedative and Preoperative anesthetic • White, scored tablet, with the word "Roche" appearing on one side • Tablet can be dissolved in a drink, where it is undetectable • Roche Pharmaceuticals has recently added a color base of royal blue to the tablet; if the drug is mixed with a drink, the color will appear	• Impaired judgment and motor skills • Loss of social inhibition • Decreased blood pressure • Drowsiness • Dizziness • Confusion • Memory loss (victim will have no memory of approximately the last 15 to 20 minutes before blacking out)	• Supportive, with possible administration of flumazenil • Naloxone (Narcan) has no effect on Rohypnol, but its administration may be considered because Rohypnol is sometimes used in conjunction with other drugs

Chapter 23: Endocrine Emergencies

Matching

1. E (page 1242)   **2.** B (page 1240)   **3.** D (page 1240)   **4.** G (page 1240)   **5.** F (page 1240)

6. A (page 1241)   **7.** C (page 1241)   **8.** N (page 1240)   **9.** K (page 1241)   **10.** M (page 1241)

11. I (page 1241)   **12.** H (page 1241)   **13.** L (page 1240)   **14.** J (page 1242)   **15.** R (page 1242)

16. P (page 1242)   **17.** O (page 1242)   **18.** Q (page 1241)

Multiple Choice

1. D (page 1212)   **2.** C (page 1212)   **3.** B (page 1216)   **4.** A (page 1213)   **5.** B (page 1214)

6. B (page 1216)   **7.** B (page 1216)   **8.** B (page 1224)   **9.** C (page 1224)   **10.** A (page 1229)

11. D (page 1230)   **12.** A (page 1232)   **13.** D (page 1233)   **14.** A (page 1234)   **15.** D (page 1235)

Labeling

1. Six-Step Process of the Body's Fight-or-Flight Response to Stress (page 1214, Figure 2)
   - **A.** Stress
   - **B.** SNS stimulation
   - **C.** Adrenal medulla response (epinephrine into the bloodstream)
   - **D.** Stress stops
   - **E.** Decreased SNS stimulation
   - **F.** Decreased epinephrine release into the bloodstream
2. The Kidney (page 1216, Figure 4)
   - **A.** Adrenal cortex
   - **B.** Adrenal medulla
3. The Endocrine System (page 1213, Figure 1)
   - **A.** Pineal
   - **B.** Pituitary
   - **C.** Thyroid
   - **D.** Adrenal
   - **E.** Stomach
   - **F.** Pancreas
   - **G.** Duodenum
   - **H.** Ovary
   - **I.** Testis
4. Diabetic Emergencies (page 1228, Figure 11)
   - **A.** Diabetic coma
   - **B.** DKA or HHNC
   - **C.** Hyperglycemia
   - **D.** Normoglycemia
   - **E.** Hypoglycemia
   - **F.** Insulin shock

Fill-in-the-Blank

1. Myxedema coma (page 1235)
2. thyroid-stimulating hormone (page 1233)
3. salt; potassium (page 1216)

4. rehydration; electrolyte (page 1229)

5. head injury; seizures; traumatic (page 1226)

6. fatigue; seizure; thirst (page 1224)

7. type 1; type 2; medical management (page 1223)

8. islets of Langerhans; glucagon; insulin (page 1216)

9. master gland; endocrine (page 1213)

10. feedback systems; negative feedback (page 1212)

Identify

1. **a.** Chief complaint: Altered level of consciousness
   b. Vital signs: Respirations are shallow and the patient is diaphoretic. Her pulse is 118 beats/min, and her blood pressure is 104/88 mm Hg.
   c. Pertinent negatives: Her blood glucose is 48 mg/dL.
   d. Nature of the endocrine disorder: Type 1 diabetes

   This patient is likely suffering from hypoglycemia. Hypoglycemia in the insulin-dependent diabetic is often the result of having taken too much insulin, too little food, or both. Her vital signs include a mental status of being unresponsive, a tachycardia of 118 beats/min, and a blood pressure of 104/88 mm Hg. Her skin indicates diaphoresis as well as blood glucose of 48 mg/dL. (page 1228)

2. **a.** Chief complaint: Shortness of breath
   b. Vital signs: Rapid breathing. He is tachycardic with a blood pressure of 108/82 mm Hg.
   c. Pertinent negatives: Fruity, acetone breath. He has poor skin turgor, and skin tenting is present.
   d. Nature of the endocrine disorder: Diabetic patient

   This patient is likely suffering from diabetic ketoacidosis. His vital signs include tachycardia, an elevated blood glucose level, and blood pressure of 108/82 mm Hg. Oxygen saturation is 95%. (page 1228)

3. **a.** Chief complaint: Altered mental status
   b. Vital signs: Bradycardic and hypotensive
   c. Pertinent negatives: Can't get a pulse oximeter reading. She is acting confused and psychotic.
   d. Nature of the endocrine disorder: Myxedema coma

   This patient is most likely suffering from myxedema coma. The hallmarks of myxedema coma include elderly females, behavioral/mental status changes, and hypothermia. (page 1234)

Ambulance Calls

1. The patient is showing characteristic signs of diabetic ketoacidosis (DKA). The steps of prehospital management are aimed primarily at stabilizing vital functions and restoring fluid. The goals of prehospital treatment are as follows:
   a. Begin rehydration and to correct the patient's electrolyte and acid–base abnormalities.
   b. Follow the procedure for any comatose patient with regard to airway maintenance and supplemental oxygen. Be particularly alert for vomiting and have suction ready.
   c. Start an IV and infuse up to 1 L of normal saline over the first half hour or at the rate suggested by protocol or online medical control.
   d. Monitor cardiac rhythm. Changes in serum potassium caused by DKA can lead to marked myocardial instability. (page 1229)

2. **a.** Probable underlying illness(es): Hypoglycemia (page 1229)
   b. Probable underlying illness(es): Diabetes
   c. The patient has an insulin pump. Consider the possibility of a malfunctioning pump, the patient not loading the insulin into the pump, or, regardless of the pump, the patient disregarding proper dietary control. Any of these scenarios could cause a hypoglycemic emergency. (page 1229)
   d. Don't let a known diagnosis of diabetes prevent you from considering other causes of coma. Diabetics are not immune to head injury, stroke, seizures, meningitis, and other traumatic injuries or conditions. Keep an open mind and assess the patient thoroughly. (page 1226)

Complete the Patient Care Report (PCR)

Show your completed PCR to your paramedic instructor and ask for feedback on how well you recorded the case you were given.

True/False

1. T (page 1229)   **2.** F (page 1216)   **3.** T (page 1234)   **4.** T (page 1233)   **5.** F (page 1232)

6. T (page 1229)   **7.** F (page 1228)   **8.** T (page 1224)   **9.** T (page 1224)   **10.** F (page 1223)

11. T (page 1212)   **12.** T (page 1216)   **13.** F (page 1216)   **14.** T (page 1214)   **15.** F (page 1212)

Short Answer

1. Vocabulary:
   a. Hypoglycemia: Hypoglycemia in the insulin-dependent diabetic is often the result of having taken too much insulin, too little food, or both. Unlike other tissues, which can usually metabolize fat or protein in addition to sugar, the tissues of the central nervous system (including the brain) depend entirely on glucose as their source of energy. If the level of glucose in the blood drops dramatically, the brain is literally starved. (page 1226)
   b. Diabetic ketoacidosis (DKA): A life-threatening condition, DKA occurs when certain acids accumulate in the body because insulin is not available. Patients who suffer from this condition tend to be young—teenagers and young adults. In DKA, the deficiency of insulin prevents cells from taking up the extra sugar. (page 1228)
   c. Thyrotoxicosis: A toxic condition caused by excessive levels of circulating thyroid hormone. Although hyperthyroidism can cause thyrotoxicosis in some patients, the two conditions are not identical. Thyrotoxicosis may also be caused by goiters, autoimmune disease (Graves disease—the most common cause of hyperthyroidism), and thyroid cancer. Graves disease, which has an incidence of 1.4 cases per 1,000 persons, has a chronic course with remissions and relapses. If left untreated, it may be fatal. (page 1234)
   d. Insulin: Hormone produced by the pancreas that is vital to the control of the body's metabolism and blood glucose level. Insulin causes sugar, fatty acids, and amino acids to be taken up and metabolized by cells. (page 1216)
   e. Cushing syndrome: A condition caused by an excess of cortisol production by the adrenal glands or by excessive use of cortisol or other similar steroid (glucocorticoid) hormones. (page 1233)
2. Treatment:
   a. Myxedema coma: Administer supplemental oxygen therapy to correct hypoxia. Intubation and ventilation are indicated for patients with diminished respiratory drive or those who are unable to protect their airway; these measures help prevent respiratory failure. Monitor the patient's cardiac status. Hypotension may respond to crystalloid therapy, and a vasopressive agent, such as dopamine (Intropin), may be necessary. Administer 25 to 50 g of D_{50} (or D_{10} if your system has switched to that concentration) if glucose levels are less than 60 mg/dL. Treat hypothermia with passive rewarming methods because aggressive rewarming may lead to vasodilation and hypotension. Hemodynamically unstable patients with profound hypothermia, however, require active rewarming. Avoid sedatives, narcotics, and anesthetics because of the delayed metabolism. (page 1235)
   b. Adrenal insufficiency: The treatment for adrenal insufficiency is based on the clinical presentation and findings, and is geared toward maintaining the airway, breathing, and circulation until arrival at the emergency department. Other goals of prehospital treatment are to begin rehydration of the patient and to correct the electrolyte and acid–base abnormalities. Follow the procedure for a patient with altered mental status or comatose patient with regard to airway maintenance and supplemental oxygen. Be alert for vomiting and have suction ready. Start an IV and infuse up to 1 L of 0.9% normal saline. If the patient is hypotensive, administer a normal saline bolus at 20 mL/kg. Remember, a patient in adrenal insufficiency may be severely dehydrated, often to the point of shock, and needs volume. Check the patient's glucose level. Administer 25 to 50 g of D_{50} (or D_{10} if your system has switched to that concentration) to correct the hypoglycemia. D_5NS is the preferred IV fluid, but a second IV administering D_5W can be used to maintain the patient's blood glucose level. Monitor cardiac rhythm because changes in serum electrolytes can lead to marked myocardial instability. (page 1232)
   c. Hyperosmolar nonketotic coma: The treatment of hyperosmolar nonketotic coma/hyperosmolar hyperglycemic nonketotic coma (HONK/HHNC) in the prehospital setting follows the pathway for dehydration and altered mental status. Airway management is the top priority. The comatose patient is often unable to maintain and protect his or her airway. For this reason, endotracheal intubation may be indicated and should be completed as early as possible. Cervical spine immobilization should be used for all unresponsive patients found down, unless witnesses can validate that no fall occurred. Large-bore IV access should be gained as soon as possible, but

do not delay transfer while initiating the IV. If necessary, obtain IV access during the transport to the emergency department. Also obtain a blood glucose level as soon as possible. After you have initiated the IV, a bolus of 500 mL 0.9% normal saline is appropriate for nearly all adults who are clinically dehydrated. In patients with a history of congestive heart failure and/or renal insufficiency, a 250-mL bolus may be a more appropriate starting point. Fluid deficits in HONK/HHNC patients may amount to 10 L or more. These patients may receive 1 to 2 L in the first hour. If the glucose level is less than 60 to 80 mg/dL, then (depending on your local protocols) administer 25 g of D_{50} as soon as possible. (page 1230)

Fill-in-the-Table

1. (page 1216, Table 2)

Hormones of the Adrenal Glands		
Hormone	Class	Functions
Cortisol	Glucocorticoid	**Increases metabolic rate, using fat and protein for energy**
Aldosterone	Mineralocorticoid	**Reabsorbs sodium and water from the urine, and excretes excess potassium**
Epinephrine/norepinephrine	Catecholamines	**Stimulates sympathetic nervous system receptors**

2. (page 1217, Table 4)

Hormones of the Gonads	
Hormone	Functions
Male	
Testosterone	**Main sex hormone in males** **Responsible for secondary sex characteristics: voice deepening, growth of facial hair, muscle development, pubic hair, growth spurts**
Female	
Estrogen	**Responsible for secondary sex characteristics: breast growth, fat accumulation at hips and thighs, pubic hair, growth spurts** **Involved in pregnancy** **Regulation of menstrual cycle**
Progesterone	**Involved in pregnancy** **Regulation of menstrual cycle** **Prevents maturation of additional egg during ovulation**

Chapter 24: Hematologic Emergencies

Matching

1. E (page 1262)   2. J (page 1262)   3. H (page 1261)   4. A (page 1261)   5. I (page 1262)
6. B (page 1261)   7. G (page 1261)   8. N (page 1262)   9. D (page 1262)   10. F (page 1262)
11. C (page 1261)   12. L (page 1261)   13. M (page 1261)   14. K (page 1261)

Multiple Choice

1. D (page 1250)   2. D (page 1250)   3. D (page 1257)   4. A (page 1246)   5. C (page 1248)
6. C (page 1248)   7. C (page 1255)   8. A (page 1256)   9. B (page 1257)   10. D (page 1245)

Labeling

1. Major Organs for Producing and Regulating the Blood (page 1246, Figure 1)
   A. Liver
   B. Bone marrow
   C. Spleen
2. Normal RBCs and Sickle Cells (page 1252, Figure 3)
   A. Sickle cell
   B. Normal red blood cell

Fill-in-the-Blank

1. life (page 1245)
2. hematopoietic (page 1245)
3. blood cells; blood cells; platelets; plasma (page 1245)
4. stem cells (page 1245)
5. RBC count; hemoglobin level; hematocrit (page 1245)
6. Platelets (page 1245)
7. Hodgkin lymphoma (page 1255)
8. sickle cell disease (page 1252)
9. fatigue; headaches; dyspnea (page 1254)
10. pain (page 1255)

Identify

1. a. Chief complaint: Extreme weakness, fatigue, and dyspnea
   b. Vital signs: Pulse is 86 beats/min, slightly irregular, and difficult to palpate; blood pressure is 92/P. Skin is pale, warm, and dry. PEARRL. Oxygen saturation is 91% on ambient air.
   c. Pertinent negatives: Denies chest pain or shortness of breath
2. a. Chief complaint: Altered mental status and possible syncope
   b. Vital signs: His radial pulses are equal bilaterally and regular at 86 beats/min. Skin is jaundiced, but cool and dry. PEARRL. Oxygen saturation is 98% on a nonrebreathing face mask.
   c. Pertinent negatives: Not sure if he lost consciousness
3. a. Chief complaint: Acute sickle cell crisis, pain
   b. Vital signs: Pulse is 112 beats/min, regular; pulse oximetry is 91%; blood pressure is 148/96 mm Hg. Skin is warm/moist. PEARRL.
   c. Pertinent negatives: None

Ambulance Calls

1. a. The patient who develops back pain, diaphoresis, cyanosis, and so forth during a blood transfusion is showing signs of a hemolytic reaction to the blood transfusion. (answer 2)
   b. To deal with this situation, you need to do the following:

(1) Stop the transfusion! Disconnect the blood bag and save it for testing.

(2) Keep the IV line open with D5W (if signs of shock develop, switch to normal saline or Ringer's).

(3) Draw a blood sample (red-top tube) from a site other than the IV line.

(4) Notify the physician and request orders.

2. a. Polycythemia is characterized by an overabundance or overproduction of RBCs. The increased RBC production can be caused by a rare disorder. It can arise in persons who live in high-altitude areas for long periods. The disease causes hyperviscosity of the circulatory system. (page 1256)

   b. Prehospital care largely consists of supportive care and transporting the patient to an appropriate facility. Administer oxygen as needed. Establish IV access for possible pharmacologic interventions for pain or pulse rate control as appropriate. (page 1256)

True/False

1. F (page 1245)   **2.** F (page 1245)   **3.** T (page 1247)   **4.** F (page 1248)   **5.** T (page 1255)

6. F (page 1256)   **7.** T (page 1257)   **8.** T (page 1250)   **9.** F (page 1251)   **10.** T (page 1252)

Short Answer

1. Blood disorders present differently from other typical injuries and diseases encountered by paramedics. Students should provide some of the following common findings: (page 1250)

   a. Level of consciousness: Alterations in level of consciousness, ranging from excitability, agitation, and combativeness, to complete unresponsiveness

   b. Skin: Uncontrolled bleeding, unexplained or chronic bruising, itching, pallor, or jaundice (yellow appearance usually indicates liver problems)

   c. Visual disturbances: Visual disturbances, including blurred vision, decreased vision, and seeing black or grey spots

   d. Gastrointestinal system: Epistaxis (bloody nose), bleeding or infected gums, ulcers, melena (blood in the stool), and liver failure (causes jaundice)

   e. Skeletal system: Chronic joint or bone pain or rigidity

   f. Cardiovascular system: Dyspnea, tachycardia, chest pain, hemoptysis (coughing up blood)

   g. Genitourinary system: Hematuria, menorrhagia, chronic or recurring infections

2. a. Leukemia (pages 1254–1255)

   (1) Depends on stage.

   (2) Patient complains of fatigue, headaches, or dyspnea.

   (3) Fever, bone pain, and diaphoresis may be present.

   (4) Vital signs may indicate shock.

   (5) Treatment includes ABCs, IV access, and pain medications.

   b. Hemophilia (page 1257)

   (1) Acute and chronic bleeding may occur at any time.

   (2) Spontaneous intracranial bleeding may be common.

   (3) Be supportive of patients and families.

   (4) Treatment includes ABCs and IV access; treat all bleeding as potentially life threatening.

   c. Polycythemia (page 1256)

   (1) Characterized by an overabundance of RBCs.

   (2) Can be caused by a rare disorder or congestive heart failure.

   (3) Can lead to strokes, TIAs, headaches, and abdominal pain.

   (4) Found more frequently in adults older than 50 years.

   (5) Clinical treatment includes phlebotomy.

   (6) Provide and support ABCs.

3. Provide definitions for the following terms: (pages 1261–1262)

   a. Leukopenia: A reduction in the number of WBCs

   b. Polycythemia: An overabundance or overproduction of RBCs, WBCs, and platelets

c. ABO system: The commonly used blood classification system, based on the antigens present or absent in the blood

d. Reticuloendothelial system: The system in the body that is primarily used to defend against infection

e. Pruritus: Unspecified itching

f. Hematocrit: The proportion of RBCs in total blood volume

g. Melena: Blood in the stool

Fill-in-the-Table

(page 1248, Table 3)

Blood Types			
Blood Type	**ABO Antigens**	**ABO Antibodies**	**Acceptable Blood Donor Types**
A	A	Anti-B	**A, O**
B	B	Anti-A	**B, O**
AB	A, B	None	**A, B, AB, O**
O	None	Anti-A Anti-B	**O**

Chapter 25: Immunologic Emergencies

Matching

Part I
(page 1265)

1. D	**2.** C	**3.** B	**4.** A	**5.** C
6. A	**7.** D	**8.** C	**9.** A	**10.** D

Part II
(page 1284)

1. E	**2.** F	**3.** K	**4.** L	**5.** A
6. B	**7.** G	**8.** H	**9.** N	**10.** M
11. C	**12.** D	**13.** J	**14.** I	

Multiple Choice

1. D (page 1266)	**2.** D (page 1277)	**3.** B (page 1277)	**4.** D (page 1277)
5. D (page 1277)	**6.** D (page 1277)	**7.** C (page 1271)	**8.** A (pages 1275–1277)
9. C (page 1269)	**10.** C (page 1269)	**11.** B (page1278)	**12.** D (page 1279)

Labeling

(page 1270, Figure 1)

1. Antigen is introduced into the body
2. Mast cells
3. Bronchospasm, vasoconstriction
4. Decreased cardiac output, decreased coronary flow
5. Vasodilation, leakiness
6. Pruritus, urticaria, edema

Fill-in-the-Blank

1. acquired immunity (page 1270)
2. natural immunity (page 1270)
3. antigen (page 1265)
4. Mast (page 1269)
5. Histamine (page 1273)
6. noisy upper (page 1271)
7. life-threatening (page 1271)
8. epinephrine (page 1273)
9. glucagon (page 1277)
10. oxygen (page 1276)

Identify

1. a. Chief complaint: This patient is probably having a localized reaction at the sting site.
   b. Vital signs: She is conscious and alert. Her skin color is normal, warm, and dry. Capillary refill is normal. Her oxygen saturation is 99%, and her blood pressure is 112/68 mm Hg. PEARRL.
   c. Pertinent negatives: No history and no medications

2. **a.** Chief complaint: This call isn't all that unusual, especially given the recent concerns about Lyme disease. This patient does not appear to be suffering from an allergic reaction.

   b. Vital signs: He is conscious and alert. His pulse is 110 beats/min and regular. Blood pressure is 142/84 mm Hg. PEARRL. Skin is warm and moist.

   c. Pertinent negatives: No previous medical history, no allergies, and no known drug allergies

3. **a.** Chief complaint: This call seems as though it is a true medical emergency. Many schools and classrooms are "peanut free." The patient presents as being in noticeable distress with a well-documented allergy history. In fact, many restaurants and bakeries have signs posted regarding their ingredients and the use of products that may cause allergic reaction.

   b. Vital signs: Pulse is 124 beats/min, oxygen saturation is 90%, and blood pressure is 90/62 mm Hg.

   c. Pertinent negatives: None indicated

4. **a.** Chief complaint: It's not uncommon to respond to a reported allergic reaction only to find the patient in minor distress. What is not really clear is the time the patient had dinner. If several hours have gone by, it is less likely that the cause is an allergic reaction. A number of ailments can cause GI upset, including bacterial and viral infections.

   b. Vital signs: Pulse is 124 beats/min, oxygen saturation is 90%, and blood pressure is 112/62 mm Hg.

   c. Pertinent negatives: None

5. **a.** Chief complaint: Once again, this is a true life-threatening emergency. It's hard to predict how babies and small children may present after receiving routine inoculations. The vast majority of small patients suffer only from minor systemic complications, such as pain and fever. But, occasionally you may encounter a child who has had serious side effects. Remember to maintain ABCs aggressively, contact medical control immediately, and follow pediatric advanced life support as well as local protocols.

   b. Vital signs: Apical pulse is 190 beats/min. Capillary refill is delayed, and skin is mottled.

   c. Pertinent negatives: None

Ambulance Calls

1. This 58-year-old man who was stung by a bee is also suffering an anaphylactic reaction, but because of his age, you have to be a little more careful in giving epinephrine.

   a. The treatment is as follows:

   (1) Ensure that his airway stays patent.

   (2) Administer high-flow oxygen by nonrebreathing mask.

   (3) Monitor the ECG throughout (keep the beep tone on).

   (4) Start a large-bore IV and run in 1 to 2 L of normal saline (according to your protocols).

   (5) Give epinephrine as follows: First, dilute 0.1 mg (0.1 mL) of 1:1,000 epinephrine in 10 mL of normal saline and inject it over 10 minutes. If the patient is not getting better by then, start an infusion at 1 μg per minute.

   (6) Remove the stinger from the patient's skin, taking care not to squeeze it. If the site is on an extremity, put a constricting band (venous tourniquet) proximal to the sting site.

   (7) Consult medical command regarding any other pharmacotherapy (eg, Benadryl, Solu-Medrol).

   (8) Transport without delay. (pages 1274–1277)

   b. Epinephrine, if given in excessive dosage, may cause the following:

   (1) Extreme hypertension

   (2) Angina

   (3) Cardiac dysrhythmias and consequent palpitations (page 1276)

2. If you want to stay out of trouble on your night off, stay out of restaurants! The lady at the next table is suffering an anaphylactic reaction, apparently to something she ate. The sensation of a lump in the throat along with her squeaky voice indicates that she is in a lot of trouble. The steps in management are as follows:

   a. Administer albuterol by a metered-dose inhaler to try to buy some time for the airway (but have your cricothyrotomy kit on hand just in case).

   b. Administer supplemental oxygen by nasal cannula.

   c. Start transport.

   d. Start an IV with a large-bore cannula.

   e. Give diphenhydramine, 50 mg IM.

   f. If you are a long way from the hospital, call for an order for a corticosteroid. (pages 1275–1277)

3. a. Patient A is showing classic signs of choking, and a shot of epinephrine will not help him a bit (except during resuscitation from the cardiac arrest he will surely suffer if you failed to diagnose his choking and act immediately).

   b. Patient B is simply experiencing a very common untoward side effect of erythromycin, about which he should have been warned by the doctor who prescribed the drug.

   c. Patient C is suffering an anaphylactic reaction.

4. Use the following steps to manage patient C:

   a. Ensure that his airway stays open. It is already in jeopardy, judging from his hoarse voice. If you are unable to quickly insert an endotracheal tube, administer 4 to 10 sprays of 1:1,000 racemic epinephrine, and get moving at once to the hospital, administering oxygen throughout.

   b. Monitor the ECG; cardiac dysrhythmias are likely.

   c. Start at least one large-bore IV and run it wide open.

   d. Unfortunately, in this particular case, you probably cannot use a constricting band to isolate the injection site because what the patient in all probability got was two shots of penicillin, one in each buttock, so there's no place to put the venous tourniquet!

   e. You can, however, give epinephrine, 0.1 mg/kg of a 1:10,000 solution (about 5–10 mL) slowly IV. (page 1277)

5. The contraindications to diphenhydramine are the following:

   a. Asthma or chronic obstructive pulmonary disease

   b. Glaucoma

   c. Prostate problems

   d. Ulcer disease

   e. Pregnancy (answer found in *Emergency Medications* chapter)

6. The dosage in this case would be 25 to 50 mg slowly IV. (page 1277)

7. Possible side effects of diphenhydramine include the following:

   a. Drowsiness

   b. Blurring of vision

   c. Dry mouth

   d. Wheezing

   e. Difficulty urinating (page 555, *Emergency Medications* chapter)

Before you finish with this case, be sure to have a word with your medical director so that he or she can have a word with the people at the Public Health Clinic. They need to be reminded that it just won't do to give a patient a parenteral antibiotic (or any other drug) and whip him out the door! Patients should remain under observation for at least 30 minutes after any parenteral medication.

Complete the PCR

Show the completed PCR to your instructor to obtain feedback on your completion of the form.

True/False

1. F (page 1275)	**2.** T (page 1280)	**3.** F (page 1276)	**4.** F (page 1276)	**5.** F (page 1275)
6. T (page 1266)	**7.** T (pages 1268–1269)	**8.** F (page 1269)	**9.** T (page 1270)	**10.** F (page 1275)

Short Answer

1. Effects produced by mast-cell mediators include the following:

   a. Systemic vasodilatation

   b. Pulmonary vasoconstriction

   c. Increased capillary permeability

   d. Bronchoconstriction

   e. Decreased coronary blood flow

   f. Decreased strength and contractility of the heart

   g. Increased tendency for dysrhythmias (pages 1269–1270)

2. Agents commonly responsible for anaphylactic reactions fall into three general categories: drugs, foods, and insect venoms. *Students should provide four of the following:*

DRUGS

Penicillin

Blood products

Horse serum products

Vaccines

Biologic extracts

FOODS

Nuts

Seafood

Egg whites

Fruits

INSECT VENOMS

Hymenoptera

Fire ants (page 1266)

Fill-in-the-Table

(page 1266)

Common Substances Associated With Anaphylaxis	
Antigen	**Examples**
Drugs	Antibiotics, colloids, enzymes, vaccines
Insect stings	Bees, yellow jackets, hornets, wasps, fire ants
Foods	Peanuts, fish, shellfish, egg, soy, milk
Latex	Gloves and other medical materials
Animals	Long-haired animals, horse serum, gamma globins

Problem Solving

1. 0.3 to 0.5 mL from a 1 mg/1 mL ampule
2. 1:10,000 epi, 0.1 mg per 10 mL, 3 to 5 mL
3. 30 gtt/minute
4. Benadryl (diphenhydramine), 25 to 50 mg (page 1277)

Chapter 26: Infectious Diseases

Matching

1. E (page 1320)   2. G (page 1320)   3. C (page 1321)   4. A (page 1322)

5. D (page 1321)   6. F (page 1321)   7. H (page 1321)   8. B (page 1320)

9. I (page 1290)   10. J (page 1320)   11. P (page 1322)   12. M (page 1322)

13. K (page 1322)   14. N (page 1322)   15. O (page 1322)   16. L (page 1322)

Multiple Choice

1. D (page 1288)   2. D (pages 1289–1290)   3. B (page 1295)   4. B (page 1293)   5. D (page 1290)

6. A (page 1292)   7. C (page 1294)   8. A (page 1290)   9. C (pages 1297, 1314–1316)   10. D (page 1303)

Fill-in-the-Blank

1. Standard precautions (page 1294)
2. handwashing (page 1290)
3. postexposure medical follow-up (page 1292)
4. Pathogenic organisms (page 1295)
5. Epstein-Barr; oral (page 1300)
6. Lyme disease (page 1309)
7. sexually transmitted diseases (page 1301)
8. viral hepatitis (page 1303)
9. patient; patient; unwashed (page 1311)
10. mammals; birds (page 1317)

Identify

1. a. Chief complaint: Flu-like symptoms that include fever, chills, dry cough.
   b. Vital signs: Respiratory rate is 20 breaths/min, oxygen saturation on ambient air is 95%, pulse is 106 beats/min and regular, and blood pressure is 128/68 mm Hg. Skin is warm and dry. Victim is conscious and alert.
   c. Pertinent negatives: He denies medication, allergies to medication, international travel, other previous medical history.
2. a. Chief complaint: Infestation of lice; patient is contaminated.
   b. Vital signs: Pulse is 88 beats/min and irregular, blood pressure is 98/72 mm Hg, oxygen saturation is 88%. He is tachypneic, and there is obvious skin tenting and delayed capillary refill.
   c. Pertinent negatives: He believes he just put on the "new clothing" this morning and rarely "needs" to take any pills.
3. a. Chief complaint: ALS interfacility transport.
   b. Vital signs: Blood pressure as noted on the noninvasive monitor is 98/54 mm Hg with a heart rate of 62 beats/min.
   c. Pertinent negatives: Patient is "stable" for transport.

Ambulance Calls

1. a. The college student with fever, headache, stiff neck, vomiting, and an altered state of consciousness is showing typical signs of meningitis, perhaps meningococcal.
   b. The paramedic can minimize the risk of catching meningitis from a patient by wearing a mask and washing hands after the call. (page 1297)
2. a. The 54-year-old man with hemoptysis, night sweats, and weight loss most probably has tuberculosis.
   b. The paramedic can minimize the risk of contracting the infection by wearing a mask and washing hands after the call. It is also a good idea to check, about 2 months later, for evidence of new tuberculosis infection by having a tuberculin test. (pages 1297–1298)

3. a. The IV drug user with yellow eyes, dark urine, anorexia, and distaste for cigarettes has classic symptoms of viral hepatitis, most likely type B in view of his IV drug use.

　b. To minimize the risk of contracting hepatitis from a patient, the paramedic should employ standard precautions, including barrier protection (mask, gown, gloves) and extreme caution with needles and IV equipment. And, as always, wash your hands after the call. (page 1304)

4. a. The 8-year-old with fever, sore throat, and swelling around the angles of the jaw most likely has mumps.

　b. The paramedic's best protection against mumps is immunization, either by mumps vaccine or by having had the illness as a child. The paramedic who is not immunized should wear a mask. And whether immune or not, wash your hands after the call. (page 1315)

5. a. The young woman with fever, conjunctivitis, and spots has measles.

　b. If you haven't had measles, or immunization against measles, you can try wearing a mask, but in all likelihood you will soon have measles, too—just wait about 10 days. Be sure to wash your hands after the call, though, to minimize the risk to the next patients you treat. (page 1314)

6. a. (1) PPE

　　(2) Leather gloves

　　(3) Face/eye protection

　　(4) Turn-out gear (pages 1290–1291)

　b. (1) Completely restock the vehicle and replace any used items.

　　(2) Clean/cold-sterilize any reusable patient contact equipment.

　　(3) Clean all exposed surfaces with disinfectant. (page 1305)

　c. Assuming that appropriate PPE was used during and after the call, there is nothing that really needs to be completed. A soiled uniform/gear should be changed and laundered at work. If there was an exposure, your designated infection control officer should be contacted. Disinfect the vehicle and its equipment. Use commercially available antiviral and antibacterial cleansers, or use a 10% bleach and water mixture. (page 1305)

Complete the PCR

Show the completed PCR to your instructor to obtain feedback on your completion of the form.

True/False

1. F (page 1306)　　**2.** T (page 1306)　　**3.** F (page 1306)　　**4.** T (page 1297)　　**5.** T (page 1305)

6. F (page 1306)　　**7.** F (page 1306)　　**8.** T (page 1301)　　**9.** F (page 1301)　　**10.** F (page 1302)

Short Answer

1. a. Students will check the illnesses they had as a child or up to this point.

　b. What did your personal immunization survey turn up? Are you completely covered, or do you have some deficits to make up?

　c. If your last tetanus booster was more than 10 years ago, or if you never had an immunization against hepatitis B, make sure you remedy those and any other immunization deficits before you take your first call. And be sure to wash your hands.

2. There is no need to be panicky about AIDS or any other communicable disease if you know something about it.

　a. There are only three ways in which AIDS can be transmitted from one person to another:

　　(1) Through sexual contact

　　(2) Through contaminated blood or blood products (eg, being stuck by a needle used on an HIV-positive person)

　　(3) From mother to fetus (page 1306)

　b. To minimize the risk of acquiring HIV from a patient, follow standard precautions. *Students should provide three of the following:*

　　(1) Wear disposable gloves for any contact with a patient's blood or body fluids.

　　(2) Use additional barrier protection (eg, mask, eye wear) for any procedures that may involve the splashing of blood or body fluids.

　　(3) Wash your hands after every patient contact!

　　(4) Handle needles and other sharp instruments with extreme caution. Do not recap needles. Dispose of them safely. (pages 1290–1292)

Fill-in-the-Table

1. (page 1290, Table 1)

Recommended Personal Protective Equipment for Preventing Transmission of Human Immunodeficiency Virus and Hepatitis B Virus in the Prehospital Setting				
Task or Activity	**Disposable Gloves**	**Gown**	**Mask**	**Protective Eyewear**
Bleeding control with spurting blood	Yes	**Yes**	Yes	**Yes**
Bleeding control with minimal bleeding	Yes	**No**	No	**No**
Emergency childbirth	Yes	**Yes**	Yes, if splashing is likely	**Yes, if splashing is likely**
Drawing blood samples	Not required by CDC, but recommended for EMS	**No**	No	**No**
Inserting an IV line	Yes	**No**	No	**No**
Endotracheal intubation, laryngeal mask airway, Combitube use	Yes	**No**	No, unless splashing is likely*	**No, unless splashing is likely***
Oral/nasal suctioning, manually cleaning airway	Yes	**No**	No, unless splashing is likely*	**No, unless splashing is likely***
Handling and cleaning instruments with microbial contamination	Yes	**No, unless soiling is likely**	No	**No**
Measuring blood pressure	No	**No**	No	**No**
Measuring temperature	No	**No**	No	**No**
Giving an injection	Not required by CDC, but recommended for EMS	**No**	No	**No**
*Splashing is often likely, so use personal protective equipment accordingly				

2. (pages 1297–1298, 1301, 1303–1307, 1314–1315, and 1317)

Disease	Mode(s) of Transmission	Protective Measures
AIDS	**Sexual contact; injection of contaminated blood products; from mother to fetus**	**Gloves, mask; extreme caution with needles and sharp objects; handwashing**
Hepatitis type A	**Fecal-oral; from ingesting contaminated water, shellfish, etc.**	**Handwashing**
Hepatitis type B	**Sexual contact; injection of contaminated blood products**	**Immunization; gloves, mask; extreme caution with needles and sharp objects; handwashing**
Meningitis	**Droplet spread**	**Mask; handwashing**
Mumps	**Saliva; droplet spread**	**Immunization; mask; handwashing**
Syphilis	**Sexual contact; infected saliva; semen, vaginal discharge**	**Gloves; handwashing**
Tuberculosis	**Droplet spread**	**Mask; handwashing**
MRSA	**Spread of material from infected wound**	**Handwashing; gloves; excellent cleaning routines**
SARS	**Direct contact with respiratory secretions or body fluids**	**Handwashing; mask that has been fit-tested (ie, N-95 or P100)**

Chapter 27: Toxicology

Matching

1. J (page 1365)   **2.** N (page 1365)   **3.** A (page 1364)   **4.** I (page 1366)   **5.** O (page 1366)

6. L (page 1365)   **7.** B (page 1365)   **8.** G (page 1365)   **9.** D (page 1364)   **10.** M (page 1365)

11. C (page 1365)   **12.** H (page 1365)   **13.** F (page 1364)   **14.** E (page 1366)   **15.** K (page 1366)

16. R (page 1365)   **17.** P (page 1364)   **18.** T (page 1365)   **19.** S (page 1365)   **20.** Q (page 1364)

Multiple Choice

1. C (pages 1325–1326)   **2.** D (page 1327)   **3.** A (page 1334)   **4.** D (pages 1334–1335)

5. D (page 1335)   **6.** D (page 1331)   **7.** B (page 1326)   **8.** B (page 1331)

9. C (page 1337)   **10.** D (pages 1342–1343)   **11.** D (page 1344)   **12.** D (page 1346)

13. A (page 1353)   **14.** C (page 1355)   **15.** C (pages 1358–1360)

Fill-in-the-Blank

1. poison; drug (page 1325)

2. Toxicologic emergencies; intentional; unintentional (pages 1325–1326)

3. ingestion; inhalation; injection; absorption (page 1327)

4. Toxidromes; clinical umbrella (page 1329)

5. malnutrition; traumatic brain (page 1334)

6. respiratory depression; gag reflex (page 1335)

7. heroin; lucid (page 1342)

8. hypotension; rhythm disturbances; breathing (page 1342)

9. poisoning; oxygen; hemoglobin (page 1345)

10. water-soluble; alkalis; alkalis (page 1348)

11. sildenafil (Viagra); nitrites; hypotension (page 1349)

12. inhalant; hearing; function; equilibrium; death (page 1351)

13. gastric irritation; pain; toxicity; death (page 1352)

14. tricyclic antidepressants; tachycardia; depression; seizures (page 1353)

15. monoamine oxidase; hyperkalemia; acidosis (page 1354)

Identify

1. a. Sedative and hypnotic
   b. *Students should provide two of the following:*
      (1) Phenobarbital
      (2) Diazepam
      (3) Thiopental (page 1340)

2. a. Stimulant
   b. *Students should provide two of the following:*
      (1) Amphetamine
      (2) Methamphetamine
      (3) Cocaine
      (4) Diet aids
      (5) Nasal decongestants (pages 1336–1337)

3. The odor of alcohol (ETOH) along with nausea and vomiting may indicate ingestion and poisoning as a result of alcohol. (pages 1333–1335)

4. A seizing patient could be consistent with amphetamines, camphor, cocaine, strychnine, arsenic, carbon monoxide (CO), or petroleum poisoning. Depressed respirations could be indicative of narcotic, alcohol, propoxyphene, CO, or barbiturate poisoning. The type of poisoning common to both symptoms might lead you to be suspicious of a narcotic overdose. CO does not seem likely because family members are able to give you some information and there is no indication that they are suffering any of the same symptoms. (pages 1329–1330)

Ambulance Calls

1. a. Questions to ask the patient's neighbors include the following:

(1) When was the patient last seen?

(2) Do you have any idea of what happened to him?

(3) Is he known to suffer any chronic illnesses (eg, diabetes, epilepsy)?

(4) Has he been injured recently?

(5) Did he complain of any symptoms when last seen?

(6) Is he a known abuser of drugs or alcohol?

b. Besides the neighbors, the scene itself may provide valuable information about what may have caused the patient's coma. Check out:

(1) The bathroom and bedroom for medicine bottles or drug paraphernalia

(2) The kitchen for insulin in the refrigerator or other medications on the counter

(3) The living room and the kitchen trash for empty liquor bottles

c. The patient's physical findings can also help narrow down the possible causes of his coma:

Finding	Possible Diagnostic Significance
Cold, dry skin	Overdose of alcohol or sedative drugs
Pulse = 110 beats/min, thready	Hypovolemia, hypoglycemia, overdose of barbiturates
Blood pressure = 90/60 mm Hg	Hypovolemia
Respirations = 12 breaths/min and shallow	Overdose with sedative drugs
Pupils dilated and not reactive to light	Cerebral anoxia, barbiturate overdose, certain eye drops
Breath smells of alcohol (ETOH)	Patient ingested alcohol
Left arm is cold and blue	Patient has been lying for a long time on his left arm

(pages 1329–1330)

d. The patient is best described as comatose, answer (3).

e. The steps in managing this patient are as follows:

(1) Ensure that the scene is safe for access and egress.

(2) Maintain the airway. (Check whether the patient accepts an OPA.)

(3) Ensure the breathing is adequate. (Assist with a bag-mask device.)

(4) Ensure that circulation is not compromised (eg, by hypoperfusion or dysrhythmia).

(5) Administer high-concentration supplemental oxygen to achieve saturation levels of 95%.

(6) Establish vascular access. (Check blood glucose and administer dextrose 50% IV if hypoglycemic.)

(7) Be prepared to manage shock, coma, seizures, and dysrhythmias. (Consider administering naloxone [Narcan] per local protocol and/or medical control.)

(8) Transport the patient as soon as possible. Place the patient in the left lateral recumbent position if there is any risk of vomiting to reduce the risk of aspiration.

(9) Other considerations specific to this patient: intubation, 12-lead ECG, frequently rechecking vitals and neurologic function (and noting any trends), splinting the patient's left arm in a position of function. (page 1333)

2. When Junior, or anyone else for that matter, swallows something he shouldn't have swallowed, it is important to obtain details of the ingestion.
   a. What was swallowed? (Bring the container to the hospital with the patient if possible.)
   b. When was it swallowed?
   c. How much was swallowed? (Check to see how much is left in the container if there is any uncertainty; doing so will give you an upper limit of the amount that could have been ingested.)
   d. What else was swallowed? Did Junior perhaps sample some washing powder as an hors d'oeuvre, or maybe a bit of furniture polish as a chaser?
   e. Did he vomit? (pages 1331–1332)

3. When a person is found unconscious and there is reason to suspect a toxic cause, the physical assessment should focus not only on the evaluation of the level of consciousness but also on parameters that might provide clues to a specific toxic agent. *Students should provide five of the following:*
   a. Unusual odors on the breath
   b. A precise assessment of the level of consciousness, charted on a patient care report (PCR)
   c. The condition of the skin (CTC: color, temperature, condition)
   d. The respirations, for signs of respiratory depression or metabolic acidosis
   e. Abnormalities of the pulse and blood pressure
   f. Abnormalities of the pupils (very dilated or very constricted) (page 1345)

4. When the teenager swallows his father's tricyclic antidepressant medications:
   a. Activated charcoal is given to absorb poisonous compounds to its surface and thereby effectively remove them from the body. (page 1341)
   b. There are poisonings in which activated charcoal is not effective. *Students should provide three of the following:*
      (1) Methanol ingestion
      (2) Acid or alkali ingestion
      (3) Organophosphate poisoning
      (4) Cyanide poisoning (pages 1344–1350)
   c. Follow local protocol and medical control regarding dosing of activated charcoal.
   d. The steps in treatment for this teenager are as follows:
      (1) Give activated charcoal as early as possible if indicated by local protocol and medical control.
      (2) Maintain ABCs and administer high-flow supplemental oxygen.
      (3) Initiate IV access.
      (4) Monitor cardiac rhythm and vital signs frequently.
      (5) Transport the patient to the hospital. (page 1353)

5. The gentleman who swallowed crystalline Drano ingested a very strong alkali that will continue burning holes in everything it touches until it is removed from the body.
   a. The objective of prehospital treatment is primarily to dilute the alkali, as follows:
      (1) Maintain ABCs and administer high-flow supplemental oxygen.
      (2) Initiate IV access.
      (3) Monitor cardiac rhythm and vital signs frequently.
      (4) Transport the patient to the hospital. (page 1348)

6. Down by the railway, some of the community's homeless population has congregated to console themselves with whatever they can find to drink. Sometimes, the substances chosen as cheap substitutes for ethanol can have disastrous consequences when ingested.
   a. The first patient is showing classic signs of ethylene glycol toxicity. The pleasant taste of the substance, the gastrointestinal symptoms some hours later, and the severe respiratory distress about 24 hours later are all characteristic. (pages 1350–1351)
   b. The steps of management are the same as that of methanol, which are as follows:
      (1) Establish and manage the airway. (Consider advanced airway placement as needed.)
      (2) Establish vascular access.
      (3) Assess the blood glucose level and administer glucose if the patient has hypoglycemia.
      (4) Consider thiamine per local protocol.

(5) Consult with medical control for consideration of sodium bicarbonate and 10 mL of 10% calcium gluconate via slow IV push.

(6) Provide immediate transport to an appropriate facility. (pages 1350–1351)

   c. The second patient, who appears drunk, is most likely suffering from methyl alcohol poisoning. (pages 1349–1350)

   d. The care plan for a patient with suspected methanol poisoning is the same as for ethylene glycol poisoning, with the exception of possibly getting an order from medical control to administer 10 mL of 10% calcium gluconate via slow IV push, which is appropriate for the ethylene glycol and not the methanol.

   (1) Establish and manage the airway (consider advanced airway placement as needed).

   (2) Establish vascular access.

   (3) Assess the blood glucose level and administer glucose if the patient has hypoglycemia.

   (4) Consider thiamine per local protocol.

   (5) Consult with medical control for consideration of sodium bicarbonate.

   (6) Provide immediate transport to an appropriate facility. (page 1350)

7. a. The woman who swallowed silver polish most probably swallowed cyanide, as evidenced by the smell of almonds on her breath, flushing of the skin, and tachycardia and hypotension. (page 1346)

   b. The drug that can buy some time is amyl nitrite, which in effect pulls cyanide away from the cellular enzymes it is poisoning. (Cyanide antidote kits also contain 50 mL of sodium thiosulfate solution.) (page 1346)

   c. Amyl nitrite is given by breaking a vial into a gauze pad and having the patient inhale through the handkerchief for 20 seconds, immediately followed by the inhalation of 100% supplemental oxygen for about 40 seconds. (page 1346)

   d. The side effects of amyl nitrite include hypotension. In anticipation of the hypotensive effects, keep the patient recumbent during amyl nitrite administration. (page 1346)

   e. The steps of management, then, for this victim of cyanide poisoning are as follows:

   (1) Maintain a patent airway; if her level of consciousness continues to deteriorate, maintaining the airway may require endotracheal intubation.

   (2) Give 100% supplemental oxygen by a tight-fitting nonrebreathing mask.

   (3) Administer amyl nitrite as just described.

   (4) Start an IV and give enough fluid to maintain the blood pressure.

   (5) Monitor ECG rhythm.

   (6) Notify the receiving hospital to ready a sodium thiosulfate kit if you do not carry one.

   (7) Transport the patient without delay; amyl nitrite is only a temporizing measure, and you cannot keep it up for very long. (page 1346)

8. There's something called too much of a good thing, and too much insulation of a cabin heated by a wood stove is definitely in the too-much-of-a-good-thing category!

   a. In the case in question, everyone inside the cabin is showing signs of carbon monoxide poisoning. (pages 1344–1345)

   b. The steps to take are as follows:

   (1) Bundle up in warm clothes and open all the windows of the cabin.

   (2) Get everyone outdoors as quickly as possible (ie, remove the patient from the exposure environment). Call for an ambulance. Don't trust yourself or anyone else under the influence of carbon monoxide to drive.

   (3) Establish and maintain the airway, inserting an advanced airway as needed.

   (4) As soon as the ambulance arrives, give 100% high-flow supplemental oxygen by a tight-fitting nonrebreathing mask to achieve and maintain a saturation level of 95% to all exposed victims, but give priority to the baby, who is clearly the most severely affected.

   (5) Establish vascular access.

   (6) Keep the patients quiet and at rest to minimize oxygen demand.

   (7) Monitor the patient's ECG rhythm and level of consciousness.

   (8) Transport to the appropriate facility. If the patient is unresponsive or has signs of serious CO poisoning, direct transport to a facility capable of providing hyperbaric medicine is preferred. (page 1345)

9. a. The patient stricken with a "possible heart attack" while sitting out on the lawn is in fact the victim of his next-door neighbor's insecticide spray. Although you must take very seriously the possibility of acute myocardial infarction in any middle-aged man who complains of weakness, nausea, and a tight feeling in his chest, the hypersalivation combined with constricted pupils and severe bradycardia all point to organophosphate poisoning. And, indeed, your partner returns from his discussion with Mr. Dimbledirt carrying the offending bottle of parathion. (page 1344)

b. The drug used to treat organophosphate poisoning is the parasympathetic blocking agent atropine. (page 1344)

c. Massive doses of atropine are often required to counteract the effects of organophosphates. Paramedics administer 1 mg IV. Thereafter, atropine is administered 1 mg IV every 3–5 minutes until the patient is atropinized. (page 1344)

d. (1) Treatment for organophosphate poisoning starts with decontamination and removal of all contaminated clothing before initiating care or loading the patient into the ambulance. Contaminated clothing should be placed in plastic bags and disposed of as hazardous materials. Ideally, the patient should be scrubbed with soap and water. After that, patient care includes the following measures:

(2) Establish and maintain the airway. Consider an advanced airway as needed.

(3) Suction as needed.

(4) Give high-flow oxygen to achieve and maintain saturation levels of 95%.

(5) Establish vascular access.

(6) Administer 1.0 mg atropine IV push, and repeat the dose every 3 to 5 minutes until symptom reversal (that is, atropinization) occurs.

(7) Administer 1 to 2 g of pralidoxime (2-PAM) infused with normal saline during 5 to 10 minutes.

(8) Apply the ECG monitor, pulse oximeter, and capnometer.

(9) Immediately transport to the appropriate facility. (page 1344)

10. The boy who suffered a seizure after inhaling typewriter correction fluid should be treated as any other postictal patient:

a. Protect his airway by positioning him on his side; suction secretions as needed.

b. Administer supplemental oxygen by nasal cannula.

c. Monitor cardiac rhythm; dysrhythmias and "sudden sniffing death" are not unheard of after inhalation of typewriter correction fluid.

d. Start an IV.

e. Transport without delay. (page 1352)

Complete the PCR

Show the completed PCR to your instructor to obtain feedback on your completion of the form.

True/False

1. T (page 1326) **2.** F (page 1344) **3.** T (page 1327) **4.** T (page 1329) **5.** T (page 1334)

6. T (page 1334) **7.** T (page 1335) **8.** F (page 1331) **9.** T (page 1336) **10.** T (page 1355)

11. T (page 1347) **12.** T (page 1351) **13.** T (page 1353) **14.** F (page 1356)

Short Answer

1. The patient whom you are tempted to write off as "just another drunk" is in fact much more vulnerable to a host of injuries and medical problems than the more sober John Q. Citizen. The conditions to which alcoholics are particularly susceptible include the following (*students should list 10 of the following*):

a. Subdural hematoma

b. Gastrointestinal bleeding

c. Pancreatitis

d. Hypoglycemia

e. Pneumonia

f. Burns

g. Hypothermia

h. Seizures

i. Dysrhythmias

j. Cancer

k. Esophageal varices (page 1335)

Fill-in-the-Table

1. You don't have to look very far to find commonly ingested poisons. Just check your own home. (pages 1347 and 1351)

Type of Poison	Examples
Strong acid	Toilet bowl cleaner, battery acid, bleach disinfectant
Strong alkali	Drain buildup remover (Drano), Clinitest tabs, chlorine bleach, dishwasher detergent
Hydrocarbons	Benzene industrial solvents, toluene spray paints and lacquer thinner, Gasoline for power tools
Toxic plants	Lantana, dieffenbachia, caladium, castor bean

2. (Pages 1356, Table 7)

Signs and Symptoms of Acetaminophen Toxicity		
Stage	Time Frame	Signs and Symptoms
I	< 24 h	Nausea, vomiting, loss of appetite, pallor, malaise
II	24-72 h	Right upper quadrant abdominal pain; abdomen tender to palpation
III	72-96 h	Metabolic acidosis, renal failure, coagulopathies, recurring GI symptoms
IV	4-14 d (or longer)	Recovery slowly begins, or liver failure progresses and the patient dies

Chapter 28: Psychiatric Emergencies

Matching

Part I

1. H (page 1399) **2.** I (page 1399) **3.** G (page 1399) **4.** J (page 1399)

5. F (page 1399) **6.** K (page 1399) **7.** E (page 1400) **8.** L (page 1400)

9. D (page 1400) **10.** M (page 1400) **11.** C (page 1400) **12.** N (page 1400)

13. B (page 1400) **14.** O (page 1400) **15.** A (page 1400) **16.** P (page 1400)

Part II

1. P (page 1372) **2.** P (page 1372) **3.** O (page 1371) **4.** B (pages 1371–1372) **5.** P (page 1372)

6. O (page 1371) **7.** O (page 1371) **8.** B (page 1372) **9.** O (page 1371) **10.** P (page 1372)

Part III
(page 1373, Table 3)

1. F **2.** B **3.** E **4.** D **5.** H **6.** G

7. A **8.** C **9.** D **10.** B **11.** E **12.** H

Multiple Choice

1. A (page 1376) **2.** D (page 1373) **3.** C (pages 1373–1374) **4.** D (pages 1375–1376)

5. A (page 1387) **6.** D (page 1385) **7.** A (page 1379) **8.** D (page 1369)

9. B (page 1371) **10.** A (page 1373) **11.** B (pages 1376–1377) **12.** C (page 1382)

Fill-in-the-Blank

1. biologic; organic; environment; illness; injury; substance-related (page 1371)

2. clearly; confused; delusional; frequent (page 1374)

3. fear; dread (page 1388)

4. bulimia nervosa; anorexia nervosa (page 1389)

5. *Students should list three of the following:* Amitril, Elavil, Endep, Asendin, Norpramin, Pertofane, Adapin, Sinequan, Imavate, Janimine, Pramine, Presamine, Tofranil, Ludiomil, Aventyl, Pamelor, Vivactil, Surmontil (page 1391)

6. orthostatic hypotension (page 1392)

7. Suicide (page 1384)

8. 100; schizophrenia (page 1387)

Identify

1. Fluoxetine (Prozac) and diazepam (Valium) (pages 1391–1392)

2. Phenelzine (Nardil) and bupropion (Wellbutrin) (page 1391)

3. Aripiprazole (Abilify) (page 1393)

Ambulance Calls

1. The shortest answer to this question is that the paramedic did just about everything wrong! Furthermore, he or she was inexcusably rude.

   a. The paramedic never identified himself (assume it was a male paramedic).

   b. The paramedic used a demeaning term to address the patient ("dearie") instead of asking her name and addressing her with respect as Miss, Ms., or Mrs. So-and-so.

   c. The paramedic stood in front of the patient, towering over her and also blocking her escape—a very threatening stance. He should have crouched down to be at the same level as the patient, and positioned himself somewhat to the side so that she wasn't trapped in the corner.

d. The paramedic passed judgment on the patient's feelings ("Big girls don't cry"). Furthermore, he belittled the patient's problem without even waiting to find out what the problem was! ("You're making a mountain out of a molehill.")

e. The paramedic gave inappropriate and premature reassurance, telling the patient in essence that everything will be all right by tomorrow without even knowing what's wrong today.

f. The paramedic tried to forestall the patient's expressions of feeling, urging her to stop crying.

g. The paramedic never gave the patient a chance to talk.

h. The paramedic then turned his back on the patient and asked if someone else could tell him what was going on, implying that the patient's version of things was of no importance. (page 1374)

2. The fact that Mr. Crosby has admitted you to his apartment, even reluctantly, is a hopeful sign.

a. You might start the interview something like this: "Your neighbors have been worried about you; that's why they called us. They thought there might be some kind of problem here. Is there any way we can help?" If the patient then says something to the effect that there's nothing anyone can do to help, you might comment on his statement: "You seem really discouraged." The object is to indicate that you are a "sympathetic ear," prepared to listen to his troubles. (page 1374)

b. The symptoms of depression that this patient is showing include the following:

   (1) A sense of worthlessness

   (2) Decreased appetite

   (3) No apparent interest in anything

   (4) Lack of energy (page 1387)

c. Other symptoms and signs of depression include:

   (1) Sleep disturbances

   (2) Difficulty concentrating

   (3) Psychomotor abnormalities (retardation or agitation)

   (4) Suicidal thoughts (page 1387)

d. The risk factors for suicide in this patient's history include:

   (1) Male, over 55 years old

   (2) Widower

   (3) Socially isolated

   (4) Depressed

   (5) Possible alcohol problem (empty bottles lying around) (page 1384)

e. Other risk factors for suicide include the following. *Students should provide four of the following:*

   (1) A previous suicide attempt

   (2) A family history of suicide

   (3) Suicidal thoughts, particularly when there are concrete plans

   (4) Clear warning of intent to commit suicide

   (5) Recent loss of a significant person

   (6) Recent job loss or financial setback (page 1384)

f. Among the questions to ask in evaluating this patient's suicide risk are the following:

   (1) Have you ever felt that life wasn't worth living?

   (2) Have you thought about harming yourself?

   (3) How would you go about it? Have you made any plans? (page 1384)

3. The young woman with a "possible heart attack" is unlikely to be suffering a heart attack (although it's not completely out of the question).

a. Her problem is most likely a panic attack. (page 1388)

b. The symptoms and signs that suggest that diagnosis include the following:

   (1) Dyspnea

   (2) Chest tightness

   (3) Feeling faint

   (4) Her feelings of unreality and impending death

   (5) Tachycardia

(6) Sweating

(7) Trembling (page 1388)

c. Yes, there certainly are other possibilities that must be taken into account, including:

(1) Pulmonary embolism, which is highest on the list of possibilities

(2) Cardiac arrhythmia

(3) A reaction to a drug

(4) An anaphylactic reaction

(5) An acute myocardial infarction, which is seen much more frequently among young people these days because of the widespread use of cocaine

d. To manage this patient, therefore:

(1) Separate her from all the panicky bystanders. Move her into a private office, or move everyone out of her office.

(2) Sit down to talk with her.

(3) Administer supplementary oxygen. Until you know that you are not dealing with a pulmonary embolism or cardiac event, you need to cover all bases.

(4) Apply monitoring electrodes, and check the rhythm on the scope.

(5) Assuming there are no abnormal findings, reassure the patient that you cannot find any indication of serious illness and that the chances are she is suffering a panic attack. Tell her that to make absolutely sure, she needs to be checked out in the hospital. If it does turn out she is having a panic attack, there are effective treatments for that condition. (pages 1388–1389)

4. The police officer who summoned you to the bar was on the right track, even if "psycho case" is not a very specific diagnosis.

a. The patient is probably in the manic phase of a bipolar disorder. (page 1387)

b. The evidence to suggest this diagnosis includes the following:

(1) His pressure of speech

(2) His grandiose ideas (big business deals, big spender)

(3) His apparently euphoric mood that is, nonetheless, very brittle (His good cheer easily turns to a less pleasant affect when he is challenged by the bartender or the police officer.)

(4) His hyperactivity, pacing up and down (page 1387)

c. In managing this patient, you will have to try to persuade him to go voluntarily to the hospital. If he will not be persuaded, and probably he will not, coercion will be necessary. Consult your medical director first. (page 1387)

5. The strangely dressed man found wandering down the middle of the street is a good example of disorganized behavior. Because walking in traffic is not a healthy activity, the patient must be assumed to be unable to care for himself and probably needs institutional care. From the description, it does not sound as if you will be able to obtain a useful history. You should simply tell the patient gently but firmly that you are going to take him to the hospital for care. He will probably go along without much fuss if you are nonthreatening about it. (page 1383)

6. The karate expert is seriously ill and probably dangerous.

a. He is showing signs of psychosis (answer 2)—hallucinations, persecutory delusions, loosening of associations. (page 1382)

b. Yes, there are indications that he might become violent.

c. Indications. *Students should provide four of the following:*

(1) His body language—sitting there like a coiled spring, gripping the armrests of the chair

(2) The fact that he is easily startled

(3) His avoidance of eye contact

(4) The fact that he views the paramedics as adversaries (He thinks you're the FBI!)

(5) His hearing voices that tell him to put up a fight

d. In managing this situation:

(1) Observe your surroundings. Keep yourself between the patient and the door to his room. Make note of any potential weapons.

(2) Maintain a safe distance, at least two arm lengths (which will keep you out of range of his foot).

(3) Identify yourself again as a paramedic.

(4) Acknowledge the patient's behavior ("You seem very worried."), and state your willingness to help. Don't sound too friendly.

(5) Encourage the patient to talk about what's bothering him.

(6) Define your expectations of his behavior.

(7) If talking to the patient isn't working, back off and get help.

(8) Explain to the patient's mother that it will be necessary to take the young man to the hospital against his will (she may be required to sign his commitment papers). Call for police backup, and consult medical command.

(9) When you have sufficient manpower, apply restraints as quickly and efficiently as you can. Once the patient is restrained, don't remove the restraints.

(10) Maintain verbal contact with the patient throughout transport. (page 1383)

True/False

1. T (page 1377) **2.** F (pages 1373–1374) **3.** F (page 1378)

4. F (page 1378) **5.** T (page 1379) **6.** T (page 1379)

Short Answer

1. The paramedic needs to develop a "nose for danger" and be able to predict which situations present a high risk for violence.

    a. Any place where alcohol is being consumed

    b. Crowd incidents

    c. Scenes of violent injury (page 1385)

2. a. Patients intoxicated with drugs or alcohol

    b. Patients withdrawing from drugs or alcohol

    c. Psychotic patients

    d. Patients with delirium (page 1385)

Fill-in-the-Table

(page 1371, Table 2)

Selected Disease States That May Produce Psychotic Symptoms	
Disease State	**Psychotic Symptoms**
Toxic and deficiency states	Drug-induced psychoses, especially from: • Digitalis • Steroids • Disulfiram • Amphetamines • LSD, PCP, and other psychedelics Nutrition disorders: • Alcohol abuse • Vitamin deficiencies Poisoning with bromide or other heavy metals Kidney failure Liver failure
Infections	Syphilis Parasites Viral encephalitis (eg, after measles) Brain abscess
Neurologic disease	Seizure disorders (especially temporal lobe seizures) Primary and metastatic tumors of the brain Dementia Stroke Closed head injury
Cardiovascular disorders	Low cardiac output (eg, in heart failure)
Endocrine disorders	Thyroid hyperfunction (thyrotoxicosis) Adrenal hyperfunction (Cushing syndrome)
Metabolic disorders	Electrolyte imbalances (eg, after severe diarrhea) Hypoglycemia Diabetic ketoacidosis

Skill Drill

1. Restraining a Patient (page 1381, Skill Drill 1)

    Step 3

    Step 5

    Step 2

    Step 4

    Step 1

Section 7: Trauma
Chapter 29: Trauma Systems and Mechanism of Injury

Matching

Part I

1. C (page 1488) **2.** B (page 1488) **3.** D (pages 1495–1496) **4.** A (page 1488) **5.** B (page 1488)

6. A–D (pages 1488, 1495–1496) **7.** A (page 1488) **8.** A (page 1488) **9.** B (page 1488) **10.** A, B (page 1488)

Part II
(pages 1515–1516)

1. K	**2.** J	**3.** L	**4.** I	**5.** M	**6.** H	**7.** N	**8.** G	**9.** O	**10.** F
11. P	**12.** E	**13.** Q	**14.** D	**15.** R	**16.** C	**17.** S	**18.** B	**19.** T	**20.** A

Multiple Choice

1. A (pages 1507–1509) **2.** C (page 1505) **3.** B (page 1483) **4.** B (page 1496) **5.** A (page 1499)

6. D (page 1499) **7.** D (page 1499) **8.** A (page 1484) **9.** D (page 1509) **10.** A (page 1491)

Labeling
(page 1500)

A. Primary blast injury (injuries due to the blast wave itself)
B. Secondary blast injury (injuries due to missiles being propelled by blast force)
C. Tertiary blast injury (injuries due to impact with another object)

Fill-in-the-Blank

1. a. The size of the explosive charge
 b. The nature of the surrounding medium
 c. The distance from the explosion
 d. The presence or absence of reflecting surfaces (page 1501)

2. anatomic; penetration (page 1498)

3. Arterial air embolism (page 1502)

4. a. Height
 b. Position
 c. Surface
 d. Physical condition
 e. Area (pages 1496–1497)

5. cervical; neck (page 1493)

Identify

1. **a.** Mechanism of injury: Rollover motor vehicle crash
    b. Chief complaint: Pain to radius/ulna, neck pain
    c. Vital signs: Pulse 110 beats/min regular, respiration 16 breaths/min unlabored, blood pressure 106/96 mm Hg, SpO_2 98%, and skin is ashen colored
    d. Pertinent negatives: Denies LOC

2. **a.** Mechanism of injury: High-speed motorcycle-versus-guardrail crash
    b. Chief complaint: Hurts all over
    c. Vital signs: Conscious and alert, skin ashen and diaphoretic, no palpable blood pressure, > 2-second capillary refill, respiration 28 breaths/min, and SpO_2 92%
    d. Pertinent negatives: None

3. **a.** Mechanism of injury: Possible fall, TIA, cardiac
    b. Chief complaint: Per patient, none; staff states she fell and has pain to hip
    c. Vital signs: Pulse 58 beats/min and irregular; blood pressure 158/110 mm Hg; SpO_2 95%; skin cool and dry; normal capillary refill
    d. Pertinent negatives: Denies chest pain, shortness of breath, neck or back pain

Complete the Patient Care Report (PCR)

Show the completed PCR to your instructor to obtain feedback on your completion of the form.

Ambulance Calls

1. Evaluate the mechanism of injury and examine the trauma scene for evidence of high-energy trauma.
    a. Speed (page 1487)
    b. Restrained versus air bag deployment (page 1493)
    c. Loss of consciousness (page 1505)
    d. Physical damage to pole and vehicle, and any intrusion into the vehicle (page 1489)
    e. Patient's chief complaint (page 1505)
    f. Secondary assessment (physical exam) (page 1505)

2. **a.** Height: The distance that he jumped. This will determine the speed at which he fell and therefore the force of impact with which he hit the ground.

    Position: How he landed. This will tell you what part(s) of the body absorbed the greatest amount of kinetic energy.

    Area: The area over which the impact is distributed—the larger the area of contact at the time of the impact, the greater dissipation of the force and the lesser the peak pressures generated.

    Surface: What kind of surface he landed on. A pile of hay has a lot more give than a concrete sidewalk. The more the surface can "give," the less the falling body will have to deform.

    Physical condition: The physical condition of the patient before the fall. Does he have any underlying physical problems—such as an ulcer or an enlarged spleen—that might predispose him to certain injuries?
    b. Spine, legs, pelvis (pages 1496–1497)

3. Children tend to fall headfirst, so head injuries are common in children as are injuries to the wrists and upper extremities when the child attempts to break the fall. The surface on which the child falls is very important. (page 1497)

4. **a.** Call the police.
    b. (1) The type of firearm used
    (2) Velocity of the projectile
    (3) Physical design of the projectile
    (4) The distance to the target from the muzzle of the firearm
    (5) The type of tissue that was struck (pages 1498–1499)

5. Explosions produce several different mechanisms of injury, and one needs to anticipate each type; otherwise, it is easy to miss the less obvious injuries.
   a. Primary blast injury: body damage caused by the explosion
   b. Secondary blast injury: damage from being struck by flying debris
   c. Tertiary blast injury: patient being hurled against a stationary object
   d. Miscellaneous blast injury: burns from hot gases or structural collapse (pages 1499–1501)
6. (page 1502)

Tissues at Risk	Evidence
1. Tympanic membrane	Blood in the ear
2. Pulmonary blast injury	Tight feeling in chest
3. Arterial air embolism	Blurry vision

True/False

1. T (page 1483)
2. F (page 1510)
3. F (page 1509)
4. T (page 1486)
5. T (pages 1490–1491)
6. F (page 1493)
7. T (page 1508)
8. F (page 1508)

Short Answer

1. In this question, you are asked to consider the forces involved when a 2,000-lb automobile traveling at 20 mph strikes a pedestrian. (pages 1485–1486)
   a. Some of the kinetic energy of the vehicle will remain energy of motion, assuming the vehicle keeps moving. (If the driver hits the brakes, the friction of the brakes will transform that kinetic energy into heat.) Some energy will be absorbed by the vehicle in the deformation of the bumper or hood, and the remainder will be absorbed by the pedestrian who has been struck by the vehicle.
   b. Had the vehicle weighed 6,000 lb instead of 2,000 lb—that is, had its weight (mass) been tripled—its kinetic energy at any given speed would also have tripled, according to the kinetic energy equation: $KE = m/2 \times V^2$.
   c. Had the vehicle been traveling at 60 mph instead of 20 mph—that is, had its velocity been tripled—its kinetic energy would have increased nine times because kinetic energy increases as the *square* of the velocity. That is why it is nearly impossible for a pedestrian to survive an impact with a vehicle, even a relatively small vehicle, going faster than about 40 mph—the kinetic energies become overwhelming.
2. When a car traveling at 50 mph slams into a concrete wall, three distinct collisions take place:
   a. Collision 1 is between the *automobile* and the concrete wall. Because the automobile is both more mobile and more deformable than the concrete wall, the majority of the kinetic energy is absorbed by the automobile in its rebound off the wall and deformity of the front end.
   b. Collision 2 is between the *occupant* and the automobile. In that collision, some of the kinetic energy is absorbed by the automobile (eg, in denting the dashboard), but the larger proportion is absorbed by the occupant.
   c. Collision 3 is between the internal *organs* of the occupant and the restraining walls of the person's body (eg, the skull, the chest cage, the pelvic girdle). The majority of the kinetic energy in that collision is absorbed by the internal organs. (page 1487)

3. When you arrive at the crash scene, a close inspection of the scene and of the damaged vehicle(s) can provide extremely important information—information that will enable the doctors who take over the patient's care to detect and manage the patient's problems much more expeditiously. Indeed, what you observe (or fail to observe) about the crash scene could make the difference between life and death for the patient—so keep your eyes open, report what you have observed to the base physician, and record your findings on the patient's PCR. (page 1488)
   a. Deformed dashboard
      (1) Ruptured spleen, liver, bowel, diaphragm
      (2) Fractured patella
      (3) Dislocated knee
      (4) Femoral fracture
      (5) Dislocated hip
   b. Deformed steering column
      (1) Sternal or rib fracture
      (2) Flail chest
      (3) Myocardial contusion
      (4) Pericardial tamponade
      (5) Pneumothorax or hemothorax
      (6) Exsanguinations from aortic tear
   c. Cracked windshield
      (1) Brain injury
      (2) Scalp, facial cuts
      (3) Cervical spine injury
      (4) Tracheal injury
   d. Door smashed in
      (1) Fractured hip
      (2) Fractured iliac wing
      (3) Fractured clavicle or ribs

4. *Students should provide six of the following:*
   a. Facial injuries
   b. Soft-tissue neck trauma
   c. Larynx and tracheal trauma
   d. Fractured sternum
   e. Myocardial contusion
   f. Pericardial tamponade
   g. Pulmonary contusion
   h. Hemothorax, rib fracture
   i. Flail chest
   j. Ruptured aorta
   k. Intra-abdominal injuries (page 1491)

Fill-in-the-Table

1. (page 1510)

Key Elements for Trauma Centers		
Level	**Definition**	**Key Elements**
Level I	A comprehensive regional resource that is a tertiary care facility. Capable of providing total care for every aspect of injury–from prevention through rehabilitation.	1. 24-hour in-house coverage by general surgeons 2. Availability of care in specialties such as orthopaedic surgery, neurosurgery, anesthesiology, emergency medicine, radiology, internal medicine, and critical care 3. Should also include cardiac, hand, pediatric, and microvascular surgery and hemodialysis 4. Provides leadership in prevention, public education, and continuing education of trauma team members 5. Committed to continued improvement through a comprehensive quality assessment program and organized research to help direct new innovations in trauma care
Level II	Able to initiate definitive care for all injured patients.	1. 24-hour immediate coverage by general surgeons 2. Availability of care in specialties such as orthopaedic surgery, neurosurgery, anesthesiology, emergency medicine, radiology, and critical care 3. Tertiary care needs such as cardiac surgery, hemodialysis, and microvascular surgery may be referred to a Level I trauma center 4. Committed to trauma prevention and continuing education of trauma team members 5. Provides continued improvement in trauma care through a comprehensive quality assessment program
Level III	Able to provide prompt assessment, resuscitation, and stabilization of injured patients and emergency operations.	1. 24-hour immediate coverage by emergency medicine physicians and prompt availability of general surgeons and anesthesiologists 2. Program dedicated to continued improvement in trauma care through a comprehensive quality assessment program 3. Has developed transfer agreements for patients requiring more comprehensive care at a Level I or Level II trauma center 4. Committed to continuing education of nursing and allied health personnel or the trauma team 5. Must be involved with prevention and have an active outreach program for its referring communities 6. Also dedicated to improving trauma care through a comprehensive quality assessment program
Level IV	Able to provide Advanced Trauma Life Support (ATLS) before transfer of patients to a higher level trauma center.	1. Include basic emergency department facilities to implement ATLS protocols and 24-hour laboratory coverage 2. Transfer to higher level trauma centers follows the guidelines outlined in formal transfer agreements 3. Committed to continued improvement of these trauma care activities through a formal quality assessment program 4. Involved in prevention, outreach, and education within its community

2. (page 1491)

"Ring" of Chest Injuries From Impact With the Steering Wheel or Dashboard

- **Facial injuries**
- Soft-tissue neck trauma
- Larynx and tracheal trauma
- **Fractured sternum**
- **Myocardial contusion**
- **Pericardial tamponade**
- Pulmonary contusion
- Hemothorax, rib fractures
- **Flail chest**
- **Ruptured aorta**
- Intra-abdominal injuries

Problem Solving

1. $KE = \dfrac{(200 + 120)}{2} \times 50^2 = 400{,}000$

(page 1486)

2. $KE = \dfrac{120}{2} \times 50^2 = 150{,}000$

(page 1486)

Chapter 30: Bleeding

Matching

(page 1542)

1. C	**2.** B	**3.** W	**4.** R	**5.** L	**6.** K	**7.** A	**8.** Q	**9.** Z	**10.** J
11. Y	**12.** I	**13.** D	**14.** BB	**15.** H	**16.** T	**17.** S	**18.** G	**19.** AA	**20.** P
21. U	**22.** O	**23.** F	**24.** V	**25.** N	**26.** X	**27.** M	**28.** CC	**29.** E	

Multiple Choice

1. B (page 1522) **2.** C (page 1521) **3.** C (page 1528) **4.** D (page 1526) **5.** D (page 1526)

6. A (page 1529) **7.** C (page 1528) **8.** B (page 1526) **9.** C (page 1532) **10.** B (page 1525)

Labeling

1. The Cardiovascular System (page 1521)
   A. Superior vena cava
   B. Right atrium
   C. Right ventricle
   D. Inferior vena cava
   E. Aorta
   F. Left atrium
   G. Left ventricle
   H. (Lower) aorta

Fill-in-the-Blank

1. MAST; PASG (page 1535)
2. hemoglobin (page 1521)
3. perfusion (page 1522)
4. Hemostatis (page 1525)
5. melena (page 1529)
6. Epistaxis (page 1531)
7. Hypoperfusion (page 1523)
8. hematochezia (page 1529)
9. clotting; hemophilia (page 1525)
10. SVR; CO; worsening (page 1526)
11. high incidence; heart; liver (page 1526)
12. compensated; decompensated; irreversible (page 1526)
13. normal saline; lactated Ringer's (page 1536)
14. anaphylactic (page 1525, Table 1)
15. crystalloids (page 1537)

Identify

1. Chief complaint: Abdominal GSW
2. Vitals signs: Sinus tachycardia rate of 120 beats/min, and equal lung sounds. Respirations are 24 breaths/min; blood pressure is 80/56 mm Hg; skin is pale, diaphoretic, and clammy. Patient is alert with oxygen administration. An eye assessment shows PEARRL (Pupils Equal And Round, Regular in size, react to Light).
3. Pertinent negatives: No pulse at wrist, little external bleeding, no ectopy on ECG

Complete the Patient Care Report (PCR)

Show the completed PCR to your instructor to obtain feedback on your completion of the form.

Ambulance Calls

1. In assessing the state of perfusion:
   a. You can judge *peripheral* perfusion by checking the radial pulse.
   b. The best indicator in the field of *perfusion of vital organs* is the patient's state of consciousness. (page 1530)

2. You are called to a bar to attend a bleeding, unconscious man. The place is full of noise and confusion—unruly customers, police, curiosity seekers. *This is the time to remember the priorities of the primary assessment:* A-B-C.

   First, before you even enter that bar, make certain that the police have the situation under control. (If you did not include that step in your answer, you do not get *any* points for your answer and, furthermore, you are a very poor risk for life insurance!) Look first to your own safety, remember?
   a. Open the patient's airway. (*Note:* If you suspect this is a cardiac arrest, the approach is CAB not ABC.)
   b. Check whether he is breathing. If not, start artificial ventilation.
   c. Check whether he has a pulse. If he does not have a pulse, start external chest compressions.
   d. Cut away the patient's trouser leg, and find the source of his bleeding. When you have found it, control the bleeding by applying direct pressure to the wound, preferably over a sterile dressing. Check quickly for other lower extremity injuries.
   e. Transfer the patient to the vehicle (he should be on a backboard by now).
   f. Get underway to the hospital and start an IV infusion en route. Complete your rapid secondary assessment as time permits. (pages 1529–1530)

3. This patient earns his "load-and-go" status by virtue of uncontrollable bleeding from the femoral artery.
   a. Steps to be taken at the scene:
      (1) Seal the open wound of the neck.
      (2) Administer supplemental oxygen.
      (3) Try at least to slow the bleeding from the groin by using direct pressure, pressure dressing, and pressure to the artery. If your system uses hemostatic dressings, they should be used on this patient.
      (4) Communicate with medical control or the receiving hospital.
   b. Steps to be taken en route:
      (1) Start two large-bore IVs with rapid infusion of fluids.
      (2) Complete a secondary assessment and physical exam.
      (3) Recheck vital and neurologic signs every 5 minutes. (pages 1530–1531)

4. Abdominal evisceration is certainly an attention-getter, but it does *not* pose an immediate threat to life.
   a. Steps to be taken at the scene:
      (1) Administer supplemental oxygen.
      (2) Complete the secondary assessment and a physical exam.
      (3) Cover the eviscerated organs with sterile dressings soaked in sterile saline and an occlusive dressing.
   b. Steps to be taken en route:
      (1) Communicate with medical control or the receiving hospital.
      (2) Start a large-bore IV with normal saline or lactated Ringer's (depending on your regional protocols).
      (3) Recheck vital and neurologic signs every 5 minutes. (pages 1530–1531)

5. An open chest wound is considered a critical injury because it prevents adequate ventilation of the lungs.
   a. Steps to be taken at the scene:
      (1) Seal off the sucking chest wound with an occlusive dressing taped on three sides.
      (2) Administer supplemental oxygen; assist ventilations as needed.
      (3) Communicate with medical control or the receiving hospital.
   b. Steps to be taken en route:
      (1) Complete a secondary assessment and physical exam.
      (2) Start an IV with fluids.
      (3) Recheck vital and neurologic signs every 5 minutes. (pages 1530–1531)

6. Your primary assessment has not given you much information regarding *where* precisely this patient has been injured, but the primary assessment *has* given you unmistakable evidence that the patient is in shock (restlessness,

profuse sweating). Don't be fooled by the slow pulse. Bradycardia occurs sometimes with intra-abdominal bleeding. *And don't wait for the blood pressure to fall before you decide the patient is in shock!*

a. Steps to be taken at the scene:

(1) Manually stabilize the head/neck and apply a cervical collar.

(2) Administer supplemental oxygen.

(3) Conduct the primary assessment.

(4) Immobilize the patient on a long backboard.

(5) Prepare for rapid transport to the appropriate facility.

b. Steps to be taken en route:

(1) Complete a secondary assessment and physical exam.

(2) Start two large-bore IVs and run a fluid challenge.

(3) Communicate with medical control or the receiving hospital.

(4) Conduct reassessment, rechecking vital and neurologic signs every 5 minutes. (pages 1530–1531)

True/False

1. F (page 1526) **2.** F (page 1527) **3.** F (page 1537) **4.** T (page 1525) **5.** T (page 1520)

6. F (page 1521) **7.** T (page 1524) **8.** T (page 1524) **9.** F (page 1534) **10.** T (page 1535)

Short Answer

1. Three components are required for a functioning regulatory system:

a. A functioning pump: the heart

b. Adequate fluid volume: the blood and body fluids

c. An intact system of tubing capable of reflex adjustments (constriction and dilation) in response to changes in pump output and fluid volume: the blood vessels (page 1519)

2. Causes of hypovolemic shock include (*students should provide four of the following*):

a. External bleeding

b. Blunt chest trauma

c. Blunt abdominal trauma

d. Fractures of the pelvis or femur

e. Ruptured ectopic pregnancy

f. Bleeding ulcer

g. Burns

h. Dehydration (page 1525)

3. Knowing the findings in hemorrhagic shock is important in being a paramedic. (page 1527)

Findings in Hemorrhagic Shock	
Heart rate	Increased
Blood pressure	Within normal limits in the early stages, then decreases as patient decompensates
Central venous pressure/renal artery pressure	Decreased
Pulmonary capillary wedge pressure	Decreased
Cardiac output/cardiac index	Decreased
Systemic vascular resistance/systemic vascular resistance index	Increased
Systemic vascular oxygen	Decreased
Urinary output	Decreased
Jugular vein distention	Flat
Hematocrit (percentage of whole blood components versus plasma)	Decreased with hemorrhage; increased with dehydration

4. It is absolutely essential that a paramedic be able to recognize the signs of shock. That is why we keep coming back to them. Symptoms and signs of shock include *(students should provide six of the following)*:
   a. Restlessness and anxiety
   b. Thirst
   c. Nausea, sometimes with vomiting
   d. Cold, clammy, pale, or mottled skin
   e. Weak, rapid pulse
   f. Rapid, shallow breathing
   g. Changes in the state of consciousness/mental status
   h. Fall in blood pressure (pages 1527–1528)

5. List four methods for the control of external hemorrhage.
   a. Apply direct pressure over the wound.
   b. Elevate the injury above the level of the heart.
   c. Apply a pressure dressing.
   d. Apply a tourniquet. *Note:* Some EMS systems also use hemostatic dressings. (pages 1530–1531)

Fill-in-the-Table

(page 1527)

Compensated Versus Decompensated Hypoperfusion	
Compensated Hypoperfusion	**Decompensated Hypoperfusion**
• **Agitation, anxiety, restlessness** • Sense of impending doom • **Weak, rapid (thready) pulse** • Clammy (cool, moist) skin • **Pallor with cyanotic lips** • Shortness of breath • **Nausea, vomiting** • Delayed capillary refill in infants and children • **Thirst** • Normal systolic blood pressure	• Altered mental status (verbal to unresponsive) • **Hypotension** • Labored or irregular breathing • **Thready or absent peripheral pulses** • Ashen, mottled, or cyanotic skin • **Dilated pupils** • Diminished urine output (oliguria) • **Impending cardiac arrest**

Skill Drills

1. Managing Hemorrhagic Shock (page 1537)

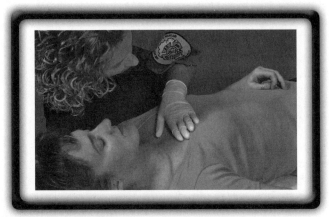

Step 1: Keep the patient supine, open the airway, and check breathing and pulse.

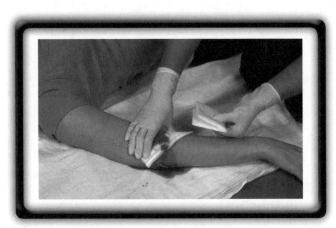

Step 2: Control obvious external bleeding.

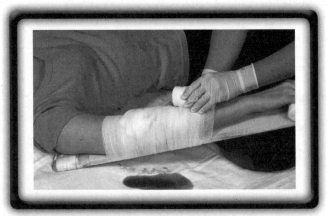

Step 3: Splint the patient on a backboard. Splint any broken bones or joint injuries during transport.

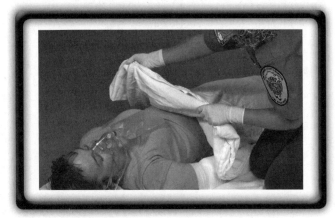

Step 4: Administer high-flow oxygen if you have not already done so, and keep the patient warm.

Chapter 31: Soft-Tissue Trauma

Matching

(pages 1571–1572)

1. L   **2.** E   **3.** M   **4.** P   **5.** N   **6.** G   **7.** O   **8.** H   **9.** K   **10.** Q   **11.** I   **12.** V

13. S   **14.** X   **15.** C   **16.** A   **17.** T   **18.** U   **19.** D   **20.** B   **21.** W   **22.** J   **23.** R   **24.** F

Multiple Choice

1. C (page 1566)   **2.** B (page 1556)   **3.** D (page 1561)   **4.** A (page 1566)   **5.** A (page 1545)

6. C (page 1547)   **7.** C (page 1551)   **8.** C (pages 1556–1557)   **9.** D (page 1559)   **10.** D (page 1550)

Labeling

1. The Skin (page 1546)
   A. Hair
   B. Pore
   C. Sebaceous gland
   D. Nerve (sensory)
   E. Sweat gland
   F. Hair follicle
   G. Blood vessel
   H. Subcutaneous fat
   I. Muscle

2. Types of Open Wounds
   (pages 1560–1563)

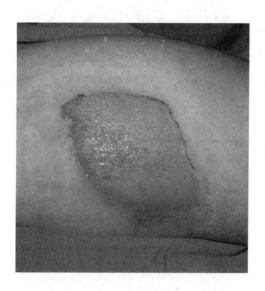

   A. Abrasion

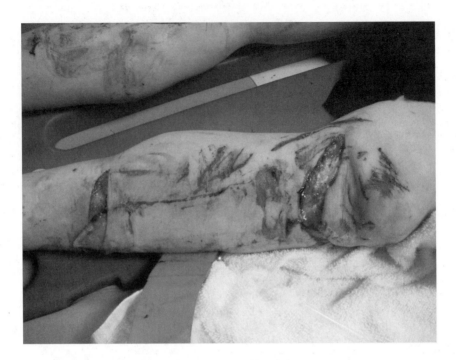

B. Laceration

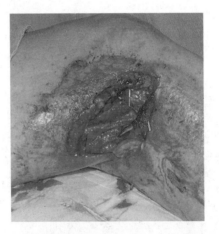

C. Avulsion

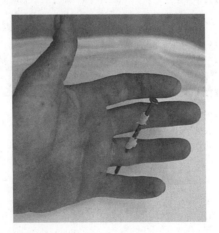

D. Puncture wound/impaled object

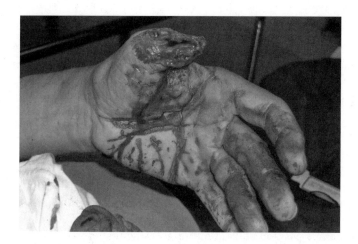

> **E.** Amputation

Fill-in-the-Blank

1. Degloving; debridement (page 1550)
2. erythema; pus; warmth; edema; local discomfort (page 1550)
3. toxin; contractions; bones (page 1551)
4. melanin (page 1546)
5. gangrene (page 1550)
6. law enforcement; safe; secondary; killed (page 1551)
7. bacteria; limited (page 1555)

Identify

1. The injury described appears to be a laceration with moderately uncontrolled bleeding. Even though this appears to be an isolated injury, a thorough primary assessment is warranted. Treatment would generally include bleeding control. Usually, this can be completed with direct pressure. Sometimes, elevation of the extremity—and in extreme cases, a tourniquet—may be needed. Perhaps splinting the extremity to minimize movement and applying a sterile dressing and roller gauze are appropriate. Don't forget to check distal capillary refill and motor neurologic (PMS) before and after bandaging. (pages 1556–1557)

2. This sounds like a classic amputation. Of immediate concern is stopping the bleeding. Doing so will require the paramedic to don PPE, which at the very least includes gloves and may include a disposable gown and blankets. Paramedics must very quickly prepare bulky trauma dressings and be prepared for the potential of uncontrolled bleeding. Bleeding control is often self-limiting in this type of situation. However, if it is not controlled, methods such as direct pressure, elevation, and use of an arterial tourniquet may be required. It may be necessary to maintain these steps all the way to the hospital. If necessary, request additional resources. Once bleeding is controlled, begin treating the patient for shock with high-flow oxygen and IV fluid replacement. It is also beneficial as soon as practical to have the patient lie down with his feet elevated. Doing so on your cot enables you to initiate transport immediately. With adequate vital signs, pain medication may also be in order. Above all, don't forget about the amputated fingers. Follow local protocols regarding wet or dry dressings and placing the parts on ice. (pages 1557, 1562–1563)

3. This patient has suffered from some type of puncture or stab wound. In her combative state she might not realize how serious the injury could be. As a paramedic you realize that she might have suffered a hemo- or pneumothorax. You rapidly treat the obvious wound with an occlusive dressing and immediately prepare for transportation with high-flow oxygen. You also prepare IVs en route. In a worst-case situation, this patient may require ventilatory assistance and intubation. (page 1567)

Ambulance Calls

1. **a.** To control the bleeding from Bugsy Butterfingers's left calf, you have several methods available to you:

    (1) Directing manual pressure over the bleeding site (likely to be the most effective)

    (2) Elevating the bleeding extremity

    (3) Splinting the left leg

    (4) As a last resort, applying a tourniquet (page 1556–1558)

    b. If Bugsy's wound had been on the forearm rather than on the leg, the brachial artery would most likely have been the cause of severe bleeding.

2. When Frank Fillet accidentally amputates two of his fingers, you have two problems—(1) to treat Mr. Fillet himself and (2) to preserve the amputated parts in optimal condition.

    a. To treat the injury, the first priority is to stop the bleeding. Probably direct pressure will be sufficient because amputations ordinarily do not bleed profusely. Apply lots of fluffed gauze to the stumps of the fingers and bandage the whole hand in a position of function (fingers slightly flexed). The patient will doubtless require a lot of calming down; if you can remain calm, it will help a great deal. (page 1563)

    b. Once you have taken care of the patient, you can turn your attention to the amputated parts. Rinse the two fingers free of contaminants with cool, sterile saline. Wrap them loosely in saline-moistened sterile gauze. Then, place them in a plastic bag, seal the bag, and place it in a cool container for transport. Do *not* place the amputated part in water or directly on ice! (pages 1562–1563)

3. Bugsy's Butcher Shop is definitely not a healthy workplace. Now poor Hercules Hamburger has also become a casualty—not only of the meat grinder that mangled his hand, but also of a Good Samaritan who was trying to help. The mistakes made in caring for Hercules include the following:

    a. No attempt was made to stop the bleeding by other means, such as direct pressure alone or in combination with elevation, splinting, and so on. *A tourniquet is a last resort*, not a first choice!

    b. A rope should not be used as a tourniquet; nor should any other narrow materials that can damage underlying tissues.

    c. The tourniquet was twisted too tightly. It is virtually never necessary to twist a tourniquet as tight as it will go; the objective is to slow the bleeding sufficiently that it can be controlled by direct pressure.

    d. A tourniquet should never be covered, lest it escape attention. The Good Samaritan covered the patient's whole arm in a butcher's apron, perhaps to spare the patient the sight of his mangled extremity. (pages 1556–1558)

4. It is, in fact, rather rare to encounter a patient with an impaled object, but considerable attention is given to the problem in EMT and paramedic courses because the consequences of mismanagement could be disastrous.

    a. When the impaled object is in the eye, the usual principle applies: Stabilize the impaled object in place. For the eye, the most efficient way to do so is usually with a stack of gauze pads that has a hole in the middle. The gauze pads are passed gently over the impaled object and bandaged in place. If the impaled object is an arrow, as in the present case, it won't be possible to cover it with a paper cup. Do not try to shorten the impaled object. Just protect it from being jarred, and be sure to patch the other eye as well to prevent the injured eye from moving every time the uninjured eye shifts its gaze. (page 1561)

    b. When an object is impaled in the cheek, you have to break the usual rule about not removing an impaled object because it will be impossible to control bleeding inside the mouth as long as the arrow is sticking through the cheek. Therefore, gently pull the arrow out of the cheek. Then, pack the inside of the cheek with sterile gauze, and apply counterpressure with a dressing secured firmly against the outside of the cheek. Keep the patient on his side so that he can more easily spit any blood out of his mouth (instruct him not to swallow blood because blood in the stomach is a stimulus to vomit). (pages 1561–1562)

5. For the man bitten by the Doberman pinscher, the treatment is as follows:

    a. Have him stop walking on the injured leg.

    b. Clean the wound with lots of soap and water; then, rinse with alcohol (there goes the rest of your gin).

    c. Send someone back along the beach to find out details about the dog (eg, name and address of owner), which must be reported to the local health authorities.

    d. See that the patient is transported to the hospital for further evaluation of his wound. (pages 1563–1564)

True/False

1. T (page 1562) 2. T (page 1545) 3. F (page 1547) 4. F (page 1547) 5. T (page 1547)

6. T (page 1563) 7. F (page 1550) 8. T (page 1551) 9. T (page 1548) 10. T (page 1554)

Short Answer

1. **a.** It protects underlying tissue from injury.
   b. It plays a major role in temperature regulation.
   c. It prevents excessive loss of water from the body.
   d. It serves as a sense organ for temperature, touch, and pain. (pages 1545–1546)

2. **a.** Hemostasis
   b. Inflammation
   c. Epithelialization
   d. Neovascularization
   e. Collagen synthesis (page 1549)

3. **a.** Contusion
   b. Ecchymosis
   c. Hematoma (page 1547)

4. **a.** A body part is trapped for more than 4 hours; then
   b. rhabdomyolysis occurs; then
   c. the trapped body part is freed; and then
   d. by-products of metabolism and harmful products from tissue destruction are released, possibly resulting in cardiac arrest and dysrhythmias. (page 1565)

Skill Drills

1. Controlling Bleeding From a Soft-Tissue Injury (Chapter 30, page 1531)

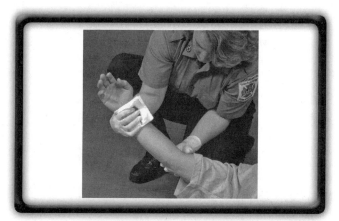

Step 1: Apply direct pressure over the wound with a dry, sterile dressing. Elevate the injury if no fracture is suspected.

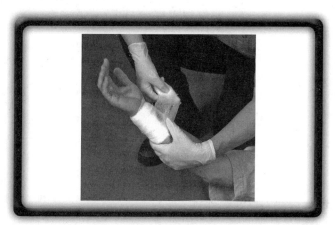

Step 2: Apply a pressure dressing.

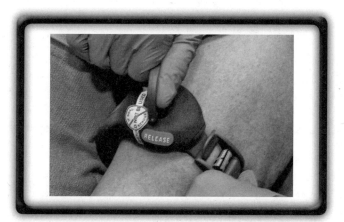

Step 3: If direct pressure with a pressure dressing does not rapidly control bleeding on an extremity, apply a tourniquet above the level of bleeding.

Chapter 32: Burns

Matching

Part I

1. (page 1585)

(1) A

(2) A

(3) B

(4) A

(5) B

(6) A

(7) A

(8) A

2. (1) D. Put out the fire.

(2) C. Open the airway manually.

(3) A. Administer supplemental oxygen.

(4) H. Intubate the trachea (if a BLS airway is not adequate).

(5) F. Pass a nasogastric tube into his stomach.

(6) B. Start an IV.

(7) J. Obtain a set of baseline vital signs.

(8) E. Remove the patient's clothing.

(9) G. Determine the extent and depth of the burn.

(10) I. Cover the burns with sterile dressings.

Part II

(page 1605)

1. F	**2.** I	**3.** J	**4.** E	**5.** H
6. D	**7.** B	**8.** C	**9.** A	**10.** G

Multiple Choice

1. D (page 1598)	**2.** B (page 1599)	**3.** A (page 1584)	**4.** C (page 1580)	**5.** B (page 1584)
6. C (page 1587)	**7.** D (page 1588)	**8.** A (page 1589)	**9.** B (page 1591)	**10.** C (page 1597)

Labeling

1. The Skin

(page 1577)

A. Hair

B. Pore

C. Sebaceous gland

D. Nerve (sensory)

E. Sweat gland

F. Hair follicle

G. Blood vessel

H. Subcutaneous fat

I. Muscle

2. Burn Severity

(page 1580)

A. Partial-thickness burn

B. Superficial burn

C. Full-thickness burn

Fill-in-the-Blank

1. skin (page 1575)
2. dermis (page 1576)
3. scald (page 1578)
4. acids; alkalis; bases (page 1590)
5. Oxidizing agents (page 1591)
6. scene is safe (page 1599)
7. alpha; beta; gamma (page 1599)
8. zone of coagulation (page 1606)
9. dry dressing (page 1590)
10. decontaminated (page 1600)

Identify

1. Chief complaint: Woman burned by oil from a hot fryer. Upon arrival, you find her with holes in her jeans on the top of both thighs. She is crying and immediately rates her pain as unbearable.
2. Vital signs: Respirations are 22 breaths/min, oxygen saturation is 97%, lungs are clear, blood pressure is 150/100 mm Hg, pulse is 114 beats/min with sinus tachycardia, skin is cool, pain is 10/10, patient is alert × 3.
3. Pertinent negatives: Airway is open, patient does not have any mental deficits, there are no burns other than on the top of her thighs.

Complete the Patient Care Report (PCR)

Show the completed PCR to your instructor to obtain feedback on your completion of the form.

Ambulance Calls

1. The patient who jumped from his bedroom window to escape a fire is in grave jeopardy. He is unconscious, so his airway is liable to be obstructed. He may have additional respiratory injury (note the burns to his face), along with head and neck injuries (note the mechanisms of injury). And he almost certainly has at least one broken bone. The steps in treating him are as follows:
    a. Put out the fire in his pants!
    b. Open his airway with cervical spine precautions (ie, chin lift or jaw thrust only).
    c. Administer supplemental oxygen—he's been in a smoky environment.
    d. Intubate the trachea. This patient is unconscious, so his airway is already in jeopardy. In addition, he has almost certainly sustained airway injury—note the singed beard and swollen lips—so don't wait until laryngeal edema closes off his airway altogether. Get the endotracheal tube in while it's still relatively easy to do so.
    e. Cut away the pants, and perform the secondary trauma assessment. In doing so, you should evaluate the extent, depth, and severity of the burn.
    f. Cover the burns with sterile dressings.
    g. Splint the left leg and any other fractures; immobilize the patient on a backboard. (He fell from 15 feet, so you have to assume until proved otherwise that he injured his spine.)
    h. Start an IV (can be done en route to hospital). *Note:* The precise time at which you start the IV will be determined by the patient's overall condition and the amount of help you have at the scene. If the patient is in shock, start the IV as soon as you have managed the airway. (pages 1587–1589)
2. Among the questions you would like answered about the burned patient are the following:
    a. When precisely did the burn occur? (That is, when did the fire break out?)
    b. Was the patient in a closed space with smoke or other products of combustion?
    c. Does the patient have any significant underlying medical problems?
    d. Does the patient take any medications regularly? Had he taken any drugs or alcohol within the past few hours?
    e. Does the patient have any allergies?
    You already know the answers to most of the other questions you would usually ask. You can assume that the patient did not lose consciousness while still in the burning building because he managed to jump out the window. You know what he was burned with (flame). And you know that nothing was done until the ambulance arrived. It would, however, be helpful to question the fire personnel regarding toxic products of combustion to which the patient might have been exposed.

3. **a.** The burn on the right arm is probably a **partial thickness (second-degree)** burn. The severe pain virtually rules out a third-degree burn, and the mottling suggests it is more serious than a superficial (first-degree) burn. The appropriate treatment is to **cover the burn with cool, wet, sterile dressings**. If the application of cool dressings is not sufficient to relieve the patient's pain, it may be necessary to give him a small dose of morphine in addition.

   b. The burn on the flank is probably a **superficial (first-degree)** burn, although it could also be partial thickness (it will be impossible to tell for sure until at least another few hours). **Treat it as you would treat a partial-thickness burn** because it might well be one.

   c. The burn on the right leg is probably a **full-thickness (third-degree)** burn. The leathery appearance, thrombosed veins, and absence of sensation are all characteristic. **Cover the burn with a dry sterile dressing.** (page 1580)

4. Electric burns can be very deceptive because the extent of injury may not be at all apparent from the burn that is visible on the surface of the body.

   a. The three types of *burns* that may occur from electricity are:

   (1) A contact burn, which usually produces a bull's-eye lesion at the point of entry and sometimes also at the point of exit

   (2) A flash burn, an electrothermal injury caused by the arcing of electric current

   (3) A flame burn, which occurs if the electricity ignites a person's clothing or surroundings (page 1596)

   b. Besides burns, electricity may cause a variety of other injuries or disorders of function, including the following:

   (1) Respiratory arrest

   (2) Cardiac arrest

   (3) Neurologic disorders (seizures, coma, paralysis)

   (4) Kidney damage

   (5) Fractures and dislocations

   (6) Cervical spine injuries (pages 1596–1597)

   c. In dealing with this electrocuted patient lying beside a live cable, you need to take the following steps:

   (1) Secure the scene. Keep all bystanders well back from the live wire. Do not get within reach of the wire if you are not fully trained and fully equipped to deal with power lines. Radio for help, and do not get within range of the wire until it has been inactivated. If you have some creative idea for extricating the patient that does not require your coming within range of the cable (eg, lassoing him and dragging him toward you), you may try such a method, but bear in mind that the patient may have a spinal injury.

   (2) As soon as it is safe to approach the patient, ensure that he has an open airway, taking precautions not to hyperextend his neck.

   (3) Provide artificial ventilation or cardiopulmonary resuscitation (CPR) as needed.

   (4) Administer supplemental oxygen.

   (5) If the patient remains unconscious, intubate the trachea (if a BLS airway is not adequate).

   (6) Start an IV, and run in normal saline solution as fast as the IV will flow.

   (7) Consult the base physician for medication orders.

   (8) Cover burns with a sterile dressing.

   (9) Splint fractures.

   (10) Immobilize the spine on a backboard. (page 1597)

5. In this question, a young man was rescued unconscious from a house fire.

   a. Signs suggestive of respiratory injury (airway involvement) in a burned patient include the following:

   (1) Hoarseness

   (2) Cough

   (3) Singed nasal or facial hairs

   (4) Facial burns

   (5) Carbon in the sputum

   (6) History of burn in an enclosed space (page 1583)

   b. The first step to take in managing this patient is to *put out the fire* in his clothing! (page 1583)

   c. (1) To calculate the extent of his burns, you need to use a combination of the rule of nines and the rule of palms (page 1584):

   Posterior surface of both legs: 18%

Whole left arm: 9%

Hand-sized patch of left flank: 1%

TOTAL: 28%

(2) Yes, the patient does have a critical burn on at least three counts:

(a) He has full-thickness burns over more than 10% of his body.

(b) He has burns of all depths or thicknesses over more than 25% of his body.

(c) He has burns involving the genitals.

d. The Consensus formula states that during the *first 8 hours* the patient should receive (page 1588):

$$8 \text{ mL/hr} = \tfrac{1}{2} \times 4 \text{ mL/kg body weight} \times \% \text{ body surface burned}$$

For this patient, that means:

$$8 \text{ mL/hr} = \tfrac{1}{2} \times 4 \text{ mL} \times 70 \text{ kg} \times 28 = 3{,}920 \text{ Ml}$$

Therefore, during each hour, the patient needs to receive

$$\text{mL/hr} = \frac{3{,}920 \text{ mL}}{8 \text{ hr}} = 490 \text{ mL/hr}$$

$$\text{mL/min} = \frac{490 \text{ mL}}{60 \text{ min/hr}} = 8 \text{ mL/min}$$

$$\text{gtt/min} = 8 \text{ mL/min} \times 10 \text{ gtt/mL} = \textbf{80 gtt/min}$$

e. (1) The dosage of morphine usually given to an adult in the field is **5 mg (may be as high as 10 to 20 mg)**.

(2) It is usually given **intravenously** because absorption after intramuscular administration may be erratic if the patient has any perfusion problems.

(3) Possible *adverse side effects* include the following (*students should provide three of the following*):

(a) Hypotension

(b) Bradycardia

(c) Respiratory depression

(d) Nausea and vomiting (pages 1588–1589)

6. a. This patient clearly has a serious chest injury. Furthermore, the chest injury is increasing venous pressure. The combination of dyspnea, shock, and distended neck veins is highly suggestive of tension pneumothorax, so you need to proceed as follows:

b. (1) Administer 100% supplemental oxygen by nonrebreathing mask.

(2) Look for deviation of the trachea, and listen for breath sounds on both sides of the chest. *If breath sounds are unequal:*

(3) Decompress the chest with a 14-gauge cannula in the second intercostal space in the midclavicular line.

(4) Immobilize the patient on a long backboard.

(5) Start transport to a trauma center.

(6) Start at least one large-bore IV en route. (Chapter 35, pages 1708–1712)

7. a. The percentage of the patient's body that is burned is (page 1584):

Entire left leg: 18%

Posterior right leg: 9%

Left forearm: 4%

TOTAL: **31%**

b. Yes, the patient has a critical burn, which we know for two reasons:

(1) The burn covers more than 25% of the body surface.

(2) The burn involves the genitals.

c. If the pedal pulses are absent in a burned leg, you have to assume that swelling from circumferential burns has cut off the circulation to the foot. If you do not act quickly in such a situation, the patient may lose his leg.

d. You need to cool the burned leg with towels that have been soaked in cold water and transport the patient immediately to the hospital.

True/False

The principles of treating chemical burns do not differ significantly from those of treating thermal burns. In both cases, the first priority is to *put out the fire*, but in a chemical burn, putting out the fire is a more difficult and time-consuming operation.

1. F (page 1592)　**2.** T (page 1592)　**3.** F (pages 1591–1592)　**4.** F (pages 1592–1593)　**5.** T (page 1594)

6. T (page 1578)　**7.** T (page 1575)　**8.** F (page 1581)　**9.** T (page 1596)　**10.** F (page 1583)

Short Answer

1. a. Rule 1: Never be the tallest object. Stay out of the middle of open fields or open areas. Don't use ladders, umbrellas, or anything else that makes you taller. Make yourself as small as possible.

b. Rule 2: Never stand under or near the tallest object that is a good conductor. Stay away from trees, metal umbrellas, or towers of any kind.

c. Rule 3: Take shelter in the most substantial structure in which you will be safe if it is hit by lighting. Try to get in an enclosed building if possible. A small metal shed probably would not be a good idea.

d. Rule 4: Avoid touching a good conductor during a lightning storm. This can apply to things inside your home such as the TV, telephone, and computer. (page 1598)

2. Suspect that a victim of flame burns has suffered respiratory injury (airway involvement) if any of the following signs are present (page 1583):

a. Hoarseness

b. Cough

c. Singed nasal or facial hair

d. Facial burns

e. Carbon in the sputum

f. History of burn in an enclosed space

3. Injury from a high-voltage electric source or from lightning may produce any of the following (pages 1596–1598):

a. Asphyxia to apnea

b. Peripheral nerve deficits

c. Cardiac arrest

d. Fracture and/or spine injury if the patient has fallen

e. Kidney damage

f. Cataracts

g. Exit wound

h. Seizures

i. Delirium, confusion, or coma

j. Severe tetanic muscle spasms

Fill-in-the-Table

(page 1589)

Consensus Formula Chart									
% Burn	**10 kg**	**20 kg**	**30 kg**	**40 kg**	**50 kg**	**60 kg**	**70 kg**	**80 kg**	**90 kg**	**100 kg**
10	25	**50**	**75**	100	125	150	175	**200**	225	250
20	50	**100**	**150**	200	250	300	350	**400**	450	500
30	75	**150**	**225**	300	375	450	525	**600**	675	750
40	100	**200**	**300**	400	500	600	700	**800**	900	1,000
50	125	**250**	**375**	500	625	750	875	**1,000**	1,125	1,250
60	150	**300**	**450**	600	750	900	1,050	**1,200**	1,350	1,500
70	175	**350**	**525**	700	875	1,050	1,225	**1,400**	1,575	1,750
80	200	**400**	**600**	800	1,000	1,200	1,400	**1,600**	1,800	2,000
90	225	**450**	**675**	900	1,125	1,350	1,575	**1,800**	2,025	2,250
20 mL/kg	200	**400**	**600**	800	1,000	1,200	1,400	**1,600**	1,800	2,000

Problem Solving

1. To calculate the patient's fluid needs, first you must assess the extent of his burns. Then, you can calculate the IV rate in the usual fashion.

   a. The percentage of the patient's body that has been burned is calculated as follows (page 1584):

      Whole right leg: 18%

      Anterior left leg: 9%

      Anterior trunk: 18%

      Whole right arm: 9%

      TOTAL: **54%**

   b. Now you have to calculate the patient's fluid needs. First, you must convert his weight from pounds to kilograms (page 1588):

      $$\frac{154\ lb}{2.2\ lb/kg} = \textbf{70 kg}$$

      Now, according to the Parkland (Consensus) formula, the patient's fluid needs over the first 8 hours will be:

      ½ × 4 mL/kg body weight × % of body surface burned

      ½ × 4 mL × 70 kg × 54 = 7,560 mL

      So his fluid needs *per hour* will be:

      $$\frac{7,560\ mL}{8\ hr} = \textbf{945 mL/hr}$$

      (Practically speaking, that figure can be regarded as equivalent to 1 liter per hour, but you should complete the calculations using the precise figures.)

      Thus, you will need to deliver:

      $$\frac{945\ mL/hr}{60\ min/hr} = 15.8\ mL/min\ (ie,\ \textbf{16 mL/min})$$

   c. If your infusion set delivers 10 gtt per milliliter, you therefore need to set the rate of the infusion at:

      10 gtt/mL × 16 mL/min = **160 gtt/min**

      We included this question to give you a little practice in computing IV rates—just in case you were getting rusty. In this particular case, however, it is an academic exercise only because to deliver the kind of volumes we are talking about—nearly 1 liter per hour—you will have to run the IV wide open, probably under pressure. Usually, when volumes of this sort are required, it makes more sense to start a second and even a third IV line.

   d. For a burned patient, give an IV fluid that will remain in the vascular space, such as normal saline solution. (page 1589)

Chapter 33: Face and Neck Trauma

Matching

(page 1639)

1. K	**2.** J	**3.** L	**4.** I	**5.** M	**6.** H	**7.** N	**8.** G	**9.** O	**10.** F
11. P	**12.** E	**13.** Q	**14.** D	**15.** R	**16.** C	**17.** S	**18.** B	**19.** T	**20.** A

Multiple Choice

1. C (page 1609)	**2.** B (page 1609)	**3.** A (page 1612)	**4.** B (page 1612)	**5.** D (page 1612)
6. B (page 1613)	**7.** A (page 1619)	**8.** B (page 1626)	**9.** C (page 1618)	**10.** B (page 1619)
11. C (page 1623)	**12.** B (page 1625)	**13.** B (page 1626)	**14.** D (page 1628)	**15.** A (page 1633)

Labeling

1. Structures of the Eye (page 1612)
   A. Iris
   B. Cornea
   C. Pupil
   D. Lens
   E. Sclera
   F. Retina
   G. Optic nerve
2. Structures of the Anterior Neck (page 1614)
   A. Thyroid cartilage
   B. Cricoid cartilage
   C. Cricothyroid membrane
   D. Trachea
   E. Sternocleidomastoid muscle
   F. Carotid arteries
3. Arteries of the Neck (page 1615)
   A. Internal carotid
   B. Carotid sinus
   C. Vertebral
   D. Subclavian
   E. Facial
   F. External carotid
   G. Superior thyroid
   H. Common carotid
   I. Brachiocephalic

Fill-in-the-Blank

1. whiplash (page 1635)
2. strain (page 1635)
3. blowout (page 1610)
4. pupil (page 1611)
5. posterior chamber (page 1611)
6. lacrimal apparatus (page 1611)
7. central; peripheral (page 1611)
8. inner ear (page 1612)

9. airway (page 1621)
10. hyphema (page 1622)
11. Chemicals; heat; light (page 1623)
12. 20 (page 1627)
13. chemical burn (page 1628)
14. hour (page 1630)
15. occlusive (page 1633)
16. spinal clearance (page 1634)
17. blood (page 1630)
18. sympathetic eye movement (page 1626)
19. never exert pressure on (page 1626)
20. craniofacial disjunction (page 1619)

Identify

1. Chief complaint: A head injury and severe facial injuries caused by the rollover and ejection from the vehicle
2. Vital signs: She presents with decerebrate posturing and unresponsiveness; GCS score is 8; respirations are 34 breaths/min and deep; oxygen saturation is 95%; pupils are sluggish; blood pressure is 160/90 mm/Hg; pulse is 72 beats/min; and skin is cool.
3. Pertinent negatives: No outward bleeding aside from the face
4. This girl has an obvious head injury. A trauma center will have a neurosurgeon on hand to treat her. A community hospital would be able only to try to stabilize her and then ship her to a trauma center. She does not have that much time. The Golden Hour rules that this patient needs surgery within an hour of the incident.
5. She has severe facial fractures, and the blood in her airway can easily be vomited or aspirated so the airway must be positioned properly (jaw thrust) and suctioned to remain clear.
6. The rising blood pressure; slowing heart rate; and deep, fast respirations are classic Cushing triad, which indicates a rising intracranial pressure.

Ambulance Calls

1. If you are able to salvage this young woman's lost tooth, you will have made a friend for life.
   a. Locate the tooth.
   b. Handle the tooth by the crown only. Do not touch the root surface of the tooth.
   c. Rinse the tooth and the empty socket with sterile saline or water (do not allow it to dry).
   d. Carefully place the tooth back in the socket.
   e. Once the tooth is in place, have the patient gently bite down on a gauze roll to maintain pressure against the tooth. (page 1631)
2. A thorough examination of an injured eye includes assessment of:
   a. The orbital rim for ecchymosis, swelling, laceration, and tenderness
   b. The eyelids for ecchymosis, swelling, and lacerations
   c. The corneas for foreign bodies
   d. The conjunctivae for redness, foreign bodies, inflammation, and pus
   e. The globes for redness, abnormal pigmentation, and lacerations
   f. The pupils for size, shape, equality, and reaction to light (PEARRL)
   g. Eye movements in all directions, for evidence of paralysis of gaze or no coordination between the movements of the two eyes
   h. Most important of all, visual acuity (page 1625)

3. a. The principal dangers associated with a laceration of the neck are massive hemorrhage from major blood vessel disruption, airway compromise secondary to soft-tissue swelling, or direct damage to the larynx or trachea. Fatal air embolism is also considered a special danger.

    b. Open neck wounds should be sealed with an occlusive dressing immediately. (page 1633)

True/False

1. F (page 1609)   **2.** T (page 1610)   **3.** F (page 1610)   **4.** T (page 1612)   **5.** F (page 1613)

6. T (page 1618)   **7.** F (page 1619)   **8.** T (page 1619)   **9.** F (page 1611)   **10.** T (page 1620)

11. F (page 1620)   **12.** T (page 1623)   **13.** F (page 1626)   **14.** T (page 1622)   **15.** T (page 1630)

16. T (page 1632)   **17.** F (page 1633)   **18.** T (page 1633)   **19.** T (page 1629)   **20.** F (page 1629)

Short Answer

1. a. Closed head injury

    b. Cervical spine injury (page 1618)

2. *Students should provide five of the following:*

    a. Swelling of the face

    b. Ecchymosis over the face

    c. Crepitus over a broken bone

    d. Pain to palpation

    e. Instability of the facial bones

    f. Impaired ocular movement

    g. Malocclusion in cases where the jaw is fractured

    h. Visual disturbances

    i. Obvious deformity of the face (eg, flattening of one side) (page 1618)

Fill-in the Table

1. Summary of Maxillofacial Fractures (page 1620)

Summary of Maxillofacial Fractures	
Injury	**Signs and Symptoms**
Multiple facial bone fractures	• Massive facial swelling • **Dental malocclusion** • **Palpable deformities** • Anterior or **posterior** epistaxis
Zygomatic and orbital fractures	• Loss of sensation below the **orbit** • Flattening of the **patient's cheek** • **Paralysis** of upward gaze
Nasal fractures	• Crepitus and instability • Swelling, tenderness, **lateral displacement** • Anterior or **posterior** epistaxis
Maxillary (Le Fort) fractures	• Mobility of the **midface** • Dental **malocclusion** • Facial swelling
Mandibular fractures	• Dental malocclusion • **Mandibular** instability

2. Signs and Symptoms of Injuries to the Anterior Part of the Neck
   (page 1633)

Signs and Symptoms of Injuries to the Anterior Part of the Neck	
Injury	**Signs and Symptoms**
Laryngeal fracture, tracheal transection	• Labored breathing or reduced **air movement** • Stridor • Hoarseness, voice changes • **Hemoptysis** (coughing up blood) • Subcutaneous emphysema • Swelling, edema • Structural irregularity
Vascular injury	• **Gross external** bleeding • Signs of shock • Hematoma, swelling, edema • **Pulse** deficits
Esophageal perforation	• **Dysphagia** (difficulty swallowing) • **Hematemesis** • **Hemoptysis** (suggests aspiration of blood)
Neurologic impairment	• Signs of a stroke (suggests air embolism or **cerebral infarct**) • **Paralysis** or paresthesia • **Cranial** nerve deficit • Signs of **neurogenic** shock

Chapter 34: Head and Spine Trauma

Matching

Part I

1. CC (page 1688)	**2.** A (page 1688)	**3.** DD (page 1688)	**4.** B (page 1688)	**5.** BB (page 1688)
6. C (page 1688)	**7.** AA (page 1689)	**8.** D (page 1689)	**9.** Z (page 1689)	**10.** E (page 1689)
11. Y (page 1689)	**12.** F (page 1689)	**13.** X (page 1689)	**14.** G (page 1689)	**15.** W (page 1689)
16. H (page 1689)	**17.** V (page 1689)	**18.** I (page 1689)	**19.** U (page 1689)	**20.** J (page 1689)
21. T (page 1689)	**22.** O (page 1690)	**23.** P (page 1690)	**24.** N (page 1690)	**25.** Q (page 1690)
26. M (page 1690)	**27.** R (page 1690)	**28.** L (page 1690)	**29.** S (page 1690)	**30.** K (page 1690)

Part II

1. C (page 1666)	**2.** A (page 1665)	**3.** B (page 1666)	**4.** D (page 1667)	**5.** C (page 1666)
6. C (page 1666)	**7.** A (page 1665)	**8.** B (page 1666)	**9.** E (page 1668)	**10.** F (page 1668)

Multiple Choice

1. D (page 1644)	**2.** C (page 1647)	**3.** B (page 1645)	**4.** B (page 1646)	**5.** D (page 1647)
6. C (page 1663)	**7.** D (page 1665)	**8.** B (page 1666)	**9.** B (page 1668)	**10.** C (page 1668)
11. D (page 1659)	**12.** A (page 1653)	**13.** B (page 1650)	**14.** C (page 1650)	**15.** A (page 1650)
16. B (page 1652)	**17.** A (page 1652)	**18.** C (page 1673)	**19.** D (page 1674)	**20.** A (page 1676)
21. B (page 1681)	**22.** D (page 1662)			

Labeling

1. Structures of the Cervical, Thoracic, and Lumbar Spine (page 1652)
   - **A.** Cervical plexus (C1–C5): Innervates the diaphragm
   - **B.** Brachial plexus (C5–T1): Controls the upper extremities
   - **C.** Lumbar plexus (L1–L4): Supplies the skin and muscles of the abdominal wall, external genitalia, and part of the lower limbs
   - **D.** Sacral plexus (L4–S4): Supplies the buttocks, perineum, and most of the lower limbs
2. Layers of the Spinal Cord (page 1651)
   - **A.** Central canal
   - **B.** Gray matter
   - **C.** White matter
   - **D.** Spinal cord
   - **E.** Pia mater
   - **F.** Subarachnoid space
   - **G.** Arachnoid
   - **H.** Ventral root
   - **I.** Dorsal root ganglion
   - **J.** Subdural space
   - **K.** Dura mater
   - **L.** Spinal nerve
3. Major Regions of the Brain (page 1647)
   - **A.** Hypothalamus
   - **B.** Thalamus
   - **C.** Meninges
   - **D.** Corpus callosum
   - **E.** Skull
   - **F.** Spinal cord
   - **G.** Medulla
   - **H.** Pons
   - **I.** Midbrain

Fill-in-the-Blank

1. axial (page 1644)
2. fontanelles (page 1644)
3. cerebrum (page 1645)
4. pons; medulla (page 1647)
5. arachnoid (page 1648)
6. coup-contrecoup (page 1664)
7. hypertension; Cushing triad (page 1665)
8. epidural (page 1666)
9. rapid sequence intubation (page 1653)
10. body temperature (page 1669)
11. lamina; pedicles (page 1649)
12. C1; C2 (page 1670)
13. brain; spinal cord (page 1644)
14. medulla; pons; midbrain (page 1647)
15. foramen magnum (page 1650)
16. hypothalamus (page 1651)
17. Complete (page 1672)
18. neurogenic shock (page 1673)
19. jaw-thrust (page 1653)
20. downward; upward (page 1661)

Identify

Part I

1. Chief complaint: A head injury caused by the rollover and ejection from the vehicle
2. Vital signs: Patient presents with decerebrate posturing and unresponsiveness; GCS score is 7; respirations are 34 breaths/min and deep; oxygen saturation is 98%; pupils are sluggish; blood pressure is 160/90 mm/Hg; pulse is 64 beats/min; and skin is cool.
3. Pertinent negatives: No outward bleeding
4. This girl has an obvious head injury. A trauma center will have a neurosurgeon on hand to treat her. A community hospital would be able only to try to stabilize her and then ship her to a trauma center. She does not have that much time. The Golden Hour rules that this patient needs surgery within an hour of the incident.
5. She is in decerebrate posturing. This indicates that she already has swelling or bleeding inside the brain that is causing this posture. The pressure is already building on the middle brainstem.
6. The rising blood pressure, slowing heart rate, and deep, fast respirations are classic Cushing triad, which indicates a rising ICP.

Part II

1. Chief complaint: Multiple trauma
2. Vital signs: Patient is V in AVPU, GCS score is 9, skin is cool, blood pressure is 100/62 mm/Hg, pulse is 124 beats/min with sinus tachycardia, oxygen saturation is 96%, respirations are 26 breaths/min.
3. Pertinent negatives: Lungs are clear, no feeling or response in lower extremities

   The chief complaint in this case study is multiple trauma caused by a rollover crash. She is responding to voice and can answer only what her name is. Thus, you can call her a V on the AVPU scale and close to a 9 on the GCS scale because of the inability to move her legs. Your patient is hypothermic by touch. Blood pressure is 100/62 mm Hg, and pulse is 124 beats/min with sinus tachycardia on the monitor. Oxygen saturation is 96% but comes up to 98% with 100% oxygen. Her breathing rate is 26 breaths/min and shallow. Lungs are clear. The absence of a pulse in either foot could be caused by the hypothermia. She has no feeling or response in her lower extremities. Blood pressure comes up slightly with a warm fluid bolus, which also helps to warm her. Second blood pressure is 108/64 mm Hg. You did your job by stabilizing her and securing her neck and body to the backboard. The physician later tells you the break was very bad, and there was nothing else you could have done to help her.

Complete the Patient Care Report (PCR)

Show the completed PCR to your instructor to obtain feedback on your completion of the form.

Ambulance Calls

1. a. The bad guy probably has a severe injury to the larynx, such as a laryngeal "fracture," as evidenced by the bruise over his throat, his hoarseness, and his subcutaneous emphysema. Furthermore, given the mechanisms of injury, one has to assume that he has a cervical spine injury as well.

   b. The steps of treatment are as follows:

      (1) Administer 100% oxygen, and instruct the patient to breathe slowly (rapid inhalation may cause an unstable trachea to collapse inward). It is preferable to avoid intubating the patient in the field, but if the airway becomes compromised further, you may have no choice.

      (2) Immobilize the spine by immobilizing the whole patient on a long backboard.

      (3) Transport the patient immediately, preferably to a major trauma center.

2. a. The boy has a sensory level around T8 and intact motor function at least from T1 upward. You can assume that his injury is no higher than T8.

   b. The boy's hypotension could mean either neurogenic shock or hypovolemic shock. It is very difficult, if not impossible, to distinguish between the two under these circumstances because if the sympathetic nervous system has been disrupted by the spinal cord injury, you will not see the usual signs of shock, such as sweating and tachycardia. Furthermore, the boy's sensory deficit may mask pain from damage to intra-abdominal structures. So, when you encounter shock in such circumstances, you have to treat it as hypovolemic shock until proved otherwise.

3. In this question about a head-injured patient, you had to review some respiratory physiology along with the pathophysiology of head injury.

   a. If the patient's respiratory rate is 8 breaths/min and his tidal volume is 500 mL, his minute volume is calculated as follows:

Minute Volume = Tidal Volume × Respiratory Rate

                   = 500 mL/breath × 8 breaths/min

                   = 4,000 mL/min (4 L/min)

   b. That minute volume is less than normal. (Normal is around 6 L/min.)

   c. Therefore, you can conclude that the patient's arterial PCO_2 will tend to **increase**, so his pH will **decrease**. The net effect will be an acid–base disorder called a **respiratory acidosis**. The way you can help correct that abnormality is to **assist the patient's ventilations and thereby increase his minute volume (which will blow off more carbon dioxide)**.

   d. The signs of increasing ICP include the following (*students should provide five of the following*):

      (1) Vomiting

      (2) Headache

      (3) Altered level of consciousness

      (4) Seizures

      (5) Hypertension with a widening pulse pressure

      (6) Bradycardia

      (7) Irregular respirations

      (8) Unequal and nonreactive pupil

      (9) Coma

     (10) Posturing (page 1659)

   e. (1) The patient's AVPU rating is P (responds only to painful stimuli).

      (2) His score on the GCS is 8 points. (page 1659)

4. It should be clear, after carrying out this exercise, that the GCS enables a much more precise description than does the AVPU rating of the patient's level of consciousness. (page 1659)

    a. AVPU: somewhere between V and P

        GCS: 10

    b. AVPU: V

        GCS: 13

    c. AVPU: somewhere between P and U

        GCS: 5

    d. AVPU: A

        GSC: 15

5. In treating the victim of the whiskey bottle, how well did you remember your priorities?

    a. Eliminate the safety hazard. So long as there are tables and chairs being launched into orbit, you and everyone else in the bar are in danger. Try to get all bystanders to leave the premises (call in police help if needed). First priority is scene safety, and then, from a safe distance, see if you can calm the patient. Explain that you are paramedics and that you have come to help him. Such an explanation is often of particular importance in municipalities where paramedics wear uniforms that could be mistaken for police uniforms (a very dangerous practice!).

    b. When you are reasonably certain that it is safe to approach the patient, encourage him to sit down, and examine his scalp by palpating the scalp wound lightly with a gloved finger to make certain that the skull beneath the wound is not fractured.

    c. If there is no evidence of skull fracture, control scalp bleeding by direct manual pressure, and apply a pressure dressing.

    d. Complete the secondary assessment, and manage any other injuries detected thereby.

True/False

    1. F (page 1644)   **2.** T (page 1644)   **3.** F (page 1647)   **4.** T (page 1645)   **5.** T (page 1646)

    6. F (page 1647)   **7.** T (page 1648)   **8.** T (page 1662)   **9.** T (page 1665)   **10.** F (page 1665)

    11. T (page 1668) **12.** T (page 1648)   **13.** F (page 1650) **14.** T (page 1651) **15.** T (page 1670)

    16. F (page 1671) **17.** F (page 1672)   **18.** T (page 1650) **19.** F (page 1654) **20.** F (page 1660)

    21. F (page 1674) **22.** T (pages 1674–1677) **23.** F (page 1676) **24.** F (page 1676) **25.** F (pages 1678–1679)

    26. T (page 1683)

Short Answer

    1. *Students should list eight of the following:*

    a. High-velocity crash (> 40 mph) with severe vehicle damage

    b. Unrestrained occupant of moderate- to high-speed motor vehicle crash

    c. Vehicular damage with compartmental intrusion (12 inches) into the patient's seating space

    d. Fall from three times the patient's height

    e. Penetrating trauma near the spine

    f. Ejection from a motor vehicle

    g. Motorcycle crash at greater than 20 mph with separation of driver from bike

    h. Diving injury

    i. Auto–pedestrian or auto–bicycle crash with greater than 5 mph impact

    j. Death of an occupant in the same passenger compartment

    k. Rollover crash (unrestrained) (page 1652)

  2. **D:** Deformity

    C: Contusion

    A: Abrasion

P: Puncture/penetration

B: Bruising

T: Tenderness

L: Laceration

S: Swelling

P: Pulse

M: Motor

S: Sensory

(page 1656)

Fill-in-the-Table

1. (page 1668)

Signs and Symptoms of Head Injury
Lacerations, contusions, or **hematomas** to the scalp
Soft area or **depression** noted on palpation of the scalp
Visible **fractures** or **deformities** of the skull
Battle sign or **raccoon** eyes
CSF rhinorrhea or **otorrhea**
Pupillary abnormalities • **Unequal** pupil size • Sluggish or **nonreactive** pupils
A period of unresponsiveness
Confusion or disorientation
Repeatedly asking the same question(s) (perseveration)
Amnesia (**retrograde** and/or **anterograde**)
Combativeness or other abnormal behavior
Numbness or tingling in the **extremities**
Loss of sensation and/or motor function
Focal **neurologic** deficits
Seizures
Cushing triad: hypertension, **bradycardia**, and irregular or erratic respirations
Dizziness
Visual disturbances, blurred vision, or double vision (**diplopia**)
Seeing "stars"
Nausea or vomiting
Posturing (**decorticate** and/or **decerebrate**)

2. (page 1659)

Glasgow Coma Scale		
Test	**Response**	**Score**
Eye opening	Spontaneous Voice **Pain stimulation** None	4 3 2 1
Verbal	**Oriented** conversation **Confused** conversation **Inappropriate** words **Incomprehensible** sounds None	5 4 3 2 1
Motor	Obeys commands Localizes pain **Withdraws from pain** Abnormal flexion (**decorticate**) Abnormal **flexion** (decerebrate) None	6 5 4 3 2 1
Score: 15 indicates no neurologic disabilities. Score: 13-14 may indicate mild dysfunction. Score: 9-12 may indicate moderate dysfunction. Score: 8 or less is indicative of severe dysfunction.		

3. (page 1662)

Landmark Dermatomes			
Nerve Root	**Anatomic Location**	**Nerve Root**	**Anatomic Location**
C2	**Occipital protuberance**	T10	Umbilicus
C3	**Supraclavicular fossa**	L1	**Inguinal** line
C5	Lateral side of **antecubital fossa**	L2	Mid anterior thigh
C6	Thumb and medial index finger (6-shooter)	L3	Medial aspect of the **knee**
C7	**Middle** finger	L5	**Dorsum of the foot**
C8	**Little** finger	S1-S3	Back of **leg**
T2	**Apex of axilla**	S4-S5	**Perianal** area
T4	**Nipple** line		

Chapter 35: Chest Trauma

Matching

Part I
(page 1724)

1. K	**2.** M	**3.** L	**4.** O	**5.** N	**6.** R	**7.** Q	**8.** P	**9.** T	**10.** S
11. I	**12.** J	**13.** G	**14.** H	**15.** E	**16.** F	**17.** D	**18.** B	**19.** C	**20.** A

Part II

1. D (page 1712)   **2.** C (page 1709)   **3.** A (pages 1706–1707)   **4.** B (page 1707)   **5.** E (page 1705)

Part III

1. C (page 1698)   **2.** B (page 1698)   **3.** A (page 1698)   **4.** E (page 1697)   **5.** D (page 1698)

Multiple Choice

1. A (pages 1703–1704) **2.** C (page 1707)   **3.** B (page 1715)   **4.** C (pages 1700–1701)   **5.** D (page 1714)

6. A (page 1697)   **7.** B (pages 1713–1714) **8.** C (page 1707)   **9.** B (page 1708)   **10.** D (page 1710)

Labeling

1. The Thorax (page 1696)
   A. Thoracic inlet
   B. Clavicle
   C. Pericardium
   D. Suprasternal notch
   E. Manubrium
   F. Angle of louis
   G. Body of sternum
   H. Xiphoid process
   I. Heart
   J. Lung
   K. Pleura
   L. Diaphragm
   M. Scapula
   N. Ribs
   O. Intercostal space

Fill-in-the-Table

1. The MOIs, or easily detected injuries, may give clues to the presence of injuries that are harder to find.

If you find:	The patient may have:
1. Steering wheel imprint on anterior chest	**Myocardial contusion (page 1715)** **Cardiac tamponade (page 1713)** **Aortic rupture (page 1716)** **Pneumothorax or hemothorax (pages 1706, 1712)** **Tracheobronchial injury (page 1719)**
2. Caved-in door on driver's side	**Diaphragmatic tear (page 1718)**
3. Fall from a height	**Thoracic aortic dissection/transaction (page 1716)** **Pulmonary contusion (page 1712)**
4. Bullet entrance wound in fifth left intercostal space	**Cardiac tamponade (page 1713)** **Injury to liver, spleen, stomach, lungs (look for exit wound)**
5. Fracture of ribs 5-7 in a young man	**Pulmonary contusion (page 1712)** **Pneumothorax and/or hemothorax (pages 1706, 1712)**
6. Fracture of first and second ribs	**Major vascular injury (page 1717)** **Hemothorax (page 1712)**

Identify

1. a. Chief complaint: Patient's chest hurts.

   b. Physical findings: Patient is verbal and has bruising on the lower chest, diaphoresis, cyanosis dyspnea, equal bilateral breath sounds, tachycardia, weak peripheral pulses, hypotension, and electrical alternans.

   c. Signs of Beck triad: Muffled heart tones, hypotension, and jugular vein distention.

   d. The patient most likely has pericardial (cardiac) tamponade. (pages 1713–1714)

2. a. Physical findings: Crackles, vital signs are within normal limits, an ECG shows ischemic changes, and no other signs of hypovolemia.

   b. Spalding effect: You believe that the pressure waves generated by the blunt trauma disrupted the capillary-alveolar membrane.

   c. Inertial effects: The tissues accelerated and decelerated at different rates, causing a tear.

   d. Implosion: The pressure created by the trauma compresses the gases within the lung.

   e. Do not run the IV wide open. If the MOI suggests pulmonary contusion, be stingy with IV fluids unless there are signs of shock. (page 1713)

Ambulance Calls

1. In this case, you have a young woman who suffered unspecified deceleration injuries serious enough to render her unconscious. The damage to the car—a caved-in dashboard and smashed windshield—also hints at significant head and chest injury. (pages 1699–1703)

   a. The major threats to this woman's airway are the following:

      (1) Her tongue, which is liable to fall back against her posterior pharynx

      (2) Blood or broken teeth in her mouth

      (3) Vomitus

      (4) Possible injury to the airway (eg, ruptured larynx)

   b. In assessing the adequacy of her breathing, you must

      (1) LOOK for:

         (a) Signs of respiratory embarrassment (nasal flaring, intercostal or supraclavicular retractions)

         (b) Tracheal deviation

         (c) Obvious bruises or open wounds of the chest

         (d) Paradoxical movement of any part of the chest

      (2) LISTEN for:

         (a) Sucking chest wound

         (b) Inequality of breath sounds

         (c) Dullness or hyperresonance to percussion

      (3) FEEL for:

         (a) Tracheal deviation

         (b) Subcutaneous emphysema

         (c) Instability of the rib cage

   c. The steps that need to be taken immediately to ensure adequate breathing are as follows:

      (1) Suction out the mouth as needed.

      (2) Administer 100% supplemental oxygen.

   d. To evaluate and manage the circulation during the primary assessment, you must do the following:

      (1) Identify and control significant external bleeding.

      (2) Check the pulse (quality, rate, regularity, presence of paradoxus).

      (3) Note the skin CTC (ie, color, temperature, condition).

      (4) Check capillary refill if pediatric patient.

      (5) Assess neck veins for distention.

2. a. The patient who has a shotgun wound to the chest in a "friendly" encounter has an open pneumothorax (answer 3), indeed a quite significant one (a 2-inch hole would be hard not to notice!). The wound inflicted by a shotgun at close range is essentially a blast injury, and so you would expect in addition a considerable amount of damage to the lung tissue beneath, probably with disruption of major blood vessels as well. (pages 1706–1709)

    b. The steps in managing this patient are the following:

        (1) Make certain that the "friend" with the shotgun has left the scene or has been "neutralized" by police.

        (2) Seal the open chest wound with an occlusive dressing as quickly as possible. Tape the dressing on three sides only, so that air can escape from it during exhalation.

        (3) Administer 100% supplemental oxygen, preferably by nonrebreathing mask. Try to avoid giving oxygen under positive pressure.

        (4) Start transport.

        (5) Start an IV en route, with lactated Ringer's solution.

3. The elderly woman struck by a car has very well localized pain over the fifth right rib as well as diminished breath sounds and hyperresonance on that side of the chest. (pages 1705–1709)

    a. This woman probably has a rib fracture together with a simple pneumothorax on the right.

    b. The principal danger associated with rib fracture is the development of atelectasis because of the patient's reluctance to breathe deeply. Atelectasis, in turn, predisposes the patient to develop pneumonia.

    c. The treatment necessary in the field is as follows:

        (1) Administer 100% supplemental oxygen by nonrebreathing mask.

        (2) Encourage the patient to take periodic deep breaths; have her splint the fractured rib against a pillow each time she does so.

        (3) Given the MOIs, it would be a good idea as well to immobilize the spine.

    d. (1) When the patient becomes suddenly "shocky," while at the same time she shows signs of increased venous pressure (neck veins distended), she has probably developed a tension pneumothorax.

        (2) If you are more than 2 to 3 minutes from the hospital when that happens, stop the vehicle and decompress the chest with a needle.

4. All that the primary assessment has revealed to you about the man ejected from his convertible is that he has a partially obstructed airway, is bleeding, and is in shock and therefore is critically injured. In fact, that is all you need to know to start appropriate treatment. Although the following steps of treatment are listed in sequence, you will, in practice, have to accomplish the first few steps almost simultaneously. (pages 1699–1700)

    a. Open the airway by jaw thrust. As soon as the equipment to do so is available, suction out the mouth and pharynx.

    b. With the hand that is maintaining jaw thrust, seal off the bleeding wound of the neck. Apply a pressure dressing as soon as possible. Then, apply a pressure dressing to the scalp wound.

    c. Administer 100% supplemental oxygen as soon as it is available.

    d. Immobilize the spine.

    e. Start transport.

    f. Start at least one large-bore IV en route. Run it wide open.

    g. Monitor cardiac rhythm.

5. The clues to this patient's tension pneumothorax are the signs of shock in the face of distended neck veins and decreased breath sounds on one side. (pages 1708–1709)

    a. Steps to take at the scene:

        (1) Administer supplemental oxygen.

        (2) Decompress the chest with a cannula in the second right intercostal space, midclavicular line.

        (3) Immobilize the patient on a long backboard.

        (4) Communicate with medical control or receiving hospital.

    b. Steps to be taken en route:

        (1) Perform a detailed secondary assessment.

        (2) Start a large-bore IV with fluids.

        (3) Recheck vital and neurologic signs every 5 minutes.

6. Assessment (pages 1719–1720)

    a. Mental status (AVPU)

    b. Airway while providing manual stabilization

        (1) Check for obstructions.

    c. Breathing

        (1) Look for abnormal respirations.

        (2) Palpate chest (evidence of instability, crepitus, subcutaneous emphysema).

        (3) Look for jugular vein distention.

      (4) Auscultate lung sounds (note absent or decreased breath sounds).

      (5) Observe for signs and symptoms of hypoxia.

      (6) Check for signs of hypocarbia.

  d. Circulation

      (1) Examine for external bleeding.

      (2) Obtain a complete set of vital signs and oxygen saturation.

      (3) Look at and feel skin.

  e. Disability

      (1) Check extremities for pulses.

  f. History taking and secondary assessment (depending on the severity of the patient)

      (1) SAMPLE history

  g. Detailed secondary assessment with head-to-toe exam

Management (pages 1719–1720)

  a. Ensure the airway is maintained.

  b. Provide oxygen (consider the need for ventilatory assistance and endotracheal intubation).

  c. Consider the need for a needle decompression.

  d. Control any external bleeding.

  e. Take frequent vital signs.

  f. Attach patient to pulse oximeter and capnography if intubated.

  g. Monitor ECG.

  h. Complete cervical spine immobilization before transport.

7. In working out the answers to this question, you may have noticed that the mechanisms and signs of various chest injuries may be very similar to one another. If it is hard to distinguish such injuries in the relative calm and quiet of your study, consider how difficult it is at midnight in a ditch by the side of the interstate highway in the pouring rain—which is where you will inevitably be making such determinations.

  a. D. This patient's distended neck veins tell you that something is increasing pressure on the venae cavae. The two most likely possibilities are air in the pleural space or blood in the pericardium. Because the breath sounds are equal, the best bet is cardiac tamponade, and the apparent pulsus paradoxus supports that diagnosis. Under ideal conditions, you might also be able to appreciate that the heart sounds are muffled, but conditions in the field are seldom ideal, and even evaluating breath sounds is usually quite challenging. Steps of management:

      (1) Provide oxygen.

      (2) Start transport.

      (3) Monitor cardiac rhythm.

      (4) Start an IV with lactated Ringer's or normal saline en route. (pages 1713–1714)

  b. E. This is the classic picture of traumatic asphyxia, the so-called bloated frog appearance, and it bespeaks massive, often fatal chest injury. Steps of management:

      (1) Provide cervical spine precautions.

      (2) Establish an airway. Don't take time at the scene for endotracheal intubation unless absolutely necessary.

      (3) Administer 100% supplemental oxygen.

      (4) Start transport.

      (5) Start at least one IV en route. (pages 1719–1720)

  c. C. If a patient has three ribs broken in two places, it's a good bet he's got a flail chest. You may not actually be able to see the paradoxical movement of the chest, especially if the patient is conscious and splinting the injured part of the chest (which he will do automatically, to reduce the pain that breathing causes him). But the nature of the injury tells you that there probably is a flail, and the asymmetry of chest movements supports the hypothesis. Steps of management:

      (1) Administer 100% supplemental oxygen by nonrebreathing mask. Be prepared to intubate and provide positive pressure ventilations.

      (2) Splint the flail segment by having the patient hold a pillow against it or by taping the unstable segment to the adjacent stable segment.

      (3) Encourage the patient to take deep breaths. If he is unable to do so, assist ventilations gently with a bag-mask device. Be alert for pneumothorax.

      (4) Start transport.

(5) Monitor cardiac rhythm.

(6) Start an IV lifeline en route, at a keep-open rate. (pages 1703–1704)

   d. A. Here again, distended neck veins point to a process that is increasing intrathoracic pressure or otherwise preventing venous return to the heart. The decrease in breath sounds on the right side tells you that the problem is in the right chest, and the hyperresonance argues for a tension pneumothorax there. Steps of management:

(1) Administer 100% supplemental oxygen by nonrebreathing mask.

(2) Obtain orders from medical control as required by protocols.

(3) Identify the second right intercostal space in the midclavicular line.

(4) Prep the point you have identified (with povidone-iodine).

(5) Use a 14-gauge long (2 inches if possible) Angiocath, or whatever other 14-gauge needle is at hand, to pop through into the pleural space and vent the pneumothorax. Secure the catheter or needle in place. Use a flutter valve if possible.

(6) Immobilize the spine.

(7) Start transport.

(8) Start an IV en route. (pages 1708–1709)

   e. B. Like the patients with cardiac tamponade and tension pneumothorax, this patient with massive hemothorax is showing signs of shock (cold, sweaty skin; rapid, weak pulse). But in contrast to the others, his venous pressure is low (neck veins not distended), which makes one suspect hypovolemia. The decreased breath sounds in the left chest indicate that something is going on there, and the dullness to percussion suggests that fluid (blood) has taken the place of air in that side of the chest. It all adds up to massive bleeding within the chest. (Given the location of the stab wound, it is not unreasonable to consider the possibility of myocardial trauma and pericardial tamponade as well.) Steps of management:

(1) Administer 100% supplemental oxygen.

(2) Start transport.

(3) Start two large-bore IVs en route. (page 1712)

True/False

   1. T (page 1697)   **2.** F (page 1707)   **3.** F (page 1713)   **4.** T (pages 1715–1716)   **5.** T (page 1699)

   6. T (page 1718)   **7.** F (page 1719)   **8.** F (page 1709)   **9.** T (page 1709)   **10.** T (page 1709)

Short Answer

What you need to remember to answer this question correctly is that any injury below the nipples is an abdominal injury as well as a chest injury. The bullet apparently took a straight line through the right upper quadrant (RUQ), and it could be expected to have hit the liver, kidney, and perhaps part of the lung. (pages 1696–1697)

Skill Drills

   1. Needle Decompression (Thoracentesis) of a Tension Pneumothorax (page 1711)

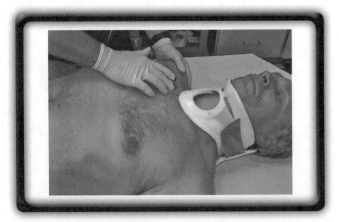

Step 1: Assess the patient.

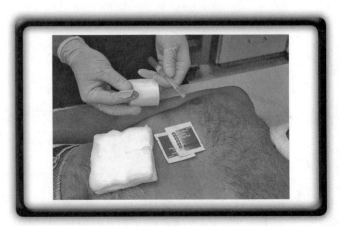

Step 2: Prepare and assemble all necessary equipment. Obtain orders from medical control.

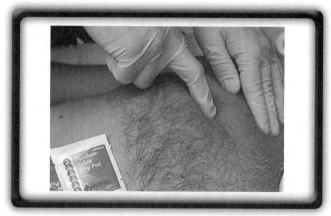

Step 3: Locate the appropriate site between the second and third rib.

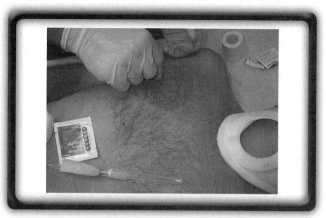

Step 4: Cleanse the appropriate area using aseptic technique.

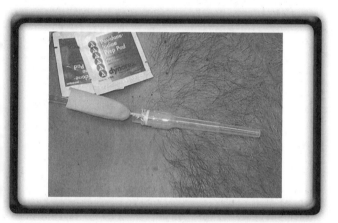

Step 5: Make a one-way valve or flutter valve.

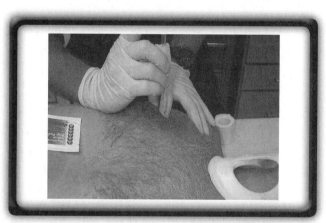

Step 6: Insert the needle at a 90° angle, and listen for the release of air.

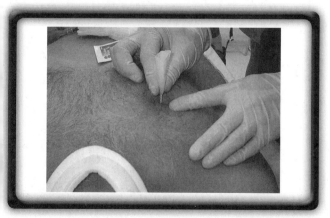

Step 7: Remove the needle. Properly dispose of the needle in the sharps container.

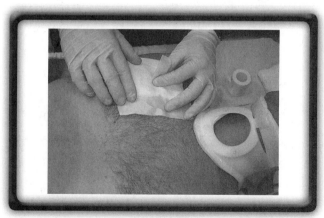

Step 8: Secure the catheter in place. Monitor the patient closely for recurrence of tension pneumothorax.

Chapter 36: Abdominal and Genitourinary Trauma

Matching

Part I
(page 1750)

1. I	2. J	3. L	4. M	5. K	6. O	7. N	8. P	9. R
10. Q	11. H	12. D	13. E	14. C	15. F	16. B	17. G	18. A

Part II

1. C (page 1742)   2. B (page 1742)   3. B (page 1742)   4. D (page 1745)   5. D (page 1745)

6. F (page 1743)   7. G (page 1741)   8. B (page 1742)   9. A (page 1743)   10. B (page 1742)

Multiple Choice

1. D (page 1739)   2. D (page 1741)   3. C (page 1731)   4. C (page 1733)   5. D (pages 1736–1737)

6. C (page 1741)   7. D (page 1729)   8. D (page 1734)   9. A (pages 1734–1735)   10. D (page 1737)

Labeling

1. Organs in the Peritoneum (page 1729)
   A. Liver
   B. Peritoneum
   C. Ascending colon
   D. Diaphragm
   E. Stomach
   F. Spleen
   G. Transverse colon

2. Organs in the Retroperitoneal Space (page 1729)
   A. Vena cava
   B. Duodenum
   C. Kidney
   D. Ureters
   E. Aorta
   F. Pancreas
   G. Kidney
   H. Descending colon

3. Organs in the Pelvis (page 1729)
   A. Iliac vessels
   B. Uterus
   C. Rectum
   D. Sigmoid colon
   E. Bladder

Fill-in-the-Blank

1. duodenum (page 1731)
2. Grey Turner sign (page 1740)
3. Cullen sign (page 1740)
4. pancreas; kidneys (page 1729)
5. liver (page 1730)
6. hollow (page 1730)
7. urinary (page 1731)
8. peritonitis (pages 1733–1734)

Identify

1. **a.** Chief complaint: Patient denies any complaint. EMS was called by police for possible stab wound.
   b. Vital signs: Pulse is 120 beats/min and regular; skin is ashen, cool, and diaphoretic; oxygen saturation is 90%; blood pressure is 86/60 mm Hg; and sinus tachycardia appears on the ECG.
   c. Pertinent negatives: He denies chest pain or other injuries.
2. **a.** Chief complaint: Evisceration, abdominal trauma
   b. Vital signs: Pulse is 100 beats/min and irregular; skin is pale, warm, and dry; oxygen saturation is 97% on room air; blood pressure is 160/90 mm Hg.
   c. Pertinent negatives: He is currently denying chest pain.

Ambulance Calls

1. The evaluation of a patient who has abdominal trauma must be systematic, keeping the entire patient in mind and prioritizing injuries accordingly. (pages 1737–1738)
   a. The mechanisms of injury, including damage to the vehicle and type of seat belt worn (if any) if the patient is the victim of a motor vehicle crash
   b. The patient's complaints referable to the abdomen, specifically complaints of nausea, vomiting, hematemesis, or abdominal pain
   c. External signs of abdominal injury, such as abrasions, contusion, seat belt marks, lacerations, or evisceration
   d. Tenderness or rigidity to palpation
2. The case of evisceration described in this question is based on an actual case (see Majernik TG, et al. Intestinal evisceration resulting from a motor vehicle accident. *Ann Emerg Med.* 1984;13:633).

   Injuries:
   a. Bruise over the right lower ribs
   b. Small bowel evisceration
   c. Avulsion in the right side of the abdomen
   d. Fractured right elbow

   The published case report does not record what care was given at the scene, but the care that should have been given at the scene is based on the fact that this patient is in shock.

   Priorities:
   a. Administer 100% oxygen.
   b. Anticipate vomiting, and have suction at hand.
   c. Assist ventilations with a bag-valve mask.
   d. Cover the eviscerated bowel with sterile dressing; use an occlusive dressing over the wet sterile dressings or use sterile universal dressings that have been soaked in sterile saline. Cover the dressings, in turn, with a towel, to minimize heat loss across the wound.
   e. Immobilize the spine, taking care not to place any straps across the eviscerated bowel. Include the right arm within the straps, to hold the fractured elbow immobile.
   f. Start transport.
   g. Start two large-bore IVs en route, and run in lactated Ringer's as rapidly as possible.
3. The principles of managing an impaled object in the abdomen are fundamentally the same as for an impaled object anywhere else: Leave the impaled object in place. (page 1741)
   a. Administer oxygen.
   b. Stabilize the impaled object in place. Buttress it on all sides with universal dressings or with triangular bandages formed into "doughnut" rings. Then, tape the buttress material securely so that the knife cannot move in any direction.
   c. Start transport.
   d. Start an IV en route.
   e. Discuss analgesia with medical control.

True/False

1. F (page 1742)   2. F (page 1743)   3. T (page 1740)   4. F (page 1741)   5. T (page 1734)
6. T (page 1743)   7. T (page 1740)   8. T (page 1746)   9. T (page 1745)   10. F (page 1746)

Fill-in-the-Table

1. Hollow and Solid Organs of the Abdominal Cavity
(pages 1730–1731)

Hollow Organs	Solid Organs
1. Stomach	1. Liver
2. Small intestine	2. Spleen
3. Pancreas	3. Kidneys
4. Large intestine	4. Adrenal glands
5. Gallbladder	
6. Ureters	
7. Urinary bladder	

Short Answer

1. a. kidneys (page 1744)
   b. liver (page 1742)
   c. bladder (page 1745)
   d. liver (page 1730)

Chapter 37: Orthopaedic Trauma

Matching

Part I

1. HH (page 1799)	**2.** LL (page 1799)	**3.** II (page 1799)	**4.** KK (page 1799)	**5.** OO (page 1799)
6. JJ (page 1799)	**7.** PP (page 1799)	**8.** YY (page 1799)	**9.** ZZ (page 1799)	**10.** WW (page 1799)
11. VV (page 1799)	**12.** SS (page 1799)	**13.** XX (page 1799)	**14.** TT (page 1799)	**15.** UU (page 1799)
16. RR (page 1799)	**17.** NN (page 1799)	**18.** QQ (page 1799)	**19.** MM (page 1799)	**20.** F (page 1800)
21. M (page 1800)	**22.** G (page 1800)	**23.** N (page 1800)	**24.** H (page 1800)	**25.** O (page 1800)
26. I (page 1800)	**27.** P (page 1800)	**28.** J (page 1800)	**29.** Q (page 1800)	**30.** K (page 1800)
31. R (page 1800)	**32.** L (page 1800)	**33.** S (page 1800)	**34.** AA (page 1800)	**35.** DD (page 1800)
36. Z (page 1800)	**37.** BB (page 1800)	**38.** Y (page 1800)	**39.** CC (page 1800)	**40.** X (page 1800)
41. EE (page 1800)	**42.** W (page 1800)	**43.** FF (page 1800)	**44.** V (page 1800)	**45.** U (page 1800)
46. GG (page 1800)	**47.** T (page 1800)	**48.** A (page 1801)	**49.** E (page 1801)	**50.** B (page 1801)
51. D (page 1801)	**52.** C (page 1801)			

Part II

1. H (page 1784)	**2.** A (page 1789)	**3.** B (page 1782)	**4.** F (page 1782)
5. D (page 1782)	**6.** E (page 1791)	**7.** G (page 1765)	**8.** C (page 1764)

Multiple Choice

1. B (page 1754)	**2.** D (page 1754)	**3.** B (page 1758)	**4.** A (page 1766)	**5.** D (page 1766)
6. D (page 1792)	**7.** B (page 1771)	**8.** D (page 1775)	**9.** A (page 1780)	**10.** B (page 1784)

Labeling

1. Bones of the Foot and Ankle (page 1757)
   A. Fibula
   B. Achilles tendon
   C. Medial malleolus
   D. Talus
   E. Navicular
   F. Medial cuneiform
   G. Phalanges
   H. Metatarsal
   I. Calcaneus
2. Types of Fractures (page 1765)
   A. Transverse fracture of the tibia
   B. Oblique fracture of the humerus
   C. Spiral fracture of the femur
   D. Comminuted fracture of the tibia
   E. Greenstick fracture of the fibula
   F. Compression fracture of a vertebral body
3. Types of Muscles (page 1761)
   A. Cardiac muscle
   B. Skeletal muscle
   C. Smooth muscle

Fill-in-the-Blank

1. **a.** atrophy (page 1759)
   b. arthritis (page 1799)
   c. articulation (page 1799)
   d. axilla (page 1799)
   e. clavicle (page 1755)
   f. diaphysis (page 1800)
   g. patella (page 1757)
   h. plantar (page 1801)
   i. pectoral girdle (page 1801)

2. The signs and symptoms of fracture are usually not terribly subtle:
   a. Unnatural shape: DEFORMITY (page 1765)
   b. Reduced length: SHORTENING (page 1765)
   c. Fracture of the small finger: BOXER'S FRACTURE (page 1783)
   d. Numbness and tingling: PARESTHESIAS (page 1771)
   e. Grating: CREPITUS (page 1766)
   f. Devastating consequence of musculoskeletal injuries: DISABILITY (page 1754)
   g. Protecting from movement: GUARDING (page 1766)
   h. Hurts to touch it: POINT TENDERNESS (page 1771)
   i. Patient with a fracture may report this: HEARD A SNAP (page 1770)
   j. Strange moves: UNNATURAL POSITION (page 1771)
   k. Clavicle: COLLARBONE (page 1755)
   l. Seen in open fracture: EXPOSED BONE ENDS (page 1766)

Identify

1. **a.** Chief complaint: Right ankle pain; severe wrist pain. He denies loss of consciousness or head or neck pain. The patient denies any respiratory distress and denies any current chest discomfort. He denies any medical condition that may have caused him to fall. He adamantly states that he simply slipped on ice and fell.
   b. Vital signs: His baseline vital signs reveal a pulse of 116 beats/min and irregular, respirations of 16 breaths/min nonlabored, oxygen saturation on room air at 98%, blood pressure of 150/90 mm Hg. ECG is rapid atrial fibrillation. PEARRL. Normal capillary refill < 2 seconds. Skin color is normal, and skin is warm and dry.
   c. Pertinent negatives: By questioning the patient, you discover that he has a previous medical history of angina, atrial fibrillation, and hypertension. He also takes one aspirin a day and an antihypertensive drug.

2. **a.** Chief complaint: The patient tripped on a curb in the parking lot. She complains of bilateral wrist injuries and is found in extreme pain. You notice that both her wrists appear bruised and deformed.
   b. Vital signs: Her initial vital signs indicate a patient that is conscious and alert. Her skin is slightly ashen and diaphoretic, and she has positive distal motor and neurologic sensations in both hands. She denies other injuries. Her capillary refill is > 2 seconds, and she has bilateral radial pulses that appear to be equal. Her blood pressure is obtainable only by palpation at 86 mm Hg. Her oxygen saturation is 96% on ambient air. She denies taking any medications or having any allergies.
   c. Pertinent negatives: The patient denies loss of consciousness or head or neck pain. She denies any respiratory distress and denies any current chest discomfort. She denies any medical condition that may have caused her to fall.

3. **a.** Chief complaint: A farm mishap where a tractor rolled on top of and is pinning a 64-year-old man. The patient is unresponsive with airway compromise.
   b. Vital signs: Patient is unresponsive, with a GCS < 8. He has delayed capillary refill and sinus tachycardia of 128 beats/min. His blood pressure is 64 mm Hg by palpation.
   c. Pertinent negatives: There are no pertinent negatives indicated.

Complete the Patient Care Report (PCR)

Show the completed PCR to your instructor to obtain feedback on your completion of the form.

Ambulance Calls

1. The presence of some injuries may also give clues to the possible presence of other injuries that share the same mechanism of injury.
   a. The young man's calcaneal fracture mandates that you check for fracture of the other calcaneus as well as fracture of the lumbar vertebrae, especially around L1–L2. (page 1789)
   b. The 50-year-old woman in the head-on collision has the classic dashboard injury. The same forces that smashed up the knee may well have acted anywhere along the femur to cause a femoral fracture or to ram the femur backward, producing fracture or dislocation of the hip. (page 1791)
   c. The 60-year-old man who fell sideways onto his outstretched hand probably has a scaphoid fracture, in which the forces are transmitted from the hand, along the radius and ulna, through the elbow, and up the humerus into the shoulder. Look for injuries anywhere along that axis, specifically fracture of the distal radius/ulna, fracture/dislocation of the elbow, fracture of the shaft of the humerus, fracture/dislocation of the shoulder, or fracture of the clavicle. (page 1783)
   d. The obvious fracture in the construction worker is the fracture of the scapula, which is a tip-off to the powerful forces involved in the injury. Thus, you need to start looking for rib fractures, vertebral fractures, and damage to underlying soft tissues (eg, pulmonary contusion, renal injury). (page 1782)

2. It's all well and good to memorize the signs and symptoms of musculoskeletal injuries, but what counts is whether you can recognize the injuries when you see them and whether you then take the appropriate action.
   a. Starting with the boy who fell off his skateboard: (page 1782)
      (1) The most likely field diagnosis is a fractured elbow. If you want to be more exact, you could specify that it's a supracondylar fracture of the humerus, but probably it won't be possible (or necessary) in the field to know exactly what is broken and what isn't. The fact that the elbow is involved in a fracture is reason enough to feel a sense of urgency.
      (2) Yes, there is a special danger in this case, the danger of the patient developing Volkmann ischemic contracture as a result of the blood supply to his forearm being jeopardized. He's already showing signs of a compromised blood supply (his hand is cool and pale), and the broken end of the humerus is probably pinching his radial nerve as well (he has a sensory loss in the distribution of the radial nerve). Those are danger signals!
      (3) If this boy is to retain the use of his right hand, urgent measures must be taken to restore the blood supply to the area. Those measures are best taken by an expert—an orthopaedic surgeon—in the hospital; so, if you are close to the hospital, splint the elbow as you found it, and hit the road—notifying the hospital of your ETA so that they can summon an "orthopod" (ie, orthopaedic surgeon) to be standing by in the ED. If you are any distance from the hospital, however, contact medical command for orders; you may be instructed to apply traction along the axis of the humerus and straighten the elbow slightly, until the patient's hand "pinks up."
   b. The boy's mother tripped over his skateboard in her haste to assist him (there's a lesson in that!). She's done something to her wrist. (page 1783)
      (1) The most likely field diagnosis is a Colles fracture—that is, a fracture of the distal radius and ulna. The "dinner-fork deformity" is classic for the Colles fracture, as is the way the woman walked over to you, holding the injured wrist in her other hand and using her body as a splint.
      (2) No, there is not ordinarily any special danger in a Colles fracture, although you must, as always, check the circulation and neurologic function distal to the injury, just to be certain.
      (3) A padded aluminum ladder splint, bent into a right angle at the elbow and supported in a sling, is probably the most comfortable splint for this woman. But you may also use an air splint (provided it comes up over the elbow) or a padded board splint. In either of those two cases, transport the woman supine, with her splinted arm supported on a pillow, to elevate the injured part.
   c. Here is another classic dashboard injury. (page 1787)
      (1) The most likely diagnosis is posterior dislocation of the hip. That is what one would expect given the mechanisms of injury (deceleration forces, femur driven backward), and the patient has characteristic signs: The affected hip is flexed, adducted, and internally rotated, and the leg appears shorter than the leg on the uninjured side.
      (2) Yes, there is a particular danger associated with posterior hip dislocation—two dangers, in fact. The most feared complication is avascular necrosis of the head of the femur, which leads to total destruction of the hip joint. There is also danger of damage to the sciatic nerve and consequent foot drop.

(3) The most important treatment for a dislocated hip is early reduction of the dislocation. If you are within 20 minutes or so of the hospital, the best thing to do is to immobilize the patient on a long backboard, generously padded with pillows, and transport immediately. If you are at a considerable distance from the hospital, contact medical control. If you are given instructions to do so, try once to reduce the dislocation.

d. The other patient from the same crash was the driver, found unconscious. (pages 1784–1786)

(1) The most likely orthopaedic field diagnosis in this case is a fractured pelvis. But this patient has some other very serious, even life-threatening injuries. Loss of consciousness in a patient with trauma means head injury until proved otherwise, and head injury in multitrauma means spinal cord injury until proved otherwise.

(2) Yes, indeed there is a particular danger in this case. There are several particular dangers. For starters, the patient is unconscious, so his airway is in jeopardy. He also seems to be in shock, perhaps from blood loss related to his pelvic fracture, but perhaps from blood loss elsewhere as well.

(3) After the scene size-up, conduct a primary assessment on this patient. The steps in the primary assessment involve a general impression and your "MS-ABC Priority Plan" searching for and managing life threats.

General impression: unconscious male trauma patient

MS: "U" unresponsive to pain

A—Open his airway (chin lift or jaw thrust); insert an oropharyngeal airway to help keep it open.

B—Determine whether he is breathing adequately; if not, assist his breathing with a bag-mask device. In any event, give supplementary oxygen.

C—Assess the circulation (pulse, capillary refill in children), and control external bleeding.

Priority: high

Given the patient's condition, you won't have time to do a lot more in the field than the following:

(a) Manage the ABCs.

(b) Secure the patient to the backboard.

(c) Start transport.

(d) En route, get a set of vital signs, if you haven't done so already.

(e) Start at least one and preferably two large-bore IVs, and run a 500-mL fluid challenge.

(f) Complete the secondary assessment and physical exam as best you can.

(g) Keep the patient warm.

e. Apparently, it's only when you get back to base that your partner mentions how much his ankle is hurting. (pages 1788–1789)

(1) The most likely diagnosis is a sprained ankle, although you can't be 100% sure without an x-ray.

(2) No, there is no particular danger associated with a sprained ankle.

(3) The treatment is to immobilize the ankle (eg, air splint, pillow splint), apply a cold pack, elevate the ankle, and transport your partner to the ED to be checked over.

f. The high school quarterback who ended up under a pile of 225-pound linemen was subject to significant crushing forces. (pages 1789–1790)

(1) The most likely diagnosis is posterior sternoclavicular dislocation.

(2) Yes, there is a particular danger in this case, and that is damage to critical underlying structures. In fact, there is already evidence that such damage has occurred, for the boy says he is "choking"—an indication of possible tracheal damage.

(3) The most important aspect of this boy's treatment will be expeditious transport to the hospital. Administer supplementary oxygen en route. If he is comfortable lying down, keep him supine, with his left arm abducted and a pillow or rolled towel under his left shoulder; that position may take the pressure off the trachea or whatever structures are being compressed by the proximal end of the clavicle.

g. The pedestrian suffered a direct blow to the shin. (pages 1780, 1788)

(1) The most likely diagnosis is an open fracture of the tibia, probably a transverse fracture.

(2) Yes, there is a particular danger associated with tibial fractures, and that is the development of a compartment syndrome. Indeed, the patient's paresthesias suggest that there may already be pressure on the sensory nerves supplying the foot.

(3) To treat the patient in the field, apply manual traction to straighten out the angulation, and splint the limb (padded board splint, long-leg air splint). Keep the patient supine so you can elevate the injured leg. Apply cold packs. Transport the patient without delay, and notify the receiving hospital to have an orthopaedic surgeon standing by.

h. In today's less-than-tranquil society, gunshot wounds are frequent sources of musculoskeletal trauma. (pages 1787–1788)

(1) The most likely diagnosis in this case is a fractured femur. The location of the wound and the shortening of the injured leg are the tip-offs.

(2) Yes, there is a particular danger in this case. Aside from the danger of shock that attends every femoral fracture, there is apparently some compromise to distal circulation (the dorsalis pedis pulse is weak). There may also be a danger to you if the person who did the shooting is still wandering around with a loaded gun. Did you bother to check on that before you ran over to attend the patient?

(3) This is another case that involves setting priorities:

(a) Administer supplemental oxygen.

(b) Cover the open wound(s) with sterile dressings.

(c) Immobilize the injured leg in a traction splint.

(d) Start transport.

(e) Start a large-bore IV en route to the hospital.

(f) Keep rechecking the dorsalis pedis pulse. Document all your findings.

(4) The purposes of splinting in general are as follows:

(a) To relieve pain

(b) To prevent further injury

(c) To help control bleeding (page 1775)

i. The skier who ended up at the bottom of a pileup doubtless suffered a hyperextension injury of the leg. (pages 1791–1792)

(1) The most likely diagnosis is dislocation of the knee (it may also be fractured).

(2) Yes, there is a particular danger associated with that diagnosis, the danger of damage to the popliteal artery and consequent ischemic damage to the lower leg.

(3) The treatment under these circumstances—where you are on the ski slopes, at some distance from a hospital—is to try once to reduce the dislocation, before muscle spasm makes it impossible to do so. Use a traction splint if you have one available. Otherwise, apply manual traction in the long axis of the leg. Then, get the patient to the hospital as quickly as possible, and notify the hospital in advance of your impending arrival.

3. a. As shown in the *Environmental Emergencies* chapter, when dealing with a severely injured patient, knowing what to do is not enough. One has to know what to do first and what to do next and what to do after that. If you remember the alphabet, you'll be in good shape.

Step 16. Start an IV.

Step 9. Take the vital signs.

Step 6. Cut away the trouser leg. (You will want to control the bleeding in the leg if it is excessive, which is part of step C, Circulation.)

Step 3. Determine whether he is breathing (he is) (step B, Breathing).

Step 14. Secure the patient to a backboard.

Step 12. Apply the PASG/MAST (if your protocols allow), while holding the right leg in traction.

Step 7. Put manual pressure on the bleeding site (part of step C, Circulation).

Step 2. Open the airway (chin lift) (step A, Airway).

Step 15. Start transport.

Step 10. Move the patient to a backboard.

Step 5. Check for a carotid pulse (pulse is present) (first part of step C, Circulation).

Steps 11 and 13. Check for a dorsalis pedis pulse on the right. (You need to do this both before and after you have applied the splint, which in this case is the PASG/MAST [if your protocols allow].)

Step 1. Do the AVPU "mental status" check (the "mental status" in the MS-ABC Priority Plan).

Step 4. Check for an open or tension pneumothorax (part of checking the adequacy of breathing, step B).

Step 8. Put a pressure dressing over the open wound on the leg. (In practice, you'll do this whenever the dressing material becomes available.)

In actual practice, you will be carrying out some of the preceding steps very nearly simultaneously. While holding the airway open and observing the movements of the chest, for instance, you will also have a finger on the carotid pulse. But it is useful to consider the actions separately to review priorities.

b. Yes, at least one step has been omitted. The patient was not given supplemental oxygen!

4. An open fracture of the tibia is a serious injury with serious potential complications (such as compartment syndrome), but it does not pose an immediate threat to life; nor are there any signs so far of other injuries that do jeopardize the patient's life.

a. Steps to be taken in the field:

(1) Conduct a rapid trauma assessment.

(2) Cover the wound on the leg with a sterile dressing.

(3) Straighten and splint the fractured leg.

(4) Start a large-bore IV (or could be done en route).

b. Steps to be taken en route:

(1) Communicate with medical control or receiving hospital.

(2) Recheck pulse and sensation distal to the fracture every 5 minutes.

(3) Start a large-bore IV (if not done yet).

5. A spinal cord injury is a tragic injury, but ordinarily it does not pose an immediate threat to life unless there is a transection high in the cervical spine that paralyzes all muscles of breathing. This patient has a traumatic paraplegia, but no evidence of spinal shock or any other life-threatening condition.

a. Steps to be taken at the scene:

(1) Manually stabilize the head/neck and apply a cervical collar.

(2) Perform the primary assessment.

(3) Immobilize the patient on a long backboard.

b. Steps to be taken en route:

(1) Communicate with medical command or receiving hospital.

(2) Start an IV with normal saline.

(3) Conduct a reassessment, rechecking vital and neurologic signs every 5 minutes.

True/False

1. T (page 1776) **2.** T (page 1777) **3.** T (page 1776) **4.** T (page 1779)

5. T (page 1776) **6.** T (page 1770) **7.** T (page 1778)

Fill-in-the-Table

1. Bones in Joints (pages 1755–1757)

Bones in Joints	
Joint	**Bones That Make Up the Joint**
Shoulder	Scapula, humerus
Elbow	Humerus, ulna
Wrist	Radius, ulna, carpals
Hip	Ilium, ischium, pubis, femur
Knee	Femur, tibia
Ankle	Tibia, fibula, tarsals

2. Potential Blood Loss From Fracture Sites
   (page 1774)

Potential Blood Loss From Fracture Sites	
Fracture Site	**Potential Blood Loss (mL)**
Pelvis	1,500–3,000
Femur	1,000–1,500
Humerus	250–500
Tibia or fibula	250–500
Ankle	250–500
Elbow	250–500
Radius or ulna	150–250

Short Answer

1. The compartment syndrome may be heralded by any or several of the six Ps, which are symptoms and signs of an ischemic limb (page 1771):
   a. Pain—the earliest and most reliable sign
   b. Pallor
   c. Pulselessness
   d. Paresthesias
   e. Paresis or paralysis
   f. Pressure

2. In examining the patient injured on the ski slope, it's a good idea to start by eliciting his chief complaint. Although his deformed right knee may be the most obvious injury to you, there may be other injuries that are bothering the patient more. If you don't ask, you may not find out. In conducting the physical assessment, pay particular attention to the following (pages 1770–1771):
   a. The position in which the extremities are found (as always, compare the injured to the uninjured limb).
   b. The circulatory status of the injured limb. Check the following:
      (1) Skin condition
      (2) Capillary refill
      (3) Distal pulses (anterior tibial and dorsalis pedis)
   c. The neurologic status of the injured limb. Check the following:
      (1) Sensation to pinprick over the heel and dorsum of the foot
      (2) Motor function: ability to plantar flex and dorsiflex the foot

3. Equipment to grab and take with you when you rush to the side of a severely injured patient should include the following:
   a. Long backboard with at least three straps
   b. Cervical collar and head immobilizer (eg, blanket roll)
   c. Portable oxygen and suction
   d. Oropharyngeal and nasopharyngeal airways
   e. Pocket mask or bag-mask device
   f. Wound kit
   g. Stethoscope, blood pressure cuff, and flashlight

Problem Solving

(page 1774)

1. 1,000 mL
2. 4,500 mL
3. 1,000 mL

Chapter 38: Environmental Emergencies

Matching

Part I

1. SS (page 1844)	**2.** RR (page 1844)	**3.** PP (page 1844)	**4.** LL (page 1844)	**5.** KK (page 1844)
6. QQ (page 1844)	**7.** EE (page 1844)	**8.** DD (page 1844)	**9.** CC (page 1844)	**10.** BB (page 1844)
11. AA (page 1844)	**12.** W (page 1844)	**13.** U (page 1844)	**14.** P (page 1844)	**15.** O (page 1844)
16. TT (page 1844)	**17.** UU (page 1844)	**18.** VV (page 1844)	**19.** WW (page 1844)	**20.** X (page 1844)
21. V (page 1844)	**22.** XX (page 1844)	**23.** ZZ (page 1844)	**24.** YY (page 1844)	**25.** NN (page 1844)
26. MM (page 1844)	**27.** JJ (page 1844)	**28.** II (page 1844)	**29.** OO (page 1844)	**30.** HH (page 1844)
31. GG (page 1844)	**32.** FF (page 1844)	**33.** Z (page 1844)	**34.** Y (page 1844)	**35.** T (page 1844)
36. Q (page 1844)	**37.** N (page 1845)	**38.** M (page 1845)	**39.** L (page 1845)	**40.** K (page 1845)
41. E (page 1845)	**42.** S (page 1844)	**43.** R (page 1844)	**44.** C (page 1845)	**45.** B (page 1845)
46. A (page 1845)	**47.** J (page 1845)	**48.** D (page 1845)	**49.** I (page 1845)	**50.** H (page 1845)
51. F (page 1845)	**52.** G (page 1845)			

Part II

(page 1809)

1. HL	**2.** HP	**3.** HL	**4.** HL	**5.** HP
6. HP	**7.** HL	**8.** HP	**9.** HL	**10.** HP

Multiple Choice

1. D (page 1810)	**2.** C (page 1807)	**3.** B (page 1808)	**4.** A (page 1809)	**5.** D (page 1812)
6. A (page 1809)	**7.** B (page 1818)	**8.** B (page 1827)	**9.** C (pages 1829–1830)	**10.** D (page 1815)

Labeling

1. Physiologic Responses to Hot and Cold Environments
   (page 1806)

   Hot Environment
   - **Hypothalamus** stimulated
   - Blood vessels **dilate**, maximizing **heat** loss from skin
   - Body **sweats**, causing evaporation and **cooling**
   - Body temperature **decreases**

   Cold Environment
   - **Hypothalamus** stimulated
   - Blood vessels **constrict**, minimizing **heat loss** from skin
   - Muscles **shiver**, generating **heat**
   - Body temperature **increases**

Fill-in-the-Blank

1. a. For the human body to maintain a nearly constant core temperature, it must balance heat loss with heat production.

Sources of Body Heat	Ways of Shedding Heat
1. Basal metabolism	1. Radiation
2. Exercise	2. Convection
3. Absorption of heat	3. Conduction
4. Evaporation of sweat	

    b. The body's mechanisms for dissipating excess heat have certain limitations. First, all of the mechanisms depend on **peripheral vasodilatation** to shunt blood from the core to the body surface. Furthermore, to be effective, three of the body's cooling mechanisms require a temperature gradient between the body and the outside. None of these three mechanisms—**radiation**, **convection**, or **conduction**—can work if the outside is not at least a few degrees cooler than the body core. Finally, one of the body's cooling mechanisms is dependent on the ambient humidity. When the humidity is high, that mechanism—namely, **evaporation of sweat**—is ineffective in lowering the core temperature.

    c. A hatless hiker standing still on a mountaintop on a windless day loses heat from his head by **radiation**. A breeze picks up. Now the hiker loses heat by **convection** as well.

    d. A white-water enthusiast who capsizes his canoe in a swift-running stream loses body heat by **conduction**.

    e. A soldier on maneuvers in the desert in ambient temperatures of more than 37.7°C (100°F) can shed heat only by **evaporation of sweat**. (pages 1807–1808)

Identify

1. a. Chief complaint: Fell through ice.

    b. Vital signs: Patient is shivering. ECG rhythm is regular with Osborn waves.

    c. Pertinent negatives: None. (page 1816)

    d. *Students should provide three of the following:*

        (1) Time in water

        (2) Patient temperature

        (3) Neurologic assessment

        (4) Amount of alcohol ingested and when

        (5) Any drugs taken

        (6) Blood glucose (page 1817)

    e. B. (Conduction) This is the transfer of heat from a hotter object to a cooler object by direct physical contact. (page 1808)

    f. A fluid bolus (unless otherwise contraindicated) (page 1819)

Complete the Patient Care Report (PCR)

Show the completed PCR to your instructor to obtain feedback on your completion of the form.

Ambulance Calls

1. a. The patient probably had a heat syncope episode that occurs in people who may be under heat stress and who experience peripheral vasodilatation that possibly may be exacerbated by dehydration. One group in which this seems prevalent is those attending mass outdoor gatherings. An additional contributing factor may be alcohol intake (beer). Some other factors that should be considered but that might not yet be identified are medical conditions such as diabetes, drug intake, and amount of physical exertion done by the patient. (pages 1810–1813)

    b. Maintain the airway and provide oxygen, place in a cool environment in the supine position, and provide fluid replacement either orally or by IV. (page 1813)

    c. If the patient does not quickly respond in the supine position, suspect heat exhaustion or heatstroke. (page 1812)

2. a. The fullback who is acting "crazy" after practicing on a hot, humid afternoon is most probably suffering from exertional heatstroke. You were fortunate to be able to record a temperature and obtain conclusive evidence. In many cases, the patient is too combative to allow you to measure the temperature, and you can only suspect the diagnosis on the basis of his symptoms and signs alone. (page 1812)

    b. The steps in managing exertional heatstroke in this patient are as follows:

        (1) Move him to a cooler environment, preferably your air-conditioned ambulance with the fans blowing.

        (2) Strip off his clothing and football gear.

        (3) Apply ice packs to his flanks while massaging his neck and torso. Spray the patient with tepid water, and keep a fan blowing in his direction.

        (4) Start an IV and administer a bolus of fluid (unless otherwise contraindicated).

        (5) Monitor temperature and cardiac rhythm.

        (6) Be prepared for seizures.

        (7) Transport without delay. (pages 1813–1814)

3. a. The running back writhing in pain is most likely suffering from heat cramps. (page 1809)

    b. The steps in treating him are as follows:

        (1) Tell the coach to stop massaging the boy's legs!

        (2) Move the boy to a cooler environment.

        (3) If he is not nauseated, give him salt-containing fluids to drink (at least a quart). If the patient is too nauseated to take the fluids by mouth, insert an IV and infuse normal saline rapidly (consult medical control for the IV rate).

        (4) Do not allow the boy to return to practice that day. He should go home and rest in a cool place. Instruct him to seek medical attention if he develops headaches, dizziness, nausea, or severe fatigue. (page 1810)

4. a. The quarterback may indeed be coming down with mononucleosis, but it could be fatal to miss a case of heat exhaustion. (pages 1810–1811)

    b. You should treat him in the field as follows:

        (1) Move the boy to a cooler environment.

        (2) Remove most of his clothing, down to his undershorts, and sponge him with cool water.

        (3) Start an IV and run it wide open.

        (4) Monitor cardiac rhythm and vital signs.

        (5) Transport to the hospital. (page 1811)

    c. By now, one would think Coach would have reached the conclusion that football practice in the searing heat is not healthy for a teenager. But you should in any case suggest to him that if he must conduct practice during the "dog days" of August, he should schedule the heavy exertion for the early morning and late afternoon hours.

5. a. The baby at the supermarket is suffering from classic heatstroke. The inside of an automobile that is parked in the sun in 37.7°C (100°F) temperatures can very quickly reach a temperature of around 82°C (180°F)—not high enough to bake a cake, perhaps, but certainly high enough to bake a baby. This infant is in severe danger and may die. (pages 1811–1812)

    b. Treatment is extremely urgent:

        (1) Open the airway. Intubate as soon as you have a chance.

        (2) Administer supplemental oxygen.

        (3) Strip off all the baby's clothing.

        (4) Spray and fan the baby continuously until you reach the hospital.

        (5) If you are able to do so, start an IV en route to the hospital with 5% dextrose in half normal saline. Consult medical control for local orders on flow rate and/or boluses of fluid.

        (6) Monitor rectal temperature.

        (7) Transport without delay. (pages 1813–1814)

6. It only happens to paramedics—a ski vacation turns into a search-and-rescue mission.

    a. The first skier has deep frostbite. You don't really have the means to rewarm his leg in the field; nor can you ensure that it won't simply freeze again during transport to the ski lodge. (page 1815)

   b. The management therefore is as follows:

     (1) Move him to a sheltered place, such as that cabin behind the trees, until the snowmobile comes.

     (2) Give him some calories, preferably a candy bar or some other carbohydrate source. Give him a hot, sweet drink if you're carrying a thermos.

     (3) Leave the frostbitten extremity frozen. Don't attempt any rewarming in the field.

     (4) Pad the frostbitten leg to prevent it from being bruised during transport.

     (5) Protect the rest of the patient's body from the cold with insulating blankets.

   c. The second skier has a more superficial frostbite. (page 1815)

   d. The management therefore is as follows:

     (1) Move him to a sheltered place, such as that cabin behind the trees, until the snowmobile comes.

     (2) Give him some calories, preferably a candy bar or some other carbohydrate source. Give him a hot, sweet drink if you're carrying a thermos.

     (3) Try to warm the frostbitten foot with your hands (or by putting it in your armpit!).

     (4) Splint the frostbitten leg to prevent it from being bruised during transport.

     (5) Protect the rest of the patient's body from the cold with insulating blankets.

   e. The third lost skier is suffering from severe hypothermia. Only his very occasional breathing tips you off that he is not (yet) in cardiac arrest. (pages 1816–1820)

   f. In managing him:

     (1) As long as his airway is not obstructed, it is best not to touch him at all until the ambulance arrives. Send someone down to the road to intercept the ambulance, help carry equipment, and guide the paramedics to the patient.

     (2) Move the patient very gently onto the stretcher, and carry the stretcher very gently to the ambulance.

     (3) Maintain the airway manually until the patient has been well ventilated with 100% oxygen by bag-mask device for at least 3 minutes. Then, intubate the trachea rapidly and smoothly.

     (4) Apply monitoring electrodes, and check the cardiac rhythm. If asystole should occur, start cardiopulmonary resuscitation (CPR), but give basic life support (BLS) only. If you see ventricular fibrillation (VF) on the monitor, give one shock, resume CPR immediately for a 2-minute cycle, and then attempt to deliver another shock. Continue until three shocks have been given. If VF persists, put the defibrillator away and just continue BLS all the way to the hospital. It is important that CPR be uninterrupted with quality compressions at a rate of at least 100 per minute. Medical control can be contacted to determine if additional shock should be provided.

     (5) If the patient's clothing is wet, gently cut away wet clothing and replace it with dry blankets.

     (6) Notify the receiving hospital of the nature of the case and your estimated time of arrival (ETA).

     (7) Keep the ambulance interior around 15.5°C (60°F).

     (8) Instruct the driver to make it a smooth ride to the hospital. (page 1820)

7. The speedboat driver who is plunged into cold lake water is a likely candidate for hypothermia by the process of conduction. Heat loss is 25% faster in water than in air and can occur after relatively short exposure because of the rapidity with which water conducts heat away from the body. In managing such a case, you should observe these guidelines:

   a. Try to prevent the victim from exerting himself. Toss him a rope and pull him to shore, or send one of the other boats over to haul him aboard and bring him ashore. But in any case, discourage him from thrashing about in the water.

   b. As soon as you have the victim ashore, carry him to a sheltered place, preferably the inside of your ambulance, and cut away his wet clothes. Be sure to keep him absolutely still.

   c. Monitor his cardiac rhythm.

   d. Cover him with insulating materials, and cover those with blankets.

   e. Wrap chemical hot packs in towels, and place them in his armpits and near the groin.

   f. Give him a hot, caffeine-free, sugary drink.

   g. Keep him recumbent.

   h. Transport him to the hospital. (pages 1817–1820)

8. The "vagrant" in the bus station represents a classic example of the kind of case that is too often misdiagnosed.
   a. Any patient found in the circumstances described must be suspected to be suffering from one of the following:
      (1) Hypothermia
      (2) Hypoglycemia
      (3) Stroke
      . . . or all of the above until proved otherwise.
   b. In view of those possibilities, the steps in management are as follows:
      (1) Administer warmed, humidified oxygen (if available).
      (2) Complete the rapid medical assessment. Obtain vital signs, and check for injuries, with particular attention to the head.
      (3) Start an IV (using warmed IV fluid).
      (4) Give 50% dextrose, 50 mL IV.
      (5) Monitor cardiac rhythm.
      (6) Cover the patient with warm blankets.
      (7) Transport to the hospital.
9. a. Ask if the headache is throbbing and worse over the temporal or occipital areas and if it is exacerbated by a Valsalva maneuver. If the answer to any of these questions is yes, there is a likelihood the patient has acute mountain sickness. (pages 1831–1832)
   b. *Students should list four of the following:*
      (1) Dyspnea at rest
      (2) Cough
      (3) Weakness or decreased exercise performance
      (4) Chest tightness or congestion
      (5) Central cyanosis
      (6) Rales or wheezing in at least one lung field
      (7) Tachypnea
      (8) Tachycardia (page 1832)
   c. (1) Give supplemental oxygen until the condition improves.
      (2) Descend as soon as possible, with minimal exertion.
      (3) A portable ventilator can be used, if available, provided descent is not possible or no oxygen is accessible. If you can't descend, give your friend nifedipine and add dexamethasone if neurologic deterioration occurs. (page 1832)
10. a. The diver ascended from his dive without exhaling constantly to vent air from the lungs or he held his breath during the ascent. The result is that he probably has sustained pulmonary overpressurized syndrome (POPS), also known as "burnt lungs," which has probably caused arterial gas embolism (AGE). (pages 1827–1828)
   b. (1) Ensure an adequate airway, intubate if a BLS airway is not effective (fill the cuff with saline if the patient is to be placed in a hyperbaric chamber).
      (2) Administer 100% supplemental oxygen.
      (3) Transport in the supine position (use ground transport if cabin pressure is an issue).
      (4) Establish an IV en route.
      (5) Place on an ECG monitor.
      (6) Have medication ready for seizures and dopamine for hypotension, and follow protocol for direct referral to a hyperbaric chamber facility. (page 1828)
   c. Decompression sickness (pages 1828–1829)

True/False

1. F (page 1816)	**2.** T (page 1815)	**3.** T (page 1816)	**4.** F (page 1816)	**5.** F (pages 1815–1816)
6. T (pages 1814–1815)	**7.** T (page 1810)	**8.** F (page 1811)	**9.** F (page 1812)	**10.** T (page 1807)

Short Answer

1. Heat is a form of cardiovascular stress because the body responds to heat by vasodilatation. Increasing the diameter of the blood vessels increases their volume so that the heart must increase its output to prevent a fall in blood pressure. The heart increases output by increasing both its rate and stroke volume, which inevitably means an increase in cardiac work. (page 1809)

2. A person's risk of suffering significant heat illness in response to heat stress can be increased by the following factors. *Students should provide five of the following:*
   a. Exertion or anything else that increases endogenous heat production (eg, fever, hyperthyroidism)
   b. High humidity
   c. Obesity
   d. Diabetes
   e. Alcoholism
   f. Dehydration
   g. Cardiovascular or cerebrovascular disease
   h. Heavy or tight clothing
   i. Drugs such as diuretics and some tranquilizers (page 1809)

3. a. The dog days of summer also put you at risk of heat illness, especially if you have to carry heat-stricken, 300-pound patients down four flights of stairs. So, take some precautions to protect yourself on very hot days. *Students should provide five of the following:*
      (1) Wear light-colored, loose-fitting clothing. If your service does not have an appropriate summer uniform, ask your union to demand one!
      (2) Stay in cool places whenever you can.
      (3) Park the ambulance in the shade.
      (4) Increase your fluid intake. Carry cold drinks with you in the vehicle, and partake frequently.
      (5) Wear a cool, damp towel around your neck.
      (6) Put a fan on the dashboard of the ambulance.
      (7) Seek medical attention at the first symptom of heat illness. (page 1814)
   b. Of course, to seek attention at the first symptom of heat illness, you have to know what the symptoms are! *Students should provide four of the following:*
      (1) Headache
      (2) Fatigue or lack of energy
      (3) Dizziness
      (4) Nausea or vomiting
      (5) Weakness
      (6) Abdominal cramping (page 1811)

4. Let's hear it for all the moms out there! They've been right all along.
   a. "Don't go out without a hat and scarf; it's freezing out there."
      Mother was right because most heat loss from the body occurs from the head and neck. By trapping some of that heat within insulating layers, a hat and scarf can reduce convective heat loss from above the shoulders.
   b. "Stop rolling around in the snow. You'll get a death of a chill."
      Mother was right because snow conducts heat away from the body faster than air does. And when the snow melts and your clothes get wet, cooling by conduction is even faster.
   c. "Get out of those wet clothes this minute."
      Mother was right because wearing wet clothing promotes heat loss by conduction while the clothes remain wet and by evaporation as the clothes dry. (page 1808)
   d. "Those skates are much too tight. Your toes will fall off."
      Mother was right because anything that interferes with the circulation to the extremities predisposes them to frostbite. (page 1817)
   e. "Make sure you wear your windbreaker. It's blowing a gale out there."
      Mother was right because exposure to the wind increases heat loss by convection. (page 1817)
   f. "Eat. Eat. You have to have something to keep you going in this weather."
      Mother was right because metabolic heat production requires fuel, so you need to maintain your caloric intake, especially in the form of carbohydrates, before anticipated exposure to cold temperatures. (page 1817)

5. It's important to follow Mother's advice because, by itself, the body does not have a lot of ways to defend itself against the cold. The three ways it can do so are as follows:

    a. By peripheral vasoconstriction, to shunt blood away from the body shell to the body core

    b. By shivering, to increase heat production by skeletal muscle

    c. By increasing the basal metabolic rate, to increase overall metabolic heat production (page 1817)

6. Some people are more likely to suffer cold injury than others are.

    a. Factors that predispose a person to frostbite include the following:

        (1) Inadequate or tight clothing, especially tight shoes or gloves

        (2) Smoking

        (3) Hunger, fatigue, or dehydration

        (4) Hypothermia (generalized cooling)

        (5) Coming in direct contact with cold objects (page 1815)

    b. Many factors predispose a person to suffer hypothermia. *Students should provide four of the following:*

        (1) Old age

        (2) Infancy

        (3) Alcoholism

        (4) Chronic illness

        (5) Poor planning for outdoor activity; unpreparedness

        (6) Trauma (page 1817)

7. Even our nursery rhyme companions were in danger of cold exposure:

    a. When the three little kittens lost their mittens, they became most vulnerable to frostbite of the paws.

    b. Sitting on an ice-cold tuffet, Miss Muffet was losing heat by conduction from her bottom to the tuffet and by radiation, mostly from her head and neck, to the surrounding atmosphere. If there was any breeze, she was losing heat by convection as well.

    c. Jack Sprat has a greater risk of hypothermia than his wife does because he has less natural insulation.

    d. Little Jack Horner had the right idea eating his Christmas pie before going out into the cold because he knew that one needs calories to increase internal heat production in cold weather.

    e. When the wind blows, the cradle rocks, and baby loses heat by convection.

Fill-in-the-Table

1. The slang expression "Cool it!" means to take it easy, to simmer down. And that is precisely what happens to the major systems of the body when cooled: They all slow down. (page 1817)

Body System	Effects of Hypothermia
Central nervous system	Apathy, lethargy Impaired reasoning Dysarthria Ataxic gait, uncoordinated movements
Cardiovascular system	Contracted intravascular space Increased blood viscosity with sludging in the capillaries Edema Bradycardia, dysrhythmias, susceptibility to ventricular fibrillation
Respiratory system	Slowing of respiratory rate Increased tracheobronchial secretions Decreased cough and gag reflexes
Muscular system	Weakness and stiffness
Metabolic system	Hypoglycemia Ketoacidosis Slowed hepatic drug metabolism

Section 8: Shock and Resuscitation
Chapter 39: Responding to the Field Code

Matching
(page 1878)

1. E　　　**2.** D　　　**3.** H　　　**4.** C　　　**5.** F　　　**6.** B　　　**7.** G　　　**8.** A

Multiple Choice

1. C (page 1851)　**2.** B (page 1852)　**3.** D (page 1853)　**4.** B (page 1853)　**5.** D (page 1856)

6. B (page 1856)　**7.** C (page 1858)　**8.** D (page 1862)　**9.** A (page 1866)　**10.** A (page 1872)

Labeling

1. CPR Devices
   (page 1871)
   A. AutoPulse load-distributing band
   B. Thumper CPR system
   C. Lucas 2 mechanical piston device
2. Resuscitation Pyramid
   (page 1853)
   A. Drugs
   B. ET tube, LMA, Combitube
   C. Ventilations (proper rate and visible chest rise)
   D. Single shock for V-fib/V-tach
   E. High-quality compressions (fast, deep, full recoil)

Fill-in-the-Blank

1. Thumper (page 1871)
2. advanced airway (page 1871)
3. impedance threshold device (page 1870)
4. asynchronous; 6; 8 (page 1870)
5. asystole; PEA (page 1869)
6. vasopressor (page 1869)

Identify

1. **a.** Chief complaint: Sudden cardiac arrest
   b. Vital signs: Initially none, then after ROSC blood pressure of 108/p and pulse of 96 regular
   c. Pertinent negatives: No prior heart attack, no allergies
   d. Epinephrine 1:10,000 and amiodarone
   e. Links in the Chain of Survival
      (1) Early access
      (2) Early CPR
      (3) Early defibrillation
      (4) Early advanced care
      (5) Post-arrest care (page 1852)

Complete the Patient Care Report (PCR)

Show the completed PCR to your instructor to obtain feedback on your completion of the form.

Ambulance Calls

1. **a.** High-quality compressions are the priority. A successful resuscitation is built around compressions with little to no interruptions. Change out the compressor every 2 minutes to assure a fresh compressor. (page 1874)
   b. The roles of the code team leader may include all of the following:
   (1) Obtaining the patient's history and performing the physical exam
   (2) Interpreting the ECG
   (3) Keeping track of the time
   (4) Making a medication decision following the algorithm
   (5) Clearly delegating tasks to code team members
   (6) Completing documentation after the resuscitation attempt
   (7) Talking with medical control
   (8) Controlling the resuscitation scene (page 1874)
   c. The code team member may be called on to perform all of the following roles (and more):
   (1) Ventilator
   (2) Active compressor
   (3) On-deck compressor
   (4) Other support personnel (page 1874)
2. **a.** As a paramedic, it is your responsibility to start CPR in all patients who are in cardiac arrest, with only two general exceptions:
   - You should not start CPR if the patient has obvious signs of death such as absence of a pulse and breathing, along with any one of the following findings: rigor mortis, dependent lividity, putrefaction, or evidence of nonsurvivable injury such as decapitation, dismemberment, or burned beyond recognition.
   - You should not start CPR if the patient and his or her physician have previously agreed not to resuscitate. If CPR has been started and a DNR or a medical orders for life-sustaining treatment (MOLST) form is presented to you by family, contact medical control for permission to terminate the resuscitation efforts. (page 1872)
   b. The significance of bystander CPR, even if only chest compressions, is that if applied properly it can double, if not triple, the chance of survival.
3. **a.** For situations where advanced life support (ALS) personnel are present to provide care for an adult with pre-hospital cardiac arrest, the ALS termination of resuscitation rule was established to consider terminating efforts before ambulance transport if all of the following criteria are met:
   (1) The arrest was not witnessed by anyone.
   (2) Bystander CPR was not provided.
   (3) There is no ROSC after complete ALS care in the field.
   (4) No AED shocks were delivered. (page 1873)
   b. The details that might lead you to ask if the patient has a DNR order or was in hospice care could best be expressed by the following quotes from the narrative:
   (1) "only 100 pounds"—Often terminal patients have lost a lot of weight and are very frail.
   (2) "hospital bed in the living room"—Those beds are large and often do not fit on the upper floors of the home. If set up on the first floor, the patient can be easily cared for while accessible to the entire family.
   (3) "been suffering for a long time"—This is an indication of a potential terminal illness.
   (4) "dad would not have wanted all this"—Hopefully he had discussed his wishes with his physician previously and has a DNR or MOLST in place!

True/False

1. T (page 1869)   **2.** T (page 1869)   **3.** T (page 1869)   **4.** F (page 1869)   **5.** T (page 1869)

6. F (page 1872)   **7.** T (page 1870)   **8.** F (page 1870)   **9.** F (page 1861)   **10.** T (page 1867)

Short Answer

1. Your initial techniques of verification of tube placement should include the following measures:
   a. Direct visualization of the tube going through the vocal cords
   b. Physical examination of the tube placement
   c. Bilateral chest expansion
   d. Five-point auscultation (two in each lung and epigastrium)
   e. Tube condensation
   f. Initial monitoring of ET_{CO_2} (waveform capnography) followed by continuous waveform capnography (page 1872)

2. A five-person team can be organized as follows:
   a. Compressor 1—Responsible for performing high-quality chest compressions, stays in position and compresses for 2 minutes and then rests for 2 minutes (for the duration of the time the patient is pulseless), may assist with application of the Thumper or other adjunct to circulation (provided Compressor 2 is continuing uninterrupted compressions).
   b. Compressor 2—Responsible for performing high-quality chest compressions, stays in position and compresses for 2 minutes and then rests for 2 minutes (for the duration of the time the patient is pulseless), may assist with application of the Thumper or other adjunct to circulation (provided Compressor 1 is continuing uninterrupted compressions).
   c. Ventilator—Responsible for providing ventilations at a ratio of 30:2, ensuring visible chest rise with each ventilation (1 second in duration). May need to briefly suction the patient as necessary, and then as appropriate will switch over to the ATV. Will assist with the transition from BLS airway to advanced airway (not a high priority). Once an advanced airway is placed, ventilate 8 to 10 times/min to achieve visible chest rise over a 1-second duration for each ventilation.
   d. Code team leader—Responsible for initial ECG analysis and defibrillation with a single shock (200 J). Responsible for overall timing of the code and reassessment after 2 minutes of cycles of CPR with the interruption not to exceed 10 seconds. After the initial shock (or ascertaining "no shock" rhythm), proceeds to establish IV or IO access, then begins administration of a vasopressor every 3 to 5 minutes, helps to transition the airway from BLS to an advanced airway, and continues with single shocks every 2 minutes if the patient is still in V-tach or V-fib. Makes the decision with input from the code team and medical control that the resuscitation should be terminated if there is no ROSC in the first 15 minutes. If there is ROSC, administers the appropriate antidysrhythmic, ensures appropriate ventilations, and assists the team in preparing for transport.
   e. EMS field supervisor—Brings in the Thumper or other adjunct to circulation and works with one of the compressors to transition the patient to mechanical CPR compressions with minimal interruption. Assists the medic with IV or IO, advanced airway placement, and preparation of medications, and contacts medical control, per local protocols. (page 1875)

Fill-in-the-Table

Paramedics should know the key elements of CPR for Adults, Children, and Infants, 2010 Guidelines. (pages 1866-1867)

Key Elements of CPR for Adults, Children, and Infants, 2010 Guidelines			
Procedure	Age 9 to Adult	Age 1 to 8 Years	Younger Than 1 Year[a]
Circulation			
Recognition	Unresponsive with no breathing, or only agonal (gasping) respirations		
Pulse check	**Carotid artery**	**Carotid artery**	Brachial artery
Compression location	In the center of the chest, in between the nipples	In the center of the chest, in between the nipples	**Just below the nipple line**
Compression area	Heel of both hands	**Heel of one or both hands**	Two fingers or two-thumb encircling-hands technique
Compression depth	At least 2 inches	At least one third of chest depth Approximately 2 inches	**At least one third of chest depth Approximately 1½ inches**
Compression rate	**At least 100/min**		
Chest wall recoil	Allow full chest recoil in between compressions Rotate professional rescuers delivering compressions every 2 minutes		
Interruptions	Limit interruptions in delivery of chest compressions to less than 10 seconds		
Ratio of compressions to ventilations (until an advanced airway is inserted)	**30:2 (one or two rescuers)**	**30:2** (one rescuer); **15:2** (two professional rescuers)	
Airway			
	Head tilt–chin lift maneuver; jaw-thrust maneuver if **spinal injury** is suspected		
Breathing			
Untrained rescuer	Compressions only		
Ventilations without advanced airway	2 breaths with a duration of **1 second** each, with enough volume to produce **chest rise**[b]		
Ventilations with advanced airway	1 breath every 6 to 8 seconds (8 to 10/min) Asynchronous with chest compressions. Duration of 1 second each with enough volume to produce chest rise		
Rescue breaths	1 breath every **5 seconds** (12 breaths/min)	1 breath every **3 seconds** (20 breaths/min)	1 breath every **3 seconds** (20 breaths/min)
Defibrillation			
Device	Adult AED	Use **pediatric dose-attenuator** unit if available; if not available, use adult unit	Use **manual defibrillator** if available; if not, use unit with pediatric dose attenuator; if neither is available, use adult unit
Procedure	Attach AED as soon as it is available. If two rescuers are available, one should immediately begin CPR while the second retrieves and applies the AED. Minimize CPR interruptions. Resume CPR immediately after shock, beginning with **chest compressions.**		
Airway Obstruction			
Foreign body obstruction	Conscious: **abdominal thrusts**	Conscious: **abdominal thrusts**	Conscious: **back slaps and chest thrusts**
	Unconscious: **CPR**[c]		

[a]Excluding newborns, in whom arrest is usually the result of asphyxiation and requires the rescue ventilations.
[b]Pause compressions to deliver ventilations.
[c]Look in the mouth for objects before delivering breaths in a patient with a known airway obstruction.

Skill Drill

The correct order for the steps in performing the CPR skills is as follows:

1. Performing Two-Rescuer Adult CPR.
(page 1857)

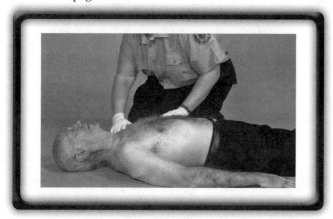

Step 1. Determine unresponsiveness and take positions.

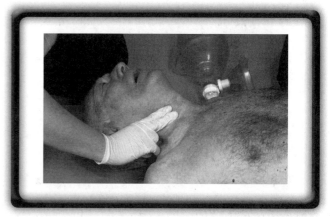

Step 2. Check for a carotid pulse (maximum of 10 seconds). If there is no pulse but an AED is available, apply it now.

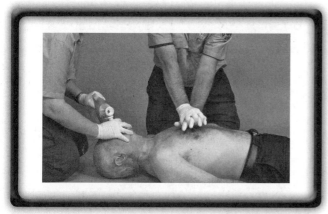

Step 3. If there is no pulse and an AED is not available or the elapsed time from collapse is greater than 4 to 5 minutes, begin chest compressions at a ratio of 30:2. Once an advanced airway is inserted, rescuers should switch from cycles of CPR to continuously delivered compressions at a rate of at least 100/min.

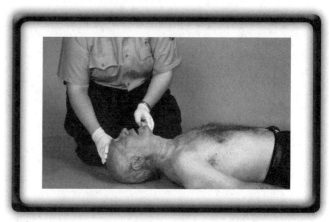

Step 4. Open the airway. Check for breathing. If breathing is adequate, place the patient in the recovery position and monitor.

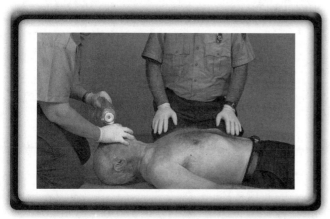

Step 5. If not breathing, give two breaths of 1 second each. After 2 minutes, switch rescuer positions to minimize fatigue. Keep switch time to 5 to 10 seconds. Depending on patient condition, continue CPR, continue ventilations only, or place in recovery position and monitor breathing and pulse.

2. Performing CPR on a Child
(page 1859)

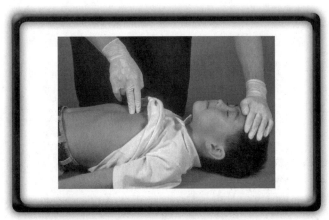

Step 1. Place the child on a firm surface. Prepare to place the heel of one or both hands in the center of the chest, in between the nipples, avoiding the xiphoid process.

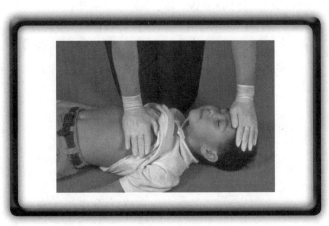

Step 2. Compress the chest one third the anterior-posterior diameter of the chest at a rate of 100/min.

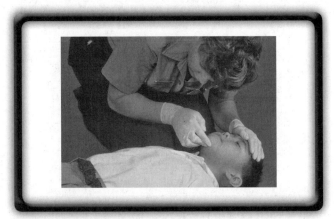

Step 3. Coordinate compressions with ventilations in a 30:2 ratio (one rescuer) or 15:2 (two rescuers). At the end of each cycle, pause for two ventilations.

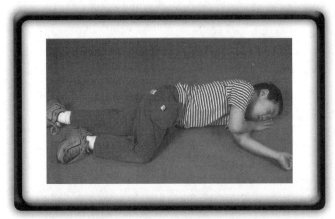

Step 4. Continue cycles of compressions and ventilations until an AED becomes available or the patient shows signs of spontaneous breathing. If the child resumes effective breathing, place him or her in a position that allows for frequent reassessment of the airway and vital signs during transport.

3. Infant CPR

(page 1860)

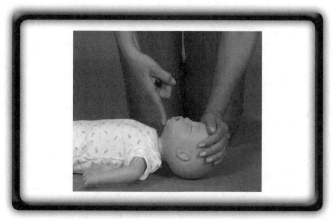

Step 1. Position the infant on a firm surface while maintaining the airway.

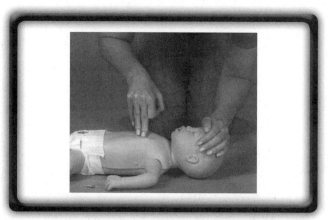

Step 2. Place two fingers in the middle of the sternum just below a line between the nipples. Use two fingers to compress the chest one third the anterior-posterior diameter of the chest at a rate of at least 100/min. Allow the sternum to return to its normal position between compressions.

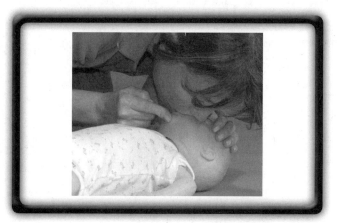

Step 3. Coordinate compressions with ventilations in a 30:2 ratio (one rescuer) or 15:2 (two rescuers), pausing for two ventilations at the end of each cycle. Continue cycles of compressions and ventilations until an AED becomes available or the infant shows signs of spontaneous breathing.

Chapter 40: Management and Resuscitation of the Critical Patient

Matching

1. Z (page 1915)	**2.** N (page 1915)	**3.** AA (page 1915)	**4.** UU (page 1915)	**5.** Y (page 1915)
6. R (page 1915)	**7.** S (page 1915)	**8.** X (page 1915)	**9.** W (page 1915)	**10.** P (page 1915)
11. Q (page 1915)	**12.** V (page 1915)	**13.** T (page 1915)	**14.** U (page 1915)	**15.** CC (page 1915)
16. BB (page 1915)	**17.** II (page 1915)	**18.** NN (page 1915)	**19.** DD (page 1915)	**20.** OO (page 1915)
21. PP (page 1915)	**22.** O (page 1915)	**23.** JJ (page 1915)	**24.** KK (page 1915)	**25.** LL (page 1915)
26. MM (page 1915)	**27.** HH (page 1915)	**28.** FF (page 1915)	**29.** QQ (page 1915)	**30.** VV (page 1915)
31. RR (page 1915)	**32.** GG (page 1915)	**33.** SS (page 1915)	**34.** TT (page 1915)	**35.** EE (page 1915)
36. D (page 1914)	**37.** E (page 1914)	**38.** F (page 1914)	**39.** M (page 1914)	**40.** L (page 1914)
41. K (page 1914)	**42.** G (page 1914)	**43.** H (page 1914)	**44.** I (page 1914)	**45.** J (page 1914)
46. C (page 1914)	**47.** B (page 1914)	**48.** A (page 1914)		

Multiple Choice

1. C (page 1881)	**2.** B (page 1882)	**3.** B (page 1882)	**4.** D (page 1883)	**5.** B (page 1883)
6. D (page 1886)	**7.** B (page 1886)	**8.** C (page 1887)	**9.** A (page 1888)	**10.** C (page 1888)
11. B (page 1888)	**12.** C (page 1891)	**13.** D (page 1894)	**14.** B (page 1896)	**15.** C (page 1900)

Labeling

1. Relationship Between the Organism and the Cells (page 1889)
   - **A.** Organism
   - **B.** Organ Systems
   - **C.** Organs
   - **D.** Tissues
   - **E.** Cells

Fill-in-the-Blank

1. anchoring (pages 1883–1884)
2. compensate; shunting (page 1889)
3. sphincters (page 1889)
4. chemoreceptors (page 1890)
5. aerobic; anaerobic (page 1891)
6. alpha 1; alpha 2; increasing (page 1891)
7. renal; necrosis; oliguria (page 1894)
8. irreversible (page 1896)
9. cardiac tamponade (page 1900)
10. Cardiogenic (page 1904)

Identify

1. Chief complaint: Chest pain
2. Vitals signs: Sinus bradycardia rate of 52 beats/min, crackles in the base of the lungs. Respirations are 24 breaths/min, blood pressure is 80/56 mm Hg, skin is diaphoretic and clammy. Patient is alert with oxygen administration and is PEARRL (Pupils Equal and Round, Regular in size, react to Light).
3. Pertinent negatives: No pulse at wrist, no ectopy on 12-lead ECG

Complete the Patient Care Report (PCR)

Show the completed PCR to your instructor to obtain feedback on your completion of the form.

Ambulance Calls

1. In assessing the state of perfusion:
   a. You can judge *peripheral* perfusion by checking capillary refill.
   b. The best indicator in the field of *perfusion of vital organs* is the patient's state of consciousness (mental status).
2. You are called to a bar to attend a bleeding, unconscious man. The place is full of noise and confusion—unruly customers, police, curiosity seekers. *This is the time to remember the priorities of the primary assessment:* A-B-C.

   First, before you even enter that bar, make certain that the police have the situation under control. (If you did not include that step in your answer, you do not get any points for your answer and, furthermore, you are a very poor risk for life insurance!) Look first to your own safety, remember?
   a. Open the patient's airway.
   b. Check whether he is breathing. If not, start artificial ventilation.
   c. Check whether he has a pulse. If he does not have a pulse, start external chest compressions.
   d. Cut away the patient's trouser leg, and find the source of his bleeding. When you've found it, control the bleeding by applying direct pressure on the wound, preferably over a sterile dressing. Check quickly for other lower extremity injuries.
   e. Transfer the patient to the vehicle (he should be on a backboard by now).
   f. Get underway to the hospital, and start an IV infusion en route. Complete your rapid secondary assessment as time permits.
3. This patient earns his "load-and-go" status by virtue of uncontrollable bleeding from the femoral artery.
   a. Steps to be taken at the scene:
      (1) Seal the open wound of the neck.
      (2) Administer supplemental oxygen.
      (3) Try at least to slow the bleeding from the groin by using pressure dressings and a hemostatic dressing if one is available.
      (4) Communicate with medical control or the receiving hospital.
   b. Steps to be taken en route:
      (1) Start two large-bore IVs with rapid infusion of fluids.
      (2) Complete a physical exam.
      (3) Recheck vital and neurologic signs every 5 minutes.
4. Abdominal evisceration is certainly an attention-getter, but it does not pose an immediate threat to life.
   a. Steps to be taken at the scene:
      (1) Administer supplemental oxygen.
      (2) Complete the physical exam.
      (3) Cover the eviscerated organs with sterile dressings soaked in sterile saline and an occlusive dressing.
   b. Steps to be taken en route:
      (1) Communicate with medical control or the receiving hospital.
      (2) Start a large-bore IV with normal saline.
      (3) Recheck vital and neurologic signs every 5 minutes.

5. An open chest wound is considered a critical injury because it prevents adequate ventilation of the lungs.
   a. Steps to be taken at the scene:
      (1) Seal off the sucking chest wound with an occlusive dressing taped on three sides.
      (2) Administer supplemental oxygen; assist ventilations as needed.
      (3) Communicate with medical control or the receiving hospital.
   b. Steps to be taken en route:
      (1) Complete a physical exam.
      (2) Start an IV with fluids.
      (3) Recheck vital and neurologic signs every 5 minutes.
6. Your primary assessment has not given you much information regarding *where* precisely this patient has been injured, but the primary *has* given you unmistakable evidence that the patient is in shock (restlessness, profuse sweating). Don't be fooled by the slow pulse—bradycardia occurs sometimes with intra-abdominal bleeding. *And don't wait for the blood pressure to fall before you decide that the patient is in shock!*
   a. Steps to be taken at the scene:
      (1) Manually stabilize the head/neck and apply a cervical collar.
      (2) Administer supplemental oxygen.
      (3) Conduct the rapid secondary assessment.
      (4) Immobilize the patient on a long backboard.
      (5) Prepare for rapid transport to the appropriate facility.
   b. Steps to be taken en route:
      (1) Complete a physical exam.
      (2) Start two large-bore IVs and run a fluid challenge.
      (3) Communicate with medical control or the receiving hospital.
      (4) Conduct a reassessment, rechecking vital and neurologic signs every 5 minutes.

True/False

1. T (page 1905) **2.** F (page 1905) **3.** T (page 1905) **4.** T (page 1905) **5.** F (page 1907)

6. T (page 1907) **7.** T (page 1907) **8.** T (page 1908) **9.** T (page 1908) **10.** F (page 1891)

Short Answer

1. M: Medication overdose/noncompliance

   T: Tumor, trauma, toxins

   S: Seizures or stroke

   H: Hypoxia, hyperthermia/hypothermia, hyperglycemia/hypoglycemia, hypertensive crisis, hypovolemia, hyperkalemia/hypokalemia

   I: Infection and uremia

   P: Psychiatric or behavioral disorders (page 1882)

2. Karl Weick's "five-step process" for communicating intuitive decisions and obtaining feedback from team members includes:
   a. Here is what I think we are dealing with.
   b. Here is what I think we should do.
   c. Here is why.
   d. Here is what we should keep our eyes on.
   e. Now talk to me. Are there any other concerns? (page 1883)

Fill-in-the-Table

1. (page 1885)

The "H and T" Questions of Cardiac Arrest	
Reversible Causes of Cardiac Arrest	Ask your team . . .
Hypovolemia	Does this patient have any evidence of internal or external bleeding or fluid loss?
Hypoxia	How well is the patient oxygenating? Could there have been a respiratory event that led to this cardiac arrest?
Hydrogen ion (acidosis)	Is there any reason for metabolic or respiratory acidosis in this patient?
Hypokalemia/hyperkalemia	Does this patient undergo renal dialysis? Might the electrolytes be altered (ie, is the patient on a liquid diet)?
Hypothermia	Does the patient feel cold to touch? If so, obtain the core body temperature.
Hypoglycemic/hyperglycemic	Is the patient a diabetic? What is the blood glucose level?
Tension pneumothorax	Does the patient have bilateral lung sounds? Is the patient becoming difficult to ventilate? Consider the need for chest decompression.
Tamponade (cardiac)	Is there penetrating trauma to the patient's heart? Consider the need for pericardiocentesis (in the ED).
Toxins	Consider substance abuse (ie, narcotics or opiates). Consider naloxone (Narcan).
Thrombosis (pulmonary)	Does the patient have a history of blood clots? Is the patient a smoker and/or take birth control? Has the patient had a recent long bone immobilization?
Thrombosis (coronary)	Does the patient have a large AMI developing? Is this patient a candidate for PCI?
Trauma	Is there a mechanism of injury for life-threatening trauma?

2. (page 1896)

Compensated Versus Decompensated Shock	
Compensated Shock	**Decompensated Shock**
• Agitation, anxiety, restlessness • **Sense of impending doom** • Weak, rapid (thready) pulse • Clammy (cool, moist) skin • **Pallor with cyanotic lips** • **Shortness of breath** • Nausea, vomiting • Delayed capillary refill in infants and children • **Thirst** • **Normal blood pressure**	• Altered mental status (verbal to unresponsive)* • **Hypotension** • **Labored or irregular breathing** • Thready or absent peripheral pulses • Ashen, mottled, or cyanotic skin • **Dilated pupils** • Diminished urine output (oliguria) • **Impending cardiac arrest**
*Mental status changes are late indicators.	

3. (page 1905)

Types of Shock			
Type of Shock	**Examples of Potential Causes**	**Signs and Symptoms**	**Assessment and Treatment**
Cardiogenic	Inadequate heart function Disease of muscle tissue Impaired electrical system Disease or injury	Chest pain Irregular pulse Weak pulse Low blood pressure Cyanosis (lips, under nails) Cool, clammy skin Anxiety Rales Pulmonary edema	**If lungs are clear and protocols allow, administer a fluid challenge of 200 mL (to increase preload)** **Consider CPAP/BiPAP**

Obstructive	Mechanical obstruction of the cardiac muscle causing a decrease in cardiac output
	1. Tension pneumothorax
	2. Cardiac tamponade
		Dependent on cause:
		• Dyspnea
		• Rapid, weak pulse
		• Rapid, shallow breaths
		• Decreased lung compliance
		• Unilateral, decreased, or absent breath sounds
		• Decreased blood pressure
		• Jugular vein distention
		• Subcutaneous emphysema
		• Cyanosis
		• Tracheal deviation toward affected side
		• Beck triad (cardiac tamponade):
		  • Jugular vein distention
		  • Narrowing pulse pressure
		  • Muffled heart tones
			Dependent on cause:
			• **Administer fluid at a keep-vein-open (KVO) rate**
			• **Consider chest decompression (injured side for suspected tension pneumothorax)**
			• **Consider pericardiocentesis for cardiac tamponade if appropriately trained and authorized by protocol**

Septic	Severe bacterial infection	Warm skin Tachycardia Low blood pressure	**Administer fluid boluses to maintain radial pulses** **Consider sepsis alert program if protocol exists in your region.** **Consider medications depending on the existence of warm versus cold shock**
Neurogenic	Cervical or thoracic spinal cord injury, which causes widespread blood vessel dilation	Bradycardia (slow pulse) or normal pulse Low blood pressure Signs of neck injury	**Administer warmed IV fluids to maintain radial pulses** **Consider vasopressors, steroids, or vagal blocker per local protocols**
Anaphylactic	Extreme life-threatening allergic reaction	Can develop within seconds Mild itching or rash Burning skin Vascular dilation Generalized edema Coma Rapid death	**Determine cause of anaphylaxis** **Administer epinephrine IM or a vasopressor** **Administer fluid at a KVO rate** **Consider bronchodilator or antihistamine**

(Continued)

Types of Shock			
Type of Shock	**Examples of Potential Causes**	**Signs and Symptoms**	**Assessment and Treatment**
Psychogenic (fainting)	Temporary, generalized vascular dilation Anxiety, bad news, sight of injury or blood, prospect of medical treatment, severe pain, illness, tiredness	Rapid pulse Normal or low blood pressure	**Determine duration of unresponsiveness** **Suspect head injury if patient is confused or slow to respond**
Hypovolemic	Loss of blood or fluid	Rapid, weak pulse Low blood pressure Change in mental status Cyanosis (lips, under nails) Cool, clammy skin Increased respiratory rate	**Control external bleeding** **Provide fluid resuscitation en route** **Consider use of vasopressors to maintain the blood pressure**
Respiratory insufficiency	Severe chest injury, airway obstruction	Rapid, weak pulse Low blood pressure Change in mental status Cyanosis (lips, under nails) Cool, clammy skin Increased respiratory rate	**Seal hole in chest** **Stabilize flail segments/impaled objects** **Administer fluid at a KVO rate**

Section 9: Special Patient Populations
Chapter 41: Obstetrics

Matching

1. EE (page 1958)	**2.** FF (page 1958)	**3.** GG (page 1958)	**4.** HH (page 1958)	**5.** LL (page 1958)
6. KK (page 1958)	**7.** CC (page 1958)	**8.** MM (page 1958)	**9.** BB (page 1958)	**10.** AA (page 1958)
11. NN (page 1958)	**12.** SS (page 1958)	**13.** QQ (page 1958)	**14.** N (page 1958)	**15.** PP (page 1958)
16. OO (page 1958)	**17.** TT (page 1958)	**18.** UU (page 1958)	**19.** VV (page 1958)	**20.** WW (page 1958)
21. RR (page 1958)	**22.** XX (page 1958)	**23.** YY (page 1958)	**24.** ZZ (page 1958)	**25.** Z (page 1958)
26. W (page 1959)	**27.** V (page 1959)	**28.** U (page 1959)	**29.** O (page 1959)	**30.** M (page 1959)
31. L (page 1959)	**32.** Y (page 1958)	**33.** X (page 1959)	**34.** II (page 1958)	**35.** K (page 1959)
36. E (page 1959)	**37.** H (page 1959)	**38.** G (page 1959)	**39.** D (page 1959)	**40.** C (page 1959)
41. B (page 1959)	**42.** A (page 1959)	**43.** R (page 1959)	**44.** Q (page 1959)	**45.** P (page 1959)
46. JJ (page 1958)	**47.** DD (page 1958)	**48.** J (page 1959)	**49.** I (page 1959)	**50.** F (page 1959)
51. T (page 1959)	**52.** S (page 1959)			

Multiple Choice

1. A (page 1936)	**2.** D (page 1938)	**3.** A (page 1927)	**4.** C (page 1939)	**5.** B (page 1943)
6. D (page 1944)	**7.** A (page 1945)	**8.** D (page 1922)	**9.** C (page 1924)	**10.** A (page 1926)

Labeling

1. Structures of the Pregnant Uterus (page 1924)
   - **A.** Placenta
   - **B.** Umbilical cord
   - **C.** Amniotic cavity
   - **D.** Uterus
   - **E.** Lumen of uterus

Fill-in-the-Blank

1. endometrium (page 1923)
2. umbilical cord (page 1924)
3. increases (page 1926)
4. Preeclampsia (page 1931)
5. spontaneous abortion (page 1936)
6. Placenta previa (page 1938)
7. Multigravida (page 1927)
8. second stage (page 1939)
9. transverse (page 1949)
10. Magnesium sulfate (page 1944)

Identify

1. Chief complaint: "I am bleeding from my vagina."
2. Vital signs: Pulse is 110 beats/min and thready, respirations are 24 breaths/min, blood pressure is 100/70 mm Hg, and the patient is pale and diaphoretic.
3. Pertinent findings: Patient is 35 years old, in her third trimester, multiparity with previous cesarean sections. The blood is bright red; she is painless and thirsty, and says she is weak. The vital signs and physical exam reveal signs of shock.

Complete the Patient Care Report (PCR)

Show the completed PCR to your instructor to obtain feedback on your completion of the form.

Ambulance Calls

1. a. The 22-year-old who has passed blood and tissue through the vagina and is showing signs of hemorrhagic shock is most likely having an **incomplete abortion** (answer C). The passage of tissue indicates some sort of abortion, and the fact that she is continuing to bleed suggests there is still tissue in the uterus. (page 1936)

   b. She should be treated for shock because her vital signs indicate that she is already in shock:

   (1) Keep the woman recumbent, lying on her left side.

   (2) Administer 100% supplemental oxygen via nonrebreathing mask at 15 L/min.

   (3) Provide rapid transport to a definitive care facility, notifying the facility of the patient's condition en route.

   (4) Start an IV lifeline of normal saline with a large-bore IV catheter. Infuse at a rate necessary to maintain blood pressure. An additional IV lifeline may be indicated.

   (5) Establish an ECG and obtain baseline vital signs. Do not attempt to examine the woman internally or pack the vagina with trauma pads.

   (6) Use loosely placed trauma pads over the vagina in an effort to staunch bleeding.

   (7) If bleeding is severe, and significant signs and symptoms of shock are present, pharmacologic management may be indicated. *Tocolytics* are drugs that are used to delay preterm labor. (page 1937)

2. a. The 32-year-old woman has good reason to be "feeling poorly": She is carrying a dead fetus in her uterus; that is, she has a **missed abortion** (answer D). Her history is typical: a threatened abortion earlier in the pregnancy that seemed to get better, but failure of the pregnancy to develop normally. By 6 months, her uterine fundus should be palpable above the umbilicus, just barely above the pelvic brim. (page 1936)

   b. The prehospital management of missed abortion is simply to transport the patient to the hospital while providing emotional support. At the hospital, surgical evacuation of the uterus will be required. (page 1937)

3. a. The primigravida with painless vaginal bleeding is experiencing a **threatened abortion** (answer A). The absence of contractions indicates that the abortion is not yet inevitable. (page 1936)

   b. The prehospital treatment of threatened abortion is simply to transport, while providing emotional support to the patient. (page 1937)

4. a. The 16-year-old who went to the backstreet abortionist has suffered one of the most common results: **septic abortion** (answer E). By the time you reach the scene, the girl already has signs of septic shock, and she may die. (pages 1936–1937)

   b. The prehospital management is to treat for shock:

   (1) Keep the woman recumbent, lying on her left side.

   (2) Administer 100% supplemental oxygen via nonrebreathing mask at 15 L/min.

   (3) Provide rapid transport to a definitive care facility, notifying the facility of the patient's condition en route.

   (4) Start an IV lifeline of normal saline with a large-bore IV catheter. Infuse at a rate necessary to maintain blood pressure. An additional IV lifeline may be indicated.

   (5) Establish an ECG and obtain baseline vital signs. Do not attempt to examine the woman internally or pack the vagina with trauma pads.

   (6) Use loosely placed trauma pads over the vagina in an effort to staunch bleeding. (page 1937)

5. a. The 26-year-old veteran of three previous miscarriages is probably correct; she seems to be having yet another, that is, an **inevitable abortion** (answer B). The severe cramping and uterine contractions that accompany her vaginal bleeding bode ill for the continuation of the pregnancy. (page 1936)

   b. The prehospital treatment of inevitable abortion is expectant treatment for shock:

   (1) Keep the woman recumbent, lying on her left side.

   (2) Administer 100% supplemental oxygen via nonrebreathing mask at 15 L/min.

   (3) Provide rapid transport to a definitive care facility, notifying the facility of the patient's condition en route.

   (4) Start an IV lifeline of normal saline with a large-bore IV catheter. Infuse at a rate necessary to maintain blood pressure. An additional IV lifeline may be indicated.

   (5) Establish an ECG and obtain baseline vital signs. Do not attempt to examine the woman internally or pack the vagina with trauma pads. (page 1937)

6. This case concerns a 36-year-old grand multipara with third-trimester bleeding.

   a. Three possible causes of third-trimester bleeding are:

     (1) Abruptio placenta

     (2) Placenta previa

     (3) Uterine rupture (pages 1937–1938)

   b. In this particular case, the most likely diagnosis is **placenta previa**. (page 1938)

   c. Among the characteristic features of placenta previa manifested by this patient are the following:

     (1) *Painless* vaginal bleeding. (There is severe pain with placental abruption or uterine rupture.)

     (2) *Bright red* blood. (In abruption, bleeding is dark.)

     (3) The *fetus remains viable.*

     (4) The *abdomen* is *soft and nontender.* (page 1938)

   d. The steps in prehospital management are (page 1938):

     (1) Keep the woman recumbent, lying on her left side.

     (2) Administer 100% supplemental oxygen via nonrebreathing mask at 15 L/min.

     (3) Provide rapid transport to a definitive care facility, notifying the facility of the patient's condition en route.

     (4) Start an IV lifeline of normal saline with a large-bore IV catheter. Infuse at a rate necessary to maintain blood pressure. An additional IV lifeline may be indicated.

     (5) Establish an ECG and obtain baseline vital signs. Do not attempt to examine the woman internally or pack the vagina with trauma pads.

     (6) Use loosely placed trauma pads over the vagina in an effort to staunch bleeding.

     (7) If bleeding is severe and significant signs and symptoms of shock are present, pharmacologic management may be indicated. *Tocolytics* are drugs used to delay preterm labor. In cases of abruptio placenta and placenta previa, magnesium sulfate may be ordered by your medical control but is not used in all areas (4 to 6 g bolus over a 20-minute period, followed by a 2 to 4 g/hr titrated drip). Oxytocin may be ordered in cases of uterine rupture, with an ordered dose of 20 to 40 units (1,000 mL at 100 mL/hour) to encourage uterine contractions.

7. a. The woman with the fainting spells is most probably suffering from **supine hypotensive syndrome** (answer E) because her pulse and blood pressure improved very quickly after she turned to her side and took the weight of her uterus off her inferior vena cava. Nonetheless, you can't take a chance on missing a concealed hemorrhage. In fact, women whose volume status is already marginal are most vulnerable to the supine hypotensive syndrome. So, you will have to treat the patient as someone who might develop hemorrhagic shock. (page 1931)

   b. The prehospital management, then, is as follows:

     (1) Administer supplemental oxygen.

     (2) Keep the patient in the recumbent position with the bulk of her uterus to the side to avoid vena cava syndrome.

     (3) Start an IV with saline.

     (4) Transport to the hospital as soon as possible.

     (5) Obtain an ECG. (page 1931)

8. a. The woman who fell in a downtown department store has a chief complaint unrelated to her pregnancy—a twisted ankle. But, in fact, a careful examination reveals a very serious problem that is related to her pregnancy, **preeclampsia** (answer B), as manifested by edema and hypertension. (page 1931)

   b. The initial prehospital treatment, therefore, is as follows:

     (1) Splint the injured ankle.

     (2) Transport the woman in the semi-Fowler's position (as long as this does not cause any dizziness).

     (3) Start an IV en route so that it will be there if you need it. Pain meds should be discussed with medical control before being administered.

   c. And, indeed, you did need that IV—when the woman proceeded to have a grand mal seizure and develop full-blown eclampsia. The steps to take at that point are:

     (1) Protect the patient from injury during the tonic-clonic phase of the seizure.

     (2) Ensure an adequate airway.

     (3) Administer supplemental oxygen.

     (4) Contact medical control for orders. You may be asked to give magnesium sulfate 10%, 2 to 4 gm IV.

(5) Notify the receiving hospital. If the woman's seizures cannot be controlled, it may be necessary to take her straight to the operating room for an emergency cesarean section. (pages 1931–1932)

9. When *two* pregnant women are involved in a motor vehicle crash, it's quadruple trouble!

    a. Some of the changes during pregnancy that make a woman more vulnerable to injury or that affect her response to injury include the following (*students should list five*):

        (1) **Elevation of the diaphragm**, which effectively pushes the abdominal contents into the chest so that abdominal organs are more apt to be injured after a blow to the chest.

        (2) **Forward, upward displacement of the bladder**, rendering it more vulnerable to injury.

        (3) The **uterus** becomes more susceptible to injury as it enlarges and occupies more space in the abdomen.

        (4) **Increase in vascular volume** by as much as 50% so that the pregnant woman can lose a lot of blood (and the fetus can be in big trouble) before she shows signs of shock.

        (5) **Relative tachycardia and hypotension** make it difficult to interpret the pregnant woman's vital signs after injury.

        (6) **Redistribution of blood flow** to the pelvic area means that a pregnant woman will bleed much more profusely from injuries such as pelvic fracture.

        (7) Delayed gastric emptying during pregnancy makes a pregnant woman more likely to vomit and aspirate after injury. (pages 1953–1954)

    b. You find the *driver* of the car conscious, but with evidence of steering wheel trauma to the abdomen and indications of impending shock (thirst, tachycardia, slight hypotension). She must, therefore, be treated for shock and regarded as a load-and-go emergency:

        (1) Manually stabilize the cervical spine.

        (2) Remove the woman from the vehicle on a long backboard, with the usual spinal precautions.

        (3) In the ambulance, keep the backboard tilted 30° to the left side.

        (4) Ensure an adequate airway; be prepared for vomiting.

        (5) Administer supplemental oxygen.

        (6) Start transport, and notify the receiving hospital.

        (7) En route, start at least one large-bore IV, and run in normal saline to maintain a normal blood pressure.

        (8) Obtain an ECG. (pages 1952–1954)

    c. The pregnant *passenger* does not seem to be seriously injured, although her complaints of neck pain ("whiplash") should prompt appropriate measures to stabilize the cervical spine. In any case, however, you cannot conclude that there is no injury to the fetus. Only careful evaluation in the hospital, and observation over several hours, can establish that fact. (pages 1953–1954)

10. Deciding whether you have time to transport a woman in active labor to the hospital is a judgment call, and there is room for debate in some of these situations. As a general rule, you will have a lot more time with nulliparas. Multiparas can progress very rapidly through labor, and so the margin for error is smaller. (pages 1939–1940)

    a. D. The urge to move the bowels indicates that the fetal head is already in the birth canal and delivery is imminent. The delivery may be complicated by fetal infection because the amniotic sac ruptured several hours ago.

    b. D. As a general rule, when a woman who has had eight babies tells you that the baby is coming, she knows what she's talking about! Complications seen more commonly in grand multiparas include uterine rupture and postpartum hemorrhage.

    c. T. In *this* case, you should have plenty of time. The woman is a beginner, and her contractions are still quite widely spaced. Don't forget to get a full set of vital signs, as there is always a potential for complications.

    d. D. No doubts here: The woman is crowning! If she's had two previous cesarean sections, she could be at increased risk for uterine rupture during labor. Also, you have to inquire why she needed the c-sections in the first place (eg, fetus in the wrong position, very large fetus, late delivery date).

    e. T. This woman may not even be in labor. Her contractions sound suspiciously like Braxton Hicks contractions. If you sit around waiting for her to deliver, you might spend several weeks at the scene! Although this is not a complication, it is a consideration in this case.

    f. D. With the contractions coming at only 2-minute intervals in a multipara, you can't afford to take a chance. The potential complications more likely in a twin birth include cord prolapse, breech presentation, and postpartum hemorrhage. The babies are also likely to be small and therefore to require the kind of special care given to premature babies.

11. Science has not yet established the precise mechanism that stimulates a woman to go into labor, but any experienced emergency medical technician (EMT) or paramedic can attest to the fact that one thing that can stimulate labor is shopping! That is why paramedics frequently find themselves delivering babies in department stores.

    a. When the baby's face is found to be covered by the intact amniotic sac, you should tear open the amniotic sac, either with your fingers or a forceps, and carefully peel it away from the baby's face. Then, suction the baby's nostrils and mouth with a bulb aspirator. (page 1942)

    b. When the umbilical cord is found *tightly* wound around the baby's neck, the only thing you can do is put two clamps on the cord, 2 inches apart, and cut the cord between the clamps. (page 1942)

    c. The steps to take from that point on are as follows:

       (1) Guide the baby's head downward to allow delivery of the upper shoulder.

       (2) Guide the baby's head upward to allow delivery of the lower shoulder.

       (3) Wipe the baby's mouth and nose free of blood and mucus, and suction out the mouth and nostrils again.

       (4) Tell the mother and all the salespersons in the lingerie department if it's a boy or a girl.

       (5) Dry the baby, cover it with a blanket, and put it on the mother's abdomen.

       (6) Record the time of birth and the Apgar score while you await the delivery of the placenta.

       (7) When the placenta separates, instruct the mother to bear down.

       (8) *After the placenta has delivered*, massage the uterus, and put the baby to the mother's breast.

       (9) Clean up, put a sanitary pad between the mother's legs, bid farewell to the women in the lingerie department, and transport. (pages 1942–1943)

12. **a.** What you are dealing with at the ski lodge is a breech presentation. That smooth presenting part with a crack down the middle is the buttocks, not a head! (page 1948)

    b. Management is as follows:

       (1) *Position the mother* with her buttocks at the edge of the bed or stretcher and her legs flexed.

       (2) Allow the buttocks and trunk of the baby to deliver spontaneously. *Do not pull on the baby.*

       (3) Once the baby's legs are clear, *support the baby's body* on the palm of your hand and volar surface of your arm.

       (4) Then, lower the baby slightly so that it very nearly hangs by its own weight downward; that will help the head pass through the pelvic outlet. You can tell when the head is in the vaginal canal because you will be able to see the baby's hairline at the nape of its neck just below the mother's symphysis pubis.

       (5) *When you can see the baby's hairline*, grasp the baby by the ankles and lift it upward in the direction of the mother's abdomen. The head should then deliver without difficulty.

       (6) If the baby's head does not deliver in 3 minutes, the baby is in danger of suffocation, and immediate action is indicated. Suffocation may occur when the baby's umbilical cord is compressed by its head against the birth canal, which cuts off the baby's supply of oxygenated blood from the placenta, and the baby's face is pressed against the vaginal wall, which prevents it from breathing on its own. Place your gloved hand in the vagina, with your palm toward the baby's face. Form a V with your fingers on either side of the baby's nose, and push the vaginal wall away from the baby's face until the head is delivered.

       (7) Do not attempt to pull the baby out forcibly or allow an explosive delivery. If the head does not deliver within 3 minutes of establishing the airway, provide rapid transport to the hospital, with the mother's buttocks elevated on pillows. If at all possible, try to maintain the baby's airway throughout transport in the manner described. En route, alert the hospital so that they can have the appropriate personnel on hand when the mother arrives. (page 1949)

13. Prolapsed umbilical cord occurs in only about 1 of every 300 deliveries, but it is more likely with a premature birth like this one. You must do the following:

    a. Position the mother supine with her hips elevated as much as possible on pillows.

    b. Administer 100% supplemental oxygen via nonrebreathing mask.

    c. Instruct the mother to pant with each contraction, which will prevent her from bearing down.

    d. If you are trained and authorized to do so, catheterize the mother's bladder; instill 500 mL of saline into the bladder through the catheter; then, clamp the catheter shut. The full bladder helps keep the presenting part off the cord.

    e. With two fingers of a gloved hand, gently *push the baby* (not the cord) back up into the vagina until the presenting part is no longer pressing on the cord.

    f. While you maintain pressure on the presenting part, have your partner cover the exposed portion of the cord with dressings moistened in normal saline.

    g. Somehow, you will have to try to maintain that position, with a gloved hand pushing the presenting part away from the cord, throughout *urgent transport* to the hospital. (page 1950)

14. a. The special measures required in delivering twins, as opposed to a single birth, are:

    (1) Wait for the second birth after the first is complete. Meanwhile, keep the first baby warm on the mother's abdomen, covered with a blanket.

    (2) Treat both babies as you would preemies, paying scrupulous attention to their warmth, prevention of bleeding, and protection from contamination. (page 1947)

    b. The mother's *risk factor for postpartum hemorrhage* was the very fact of her twin pregnancy. The placenta covers a larger area in a twin pregnancy, and the uterine muscles become overstretched so that they contract less efficiently. (page 1950)

    c. Other risk factors for postpartum hemorrhage include (*students should list three of the following*):

    (1) Prolonged labor

    (2) Retained products of conception

    (3) Grand multiparity

    (4) Multiple pregnancy

    (5) Placenta previa

    (6) A full bladder

    (7) Lacerations

    (8) Uterine atony (page 1951)

    d. The steps that should be taken to manage postpartum hemorrhage in the field are as follows:

    (1) Continue uterine massage.

    (2) Put either or both babies to the breast to start nursing.

    (3) Contact medical control to consider administration of oxytocin.

    (4) Begin transport, and notify the receiving hospital.

    (5) Start another IV with a large-bore catheter to infuse crystalloid rapidly.

    (6) Manage external bleeding from perinatal tears with a sanitary napkin and direct pressure. (page 1951)

True/False

1. F (pages 1929–1930)   **2.** T (page 1930)   **3.** F (page 1940)   **4.** T (page 1940)

5. F (page 1943)   **6.** F (page 1943)   **7.** T (page 1949)

Short Answer

1. The functions of the placenta include (*students should list four of the following*):

    a. Respiratory gas exchange

    b. Transport of nutrients

    c. Excretion of wastes

    d. Transfer of heat

    e. Hormone production

    f. Formation of a barrier (page 1924)

Fill-in-the-Table

1. (page 1939)

The Stages of Labor: Nullipara Versus Multipara		
Stages of Labor	Nullipara	Multipara
First stage	8 to 12 hours	6 to 8 hours
Second stage	1 to 2 hours	30 minutes
Third stage	5 to 60 minutes	5 to 60 minutes

2. (page 1929)

False Labor Versus True Labor		
Parameter	True Labor	False Labor
Contractions	Regularly spaced	Irregularly spaced
Interval between contractions	Gradually shortens	Remains long
Intensity of contractions	Gradually increases	Stays the same
Effects of analgesics	Do not abolish the pain	Often abolish the pain
Cervical changes	Progressive effacement and dilation	No changes

Chapter 42: Neonatal Care

Matching

1. S (page 1998)   **2.** AA (page 1999)   **3.** W (page 1999)   **4.** I (page 1998)   **5.** J (page 1998)

6. Q (page 1998)   **7.** L (page 1998)   **8.** K (page 1998)   **9.** N (page 1998)   **10.** T (page 1998)

11. M (page 1998)   **12.** O (page 1998)   **13.** P (page 1998)   **14.** U (page 1999)   **15.** EE (page 1999)

16. FF (page 1999)   **17.** E (page 2000)   **18.** V (page 1999)   **19.** BB (page 1999)   **20.** X (page 1999)

21. GG (page 1999)   **22.** D (page 2000)   **23.** DD (page 1999)   **24.** HH (page 1999)   **25.** Z (page 1999)

26. Y (page 1999)   **27.** H (page 1998)   **28.** CC (page 1998)   **29.** II (page 1999)   **30.** C (page 2000)

31. B (page 2000)   **32.** R (page 1998)   **33.** A (page 2000)   **34.** G (page 2000)   **35.** F (page 2000)

Multiple Choice

1. D (page 1964)   **2.** A (page 1964)   **3.** C (page 1967)   **4.** C (page 1969)   **5.** D (page 1981)

6. A (page 1978)   **7.** D (page 1969)   **8.** C (page 1982)   **9.** A (page 1980)   **10.** D (page 1983)

Labeling

1. Algorithm for resuscitation.
(page 1969)

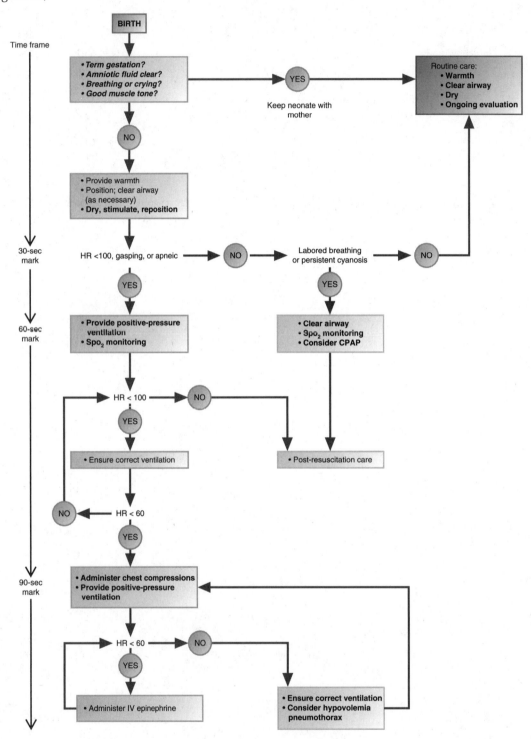

Fill-in-the-Blank

1. transition; pulmonary; oxygen (page 1964)
2. 37; 38; 42; 42 (page 1964)
3. umbilical cord; blood supply; pressure (page 1967)

4. cyanotic; vigorous; thermoregulation (page 1967)

5. pneumothorax; compressions; palpable (pages 1968–1969)

6. rarely; obstruction; choanal atresia (page 1970)

7. decompression; orogastric; diaphragmatic (page 1975)

8. seizure; newborn (page 1984)

9. infections; temperature; hypoglycemia; metabolic (page 1988)

10. hypoglycemia; apnea; feeding; lethargy; seizures (page 1986)

11. mucus; blood; uncommon (page 1986)

12. Antiemetics; resuscitation; fontanelle (page 1987)

13. Bradycardia; inadequate; hypoxia (page 1977)

14. community hospital; equipment; regional center (page 1979)

15. viral infection (page 1987)

Identify

1. **a.** If the umbilical cord comes out ahead of the baby, the blood supply through the umbilical cord may be cut off. In this case:

   (1) Relieving pressure on the cord (by gently moving the presenting part of the body off the cord and pushing the cord back) can be lifesaving.

   (2) When the baby's head is delivered, suction the mouth and nose with a bulb syringe, as needed.

   (3) After the infant is delivered, keep the baby at the level of the mother, with the head slightly lower than the body.

   (4) Clamp the umbilical cord in two places, and then cut between the clamps.

   (5) Your primary assessment of the newborn may be done simultaneously with any treatment interventions.

   (6) Note the time of delivery, and monitor the ABCs.

   (7) In particular, assess respiratory rate, respiratory effort, pulse rate, color, and capillary refill. (page 1967)

2. **a.** If the baby is apneic (ie, has a 20-second or longer respiratory pause) or has a pulse rate less than 100 beats/min after 30 seconds of drying and stimulation and supplemental free-flow (blow-by) oxygen:

   (1) Begin PPV by bag-mask device, being sure to use a newborn-sized bag mask.

   (2) You should use caution when squeezing the bag to avoid inadvertently delivering too much volume, potentially resulting in a pneumothorax. (page 1968)

   b. Chest compressions are indicated if the pulse rate remains less than 60 beats/min despite positioning, clearing the airway, drying and stimulation, and 30 seconds of effective PPV:

   (1) With the thumb (two-rescuer) technique, two thumbs are placed side by side over the sternum between the nipples, and the hands encircle the torso. With the two-finger (one-rescuer) technique, the tips of the index and middle fingers are placed over the sternum between the nipples and the sternum is compressed between the fingers and a hand behind the baby's back.

   (2) The depth of compression is one third of the anteroposterior diameter of the chest. Your fingers should remain in contact with the chest at all times but allow full chest recoil.

   (3) In neonates, the chest compressions occur in synchrony with artificial ventilation, which you continue during chest compressions. (pages 1968–1969)

Ambulance Calls

1. If you were expecting problems in delivering this 38-year-old multipara, you were right. (page 1964)

   a. Yes, there are several indications that this may be a complicated delivery or that you may have problems with the baby afterward:

   (1) Maternal age greater than 35 years

   (2) No prenatal care

   (3) Prolonged labor

   (4) Meconium staining of the amniotic fluid

   (5) Probable post-term baby (It's hard to know how much to trust the mother's estimate of the gestational age.)

    b. Other risk factors for obstetric and neonatal complications include *(students should provide four of the following)*:

        (1) Maternal diabetes

        (2) Maternal drug or alcohol abuse

        (3) Antepartum hemorrhage

        (4) Twin pregnancy

        (5) Abnormal presentation

        (6) Prolapsed umbilical cord

        (7) Fetal distress (page 1964)

    c. When the baby's head delivers and is found to be covered with meconium:

        (1) Clean the mouth and nostrils with sterile gauze.

        (2) Use a bulb aspirator to suction the mouth and nostrils as needed. (page 1981)

    d. Once the baby is fully delivered:

        (1) Quickly dry off the baby.

        (2) Clamp and cut the cord.

        (3) Hand off the baby to your partner to intubate and suction as needed.

        (4) If the baby does not breathe spontaneously, give several breaths with bag-mask device and oxygen.

        (5) Finish drying the baby, and cover with warm blankets. (page 1981)

2. *Return of the Spider Monster* is not recommended viewing for an impressionable woman in the third trimester of pregnancy. Look what can happen!

    a. When you find yourself holding a newborn premature infant that had the temerity to be born before you could even open your obstetrics (OB) kit, take the following steps:

        (1) Suction the mouth and nostrils with a bulb syringe.

        (2) Quickly dry the baby with whatever you have available.

        (3) As soon as possible, wrap the baby in something warm.

        (4) When your partner brings the OB kit, clamp and cut the cord. (page 1967)

    b. Hypothermia represents an increased risk for morbidity and mortality. However, if the newborn appears otherwise healthy, it is appropriate to clamp and cut the cord. It may also be necessary to cut and clamp the cord to resuscitate in the prehospital setting. (page 1989)

    c. The things you can do to try to prevent the baby from becoming hypothermic are the following:

        (1) Dry the baby thoroughly.

        (2) Place a cap on the baby's head.

        (3) Cover the baby with a warm blanket.

        (4) Keep the baby on the mother's body.

        (5) In the ambulance, turn on the heaters full blast until the ambient temperature increases to around 35°C (95°F), even if it's summer! (page 1989)

    d. Besides keeping the baby warm, you need to do the following:

        (1) Take particular care to maintain a patent airway.

        (2) Administer supplemental oxygen into a tent or by blow-by.

        (3) Wear a surgical mask and gown to protect the baby from infection. (page 1967)

3. You think this case is exaggerated? You don't believe that teenage girls give birth on the toilet? In fact, this scenario is based on an actual case managed by real paramedics.

    a. Immediately upon rescuing the infant from the toilet, you must do the following:

        (1) Dry off the baby, preferably with warm towels, and cover with a warm blanket.

        (2) Suction the mouth and nostrils.

        (3) Stimulate the baby to breathe.

        (4) Clamp and cut the umbilical cord.

        (5) Administer supplemental oxygen. (page 1967)

    b. The indications for starting artificial ventilation are as follows:

        (1) Apnea

        (2) A heart rate less than 100 beats/min

        (3) Persisting central cyanosis despite 100% supplemental oxygen (page 1973)

    c. After a minute of artificial ventilation, you find the heart rate to be 84 beats/min. You should continue artificial ventilation only. (page 1973)

    d. When you check again, however, the pulse rate has dropped below 60 beats/min, so at that point you should start external chest compressions at 120 per minute. (page 1973)

    e. The indications for epinephrine are:

        (1) Asystole

        (2) A heart rate persistently below 80 beats/min despite adequate artificial ventilation with 100% supplemental oxygen and high-quality external chest compressions (page 1977)

    f. The recommended concentration for newborns is 1:10,000. The recommended dose is 0.1 to 0.3 mL/kg of 1:10,000. (page 1977)

True/False

1. T (page 1980)   **2.** F (page 1981)   **3.** T (page 1965)   **4.** T (page 1977)   **5.** T (page 1989)

6. F (page 1969)   **7.** F (page 1977)   **8.** F (page 1990)   **9.** T (page 1987)   **10.** T (page 1981)

Short Answer

1. Catheterization of the umbilical vein (page 1977)

    a. Clean the cord with alcohol or another antiseptic. Place a sterile tie firmly, but not too tightly, around the base of the cord to control bleeding. Place a sterile drape over the site. Maintain sterile technique as much as possible.

    b. Prefill a sterile 3.5F to 5F umbilical vein line catheter (a comparable-size sterile feeding tube can be used in an emergency) with normal saline using a 3-mL syringe.

    c. Cut the cord with a scalpel below the clamp placed on the cord at birth about 1 to 2 cm from the skin (between the clamp and the cord tie).

    d. The umbilical vein is a large, thin-walled vessel usually found at the 12 o'clock position, as compared to the two thick-walled umbilical arteries usually found at 4 and 8 o'clock. Insert the catheter into this vein for a distance of 2 to 4 cm (less in preterm infants) until blood can be aspirated. If the catheter is advanced into the liver, the infusion of hypertonic solutions may lead to irreversible damage. If the catheter is advanced into the heart, dysrhythmias may develop.

    e. Flush the catheter with 0.5 mL of normal saline and tape it in place.

2. Intubate a neonate (pages 1974–1975)

    a. Be sure the newborn is preoxygenated by bag-mask ventilation with 100% supplemental oxygen prior to making an intubation attempt.

    b. Suction the oropharynx to remove any secretions.

    c. Place the laryngoscope blade in the oropharynx, and then visualize the vocal cords. Place the ET tube between the vocal cords until the black line on the tube is at the level of the cords.

Fill-in-the-Table

1. (page 1984)

Causes of Neonatal Seizures
• Hypoxic ischemic encephalopathy
• **Intracranial infections (meningitis)**
• **Hypoglycemia**
• **Other metabolic disturbances**
• **Epileptic syndromes**
• **Intracranial hemorrhage**
• Development defects
• Hypocalcemia
• **Meningitis**
• **Encephalopathy**
• **Drug withdrawal**

Problem Solving

1. The Apgar score is 4.
2. The Apgar score is 13. (page 1968)

Skill Drill

1. Intubating a Newborn (page 1974)

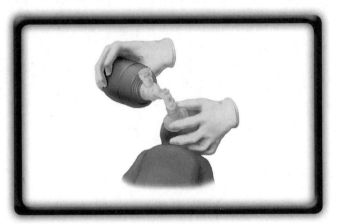

Step 1: Preoxygenate the newborn by bag-mask ventilation to an oxygen saturation greater than 95%.

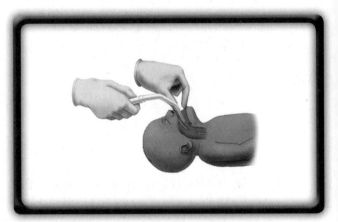

Step 2: Suction the oropharynx if there are copious secretions that prevent adequate ventilation. Avoid deep suctioning and provide bag-mask ventilation if bradycardia results.

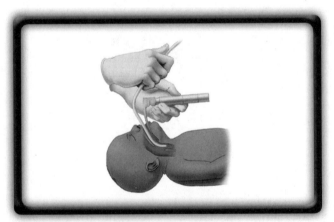

Step 3: Place the laryngoscope blade in the oropharynx. Visualize the vocal cords. Place the ET tube between the vocal cords until the black line on the ET tube is at the level of the cords.

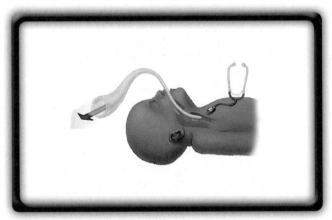

Step 4: Confirm placement. Observe chest rise, auscultate laterally and high on the chest, note mist in the ET tube, note equal breath sounds on both sides, and observe for clinical improvement. Monitor $ETco_2$ via waveform capnography and consider using pulse oximetry.

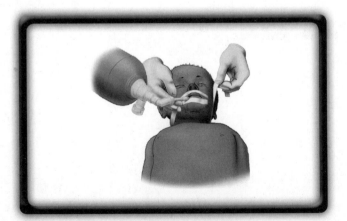

Step 5: Tape the ET tube in place. Monitor the newborn closely for complications.

Chapter 43: Pediatric Emergencies

Matching

Part I
(pages 2005–2007)

1. E	**2.** A	**3.** D	**4.** B	**5.** A, B
6. D, E	**7.** A	**8.** A, B, C, D, E	**9.** E	**10.** A, B, C, D, E
11. D	**12.** B	**13.** A	**14.** E	**15.** D

Part II

1. R (page 2075)	**2.** M (page 2075)	**3.** K (page 2075)	**4.** W (page 2075)	**5.** B (page 2075)
6. V (page 2075)	**7.** S (page 2075)	**8.** CC (page 2075)	**9.** Z (page 2075)	**10.** Y (page 2075)
11. X (page 2075)	**12.** P (page 2075)	**13.** Q (page 2075)	**14.** ZZ (page 2076)	**15.** L (page 2075)
16. I (page 2075)	**17.** J (page 2075)	**18.** H (page 2075)	**19.** G (page 2075)	**20.** F (page 2075)
21. BB (page 2075)	**22.** AA (page 2075)	**23.** LL (page 2076)	**24.** II (page 2076)	**25.** E (page 2075)
26. D (page 2075)	**27.** U (page 2075)	**28.** T (page 2075)	**29.** C (page 2075)	**30.** A (page 2075)
31. HH (page 2076)	**32.** EE (page 2076)	**33.** GG (page 2076)	**34.** FF (page 2075)	**35.** N (page 2075)
36. O (page 2075)	**37.** QQ (page 2076)	**38.** PP (page 2076)	**39.** DD (page 2076)	**40.** OO (page 2076)
41. NN (page 2076)	**42.** MM (page 2076)	**43.** JJ (page 2076)	**44.** TT (page 2076)	**45.** SS (page 2076)
46. UU (page 2076)	**47.** VV (page 2076)	**48.** WW (page 2076)	**49.** YY (page 2076)	**50.** KK (page 2076)
51. RR (page 2076)	**52.** XX (page 2076)			

Multiple Choice

1. C (page 2061)	**2.** C (page 2063)	**3.** D (page 2063)	**4.** D (page 2011)	**5.** B (page 2012)
6. D (page 2013)	**7.** A (page 2011)	**8.** D (page 2069)	**9.** C (page 2071)	**10.** C (page 2027)
11. C (page 2060)	**12.** D (page 2060)	**13.** A (page 2060)	**14.** D (page 2061)	**15.** D (page 2060)

Labeling
(page 2035)

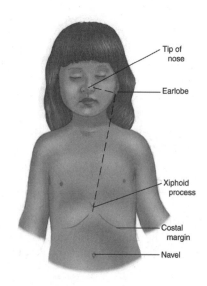

Fill-in-the-Blank

1. tolerated; oropharyngeal (page 2027)
2. blow-by technique (page 2028)
3. always; ventilation; airway management (page 2029)
4. teeth; aspiration; placement (page 2034)
5. parasympathetic; bradycardia; cardiac; pulse oximeter (page 2032)
6. hypovolemic; distributive; cardiogenic. (page 2035)
7. hypovolemic; tachypnea; pale; mottled; cyanotic (page 2036)
8. sunken eyes, mucous membranes; turgor; delayed (pages 2036–2037)
9. compartment syndrome; injury; infection (page 2038)
10. uncommon; congenital; rhythm (page 2040)

Identify

1. a. Chief complaint: Respiratory distress (probably the croup)
    b. Vital signs: Normal capillary refill, oxygen saturation of 95%, conscious and alert, audible stridor
    c. Pertinent negatives: Age-appropriate behavior, recognizes her mother
2. a. Chief complaint: Infant unrestrained and ejected during fatal motor vehicle crash
    b. Vital signs: Age-appropriate LOC, skin color normal, skin is warm and dry. Normal capillary refill, oxygen saturation of 96%, pulse rate of 150 beats/min.
    c. Pertinent negatives: No obvious external bleeding; assessment is unremarkable
3. a. Chief complaint: Seizure, probably a febrile seizure.
    b. Vital signs: Skin ashen, warm, and dry. A rectal temperature of 100.3°F. Patient responds to pain. Her oxygen saturation is 98%. Pupils are sluggish but equal. Patient has equal bilateral breath sounds. The remainder of exam is unremarkable.
    c. Pertinent negatives: The patient's mother denies any other medications, history, or allergies to medications. She further denies any recent injury or trauma to the child.

Complete the Patient Care Report (PCR)

Show the completed PCR to your instructor to obtain feedback on your completion of the form.

Ambulance Calls

1. The scene of a collision where a child has been injured is probably the most stressful environment that a paramedic will enter.
    a. (1) Fracture of the left femur
       (2) Ruptured spleen
       (3) Injury to the right side of the head (page 2063)
    b. Perhaps the hardest element to deal with at a collision scene like the one described is the feelings and behaviors of the child's parents.
       (1) Obviously, there is no "correct" answer to the question of how you feel when assaulted by an angry parent. The average paramedic, however, will probably feel angry.
       (2) What you do with your feelings is another matter, and there is a correct way to handle the situation and an incorrect way. The correct way is as follows:
          (a) Mentally count to 10 before you reply to the angry father.
          (b) Stay calm.
          (c) Don't raise your voice.
          (d) Try to enlist the father's help in caring for the child; give him something constructive to do, such as fetching the backboard from the ambulance or folding triangular bandages into cravats. (page 2010)
    c. The child's vital signs are normal for his age (answer 3). The slight tachycardia is easily explained by the pain and excitement of the situation.

2. When 2-year-old Tammy starts barking in the middle of the night, it's a great attention-getter.

   a. The vital signs are abnormal for her age. There is tachycardia and tachypnea.

   b. The most likely diagnosis is croup. (page 2022)

   c. The steps of prehospital management are as follows:

      (1) Give humidified supplemental oxygen while you set up a nebulizer.

      (2) Nebulized epinephrine is available in two formulations: racemic epinephrine and L-epinephrine. The dose for racemic epinephrine (2.25%) is 0.5 mL mixed in 3 mL of normal saline. The dose for L-epinephrine is 0.25 to 0.5 mg/kg of the 1:1,000 solution (maximum, 5 mg per dose); this form can be diluted with normal saline to bring the volume to 3 mL. (page 2023)

      (3) Place the child in a position of comfort.

      (4) Notify the receiving hospital of the case.

      (5) Transport without delay.

3. Diffuse wheezing and respiratory distress in a child under a year of age are the tip-offs in this case.

   a. The vital signs are abnormal. The baby has tachycardia, tachypnea, and a slight elevation in blood pressure. (page 2025)

   b. The most likely diagnosis is bronchiolitis.

   c. The steps of prehospital management are as follows:

      (1) Give humidified oxygen.

      (2) Assist ventilations gently with a bag-mask ventilator.

      (3) Consult medical command as to whether to give a trial of bronchodilators.

      (4) Keep the intubation kit handy in case of apnea.

      (5) Monitor cardiac rhythm.

      (6) Transport without delay. (page 2025)

4. a. When little Bobby develops severe respiratory distress and signs of airway obstruction over a very short time, and he does not have a high fever, the most likely diagnosis is foreign body obstruction of the airway—that is, choking.

   b. The steps of managing a choking child are as follows:

      (1) Kneel on one knee behind the child, and circle his or her body by placing both arms around the child's chest. Prepare to give abdominal thrusts by placing your fist just above the patient's umbilicus and well below the xiphoid process. Place your other hand over that fist.

      (2) Give the child rapid, distinct abdominal thrusts in an upward direction. Be careful to avoid applying force to the lower rib cage or sternum.

      (3) Repeat this standing technique until the child expels the foreign body or becomes unresponsive.

      (4) If the child becomes unresponsive, place him or her supine on a firm, flat surface and inspect the airway using the head tilt–chin lift. If you can see the foreign body, try to remove it. Do not perform blind finger sweeps.

      (5) Attempt rescue breathing. If the first attempt fails, reposition the head and try again.

      (6) If the airway remains obstructed, begin cardiopulmonary resuscitation (CPR) with chest compressions at the 30:2 compression/ventilation ratio and prepare for immediate transport. If you manage to clear the airway obstruction in an unresponsive child (older than 1 year), but he or she remains apneic and pulseless, begin CPR and attach the automated external defibrillator (AED) as soon as possible, using appropriately sized AED pads. If you are unable to relieve the obstruction after several attempts, transport immediately.

      (7) If the child loses consciousness, start CPR. Initiate transportation. Consider direct laryngoscopy to remove the foreign body under direct vision. (page 2022)

   c. Compress the chest about one third to one half its total depth. Push hard and fast (at least 100 compressions/min), and allow full chest recoil. (pages 2021–2022)

   d. Check the femoral pulse in infants and young children and the carotid pulse in older children and adolescents (covered in the chapter *Responding to the Field Code*).

   e. Place the heel of your hand over the middle of the sternum (between the nipples). Avoid compression over the lower tip of the sternum, which is called the xiphoid process. (page 2043)

   f. The defibrillation dosage for a 12-kg child is 24 joules (2 joules/kg). (page 2042)

   g. Anything that can be administered IV can be administered through an IO line (such as isotonic fluids, medications). (page 2038)

5. A sudden, severe sore throat along with a high fever should start some warning lights blinking in your brain.
   a. The vital signs are abnormal. The child has both tachycardia and tachypnea, not to mention his very high fever.
   b. The most likely diagnosis is epiglottitis. (page 2023)
   c. The steps in prehospital management are as follows:
      (1) Approach the child very gently so as not to disturb him.
      (2) Give humidified supplemental oxygen.
      (3) Place the child in a position of comfort.
      (4) Notify the receiving hospital to have the appropriate specialists standing by.
      (5) Transport without delay. (page 2023)
   d. The special danger threatening this child is complete airway obstruction from epiglottal swelling, which may occur within minutes. (page 2023)
6. The little boy having an asthmatic attack during nature study is already in bad shape by the time you arrive on the scene.
   a. Five signs that suggest he is in bad shape are his:
      (1) Drowsiness (a sign of carbon dioxide retention)
      (2) Pulsus paradoxus of 40 mm Hg
      (3) Cyanosis, indicating hypoxemia
      (4) Hyperinflated chest, indicating obstruction to exhalation
      (5) Silent chest, indicating that practically no air is moving in and out (page 2024)
   b. The steps in managing this case are as follows:
      (1) Give humidified supplemental oxygen by mask while preparing the nebulizer.
      (2) Start an IV.
      (3) Give a nebulized bronchodilator, such as albuterol, 0.5 mL in 3 mL of normal saline, with oxygen as the carrier gas.
      (4) Monitor cardiac rhythm.
      (5) Ask your dispatcher to notify the child's parents and request that they meet you in the emergency department.
      (6) Transport the child in a position of comfort.
7. Most calls you receive for asthmatic attacks will be for patients already known to have asthma. Such patients will not call for help unless there is something different about this particular attack.
   a. Questions to ask in taking the history of a child having an acute asthmatic attack include the following:
      (1) How long has the attack been going on?
      (2) What medications has the child already taken? When? In what dosage?
      (3) How much fluid has the child managed to take?
      (4) Does the child have any allergies?
      (5) Has the child had any hospitalizations for asthma? If so, when? (page 2024)
   b. It's easier to remember medications to give in an acute asthmatic attack if you know what you are giving them for. When giving albuterol, you need to know:
      (1) The contraindication in children: diabetes
      (2) The possible adverse side effects: palpitations, tremors, nervousness, dizziness, nausea
      (3) Administration and dosage: Metered-dose inhaler (MDI) with a spacer-mask device. Unit doses of 2.5 mg of albuterol premixed with 3 mL of normal saline are often used for nebulization and represent an acceptable starting dose for most young children. (page 2024)
8. There is no easy answer to the question of how to respond in a case of sudden infant death syndrome (SIDS). Each case will be a little different, and your response should be guided by local protocols and personal judgment. You need to make a quick appraisal to decide whether the mother already realizes that the baby is dead. If not, it might be worth starting CPR, so that she can feel, afterward, that everything possible was done. If you do start CPR, do it right; go through all the steps as you would for a baby you expected to survive. If, on the other hand, you feel that the mother already knows that her baby is dead, it may be better to take the more difficult option, and that is to confirm her worst fears. Should you do so, you must be prepared to spend time with the mother and to deal with her grief.

As this case illustrates, when you do confront a case of crib death, you will have to make an instant decision on the spot regarding how to proceed. If you haven't prepared yourself ahead of time for such decisions, it could be one of the longest instants of your experience. (page 2062)

9. Seizures in children are a lot like seizures in adults, but they tend to be considerably more upsetting to all concerned.

    a. Seizures in children result from the following causes (*students should provide five of the following*):

        (1) Head trauma

        (2) Meningitis

        (3) Fever

        (4) Hypoglycemia

        (5) Hypoxia

        (6) Failure of a known epileptic to take prescribed medications

        (7) Abuse of drugs (yes, in children) (page 2046)

    b. There are specific questions to ask in taking the history of a child who has had a seizure (*students should provide five of the following*):

        (1) Is this the child's first seizure?

        (2) How many seizures has the child had today?

        (3) Has the child had a fever? Stiff neck? Headache?

        (4) Might the child have ingested a toxic product?

        (5) Is there a family history of seizures?

        (6) If the child is known to have seizures, did the child take his or her medication today?

        (7) What did the seizure look like? (page 2047)

    c. In performing the physical assessment of a child who has had a seizure, look in particular for the following signs (*students should provide five of the following*):

        (1) Changes in the state of consciousness

        (2) Skin temperature and moisture (febrile seizure?)

        (3) Evidence of head trauma

        (4) Equality and reactivity of the pupils

        (5) Stiff neck

        (6) Signs of injury sustained during the seizure (eg, dislocation of the shoulder) (page 2047)

    d. From all of the information you obtain about this child, you conclude that he probably had a febrile seizure. The prehospital treatment is as follows:

        (1) Maintain the airway.

        (2) Transport him to the hospital. (page 2047)

10. The 14-year-old, unlike the previous patient, is in status epilepticus.

    a. The steps in treatment are as follows:

        (1) Treatment at the scene will be limited to supportive care if the seizure has stopped by the time of your arrival.

        (2) Status epilepticus requires more extensive intervention. For a child with ongoing seizure activity, open the airway using the chin-lift or jaw-thrust maneuver. Very proximal airway obstruction is common during a seizure or postictal state because the tongue and jaw fall backward as a result of the decreased muscle tone associated with altered mental status.

        (3) If the airway is not maintainable with positioning, consider inserting a nasopharyngeal airway.

        (4) Suction for secretions or vomitus, and consider the lateral decubitus position in case of ongoing vomiting. Do not attempt to intubate during an active seizure because endotracheal intubation in this setting is associated with serious complications and is rarely successful. You are better off using BLS airway management, stopping the seizure, and then considering the child's need for ALS airway support.

        (5) Provide 100% supplemental oxygen to the patient, and start bag-mask ventilation as indicated for hypoventilation. Consider placing a nasogastric (NG) tube to decompress the stomach if the patient requires assisted ventilation.

(6) Assess the child for IV sites. Measure the serum glucose level, and treat any documented hypoglycemia.

(7) Consider your options for anticonvulsant administration. (page 2047)

  b. Diazepam is used to treat repeated seizures. The contraindications to giving diazepam are pregnancy, respiratory depression, hypotension, and previous ingestion of alcohol or sedative drugs.

  c. The possible side effects include apnea, hypotension, and even cardiac arrest. (page 2047)

11. Whenever you are called to deal with injury in an infant or very young child, you must always keep the possibility of child abuse in the back of your mind.

  a. What's fishy about this particular story is the claim that the 10-month-old "stepped on a cigarette." At the age of 10 months, most babies are just beginning to stand up (while holding on) and are not yet walking, so it's hard to imagine how a 10-month-old would manage to step on a cigarette.

  b. Clues to child abuse include the following:

  (1) Parental behavior: vague, evasive, hostile

  (2) Discrepancies in the history

  (3) Delay in seeking care

  (4) A child who looks generally neglected (dirty, unkempt)

  (5) A child who does not turn to his or her parents for comfort

  (6) A child who does not cry

  (7) The presence of multiple bruises in different stages of healing

  (8) Injuries in and around the mouth

  (9) Suspicious burns (as in the present case; or scald burns without splash marks)

  (10) Fractures in an infant less than a year old (page 2060)

  c. The steps in caring for this particular child are as follows:

  (1) Put a sterile dressing on the burn.

  (2) Transport the child to the hospital.

  (3) Notify the physician in private of your suspicions.

  (4) Fill out whatever legal forms are required.

  (5) Document everything on your PCR. (pages 2060–2061)

  d. What if the parent refuses to permit you to transport the child? Your service should have a policy established in advance to deal with such situations. Here are some suggestions:

  (1) Try to persuade the parent to change his or her mind. Do so in a calm, professional manner.

  (2) Call for law enforcement.

  (3) Document the entire call, including a list of whom you notified, on your PCR.

  Remember, the abused child may be in life-threatening danger. If you fail to report a suspected case of child abuse, the next call to the same address may be for a dead child. (pages 2060–2062)

12. The baby who fell from the balcony has sustained a serious head injury. (Did you notice the signs of increasing intracranial pressure?) The prehospital treatment is as follows:

  a. Maintain an open airway (use an oropharyngeal airway if the baby becomes unconscious). Anticipate vomiting, and have suction at hand.

  b. Administer supplemental oxygen.

  c. Immobilize the spine with a baby backboard or a pediatric backboard with folded towels to elevate the baby's back slightly.

  d. Start transport.

  e. Ventilate the baby with a bag-mask device.

  f. Notify the receiving hospital. (page 2065)

13. You have two injured children in this collision.

  a. The first child has an abdominal injury and early shock. He is therefore in the load-and-go category. His prehospital treatment is as follows:

  (1) Maintain an open airway. Anticipate vomiting, and keep suction at hand.

  (2) Administer oxygen.

  (3) Immobilize the child on a backboard.

  (4) Start transport.

(5) Notify the receiving hospital.

(6) Start an IV en route to the hospital.

(7) Splint the broken arm. (pages 2035–2037)

b. The second child has a tension pneumothorax (the clues were his extreme respiratory distress, tracheal deviation, and a point of maximal impulse [PMI] shifted to the left). He is also in the load-and-go category, but only after critical interventions, including decompression of the pneumothorax, have been carried out.

(1) Ensure a patent airway.

(2) Administer supplemental oxygen.

(3) Decompress the pneumothorax by inserting a 14-gauge angiocath into the third intercostal space in the midclavicular line on the affected side.

(4) Immobilize the child on a backboard.

(5) Start transport.

(6) Notify the receiving hospital.

(7) Monitor cardiac rhythm (myocardial contusion is likely).

(8) Start an IV lifeline en route to the hospital. (pages 2037, 2064)

14. a. The infant removed from the smoky house fire should be intubated because he was unconscious in a smoky environment and therefore at high risk for respiratory complications.

b. Other factors that put a pediatric fire victim at high risk for airway obstruction and that are therefore indications for early intubation include the following (*students should provide five of the following*):

(1) Stridor

(2) Wheezing

(3) Signs of respiratory distress

(4) Facial burns

(5) Singed eyebrows

(6) Red, edematous mouth

(7) Carbonaceous sputum (pages 1580–1581, 2068)

15. a. Abdominal thrusts (Heimlich maneuver) are recommended to relieve a severe airway obstruction in a conscious child. Have little Johnny's mom call 9-1-1. Hopefully, you can dislodge the peanuts and uneventfully return to the football game. But what if you can't?

b. Follow these steps to remove a foreign body obstruction from a conscious child who is in a standing position:

(1) Kneel on one knee behind the child, and circle his or her body by placing both arms around the child's chest. Prepare to give abdominal thrusts by placing your fist just above the patient's umbilicus and well below the xiphoid process. Place your other hand over that fist.

(2) Give the child rapid, distinct abdominal thrusts in an upward direction. Be careful to avoid applying force to the lower rib cage or sternum.

(3) Repeat this standing technique until the child expels the foreign body or becomes unresponsive.

(4) If the child becomes unresponsive, place him or her supine on a firm, flat surface and inspect the airway using the head tilt–chin lift. If you can see the foreign body, try to remove it. Do not perform blind finger sweeps.

(5) Attempt rescue breathing. If the first attempt fails, reposition the head and try again.

(6) If the airway remains obstructed, begin CPR with chest compressions at the 30:2 compression-to-ventilation ratio and prepare for immediate transport. If you manage to clear the airway obstruction in an unresponsive child (older than 1 year), but he or she remains apneic and pulseless, begin CPR. (pages 2021–2022)

True/False

1. F (page 2004) **2.** F (page 2048) **3.** F (page 2005) **4.** T (page 2013) **5.** T (page 2063)

6. F (page 2026) **7.** F (page 2027) **8.** F (page 2036) **9.** F (page 2032) **10.** T (page 2031)

11. T (page 2031) **12.** F (page 2007) **13.** T (page 2068) **14.** F (page 2065) **15.** T (page 2041)

Short Answer

1. Signs of hypovolemia and shock in infants and children include the following (*students should list six of the following*):
    a. Listlessness or lethargy
    b. Pale, mottled, or cyanotic skin
    c. Delayed capillary refill (longer than 2 seconds)
    d. Collapsed veins
    e. Poor skin turgor
    f. Compensatory tachypnea
    g. Cool extremities
    h. Sunken eyes
    i. Dry mucous membranes (page 2036)

2. Load-and-go situations in children include the following (*students should provide 10 of the following*):
    a. Fall from a height of more than two times the height of child
    b. Child involved in a collision with fatalities
    c. Child ejected from a car in a motor vehicle crash
    d. Child who was struck by a car while walking or biking
    e. Child in whom you are unable to secure an airway
    f. Respiratory arrest
    g. Open pneumothorax
    h. Tension pneumothorax
    i. Cardiac arrest
    j. Shock
    k. Uncontrollable bleeding
    l. Coma or deteriorating level of consciousness
    m. Signs of increasing intracranial pressure (page 2014)

Fill-in-the-Table

1. (pages 2017–2018)

Pediatric Physical Examination	
Body Area	**What I Am Looking for in Particular**
Head	• Bulging or sunken fontanelles in infants • Battle's sign, raccoon's eyes, blood or clear fluid draining from the nose or ears • Unequal pupils
Neck	• Tenderness • Tracheal deviation
Chest	• Location of the point of maximal impulse (PMI) • Bruises, instability • Inequality of breath sounds
Abdomen	• Bruises, seat belt marks • Distention, tenderness, rigidity
Extremities	• Deformity, bruises • Peripheral pulses • Movement and sensation

2. (page 2008)

Pediatric Respiratory Rates	
Age	**Respiratory Rate (breaths/min)**
Infant	25 to 60
Toddler	20 to 30
Preschool-aged child	20 to 25
School-aged child	15 to 20
Adolescent	12 to 20

3. (page 2008)

Pediatric Pulse Rates	
Age	**Pulse Rate (beats/min)**
Infant	100 to 180
Toddler	90 to 150
Preschool-aged child	80 to 140
School-aged child	70 to 120
Adolescent	60 to 100

4. (page 2018)

Normal Blood Pressure for Age	
Age	**Minimal Systolic Blood Pressure (mm Hg)**
Infant	> 70
Toddler	> 80
Preschool-age child	> 80
School-age child	> 80
Adolescent	> 90

5. (page 2060)

CHILD ABUSE Mnemonic	
Mnemonic	**What the Letter Represents**
C	**Consistency of the injury with the child's developmental age**
H	History consistent with injuries
I	**Inappropriate parental concerns**
L	Lack of supervision
D	**Delay in seeking care**
A	Affect
B	**Bruises of varying stages**
U	Unusual injury patterns
S	**Suspicious circumstances**
E	Environmental clues

Problem Solving

1. Minimal systolic blood pressure = 80 + (2 × age in years)
   a. 92 mm Hg
   b. 100 mm Hg
   c. 90 to 92 mm Hg (page 2018)
2. a. 5.5 mm
   b. 6.25 mm (page 2031)
3. a. The initial energy setting is 2 J/kg or 36 joules. (page 2042)
   b. Subsequent defibrillations should occur at 4 J/kg or 72 joules. (page 2042)
4. a. Epinephrine should be given by the subcutaneous (SQ) or intramuscular (IM) route at a dose of 0.01 mg/kg of the 1:1,000 solution, to a maximum dose of 0.3 mg. This patient should be given 0.01 mg/kg or the maximum dose of 0.3 mg of 1:1,000 solution.
   b. Diphenhydramine (dose: 1 to 2 mg/kg IV to a maximum of 50 mg), or 27 to 50 mg IV
   c. Bronchodilators may be delivered by nebulizer or MDI with a spacer-mask device. Unit doses of 2.5 mg of albuterol premixed with 3 mL of normal saline are often used for nebulization and represent an acceptable starting dose for most young children.

Skill Drills

1. One-Person Bag-Mask Ventilation for a Child (page 2030)

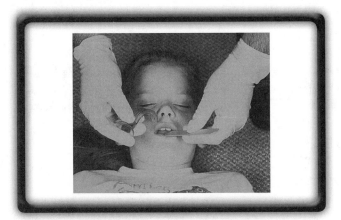

Step 1: Open the **airway**, and **insert** the appropriate airway adjunct.

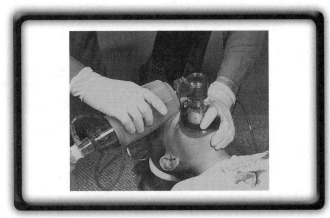

Step 2: Hold the **mask** on the patient's face with a one-handed **head tilt–chin lift** technique (E-C clamp). Ensure a good **mask-to-face** seal while maintaining the airway.

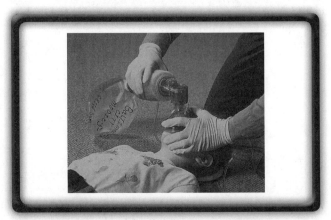

Step 3: Squeeze the bag using the correct **ventilation** rate of **12** to **20** breaths/min for children. Allow adequate time for exhalation.

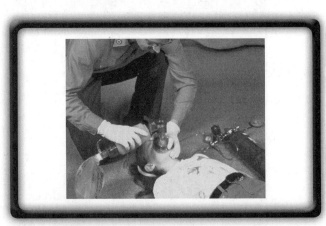

Step 4: Assess effectiveness of ventilation by assessing the **bilateral** rise and fall of the **chest**.

Chapter 44: Geriatric Emergencies

Matching

(page 2118)

1. B	**2.** J	**3.** E	**4.** L	**5.** Q	**6.** S	**7.** K
8. P	**9.** AA	**10.** C	**11.** R	**12.** U	**13.** D	**14.** V
15. G	**16.** H	**17.** T	**18.** I	**19.** X	**20.** W	**21.** O
22. Y	**23.** F	**24.** BB	**25.** Z	**26.** M	**27.** N	**28.** A

Multiple Choice

1. B (page 2080)	**2.** A (page 2081)	**3.** C (page 2082)	**4.** A (page 2082)	**5.** D (page 2101)
6. C (page 2084)	**7.** D (page 2086)	**8.** D (page 2092)	**9.** A (page 2108)	**10.** D (page 2090)

Labeling

1. Lower Gastrointestinal (GI) System (page 2100)
    A. Liver
    B. Gallbladder
    C. Duodenum
    D. Pancreas
    E. Jejunum
    F. Colon*
    G. Esophagus
    H. Stomach
    I. Ileum
    J. Rectum*
2. Upper GI System (page 2099)
    A. Liver
    B. Gallbladder
    C. Duodenum*
    D. Pancreas
    E. Jejunum
    F. Colon
    G. Esophagus*
    H. Stomach*
    I. Ileum
    J. Rectum

Fill-in-the-Blank

1. Elderly; emergency (page 2080)
2. just getting old (page 2082)
3. hypertrophies (page 2082)
4. respiratory; reductions (page 2082)
5. nephron units; filtering (page 2085)
6. appetite; saliva; dryness (page 2084)
7. intervertebral; compression; height (page 2086)
8. Meniere disease; cycles; months (page 2084)
9. Wrinkling; resiliency; drier; fragile (page 2085)
10. morbidity; mortality; 70 (page 2093)

Identify

1. a. Chief complaint: Right-sided midthigh pain

   b. Vital signs: Her pulse is 84 beats/min and very irregular. Her oxygen saturation is 88% on room air. Blood pressure is 106/86 mm Hg. The patient's skin turgor is poor, with delayed capillary refill of > 2 seconds. Pupils are Equal and Round, Regular in size, and react to Light (PEARRL). An ECG shows a sinus rhythm with frequent premature ventricular contractions (PVCs) and short runs of ventricular tachycardia (with a pulse).

   c. Pertinent negatives: She denies chest pain, shortness of breath, dizziness, nausea, or vomiting. She also denies a trip and fall. The area appears to be clear of obstacles, rugs, or other obvious trip hazards.

2. a. Chief complaint: Patient is conscious but not alert to person, place, or day, so his mental status is "V."

   b. Vital signs: Blood glucose of 66 mg/dL. His pulse rate is 92 beats/min and regular, blood pressure is 160/72 mm Hg. His skin is warm and moist, and his oxygen saturation is 96% on room air.

   c. Pertinent negatives: There is minimally detectable damage to the vehicle as well as the vehicles that were struck.

Complete the Patient Care Report (PCR)

Show the completed PCR to your instructor to obtain feedback on your completion of the form.

Ambulance Calls

1. As noted, one way to try to make sure you don't miss any important symptoms is to conduct a review of systems, which should include questions such as the following (*students should list 10 of the following*): (page 2090)

   a. Have you had any pain or discomfort in your chest (cardiovascular system)?

   b. Have you had any palpitations (cardiovascular system)?

   c. Have you been short of breath (cardiovascular/respiratory systems)?

   d. Have you been coughing (respiratory system)?

   e. Have you had any dizzy spells (nervous system)?

   f. Have you fainted (nervous system)?

   g. Can you explain the reason for calling 9-1-1 (nervous system)?

   h. Have you had any difficulty speaking (cardiovascular/nervous systems)?

   i. Have you had any severe headaches recently (nervous system)?

   j. Have you noticed any unusual weakness or odd sensations in your arms or legs (nervous system)?

   k. Have you had any changes in your appetite (digestive system)?

   l. Have you gained or lost any weight (GI system)?

   m. Has there been any change in your bowel movements (digestive system)?

   n. Have you had any nausea or vomiting (GI system)?

   o. Have you had any pain or difficulty in urinating (urinary system)?

   p. Have you noticed any change in the color of your urine (genitourinary system)?

   q. Have you noticed any changes in the frequency of urination (genitourinary system)?

2. One of the most frequent geriatric calls is for a patient who has fallen.

   a. Questions to ask in taking the history might include the following:

   (1) How did it happen?

   (2) Did you feel dizzy before you fell, or have any other similar warning symptoms?

   (3) Did you feel anything snap before you fell?

   (4) Are you taking any new medications?

   (5) Where does it hurt?

   b. The past medical history of an elderly patient may be quite extensive, and there isn't enough time in the field to elicit all the details. The things you need to know to render appropriate emergency care are:

   (1) Major underlying illnesses (eg, diabetes, angina)

   (2) Recent hospitalizations (Where? What doctor?)

   (3) Allergies

   (4) Current medications (That means all medications—prescribed and over-the-counter varieties. Collect them all in a bag and take them with the patient to the hospital.)

c. In performing the physical assessment, one should look in particular for (*students should provide six of the following*):

    (1) The patient's state of dress and grooming, as an indication of her general ability to care for herself

    (2) The level of consciousness (AVPU and then the Glasgow Coma Scale)

    (3) The position in which the patient is found

    (4) An elevated blood pressure, which might signal increasing intracranial pressure, or a decreased blood pressure, which might suggest shock

    (5) A very slow pulse, suggesting either increasing intracranial pressure or the source of a syncopal episode

    (6) An increased respiratory rate, which may signal shock or a variety of other serious conditions

    (7) Signs of head injury (eg, cerebrospinal fluid leak, Battle's sign)

    (8) Neck tenderness

    (9) Instability or tenderness of the ribs

    (10) Deformity in the limbs

    (11) The state of the surroundings, another indication of the patient's overall ability to care for herself (page 2090)

d. The elderly are more susceptible than younger people to (*students should provide three of the following*):

    (1) Subdural hematoma (page 2110)

    (2) Compression of the cervical spinal cord (page 2111)

    (3) Rib fracture (page 2110)

    (4) Hip fracture (page 2110)

3. Factors related to geriatric suicide:

a. If depression goes unrecognized or untreated, it is associated with a higher suicide rate in the elderly population than in any other age group.

b. The majority of elder suicides occur in people who have recently been diagnosed with depression.

c. The majority of suicide victims have seen their primary care physician within the month before the event.

d. Geriatric patients typically do not make suicidal gestures or attempt to get help.

e. The rate of completed suicide is disproportionately high in the geriatric population. (page 2106)

True/False

1. T (page 2081)   **2.** F (page 2087)   **3.** F (page 2090)   **4.** T (page 2083)   **5.** T (page 2083)

6. F (page 2086)   **7.** T (page 2087)   **8.** F (page 2107)   **9.** F (page 2112)   **10.** T (page 2113)

Short Answer

1. Among the attributes that make caring for the elderly particularly challenging are the following (*students should provide five of the following*):

a. Many physiologic functions are diminished. (pages 2081–2082)

b. Typical symptoms and signs of disease may be absent, altered, or delayed. (page 2082)

c. Physical illness often presents as a mental disorder. (page 2083)

d. Multiple problems coexist in the same patient, producing multiple symptoms. (page 2080)

e. Adverse reactions to drugs occur frequently. (page 2104)

f. Psychosocial factors have an increased impact on health. (page 2081)

2. Among the psychosocial stresses that accompany advancing age are the following:

a. Retirement from work, with the attendant loss of community status, sense of usefulness, and the structure that a job gives to one's daily life. (page 2081)

b. Bereavement, as more and more friends (and often a spouse) die. (page 2081)

3. A number of changes in the body occur as part of the normal aging process (*students should provide two changes per organ system*).

a. Cardiovascular (page 2082)

    (1) Increase in blood pressure

    (2) Decrease in cardiac output

    (3) Cardiac hypertrophy

    (4) Electric conduction system atrophy

b. Respiratory (page 2082)

    (1) Decreased vital capacity

    (2) Increased residual volume

    (3) Decreased airflow

    (4) Decreased arterial PO_2

    (5) Decreased cough, gag, and ciliary clearance

c. Renal (page 2085)

    (1) Decreased renal blood flow

    (2) Decreased nephron mass

    (3) Impaired thirst mechanism

    (4) Decreased ability to maintain salt and fluid balance

d. Digestive (pages 2084–2085)

    (1) Decreased sense of taste

    (2) Decreased secretion of saliva and gastric juice

    (3) Less efficient hepatic detoxification

e. Musculoskeletal (page 2086)

    (1) Decreased bone mass

    (2) Decreased muscle mass

f. Nervous (pages 2083–2084)

    (1) Decreased visual acuity

    (2) Loss of high-tone hearing

    (3) Impaired proprioception

g. Homeostatic (page 2086)

    (1) Impaired temperature regulation

    (2) Blunted febrile response to infection

    (3) Impaired blood glucose control

4. Responses to illness common among the elderly include (*students should provide four of the following*): (pages 2090–2091)

  a. Acute confusion or other change in mental status

  b. Weakness

  c. Dizziness

  d. Dyspnea

  e. Fatigue

5. A number of problems are involved in taking a history from an elderly patient, but most of those obstacles can be overcome with a little patience, tact, and ingenuity.

  a. Obstacle: The patient has trouble hearing you.

    What you can do about it: Sit facing the patient, in good light, and speak slowly and clearly.

  b. Obstacle: Patient may not report important symptoms.

    What you can do about it: Conduct a review of systems to screen the major organ systems for serious abnormality.

  c. Obstacle: The patient has several chief complaints.

    What you can do about it: Ask, "What happened *today*?" or "What is bothering you the most?" and "How is it different from the way it was yesterday?"

  d. Obstacle: The patient is too confused to give a history.

    What you can do about it: Try to obtain information from the family or other caregivers.

6. Acute myocardial infarction and congestive heart failure occur commonly in the elderly, but are as likely as not to present with atypical signs and symptoms: (page 2093)

Condition	Possible Signs and Symptoms in the Elderly
Acute myocardial infarction	**Confusion, weakness, dyspnea, stroke, syncope, incontinence**
Congestive heart failure	**Fatigue**

7. Conditions that may present as delirium in the elderly include the following: (page 2097)

    D: Drugs or toxins (including intoxication or withdrawal)

    E: Emotional (psychiatric)

    L: Low PaO_2 (carbon monoxide poisoning, COPD, CHF, acute myocardial infarction, pneumonia)

    I: Infection (pneumonia, urinary tract infection, sepsis)

    R: Retention of stool or urine

    I: Ictal (seizures)

    U: Undernutrition (including vitamin deficiencies) or underhydration

    M: Metabolism (thyroid or endocrine, electrolytes, kidneys)

    S: Subdural hematoma

Fill-in-the-Table

1. (page 2110)

Causes of Falls in the Elderly	
Cause	**Clues to Suggest This Cause**
Extrinsic (accidental)	Obvious environmental hazard at the scene, such as poor lighting, scatter rugs, uneven sidewalk, ice or other slippery surface
Intrinsic drop attacks	Sudden fall; patient found on the ground somewhat confused, often temporarily paralyzed and unable to get up; no premonitory symptoms
Postural hypotension	Fall when getting up from a recumbent or sitting position (Check medications the patient is taking, and ask about occult blood loss, such as presence of black stools. Measure blood pressure in recumbent and sitting positions.)
Dizziness or syncope	Marked bradycardia or tachydysrhythmias
Stroke	Other characteristic signs of stroke, such as hemiparesis, hemiplegia, or aphasia
Fracture	Patient felt something snap before falling

2. (page 2105)

Drugs Most Commonly Causing Toxic Reactions in Elderly People	
Medication	**Symptoms**
Anti-inflammatory agents (NSAIDs, steroids)	Drowsiness, dizziness, confusion, anxiety, bradypnea, tachypnea, GI bleeding
Antibiotics	GI signs, altered mental status, seizures, coma
Anticholinergics and antihistamines	Urination difficulty, constipation, drowsiness, restlessness, irritability, hypertension
Anticoagulants (warfarin)	Ecchymosis, epistaxis, hematuria, abdominal pain, vomiting, fecal blood
Antidysrhythmics (amiodarone, lidocaine)	Restlessness, hypotension, bradycardia, tachycardia, palpitations, angina
Antidepressants (tricyclics, long-acting selective serotonin reuptake inhibitors)	Confusion, delirium, disorientation, memory impairment
Antihypertensives (diuretics, alpha blockers, beta blockers; angiotensin-converting enzyme inhibitors)	Hypotension, palpitations, angina, fluid retention, headache
Antipsychotics (phenothiazines, atypicals)	Drowsiness, tachycardia, dizziness, restlessness
Digoxin	Headache, fatigue, malaise, drowsiness, depression
Insulin and oral antidiabetic medications	Hypoglycemia presenting as confusion
Narcotics	Delirium, respiratory depression, apnea, involuntary muscle movements
Sedative-hypnotics (benzodiazepines, barbiturates)	Incoordination, dizziness, disturbances in cognitive function

Chapter 45: Patients With Special Challenges

Matching

1. G (page 2166)
2. F (page 2166)
3. YY (page 2166)
4. C (page 2166)
5. FF (page 2168)
6. XX (page 2166)
7. B (page 2166)
8. O (page 2167)
9. DDD (page 2168)
10. X (page 2168)
11. CCC (page 2168)
12. UU (page 2167)
13. N (page 2167)
14. VV (page 2167)
15. M (page 2167)
16. BBB (page 2166)
17. L (page 2167)
18. SS (page 2167)
19. K (page 2167)
20. RR (page 2167)
21. TT (page 2167)
22. J (page 2167)
23. ZZ (page 2166)
24. D (page 2166)
25. I (page 2167)
26. PP (page 2167)
27. H (page 2167)
28. P (page 2167)
29. OO (page 2167)
30. WW (page 2166)
31. A (page 2166)
32. Q (page 2167)
33. NN (page 2167)
34. R (page 2167)
35. MM (page 2167)
36. S (page 2167)
37. LL (page 2167)
38. AAA (page 2166)
39. E (page 2166)
40. V (page 2167)
41. JJ (page 2167)
42. T (page 2167)
43. DD (page 2168)
44. EE (page 2168)
45. KKK (page 2168)
46. QQ (page 2167)
47. LLL (page 2168)
48. GG (page 2168)
49. MMM (page 2168)
50. HH (page 2168)
51. NNN (page 2168)
52. II (page 2168)
53. CC (page 2168)
54. JJJ (page 2168)
55. BB (page 2168)
56. HHH (page 2168)
57. III (page 2168)
58. AA (page 2168)
59. FFF (page 2168)
60. Z (page 2168)
61. KK (page 2167)
62. U (page 2167)
63. GGG (page 2168)
64. EEE (page 2168)
65. Y (page 2168)
66. W (page 2168)

Multiple Choice

1. D (page 2155)
2. D (pages 2155–2156)
3. D (page 2124)
4. C (page 2156)
5. C (page 2131)
6. D (pages 2151–2152)
7. D (page 2129)
8. D (page 2158)
9. B (page 2132)
10. D (page 2137)

Labeling

1. American Sign Language Signs (page 2154)
   A. Sick
   B. Hurt
   C. Help
2. Vessels and Structures in the Extremity of a Dialysis Patient (page 2146)
   A. Fistula
   B. Vein
   C. Artery
   D. Looped graft
   E. Vein
   F. Artery

Fill-in-the-Blank

1. conductive; sensorineural (page 2153)
2. impairment; congenital (page 2153)
3. language; production; articulation (page 2155)
4. semantic-pragmatic (page 2155)
5. Osteoarthritis; cartilage; trauma (page 2157)
6. bariatrics; obesity (page 2130)
7. spina bifida; fetal neural (page 2161)

8. cystic fibrosis (CF); defective recessive (page 2159)

9. altered skeletal; contraction (page 2158)

10. birth defect; pregnancy; column; develop (page 2161)

Identify

1. a. Chief complaint: Terminally ill patient
   b. History of the present illness: Irregular breathing, apnea, unconscious
   c. Other medical history: Do not resuscitate (DNR) order

2. a. Chief complaint: Seizures
   b. History of the present illness: Seizures that haven't responded to rectal diazepam
   c. Other medical history: Down syndrome, multiple medications, seizures

3. a. Chief complaint: Fever
   b. History of the present illness: Cloudy urine, has a Foley catheter
   c. Other medical history: Quadriplegic, tracheotomy, colostomy, feeding tube, can't verbalize his complaints and concerns, uses a writing board, taking a steroid and antibiotic

Complete the Patient Care Report (PCR)

Show the completed PCR to your instructor to obtain feedback on your completion of the form.

Ambulance Calls

1. a. It's best to ask the patient how to move her in the safest and most comfortable manner. She may have a special lift or assist devices that will make the transfer easier for both the crew and herself. It is important to try to protect her dignity and privacy. Calling emergency medical services (EMS) can sometimes be embarrassing for a patient, especially when his or her deformity is revealed. It is often better to work as a team. If more assistance is required, it should be requested. The goal is to provide movement that is safe for the patient and the crew.
   b. The patient may have some level of paralysis, especially in her lower trunk and extremities (if present). The patient may have bowel control issues and may have a Foley catheter. Some patients have shunts placed in their brain to relieve excess cerebrospinal fluid. If the patient has suffered other injuries, she might not even know. (pages 2156, 2161)

2. a. As with any patient who has had a seizure, your concern is to maintain adequate ABCs. Based on the primary assessment, it is obvious that this patient probably needs aggressive airway and breathing support. This should be accomplished by opening the airway with a head tilt–chin lift maneuver. Suctioning is also important, as is high-flow oxygen. If the patient needs ventilatory assistance, using a bag-mask device would be indicated. It would also be appropriate to transport the patient away from the crowd and concert to avoid an embarrassing episode when she regains consciousness. The patient's mom is probably well versed in her medical history and care. It is important to include the mother in any treatment decisions and have her assist as appropriate. If the patient doesn't recover in a reasonable period of time, transport to an appropriate hospital is required. (pages 2156–2157)
   b. The patient may present with a round head with a flat occiput; an enlarged, protruding tongue; wide-set eyes; and folded skin on either side of the nose. (page 2151)

True/False

1. T (page 2122) **2.** F (page 2144) **3.** F (page 2155) **4.** T (page 2155) **5.** T (page 2155)

6. F (page 2157) **7.** F (page 2157) **8.** T (page 2159) **9.** F (page 2160) **10.** T (page 2160)

Short Answer

1. a. Oftentimes, it is most beneficial to focus on the prevailing health condition of the patient and the need to seek treatment. A frank discussion regarding the risk/benefit of refusing treatment can often convince a patient to seek treatment. Properly documenting a patient's refusal, including exam findings, chief complaint, and risks of refusal, will usually convince a patient to be transported, especially when you ask the patient to sign this document.

b. This is something that you need to reference and investigate in your response area. Each location has its own specific rules, regulations, laws, and customs. Discuss your concern with your medical director and develop a preplan to handle these cases.

c. You should research the location of free clinics and health care resources in your community for those patients who may benefit from an alternative in a nonemergency situation. Each state has its own rules and regulations. However, it is important to note that no patient should be refused transport to an emergency care facility based on his or her ability to pay.

d. Federal laws allow patients to be seen and evaluated regardless of their ability to pay. (page 2122)

2. Many of the patients a paramedic encounters have a hearing impairment. Sometimes this impairment is readily noticeable. (page 2153)

a. The following clues would indicate to you that your patient has a hearing impairment:

(1) Presence of hearing aids

(2) Poor word pronunciation

(3) Failure to respond to your questions

b. How would you go about communicating with someone who has a hearing impairment?

(1) Face the patient; position yourself about 18 inches directly in front of the patient.

(2) Ask the patient how he or she would like to communicate with you, such as by using American Sign Language.

(3) Use written communication.

(4) Speak slowly.

(5) Use a low-pitched voice.

(6) Try the "reverse stethoscope" technique.

(7) Have only one person interview the patient to avoid confusion.

(8) Make sure the patient is using his or her hearing aid and that it is turned on. (page 2153)

3. a. Request and plan for extra help.

b. Plan the safest and easiest exit route.

c. Avoid lifting the patient by one limb.

d. Use a team approach to coordinate and preplan each move.

e. Use specialized equipment if available.

f. Notify the receiving hospital.

g. Be respectful of the patient's dignity. (page 2131)

4. a. What are some of the causes of visual impairments?

(1) Congenital defects

(2) Disease

(3) Injury

(4) Infection

(5) Degeneration of the eyeball, optic nerve, or nerve pathways (pages 2153–2155)

b. What can paramedics do to alleviate some of the fears felt by patients with visual impairments?

(1) Make yourself known when entering the room and introduce yourself and others.

(2) Tell the patient what is happening.

(3) Identify noises.

(4) Describe the situation and surroundings. (page 2155)

Fill-in-the-Table

1. (pages 2151–2162)

Care Needs for Special Needs Patients	
Special Need	**Associated Patient Care Need**
Speech impairments	**Talk to patients as adults. Patience is important. Ask the patient how he or she prefers to communicate. (page 2155)**
Visual impairments	**Introduce yourself; use visual aids if helpful; identify noises, the situation, and surroundings. (page 2154)**
Paralysis	**Patients may rely on a ventilator and other specialized equipment, and they may have feeding tubes, Foley catheters, and colostomies. Be aware of potential complications. (page 2156)**
Obesity	**Put the patient at ease. Communicate your plan to help. Request extra assistance for moving and transport. (page 2131)**
Developmental disabilities	**Treatment should be based on the complaint, unless the illness is related to the mental disability. (page 2151)**
Pathologic challenges	**Formulate your treatment plan with special consideration of these patients. Pathologies may include cancer, arthritis, cerebral palsy, muscular dystrophy, polio, previous head injury, and myasthenia gravis. (pages 2151-2162)**

2. (page 2131)

Causes of Obesity	
Primary Causes	• Poor dietary choices • **Excessive food intake** • **Lack of exercise**
Secondary Causes	• Hormonal changes • **Inadequate sleep** • Low basal metabolic rate • **Environmental toxins** • **Genetic predisposition** • Declining smoking • **Widespread dependence on air conditioning**

Section 10: Operations
Chapter 46: Transport Operations

Matching

Part I
(page 2188)

1. G   **2.** G   **3.** A   **4.** A   **5.** G   **6.** G   **7.** A   **8.** A   **9.** G   **10.** G

Part II

1. U (page 2195)   **2.** D (page 2196)   **3.** C (page 2196)   **4.** Q (page 2195)   **5.** Y (page 2195)

6. O (page 2195)   **7.** T (page 2195)   **8.** Z (page 2195)   **9.** N (page 2195)   **10.** F (page 2196)

11. I (page 2196)   **12.** AA (page 2195)   **13.** L (page 2195)   **14.** R (page 2195)   **15.** S (page 2195)

16. X (page 2195)   **17.** P (page 2195)   **18.** W (page 2195)   **19.** V (page 2195)   **20.** BB (page 2195)

21. K (page 2195)   **22.** E (page 2196)   **23.** G (page 2196)   **24.** B (page 2196)   **25.** H (page 2196)

26. J (page 2196)   **27.** M (page 2195)   **28.** CC (page 2195)   **29.** A (page 2196)

Multiple Choice

1. B (page 2173)   **2.** B (pages 2173–2174)   **3.** C (page 2186)   **4.** B (page 2183)   **5.** C (page 2182)

6. C (page 2188)   **7.** C (page 2189)   **8.** A (page 2189)   **9.** C (page 2189)   **10.** D (pages 2176–2177)

Labeling

1. Landing Zone (LZ) (page 2190)

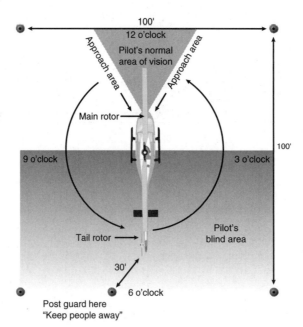

2. Helicopter Hand Signals
(page 2191)
   A. Move right
   B. Move forward
   C. Move rearward
   D. Move upward
   E. Move downward
   F. Move left

Fill-in-the-Blank

1. There's room for some discussion regarding what things are absolutely essential during the first few minutes with a patient who has been critically injured in a road collision. With experience, you may want to modify your list. In general, you will have to make a trade-off between all the equipment you would like to have immediately at hand and what you can carry comfortably during your first, hurried dash—often over difficult terrain—to the patient.

_____	Long-leg air splint
_____	Drug box
___X___	Portable suction unit
___X___	Oxygen cylinder
_____	OB kit
___X___	Pocket mask
___X___	Oropharyngeal airways
_____	Intravenous fluid bags
___X___	Dressing materials
___X___	Large-bore IV cannulas
___X___	Head immobilizer
___X___	Self-adhering roller bandage
_____	Selection of board splints
_____	Wheeled cot stretcher
_____	ECG monitor
_____	Contact lens remover
___X___	Stethoscope
___X___	Flashlight
___X___	Triangular bandages
_____	Chemical cold packs
___X___	Cervical collar
_____	Traction splint
___X___	Nonrebreathing mask
___X___	Long backboard/straps
_____	Oral thermometer
___X___	Fire extinguisher
_____	Bed pan
___X___	Heavy-duty scissors
_____	Emesis basin
___X___	Handheld radio
_____	Adhesive bandages

Other equipment that might be needed: Depending on the circumstances, you might require some light rescue and extrication equipment. And you may prefer a bag-mask device to a pocket mask. Finally, emergency medical technicians and paramedics should, in this era of acquired immune deficiency syndrome (AIDS) and other bloodborne diseases, don plastic or rubber gloves when they have to come in contact with a patient's blood or secretions.

Identify

a. Chief complaint: Deformity to left collarbone, possible internal trauma

b. Vital signs: Alert; respirations are 22 breaths/min, shallow; decreased left lung sounds. Pulse is 114 beats/min, heart monitor shows sinus tachycardia with PVCs, blood pressure is 132/84 mm Hg. Pain is 9/10, PEARRL, skin is warm.

    c. Pertinent negatives: No loss of consciousness, right lung sounds clear.

Walt and Dave did a great job in thinking on their feet. Because of the collar bone, a rigid C-collar will not work. The use of the towels and tape is the next best thing. They also went to the regional trauma center. The patient has a few PVCs and decreased lung sounds on the left, which is consistent with the seat belt injuries. They should be watching the left chest for a possible pneumothorax and the pericardial tamponade.

Complete the Patient Care Report (PCR)

Show the completed PCR to your instructor to obtain feedback on your completion of the form.

Ambulance Calls

1. a. Cory and Bill should have worked out their differences before arriving on the scene. They should know who is going to act as lead, and both of them should know what equipment to grab before leaving the squad. It is not a good idea to have a layperson digging through your squad looking for your equipment. Their actions on scene were very unprofessional and detrimental to the patient's outcome.

    b. There are many questions that could be asked on scene. Here are six that would be beneficial at this scene:

       (1) How far did the patient fall?

       (2) How did he land?

       (3) Has he been unconscious the whole time or has he made any noises or movements since he fell?

       (4) Do you know any of his medical history?

       (5) What is his name and who will be contacting family?

       (6) What made him fall?

    c. What kind of transport decision would you make right away? This patient needs to be at a trauma center. Most likely he has a head injury, and because he is unconscious as a result of a fall from a second-story roof, he is a definite regional trauma center candidate. If air medical is available and able to get the patient to the trauma center more quickly than by ambulance, they should be called within the first minute of arriving on the scene. Cory and Bill should be thinking of the "platinum 10 minutes" and the "golden hour" when treating this patient. (page 2188)

2. a. Jeff and Larry should know better than to skip checking the squad. You should always recheck after every change in crews. Tires can leak during downtime; people forget to refuel. A turn signal may be working in the morning but may quit sometime during the day. Checking the squad also mentally prepares you for the coming shift. It gives you confidence in your equipment because *you* know that it is ready to go, instead of relying on someone else. Everything should be checked once a day. (pages 2173–2174)

    b. A visual check should include a quick walk around to ensure that there are no flat tires or fluids dripping from the engine. Many services have a checklist beside the squad so that you can see when the last check was made on the unit and the equipment. The responding crew could have someone in the back check other equipment on the way to the scene. Every department is different, so make sure you understand the checks that are designed for your unit, and make sure when your call is over that all supplies are stocked and ready for the next call. (pages 2173–2175)

True/False

1. F (page 2173)   **2.** T (page 2173)   **3.** T (page 2173)   **4.** F (page 2174)   **5.** F (page 2175)

6. T (page 2177)   **7.** F (page 2177)   **8.** T (page 2178)   **9.** F (page 2185)   **10.** T (page 2188)

Short Answer

There are many ways to save time without cutting corners in the management of the critically injured. Among them are the following:

1. Get rolling at once when dispatched. Don't wait until you have all the details; all you need to get on the road is the *address*—you can find out the rest en route.

2. Know the map, and take the shortest route to the scene.

3. While en route to the scene, assemble the equipment you will need when you get there. (page 2180)

What other ideas did you come up with for saving time? It is always possible to find a more efficient way to do a job.

Fill-in-the-Table

(Tables 3 and 4, page 2188)

Advantages and Disadvantages of Using an Air Ambulance	
Advantages	**Disadvantages**
• Specialized skills or equipment is needed • **Rapid transport is possible** • **Can provide access to remote areas** • Helicopter hospital helipads are available • **Availability of medical crew with advanced skills**	• **Weather/environment** • Altitude limitations • **Airspeed limitations** • Aircraft cabin size • Terrain • **Cost** • Patient's condition • Restrictions on the number of caregivers • **Potential for crash**

Chapter 47: Incident Management and Multiple-Casualty Incidents

Matching

1. M (page 2217)	**2.** J (page 2217)	**3.** DD (page 2218)	**4.** BB (page 2218)	**5.** Y (page 2218)
6. AA (page 2218)	**7.** G (page 2217)	**8.** II (page 2217)	**9.** KK (page 2217)	**10.** JJ (page 2217)
11. B (page 2218)	**12.** Q (page 2218)	**13.** C (page 2218)	**14.** R (page 2218)	**15.** T (page 2218)
16. X (page 2218)	**17.** K (page 2217)	**18.** HH (page 2217)	**19.** L (page 2217)	**20.** H (page 2217)
21. N (page 2217)	**22.** O (page 2217)	**23.** LL (page 2218)	**24.** S (page 2218)	**25.** E (page 2218)
26. I (page 2218)	**27.** V (page 2218)	**28.** W (page 2218)	**29.** CC (page 2218)	**30.** NN (page 2218)
31. MM (page 2218)	**32.** FF (page 2217)	**33.** GG (page 2217)	**34.** D (page 2218)	**35.** EE (page 2218)
36. Z (page 2218)	**37.** F (page 2218)	**38.** A (page 2218)	**39.** U (page 2218)	**40.** P (page 2218)

Multiple Choice

1. C (page 2200)	**2.** B (page 2200)	**3.** C (page 2203)	**4.** C (page 2205)	**5.** D (page 2206)
6. A (page 2209)	**7.** C (page 2212)	**8.** D (page 2211)	**9.** A (page 2211)	**10.** B (page 2204)

Labeling

1. Diagram of an MCI (page 2208)

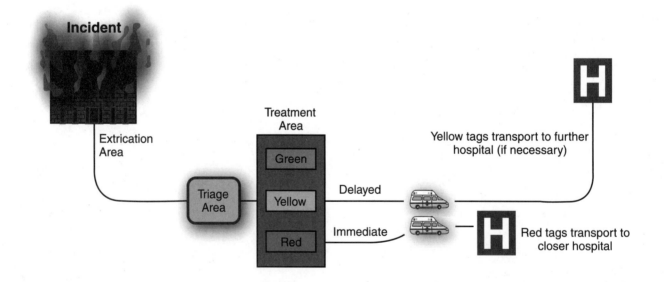

2. The JumpSTART Pediatric MCI Triage Algorithm (page 2212)

JumpSTART Pediatric MCI Triage©

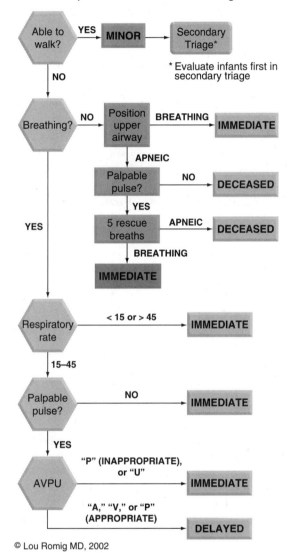

© Lou Romig MD, 2002

Fill-in-the-Blank

1. multiple-casualty incident; mutual aid response (page 2207)
2. closed (page 2207)
3. finance (page 2201)
4. safety; PIO; liaison (pages 2202–2203)
5. Preparedness (page 2199)
6. transportation (page 2205)
7. primary; secondary (page 2209)
8. rapid (page 2211)
9. Jump (page 2212)
10. staging (page 2206)

Identify

1. Chief complaint: Impaled object in left buttock

2. Vital signs: Respirations are 20 breaths/min, oxygen saturation is 97%, lungs are clear, pulse is 98 beats/min, sinus rhythm is normal, blood pressure is 136/88 mm Hg, patient is 7/10 on scale for pain, skin is warm and dry.

3. Pertinent negatives: Remained alert the whole time, not a lot of bleeding, which indicates a tamponade effect inside where the wood is pressing against the veins and arteries.

   Your patient provides a small challenge because of the need to stabilize him to a backboard as a result of the blast knocking him down. However, the impaled object is not letting you lay him flat. This is where you do the best job possible and move him as little as possible. A scoop stretcher may be a better tool to use to "pick up" the patient.

Ambulance Calls

1. This call may be the most stressful event you ever respond to. Remember to take care of yourself as soon as possible, and debrief. Don't be a hero; take your turn in the rehab section. Don't become a victim! Stay on top of scene safety and don't get lulled into a false sense of security. Stay on your toes!

   a. Everyone's answers may be different because there are no right or wrong answers here. Work as a group to develop a list of the best items to carry.

      (1) Communication radio

      (2) Multi tool

      (3) Gloves

      (4) Pen and paper

      (5) Flashlight

      (6) AM/FM radio

      (7) Trauma bandages

      (8) Pocket face mask

      (9) Leather gloves

      (10) Orange vest (page 2202)

   b. Once again there will be a lot of different answers. Two heads are always better than one. Tell them help will be coming soon, to stay away from downed power lines, and not to move patients unless they are in extreme danger. Try to account for everyone in the area. Stay in a group. Do not go back into a destroyed building.

   c. Remember, anything can become a hazard during a disaster, including people, animals, burst water and gas mains, downed electrical lines, fires, falling debris, sewage, and the weather. Can you think of any others?

2. a. If you have emergency management people that are trained for this, they should take command. If the fire station is unharmed, it would make a great central command post. The nursing home should also have a command post that reports back to central command because of the large volume of people in that area. The fire station can also serve as a rehab center or staging area because a lot of supplies are already there. The fire station will be a logical gathering area for incoming help.

   b. Because the high school has not been touched it would be a logical place to go. It has large open spaces and a large kitchen that could be used to feed people. Churches, community buildings, libraries, and senior citizen centers are all good places to use. Check to see if the local grocery store is able to start bringing food and water to your chosen site.

3. a. Your emergency response team should have a list of these agencies and phone numbers to call for help right away. If your dispatch center is still operating, it may have already alerted these agencies. Red Cross Disaster Services will probably be the first to arrive. You may have church agencies and state and local governmental agencies that will also respond.

True/False

1. F (page 2206)   2. T (page 2202)   3. T (page 2202)   4. T (page 2207)   5. F (page 2205)

6. T (page 2202)   7. T (page 2202)   8. T (page 2205)   9. F (pages 2208–2209)   10. T (page 2211)

Short Answer

1. In the first stage of the START triage system, you will use a strong, commanding voice to shout out to the victims. You need to tell them that if they can walk or are uninjured, they should move to a specific landmark away from the disaster site. In this way, you have just effectively triaged all the walking wounded into one area without actually looking at each patient. (page 2211)

2. In the second stage of START, you begin with the first patient you reach. Assess the respiratory status by opening the airway. If the patient is not breathing, tag the person black and move to the next patient. A patient breathing faster than 30 breaths/min should be tagged red. If the breathing rate is less than 30 breaths/min, move on to the assessment of the circulatory system. If the person has no radial pulse, tag him or her red; if not, move again to the neurologic assessment. If the patient is unconscious or unable to follow a simple command, tag him or her red. If the person can follow the command, tag the person yellow and move on to the next patient. (page 2211)

3. Children and infants may not be able to understand your commands. Children with special needs will be confused and need to be taken to the treatment center as soon as possible. Remember that children go into cardiac arrest because of respiratory arrest; therefore, the assessment process is a little different for children. (page 2212)

4. Always take advantage of a debriefing after a large incident. It can really help to manage stress after the initial event. Encourage participation, but do not force people to attend. The quicker you can return to active work after an incident, the better off you will be in the long run. (page 2213)

Fill-in-the-Table

(page 2202)

MCI Equipment and Supplies*	
Airway control	PPE (gloves, face shield, HEPA or N-95 mask) **Oral airways, nasal airways** **Suction units (manual units)** Rigid-tip Yankauer and flexible suction catheters LMA, Combitube, King- LT, ET tubes* **Laryngoscope and blades*** Tube check, tube restraint, tape, syringes, stylet* End-tidal CO_2 device
Breathing	**Pocket mask and one-way valve** Bag-mask device(s) (adult and child), spare masks Oxygen delivery devices (nonrebreathing mask, cannula, extension tubing) **Oxygen tank, regulator** **Occlusive dressings** Large-bore IV catheter for thoracic decompression*
Circulation	**Dressings, bandages, tape** Sphygmomanometer, stethoscope Burn dressings, burn sheets, sterile water for irrigation **One-handed tourniquets** 1,000-mL bags of normal saline, IV start kits, catheters*
Disabiltiy	**Rigid collars (one size fits all)** Head beds, wide tape, backboard straps **Flashlights, spare batteries**
Exposure	Space blanket to cover patients Scissors
Logistic/Command	Sector vests (triage, treatment, transport, staging, command, rescue) Pads of paper, pencils, pens, markers **Triage tags or kits used by your regional system** Assessment cards
Note: The items denoted by * could be packaged in an ALS pod.	

Chapter 48: Vehicle Extrication and Special Rescue

Matching

1. K (page 2253)	**2.** O (page 2253)	**3.** AA (page 2254)	**4.** B (page 2254)	**5.** G (page 2254)
6. M (page 2253)	**7.** I (page 2253)	**8.** R (page 2253)	**9.** S (page 2253)	**10.** T (page 2253)
11. E (page 2254)	**12.** V (page 2254)	**13.** II (page 2253)	**14.** HH (page 2253)	**15.** KK (page 2253)
16. N (page 2253)	**17.** L (page 2253)	**18.** JJ (page 2253)	**19.** BB (page 2253)	**20.** P (page 2253)
21. EE (page 2253)	**22.** FF (page 2253)	**23.** GG (page 2253)	**24.** J (page 2253)	**25.** H (page 2254)
26. F (page 2254)	**27.** LL (page 2253)	**28.** CC (page 2253)	**29.** Z (page 2254)	**30.** D (page 2254)
31. W (page 2254)	**32.** C (page 2254)	**33.** X (page 2254)	**34.** Y (page 2254)	**35.** U (page 2254)
36. Q (page 2253)	**37.** DD (page 2253)	**38.** A (page 2254)		

Multiple Choice

1. B (page 2222)	**2.** D (page 2222)	**3.** A (page 2222)	**4.** C (page 2224)	**5.** A (page 2223)
6. B (page 2225)	**7.** B (page 2225)	**8.** C (page 2228)	**9.** D (page 2230)	**10.** D (page 2232)

Labeling

1. Posts of a Vehicle (page 2228)

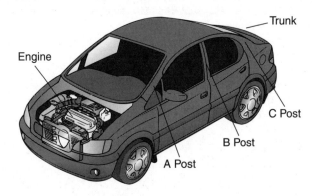

2. Wood Cribbing Designs (page 2231)
   A. Box crib
   B. Step chocks
   C. Wedges
   D. Shims

Fill-in-the-Blank

1. protect (page 2233)
2. hazard (page 2235)
3. A (page 2236)
4. confined space (page 2238)
5. Hydrogen sulfide (page 2238)
6. shoring (page 2239)
7. self-rescue position (page 2240)
8. reach out (page 2242)
9. recovery (page 2242)
10. low-angle (page 2244)

Identify

1. Chief complaint: Decreased level of consciousness, trauma to left side region

2. Vital signs: Verbally responsive, blood pressure 102/68 mm Hg, pulse of 116 beats/min and thready at the wrist, sinus tachycardia. Skin is pale and cool. Oxygen saturation is 96%. Respirations are 24 breaths/min and shallow with diminished lung sounds in left side. Pupils Equal And Round, Regular in size, but are slow to react to Light.

3. Pertinent negatives: Negative halo test

Complete the Patient Care Report (PCR)

Show the completed PCR to your instructor to obtain feedback on your completion of the form.

Ambulance Calls

1. To answer this question, you need to apply a lot of the information you have learned in the past chapters. How well did you do?
   a. The steps to take are as follows:
      (1) Assess the scene for
         (a) Hazards
         (b) Missing patients (Could a front-seat passenger who was not wearing a seat belt have been thrown through that shattered front windshield?)
      (2) Call for help. At the least, you will need the police, the fire department, and perhaps additional help in the extrication.
      (3) Once the hazards have been dealt with, gain access to the patient. Try all the doors first.
      (4) Enter the vehicle and start care. Specifically:
         (a) Open the airway by lifting the head into neutral position; if possible, have one of your crew take up a position in the back seat where he or she can apply a cervical collar and hold the patient's head in neutral position.
         (b) Administer supplemental oxygen.
         (c) Quickly check the chest for signs of pneumothorax or sucking chest wound.
         (d) Control external hemorrhage by direct pressure.
         (e) Start a large-bore IV with lactated Ringer's or normal saline.
         (f) Cover open wounds.
         (g) Splint fractures.
      (5) As soon as disentanglement is complete, remove the patient on a long backboard, and transfer the patient to the ambulance.
      (6) Notify the receiving hospital.
      (7) Transport. This is a "load-and-go" situation.
      (8) If possible, start another IV en route.
   b. (1) Once the patient has been transferred to the hospital, you have to clean up the ambulance and equipment.
      (2) Restock all kits used.

True/False

A lot of extrication is common sense.

1. F (page 2223)
2. F (page 2226)
3. T (page 2225)
4. T (pages 2224–2225)
5. T (page 2224)
6. T (page 2131)
7. F (page 2232)
8. F (pages 2232–2233)
9. F (page 2234)
10. T (page 2235)

Short Answer

1. **a.** Awareness: You need to be trained in recognizing hazards at the scene and being able to call for the appropriate assistance, such as the power company, or calling for the correct rescue team.
   b. Operations: You will be working in the area directly outside of the rescue zone. This area helps to assist the people working on the rescue. An example would be a rehab zone for a diving team.
   c. Technician: This is where you are directly involved in the rescue operation. It could be high-angle rappelling or swift-water rescue. You will be the person saving the patient from the incident. (page 2222)
2. **a.** Be safe: Your safety and your team's safety should *always* be your number one priority. Check for hazards before entering the scene! Live to work another day!
   b. Follow orders: Don't do anything without checking for orders. Orders stop the duplication of work and provide for the most qualified personnel working in the right area.
   c. Work as a team: Team effort is essential, and it is the quickest way to get the job done. Every link of the chain is strong, but the chain is strongest when linked together.
   d. Think: You must have your head in the game. You should constantly be assessing and reassessing the scene safety. You should report anything that changes on the scene to the appropriate person.
   e. Follow the golden rule of public service: Keep your patient calm by letting the patient know what is going on around him or her and what you are trying to accomplish. There should be one person who is there for emotional support of the patient if possible. (page 2222)
3. Gear that is standard for a water rescue is a personal flotation device, a lightweight helmet made for water rescue, a cutting device, a whistle, and some type of contamination protection. Remember, you must be trained for the correct water rescue before attempting a rescue. (page 2240)
4. Side glass vs. windshield. Tempered glass is used in the windows and the rear window. This glass will break in small pieces by using a spring-loaded punch in the corner. A windshield will not break because of the plastic that is between the layers of the glass, and it must be removed in one large piece. This is done by using an axe or a saw. The windshield will need to be removed before displacing the roof on a vehicle. Remember to cover your patient and to tell the patient before attempting to remove or break glass around him or her. (pages 2232–2233)

Fill-in-the-Table

(page 2222)

FAILURE Mnemonic	
F	Failure to understand or underestimating the environment
A	Additional medical problems not considered
I	Inadequate rescue skills
L	Lack of teamwork or experience
U	Underestimating the logistics of the incident
R	Rescue versus recovery mode not considered
E	Equipment not mastered

Skill Drills

Stabilizing a Suspected Spinal Injury in the Water (page 2243)

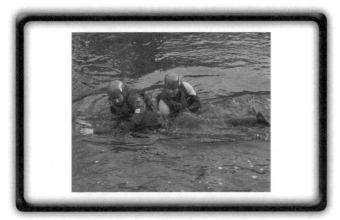

Step 1: Turn the patient supine by rotating the entire upper half of the patient's body as a single unit.

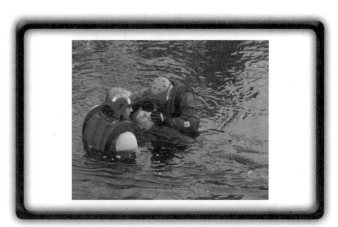

Step 2: As soon as the patient is turned, begin artificial ventilation using the mouth-to-mouth method or a pocket mask.

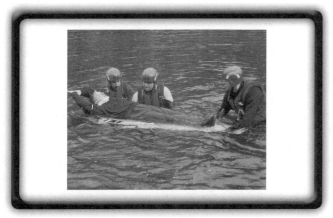

Step 3: Float a buoyant backboard under the patient as you continue ventilation.

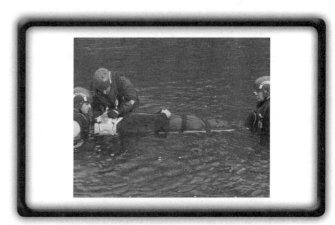

Step 4: Secure the trunk and head of the patient to the backboard to eliminate motion of the cervical spine.

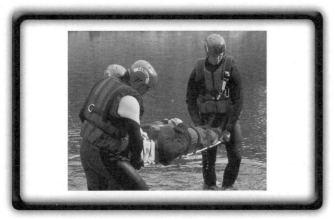

Step 5: Remove the patient from the water, on the backboard.

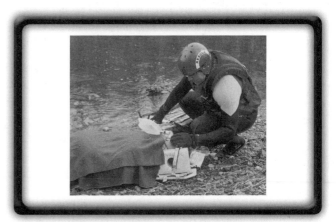

Step 6: Remove the patient's wet clothes and cover the patient with a blanket. Apply oxygen if breathing adequately; apply positive-pressure ventilation if apneic or breathing inadequately. Begin CPR if breathing and pulse are absent.

Chapter 49: Hazardous Materials

Matching

1. W (page 2283)	**2.** BB (page 2283)	**3.** X (page 2283)	**4.** AA (page 2283)	**5.** Y (page 2283)
6. Z (page 2283)	**7.** V (page 2283)	**8.** CC (page 2284)	**9.** MMM (page 2284)	**10.** DD (page 2284)
11. NNN (page 2284)	**12.** EE (page 2284)	**13.** OOO (page 2284)	**14.** FF (page 2284)	**15.** PPP (page 2284)
16. II (page 2284)	**17.** QQQ (page 2284)	**18.** HH (page 2284)	**19.** RRR (page 2284)	**20.** GG (page 2284)
21. PP (page 2284)	**22.** LLL (page 2284)	**23.** OO (page 2284)	**24.** KKK (page 2284)	**25.** MM (page 2284)
26. JJJ (page 2284)	**27.** LL (page 2284)	**28.** III (page 2284)	**29.** KK (page 2284)	**30.** HHH (page 2284)
31. JJ (page 2284)	**32.** I (page 2285)	**33.** VV (page 2285)	**34.** J (page 2285)	**35.** UU (page 2285)
36. K (page 2285)	**37.** TT (page 2285)	**38.** L (page 2285)	**39.** SS (page 2285)	**40.** T (page 2285)
41. RR (page 2285)	**42.** U (page 2285)	**43.** QQ (page 2285)	**44.** O (page 2285)	**45.** WW (page 2285)
46. N (page 2285)	**47.** XX (page 2285)	**48.** M (page 2285)	**49.** S (page 2285)	**50.** YY (page 2285)
51. R (page 2285)	**52.** ZZ (page 2285)	**53.** Q (page 2285)	**54.** AAA (page 2285)	**55.** P (pages 2285–2286)
56. A (page 2286)	**57.** BBB (page 2286)	**58.** B (page 2286)	**59.** CCC (page 2286)	**60.** C (page 2286)
61. SSS (page 2286)	**62.** D (page 2286)	**63.** DDD (page 2286)	**64.** E (page 2286)	**65.** FFF (page 2286)
66. F (page 2286)	**67.** GGG (page 2286)	**68.** G (page 2286)	**69.** NN (page 2286)	**70.** H (page 2286)
71. EEE (page 2286)				

Multiple Choice

1. B (page 2266)	**2.** A (page 2278)	**3.** D (page 2274)	**4.** C (page 2275)	**5.** D (page 2279)
6. B (page 2258)	**7.** C (page 2263)	**8.** D (page 2269)	**9.** A (page 2259)	**10.** A (page 2277)

Fill-in-the-Blank

1. awareness level (page 2258)
2. ensure your safety (page 2258)
3. authority having jurisdiction (page 2258)
4. information (page 2258)
5. agricultural; insecticides (page 2258)
6. bill of lading; waybill (page 2261)
7. primary; secondary (page 2272)
8. Primary contamination (page 2272)
9. Secondary contamination (page 2272)
10. local effect; systemic (page 2272)

Identify

1. **a.** Based on the information provided in the *ERG*, this product is highly toxic and may be fatal if inhaled or absorbed through the skin.
   b. Specialized protective clothing with SCBA is required. Structural fire fighter clothing will provide only a limited amount of protection. Most paramedics and ambulances don't carry the proper clothing unless it is a specialized unit with specially trained personnel.
   c. Based on the information given, the ambulance and stopped nearby traffic are in immediate danger. It's important to relocate upwind and to set up a staging area a safe distance as determined by incident command and the parameters of the guidebook. It's also advisable to begin requesting the allocation of additional resources and personnel based on the life-threatening nature of the incident.

2. The photos show the four levels of protection in the following order: level B, level A, level D, level C.

Level A provides the greatest protection from exposure to hazardous substances. These suits look like an astronaut's suit because they are fully encapsulating. These suits fully cover and protect the SCBA worn by hazardous materials technicians. The suits are rigorously tested by the manufacturers to determine resistance and permeability to many chemicals.

Level B is called for when the technician needs protection from splashes and inhaled toxins. It is not fully encapsulating like Level A is, and it is worn with SCBA. Level B suits are typically worn by the hazardous materials decontamination team in the warm zone.

Level C is designed to protect against a known agent. The equipment provides splash protection and is worn with an air-purifying respirator that must have filters specifically chosen to provide protection against the known agent. Offering eye and hand protection and foot coverings, Level C protection could be used during transport of patients with the potential of secondary contamination.

Level D is the level of PPE offered by fire fighters' turnout gear. It is typically not worn in hazardous materials incidents but may be used by some personnel in the cold zone. (pages 2269, 2271–2272)

Ambulance Calls

1. **a.** What safety precautions are necessary in handling and decontaminating this patient? List three considerations. (page 2275)

    (1) Your safety comes first.

    (2) You must work as part of a team to prevent more casualties.

    (3) Use the incident command system, which permits only properly trained and equipped hazardous materials personnel to enter the hot zone.

2. **a.** Three potential sources of information regarding the nature of the train's cargo are the following:

    (1) The USDOT placard on the side of each car

    (2) The waybill and the consist carried by the conductor

    (3) The conductor (pages 2260–2261)

   b. Once you know that you are dealing with a hazardous cargo, you should radio your dispatcher with details of the incident and request help from the following sources:

    (1) Hazardous materials team

    (2) Fire department with heavy rescue gear

    (3) Police for crowd and traffic control

    (4) At least one ambulance for every two estimated casualties on the road

True/False

1. Transport accidents involving radioactive materials are likely to increase in frequency, so it is important to have a clear plan of action for such events and to know what you should and should not do at the scene.
    a. T (page 2259)
    b. F (page 2279)
    c. F (page 2278)
    d. T (page 2262)
    e. T (page 2261)

2. It is just as important to know what *not* to do at a hazardous materials incident as to know what *to* do.
    a. F (page 2259)
    b. T (page 2272)
    c. F (page 2275)
    d. F (page 2279)
    e. T (page 2279)

Short Answer

1. **a.** Name of substance
    b. Specific properties and hazards of substances
    c. Evacuation and isolation distances (pages 2259–2260)

2. a. CHEMTREC
  b. Bill of lading
  c. Waybill
  d. Hazardous materials warning labels, placards, and markings
  e. Material safety data sheet (pages 2261–2262)

3. The most important step in dealing with a hazardous materials incident is recognizing that a hazardous materials situation exists in the first place. If you have to wait until you start to feel sick from your own exposure to a poisonous material before you figure out that the situation might be dangerous, you've waited too long.

  a. Two-car collision downtown: If either of those cars is on fire, you may be dealing with toxic products of the combustion of automobile upholstery, including phosgene, chlorine, and hydrogen chloride.
  b. Apartment-house fire: Not immediately likely, but the products of combustion do contain soot, carbon monoxide, carbon dioxide, water vapor, formaldehyde, cyanide compounds, and many oxides of nitrogen. (page 2278)
  c. Three municipal workers collapsed in a sewer: The sewer could be a low-oxygen environment, and there is a lot of potential for chemical inhalation.
  d. Two police officers injured in a riot: The presence of hazardous materials would depend on whether tear gas or pepper spray was used.
  e. Fire in a garden supply store warehouse: There are many dangerous chemicals stored and sold at a garden supply company. Was there any exposure to pesticides? (page 2278)
  f. Semitrailer overturned on the interstate. If the semitrailer is carrying hazardous materials, they could have leaked and there may be an increased risk of fire.
  g. Two "men down" on the maintenance staff of the municipal swimming pool. This scene could include a chlorine leak.
  h. Freight train struck car on level crossing. Until you know what freight the train was carrying, you should suspect a possible hazardous materials situation.
  i. Fire in a furniture factory. A furniture factory not only carries a big wood fire load, but also stains and finishes that may be hazardous.

Chapter 50: Terrorism

Matching

1. G (page 2314)
2. M (page 2314)
3. FF (page 2314)
4. N (page 2314)
5. EE (page 2314)
6. O (page 2314)
7. DD (page 2314)
8. GG (page 2315)
9. OOO (page 2315)
10. HH (page 2315)
11. SS (page 2315)
12. J (page 2315)
13. TT (page 2315)
14. II (page 2315)
15. UU (page 2315)
16. JJ (page 2315)
17. VV (page 2315)
18. KK (page 2315)
19. DDD (page 2315)
20. LL (page 2315)
21. WW (page 2315)
22. A (page 2315)
23. XX (page 2315)
24. MM (page 2315)
25. YY (page 2315)
26. NN (page 2315)
27. K (page 2315)
28. PPP (page 2315)
29. TTT (page 2315)
30. F (page 2315)
31. B (page 2315)
32. QQQ (page 2315)
33. VVV (page 2315)
34. RRR (page 2315)
35. SSS (page 2315)
36. I (page 2315)
37. UUU (page 2315)
38. CCC (page 2315)
39. X (page 2315)
40. RR (page 2315)
41. BBB (page 2315)
42. QQ (page 2315)
43. AAA (page 2315)
44. PP (page 2315)
45. ZZ (page 2315)
46. OO (page 2315)
47. L (page 2315)
48. R (page 2316)
49. NNN (page 2316)
50. U (page 2316)
51. LLL (page 2316)
52. MMM (page 2316)
53. T (page 2316)
54. KKK (page 2316)
55. S (page 2316)
56. JJJ (page 2316)
57. H (page 2316)
58. D (page 2316)
59. III (page 2316)
60. W (page 2316)
61. CC (page 2316)
62. V (page 2316)
63. BB (page 2316)
64. HHH (page 2316)
65. AA (page 2316)
66. Z (page 2316)
67. GGG (page 2316)
68. FFF (page 2316)
69. C (page 2316)
70. Y (page 2316)
71. E (page 2316)
72. EEE (page 2316)
73. Q (page 2316)
74. P (page 2316)

Multiple Choice

1. C (page 2303)
2. D (page 2294)
3. A (pages 2298–2299)
4. C (page 2299)
5. B (page 2299)
6. A (page 2301)
7. B (page 2304)
8. D (page 2306)
9. C (page 2307)
10. A (page 2310)

Labeling

1. Alpha, Beta, and Gamma Radiation
   (page 2310)
   A. Gamma
   B. Beta
   C. Alpha

Fill-in-the-Blank

1. Weapon of mass destruction (page 2297)
2. covert (page 2293)
3. secondary (page 2297)
4. Route of exposure (page 2298)
5. Nerve agents (page 2300)
6. German (page 2300)
7. lymphatic (page 2306)
8. Anthrax (page 2306)
9. castor bean (page 2307)
10. Points of distribution (page 2309)

Identify

1. Chief complaint: Trauma, organophosphate poisoning
2. Vital signs: Alert to start, but loses consciousness as the poisoning progresses. Heart rate is 50 beats/min, blood pressure is 98/66 mm Hg, oxygen saturation is 88%, respirations are 9 breaths/min.

3. Pertinent negatives: There are no pertinent negatives.

Always look around before running into the scene. You never know what people are carrying in the truck. It is no fun to become a patient yourself!

Complete the Patient Care Report (PCR)

Show the completed PCR to your instructor to obtain feedback on your completion of the form.

Ambulance Calls

1. a. This train derailment could be a terrorist attack. You need to be thinking about what kind of attack it was and be prepared for the type of scene you will be entering.

   (1) Chemical—Not very likely at this scene.

   (2) Biological—Probably not this scene, but you never know what the train is carrying.

   (3) Radiologic—Not very likely at this scene.

   (4) Nuclear—No signs of radiation, so you should be okay here.

   (5) Explosives—This is the best bet here; either the tracks were blown up or something inside the train blew to cause the derailment. Be careful because there may be some secondary explosions. (page 2289)

b. You can designate someone to walk toward the vehicles, but have the person stay clear of the vehicles. It is a good idea for the person to be wearing a bright color because people will be able to see him or her. Appoint that person and tell the person he or she is the leader. Have the person remain standing so the walking wounded have someone to walk toward. If you have enough responders, you can designate one of them. They can wave a white towel or some type of flag; whatever your solution, get the walking wounded cleared out of the wreckage as soon as possible! (page 2296)

2. a. Chlorine, which is used a lot in swimming pools, is what is leaking and causing the green haze. It will have the smell of bleach. (page 2299)

b. Before getting out, you'd better call for help. First, you need a hazardous materials team or at least the fire department to go into the pool area with their self-contained breathing apparatus (SCBA) gear and bring out the missing lifeguards. Leave all your windows up and use your external public address (PA) system to direct the children standing around to walk upwind and away from the pool. Have them follow the ambulance until you are a safe distance away.

c. With chlorine gas, complete airway obstruction can occur as a result of pulmonary edema. Be prepared to intubate if necessary. Oxygen is a must! (page 2299)

True/False

1. F (page 2311)   **2.** T (page 2310)   **3.** F (page 2305)   **4.** F (page 2304)   **5.** T (page 2303)

6. T (page 2304)   **7.** F (page 2301)   **8.** F (page 2292)   **9.** T (page 2292)   **10.** T (page 2295)

Short Answer

1. Three *reactions* sometimes seen in bystanders at an MCI are the following:

   a. Overreaction

   b. Conversion hysteria

   c. Depression

   If you mentioned anxiety, that is also correct.

2. Triage tags are usually not very large and cannot accommodate a lot of information. But they should at least contain the most essential facts about the patient, especially if the person is unconscious or for any other reason is unable to provide information to the emergency department staff:

   a. Identifying information: name, age, address, next of kin's name and telephone number

   b. Information about the scene: anything that will help the emergency department staff understand the mechanisms of injury

   c. Pertinent (SAMPLE) medical history

   d. Physical findings: vital and neurologic signs, any positive findings on physical examination

   e. Any treatment given (if a drug, the dose given, the time it was given, and the route by which it was given)

   f. Priority (will usually be indicated by the color of the triage tag) (page 2313)

Fill-in-the-Table

1. (page 2302)

Nerve Agents						
Name	**Code Name**	**Odor**	**Special Features**	**Onset of symptoms**	**Volatility**	**Route of exposure**
Tabun	GA	Fruity	Easy to manufacture	Immediate	Low	Both contact and vapor hazard
Sarin	GB	None (if pure) or strong	Will off-gas while on victim's clothing	Immediate	High	Primarily respiratory vapor hazard; extremely lethal if skin contact is made
Soman	GD	Fruity	Ages rapidly, making it difficult to treat	Immediate	Moderate	Contact with skin; minimal vapor hazard
V agent	VX	None	Most lethal chemical agent; difficult to decontaminate	Immediate	Very low	Contact with skin; no vapor hazard (unless vaporized)

2. (page 2304)

Chemical Agents						
Class	**Military Designation**	**Odor**	**Lethality**	**Onset of Symptoms**	**Volatility**	**Primary Route of Exposure**
Vesicants	Mustard (H) Lewisite (L) Phosgene oxime (CX)	**Garlic (H) Geranium (L)**	Causes large blisters to form on victims; may severely damage upper airway if vapors are inhaled; severe intense pain and grayish skin discoloration (L, CX)	**Delayed (H) Immediate (L, CX)**	Very low (H, L) Moderate (CX)	Primarily contact; with some vapor hazard
Pulmonary agents	Chlorine (CL) Phosgene (CG)	**Bleach (CL) Cut grass (CG)**	Causes irritation; choking (CL); severe pulmonary edema (CG)	**Immediate (CL) Delayed (CG)**	Very high	Vapor hazard
Nerve agents	Tabun (GA) Sarin (GB) Soman (GD) V agent (VX)	**Fruity or none**	Most lethal chemical agents can kill within minutes; effects are reversible with antidotes	**Immediate**	Moderate (GA, GD) Very high (GB) Low (VX)	Vapor hazard (GB) Both vapor and contact hazard (GA, GD) Contact hazard (VX)
Cyanide agents	Hydrogen cyanide (AC) Cyanogen chloride (CK)	**Almonds (AC) Irritating (CK)**	Highly lethal chemical gases; can kill within minutes; effects are reversible with antidotes	**Immediate**	Very high	Vapor hazard

3. (page 2301)

SLUDGEM and DUMBELS	
Military Mnemonic: SLUDGEM	
S	Salivation
L	**Lacrimation**
U	Urination
D	**Defecation**
G	GI distress
E	**Emesis**
M	Miosis
Medical Mnemonic: DUMBELS	
D	**Defecation**
U	Urination
M	**Miosis**
B	Bradycardia, Bronchorrhea
E	**Emesis**
L	Lacrimation
S	**Salivation**

Chapter 51: Disaster Response

Matching

1. G (page 2341)	**2.** W (page 2341)	**3.** H (page 2341)	**4.** L (page 2341)	**5.** V (page 2341)
6. F (page 2341)	**7.** U (page 2341)	**8.** K (page 2341)	**9.** J (page 2341)	**10.** T (page 2341)
11. I (page 2341)	**12.** S (page 2341)	**13.** E (page 2341)	**14.** O (page 2342)	**15.** X (page 2342)
16. AA (page 2342)	**17.** N (page 2342)	**18.** Z (page 2342)	**19.** Q (page 2342)	**20.** B (page 2342)
21. Y (page 2342)	**22.** P (page 2342)	**23.** C (page 2342)	**24.** BB (page 2342)	**25.** D (page 2342)
26. CC (page 2342)	**27.** DD (page 2342)	**28.** A (page 2342)	**29.** R (page 2342)	**30.** M (page 2342)

Multiple Choice

1. D (page 2319)	**2.** B (page 2320)	**3.** B (page 2321)	**4.** A (page 2322)	**5.** C (pages 2325–2326)
6. B (page 2326)	**7.** A (page 2330)	**8.** C (page 2333)	**9.** D (page 2333)	**10.** B (page 2334)

Fill-in-the-Blank

1. preplanning; all-hazards (page 2319)
2. mutual aid agreement (page 2321)
3. transportation; log (page 2324)
4. hospitals; readjust (page 2324)
5. briefing; briefing; media (page 2325)
6. after-action report (page 2326)
7. casualty collection points (page 2328)
8. emergency operations center (page 2328)
9. heavy; vegetables (page 2333)
10. epidemic; pandemic (page 2334)

Identify

1. Chief complaint: Critical thermal burns and potential respiratory involvement
2. Vital signs: Respiration is 24 breaths/min and shallow; oxygen saturation is 96%; lungs are clear; pulse is 110 beats/min; heart monitor shows sinus tachycardia; blood pressure is 108/68 mm Hg; PEARRL; patient is 10/10 on scale for pain; skin is pale, cool, and moist.
3. Pertinent negatives: He denies taking any drugs and has no allergies. He has no ectopy on his ECG.

   In addition to almost losing his life and spending a month in the burn unit, he is ultimately convicted of arson for destroying over a million dollars in property. Fortunately, no one else was injured in the blaze.

Ambulance Calls

1. This call may be one of the most stressful events you have responded to in your EMS career thus far. Remember to take care of yourself and your crew during the entire response so you do not become a patient also. It is hot in there for the patients and will become exhausting for you, too. Keep drinking fluids! As for those patients "trapped" in the hot environment: remove their hot clothing, give them water, and undo the restraints as long as there is no potential for the patients to fall down.

   a. There are many correct responses to this question. Here are six (*students should list four*):

      (1) Vigilance is the key. If possible, work in pairs, monitoring each other for heat-related problems.

      (2) Water must be consumed at all times. Small, constant sips of water throughout the day are best. You may also consider some electrolyte fluid replacement in addition to the water.

      (3) Small, more frequent meals are better than large ones. Eat foods that are heavy in fluids, such as vegetables and fruits.

      (4) Set up "water trains." As you empty water bottles, have them refilled. Your agency must ensure that it has a good, clean source of water. Use of water buffalo trailers, lister bags, and portable water backpacks is advisable if outdoors.

(5) If you have air conditioning in your buildings or vehicles, use it.

(6) Wet towels placed on the head or on the body can help reduce body temperature. (pages 2333–2334)

b. Many medical problems are exacerbated by extreme heat. The following list provides examples but is not exhaustive (*students should list five examples*):

(1) Circulatory problems

(2) Diabetes

(3) Cardiovascular problems

(4) COPD

(5) Asthma

(6) Cardiac dysrhythmias

(7) The "traditional" heat emergencies such as heat exhaustion and heatstroke

True/False

1. F (page 2334)   **2.** F (page 2334)   **3.** T (page 2333)   **4.** F (page 2333)   **5.** T (page 2329)

6. T (page 2330)   **7.** T (page 2331)   **8.** F (page 2322)   **9.** T (page 2322)   **10.** T (page 2324)

Short Answer

1. The three phases of any plan of response:
   a. Before the event (preplanning)
   b. During the event
   c. After the event (page 2319)

2. Considerations during a disaster should include inventory, mobilization of personnel, command setup or response, unification of command, personal protective and safety equipment, equipment resupply, triage and classification, patient tracking, assignment of personnel, personnel mental needs, personnel physical needs, hospital updates, providing and accepting relief, surveillance, media, legal issues, and unit leadership reinforcement. (page 2322)

Fill-in-the-Table

1. Examples of Natural and Man-Made Disasters
(pages 2326, 2334)

Examples of Natural and Man-Made Disasters	
Natural Disasters	**Man-Made Disasters**
Forest and brush fires	**Structural fires**
Snow and ice storms	Construction failures and building collapse
Tornadoes	**Power failures or disruptions**
Hurricanes	Riots, civil disturbances, and stampedes
Tsunamis	**Strikes and labor disputes**
Earthquakes	Sniper, shooter, and hostage situations
Landslides, avalanches, mudslides	**Explosions (intentional and unintentional)**
Cave-ins	IT (cyber) disruptions
Volcanoes	**Incidents involving weapons of mass destruction**
Flooding	Hazardous materials incidents
Sandstorms and dust storms	
Prolonged cold weather	
Drought	
Heat wave	
Meteors and space debris	
Pandemics	

Chapter 52: Crime Scene Awareness

Matching

(page 2364)

1. C   **2.** K   **3.** G   **4.** A   **5.** B   **6.** F   **7.** E   **8.** L   **9.** D   **10.** J   **11.** H   **12.** I

Multiple Choice

1. C (page 2347)   **2.** C (page 2348)   **3.** A (page 2350)   **4.** C (page 2350)   **5.** D (page 2358)
6. B (page 2350)   **7.** B (page 2351)   **8.** C (page 2356)   **9.** D (page 2353)   **10.** A (page 2359)

Fill-in-the-Blank

1. tunnel vision (page 2347)
2. 21; 10 (page 2347)
3. incident commander (IC) (page 2348)
4. A (page 2349)
5. primary; secondary (page 2350)
6. contact; cover (page 2351)

Identify

1. Errors in handling scene safety: Paramedics did not announce themselves at front, stood in front of door to knock, did not identify a secondary exit, did not look for visible weapons (drawers in tables can conceal weapons, and the poker in the fireplace stand is a potential weapon), and both approached the patient (should have considered using contact and cover technique).
2. Warning signs of danger: Loud conversation inside (possible domestic violence), the patient arguing with the other person, and the person getting between you and a means of egress.
3. Potential evidence: Ceramic object is possible evidence and should not be brushed away with shoe. Also, the patient's shirt is potential evidence that should not be cut or ripped unless absolutely necessary to provide care and no alternative is available to access injuries. (pages 2359–2361)

Ambulance Calls

1. Listen for loud or threatening voices, glance through available windows for signs of a struggle, and look for visible weapons. Once at the door, stand to the doorknob side before knocking and announce yourself. Once inside, ask the person who answers to lead you to the patient. (page 2346)
2. **a.** The ambulance should be positioned a minimum of 21 feet behind the car at a 10° angle to the driver's side facing the shoulder. (page 2347)
   b. Before leaving the ambulance, the license plate number and state-issued registration of the car should be recorded and left by the radio (some experts recommend giving it to the dispatcher). Also, notify the dispatcher of this information along with any additional information that might be helpful, such as the precise location. (pages 2347–2349)
   c. The incident commander, the person in the right front seat of the ambulance, should approach the rear passenger side of the car from the trunk to see that it is properly closed. Use a belly-in toward the motor vehicle and stop at the C column to look in the rear and side windows. Notice the number of people and pay close attention to their hands. Look for weapons. At any sign of a weapon or other danger, retreat immediately to a safe area. (pages 2347–2349)
3. **a.** *Contact and cover* means you make contact with the patient to assess and provide care and your partner obtains patient information, gauges the level of tension, and warns you at the first sign of trouble. (page 2351)
   b. If you suspect that the location is a clandestine drug laboratory, immediately leave the house with the patient. Do not touch anything! Once clear of the lab, leave the area and notify the police as soon as possible without placing yourself in harm's way. (page 2351)

c. Safety is a major issue for everyone because of the toxic nature of the material used, the highly flammable agents used, and the possibility of booby traps that are sometimes used to safeguard the illegal operations. (page 2351)

4. Alter the scene as little as possible while providing care. Be mindful of physical evidence such as bullet casings, weapons, and blood. Do not move or pick up items that might be evidence. When you remove a patient's clothes to expose wounds, do not cut through bullet holes. Once you have removed the patient's clothes, do not shake the clothing because valuable evidence, including trace evidence, may fall off the clothing or from the pockets. (pages 2359–2361)

True/False

1. F (page 2359) **2.** T (page 2355) **3.** F (page 2350) **4.** F (page 2350) **5.** F (page 2348)

6. T (page 2347) **7.** T (page 2348) **8.** F (page 2347) **9.** T (page 2349) **10.** F (page 2351)

Short Answer

1. **a.** Number of aggressors involved
   b. Number and type of injuries
   c. Number and type of weapons involved
   d. Make, color, body style, and license number of any vehicle involved
   e. Direction of travel if vehicle leaves scene (pages 2349–2350)
2. **a.** Highly flammable properties of materials
   b. Toxic nature of chemicals and materials used
   c. Booby traps (fragmentation and incendiary devices) (page 2351)
3. **a.** Glove box
   b. Top of sun visor
   c. Arm rest
   d. Under the seats
   e. In the center console
   f. Side door pocket
   g. Next to driver's right thigh (page 2349)
4. A secondary exit could be used if the primary exit is blocked or an alternate means of egress is needed because of a threat or danger. A rear door or, in an emergency, a window can be used as a secondary exit. (page 2350)
5. *Cover* includes objects that are usually impenetrable by bullets. *Concealment* includes objects that hide you until you can assess the situation and find cover. (page 2355)
6. **a.** Cover (*students should list three of the following*)
      (1) Trees
      (2) Mail collection boxes
      (3) Dumpsters
      (4) Utility poles
      (5) Curbs
      (6) Vehicles
      (7) Depressions in the ground
   b. Concealment
      (1) Tall grass
      (2) Shrubbery
      (3) Dark shadows (page 2355)
7. At this stage, you are in grave danger. You must assume that the person on the other end of the gun will use violence if you do not follow instructions. (pages 2355–2356)
8. **a.** Testimonial evidence is oral documentation by a witness of the facts.
   b. Physical evidence ties a suspect to a crime and includes body materials, objects, and impressions. (page 2359)

Photo Credits

Chapter 17

Page 141 (top) Adapted from 12-Lead ECG: The Art of Interpretation, courtesy of Tomas B. Garcia, MD.; **Page 153 (top)** From 12-Lead ECG: The Art of Interpretation, courtesy of Tomas B. Garcia, MD.; **Page 153 (bottom)** From 12-Lead ECG: The Art of Interpretation, courtesy of Tomas B. Garcia, MD.; **Page 154 (top)** From 12-Lead ECG: The Art of Interpretation, courtesy of Tomas B. Garcia, MD.; **Page 154 (bottom)** From 12-Lead ECG: The Art of Interpretation, courtesy of Tomas B. Garcia, MD.; **Page 155 (top)** From 12-Lead ECG: The Art of Interpretation, courtesy of Tomas B. Garcia, MD.; **Page 155 (bottom)** From 12-Lead ECG: The Art of Interpretation, courtesy of Tomas B. Garcia, MD.; **Page 156 (top)** From 12-Lead ECG: The Art of Interpretation, courtesy of Tomas B. Garcia, MD.; **Page 156 (bottom)** From 12-Lead ECG: The Art of Interpretation, courtesy of Tomas B. Garcia, MD.; **Page 157 (top)** From 12-Lead ECG: The Art of Interpretation, courtesy of Tomas B. Garcia, MD.; **Page 157 (bottom)** From 12-Lead ECG: The Art of Interpretation, courtesy of Tomas B. Garcia, MD.; **Page 158 (top)** From 12-Lead ECG: The Art of Interpretation, courtesy of Tomas B. Garcia, MD.; **Page 158 (bottom)** From 12-Lead ECG: The Art of Interpretation, courtesy of Tomas B. Garcia, MD.; **Page 159 (top)** From 12-Lead ECG: The Art of Interpretation, courtesy of Tomas B. Garcia, MD.; **Page 159 (bottom)** From 12-Lead ECG: The Art of Interpretation, courtesy of Tomas B. Garcia, MD.; **Page 160 (top)** From 12-Lead ECG: The Art of Interpretation, courtesy of Tomas B. Garcia, MD.; **Page 160 (bottom)** From 12-Lead ECG: The Art of Interpretation, courtesy of Tomas B. Garcia, MD.; **Page 161 (top)** From 12-Lead ECG: The Art of Interpretation, courtesy of Tomas B. Garcia, MD.; **Page 161 (bottom)** From 12-Lead ECG: The Art of Interpretation, courtesy of Tomas B. Garcia, MD.; **Page 162 (top)** From 12-Lead ECG: The Art of Interpretation, courtesy of Tomas B. Garcia, MD.; **Page 162 (bottom)** From 12-Lead ECG: The Art of Interpretation, courtesy of Tomas B. Garcia, MD.

Chapter 23

Page 207 Courtesy of Leonard Crowley.

Chapter 24

Page 217 Courtesy of Bill Branson/National Cancer Institute.

Chapter 26

Page 241 Adapted from: Centers for Disease Control and Prevention (CDC): Morbidity and Mortality Weekly Report (MMWR). Vol. 38, No. S-6. Table 4. Available at: http://wonder.cdc.gov/wonder/prevguid/p0000114/p0000114.asp. Published June 23, 1989. Accessed November 10, 2011.

Chapter 31

Page 292 Courtesy of Rhonda Beck; **Page 293** © E. M. Singletary, M.D. Used with permission.

Chapter 32

Page 303 (top) © E. M. Singletary, M.D. Used with permission.; **Page 303 (middle)** © Amy Walters/ShutterStock, Inc.

Chapter 39

Page 392 (top) Courtesy of ZOLL; **Page 392 (middle)** Courtesy of Michigan Instruments, Inc.; **Page 392 (bottom)** Courtesy of Physio-Control, Inc.

Chapter 47

Page 499 © Lou Romig MD, 2002.

Chapter 48

Page 507 Courtesy of David Sweet; **Page 508 (top)** Courtesy of David Sweet; **Page 508 (middle)** Courtesy of David Sweet; **Page 508 (bottom)** Courtesy of David Sweet.

Chapter 49

Page 523 © Huntstock/age fotostock.

Answer Key

Page 611 Source: National Center for Health Statistics/National Vital Statistics Reports, 2007, United States.; **Page 700** Adapted from: Centers for Disease Control and Prevention (CDC): Morbidity and Mortality Weekly Report (MMWR). Vol. 38, No. S-6. Table 4. Available at: http://wonder.cdc.gov/wonder/prevguid/p0000114/p0000114.asp. Published June 23, 1989. Accessed November 10, 2011.; **Page 724** Courtesy of Rhonda Beck; **Page 725** © E. M. Singletary, M.D. Used with permission.; **Page 817** © Lou Romig MD, 2002.